Recent Progress in Ovarian Research

Recent Progress in Ovarian Research

Edited by Margaret Booth

hayle
medical

New York

Hayle Medical,
750 Third Avenue, 9th Floor,
New York, NY 10017, USA

Visit us on the World Wide Web at:
www.haylemedical.com

ISBN: 978-1-63241-622-3

Cataloging-in-Publication Data

Recent progress in ovarian research / edited by Margaret Booth.
p. cm.
Includes bibliographical references and index.
ISBN 978-1-63241-622-3
1. Ovaries--Research. 2. Ovaries--Abnormalities. 3. Ovaries--Diseases.
I. Booth, Margaret.
QP261 .R43 2019
612.62--dc23

Table of Contents

Permissions

List of Contributors

Index

Preface

Every book is initially just a concept; it takes months of research and hard work to give it the final shape in which the readers receive it. In its early stages, this book also went through rigorous reviewing. The notable contributions made by experts from across the globe were first molded into patterned chapters and then arranged in a sensibly sequential manner to bring out the best results.

Ovary refers to the organ in the female reproductive system which produces an egg cell or ovum. After the release, the ovum reaches the uterus by traveling down the fallopian tube, where it may get fertilised by a sperm. There are two ovaries in a female body, i.e., one on the left, and the other on the right. Ovaries secrete hormones which play a significant role in fertility and the menstrual cycle. They are considered to be female gonads. The changes in the structure and function of the ovaries begin at puberty. Some of the common conditions associated with ovaries include ovarian cyst, polycystic ovary syndrome, premature ovarian failure and ovarian cancer. The book studies, analyzes and upholds the pillars of ovarian research and its utmost significance in modern times. It presents researches and studies performed by experts across the globe. From theories to research to practical applications, case studies related to all contemporary topics of relevance to ovarian research have been included in this book.

It has been my immense pleasure to be a part of this project and to contribute my years of learning in such a meaningful form. I would like to take this opportunity to thank all the people who have been associated with the completion of this book at any step.

Editor

Circular RNAs: biogenesis, expression and their potential roles in reproduction

Guobo Quan[1,2] and Julang Li[2,3]*

Abstract

Unlike other non-coding RNAs (ncRNAs), circular RNA (circRNA) is generally presented as a covalently linked circle lacking both a 5′ cap and a 3′ tail. circRNAs were thought to be spliced intermediates, byproducts, or products of abnormal RNA splicing events. However, the high-throughput sequencing technology coupled with bioinformatics has recently uncovered thousands of endogenous circRNAs in cells of many different species. These circRNAs show various features, such as abundant expression, evolutionary conservation, cell- or tissue-specific expression, and a higher resistance to degradation caused by exonuclease or ribonuclease (RNase), suggesting their potentially biological significance. However, the function of these circRNAs, their mechanism of action, and the regulation of their biogenesis and degradation remains largely unclear. The current research and findings of circRNA in the context of reproduction will be reviewed. Additionally, the perspectives of circRNAs in the field will be discussed.

Keywords: Circular RNA, Reproduction, Gene regulation, miRNA, lncRNA

Background

As a subclass of ncRNAs, circRNAs are not novel because of their natural existence in some low grade organisms or plants. A typical circRNA class has been detected in some viruses, such as the hepatitis D virus [1]. HDV was initially discovered in some Italian patients infected with the hepatitis B virus [2]. Its structure was proven to be a covalently-linked circle based on its biomedical and electron microscopic analysis [1]. In addition, some plant viroids are presented as a covalently bound circular RNA molecule [3, 4]. The existence of circRNAs in mammalian cells, however, was heavily debated. An important finding was reported in 1979 when some interesting RNAs with a circular structure in the eukaryotic cytoplasm were identified using an electron microscope [5]. However, due to their low abundance and uncommon features, these RNAs were only regarded as byproducts of abnormal splicing and did not receive much attention at the time. Later in 1991, when studying the expression of a tumor suppressor gene, some circular transcripts were detected in human cells

although the significance of these circRNAs remained unclear [6].

With the advancement of high-throughput sequencing technologies and bioinformatics, an important breakthrough discovery in circRNA research appeared in 2012. In a study initially designed to screen genomic rearrangements associated with cancer, the global expression of circRNAs was accidentally discovered in the RNA sequencing (RNA-seq) data of human pediatric acute lymphoblastic leukemia samples. Additionally, the existence of circRNAs was further confirmed in both healthy and cancerous cells [7]. Based on the RNA-seq data, it is estimated that approximately 100,000 circRNAs are expressed in humans [7]. The higher abundance and diversity of circRNA expression may be associated with the alternative splicing of RNA transcripts [8–11]. Additionally, most circRNAs are presented in the cytoplasm, which is consistent with their regulatory role in the post-transcriptional function [7, 12, 13]. However, the newly discovered circular intron circRNAs (ciRNAs) or exon–intron circRNAs (EIciRNAs) are primarily located in the nucleus, which may correlate with their regulatory roles in their parental gene transcription [14, 15].

Although thousands of circRNAs have now been discovered, the ability to utilize the vast amount of circRNAs in the database poses a great challenge. At

* Correspondence: jli@uoguelph.ca
[2]Department of Animal Biosciences, University of Guelph, 50 Stone Road East, Building #70, Guelph, ON N1G 2W1, Canada
[3]College of Life Science and Engineering, Foshan University, Foshan, Guangdong province, China
Full list of author information is available at the end of the article

present, some features of circRNAs, such as high abundance, diverse structures, high resistance to degradation by exonuclease or RNase, cell- or tissue-specific expression, and highly evolutionary conservation, have been confirmed [11, 16, 17]. However, the mechanisms regulating their biogenesis, function, degradation, and cellular localization remain largely unclear [18, 19].

In the field of reproduction, investigations about circRNAs in the ovary, testis, and placenta have been reported. However, these reports mainly focus on circRNA screening and expression pattern [20–22]. Some of the studies suggested that circRNA may be engaged in epigenetic regulation and embryonic development [20, 21, 23]. These studies shed light on the role of circRNAs in the reproductive system.

The putative mechanism regulating circRNA biogenesis

Most circRNAs consist of protein-coding exons and are covalently circulated by canonical splicing sites. The canonical spliceosomal splicing mechanism is thus believed to be engaged in the regulation of circRNA biogenesis [11, 16, 24, 25]. A support for the involvement of a canonical spliceosomal splicing mechanism in circRNA biogenesis is that isoginkgetin, a splicing inhibitor, simultaneously blocks the formation of both linear and circular RNAs [11, 24]. Additionally, the induced mutation of canonical splicing sites interfered with exon circularization, subsequently prohibiting circRNA biogenesis [16, 26].

The current mainstream opinions tend to approve the regulatory roles of the backsplicing mechanism during circRNA biogenesis [7, 13, 19, 27]. The backsplicing mechanism is different from the canonical linear splicing mechanism based on the sequence of its splicing donors and acceptors [16, 25]. In canonical splicing, an upstream (5′) splice donor site is linked to a downstream (3′) splice acceptor site. Coupled with other transcriptional and post-transcriptional processes including 5′ capping and 3′ polyadenylation, canonical splicing produce a linear RNA transcript with 5′ to 3′ polarity [28]. By contrast, in backsplicing, a downstream (3′) splice donor site reversely accesses an upstream (5′) splice acceptor site, consequently forming a covalently linked circRNA and a linear RNA with skipped exons [28]. However, circRNA biogenesis regulated by the backsplicing mechanism is still influenced by both canonical splicing signals and spliceosomal machinery [11, 24]. Since most of the highly expressed circRNAs are generally derived from internal exons of pre-mRNAs, backsplicing is generally coupled with canonical splicing [28].

Meanwhile, there is a competitive relationship between the canonical linear splicing and circRNA biogenesis. The mechanism regulating this competition is tissue-specific and highly conserved between flies and

humans [24]. Moreover, circRNA generation has been shown to be influenced by the transcriptional elongation velocity. In a recent study, 4-thiouridine labeling was used to identify newly produced circRNAs, suggesting a faster transcribing velocity (2.9 kb/min) when compared to non-circRNA transcriptions (2.29 kb/min) [29]. Therefore, the backsplicing efficiency is positively influenced by the elongation velocity of RNA polymerase II [29]. For example, a mutation of a large subunit of the RNA polymerase II can greatly reduce the elongation velocity of RNA polymerase II, subsequently leading to a lower backsplicing efficiency in flies or mammals [30–32]. Additionally, according to the ratio between linear and circular RNAs, the circRNA expression level in flies with the mutation was significantly reduced [24], further supporting the effects of canonical splicing on circRNA formation.

circRNA biogenesis can be promoted by inverted repeats existing on both sides of exons. The base-pairing formation between these inverted repeats contributes to RNA circularization due to the induced spatial reduction among the splice signals involved in backsplicing [13, 15, 33]. Additionally, the existence of inverted ALU repeat elements (IAREs) can promote exon circularization [13]. In humans, IAREs, as critical components of complementary sequences and flanking introns, play an important role during exon circularization [34].

Some RNA binding proteins (RBPs), such as muscleblind (MBL) and quaking (QKI), are believed to promote circRNA biogenesis. MBL strongly and specifically binds to the circRNA derived from its own RNA. Owing to the regulation by MBL, a circRNA derived from the second exon circulation of Mbl pre-mRNA (circMbl) can be formed, which relies on the presence of conservative binding sites for MBL in the introns flanking the circularized exons [24, 35]. In addition, the exogenous expression of fly MBL enhances circRNA biogenesis from endogenous fly and human muscleblind transcripts. Down-regulation of MBL in mammalian cell culture or fly neural tissue significantly reduced the expression level of circMbl [24]. QKI, another important RBP, can also positively regulate circRNA formation. QKI contributes to circRNA biogenesis during the epithelial-to-mesenchymal transition (EMT) in human immortalized mammary epithelial cells [26]. The evidence that the knockdown of QKI blocks the expression of circRNAs related to the EMT further verifies the positive roles of QKI during circRNA biogenesis [26]. It should be noted that the regulatory roles of QKI require the involvement of putative binding sites in the flanking introns of circularized exons [26]. However, whether MBL or QKI can form base-pairing between two introns during circRNA biogenesis still lacks direct evidence.

The circRNA subclasses and their biogenesis

As illustrated in Fig. 1, circRNAs consist of three sub-classes based on their generating pathways. The most popular circRNA is the exon-derived circRNA (ecRNA), containing only exons and completely lacking introns [16]. Two mechanisms, including both exon skipping and direct backsplicing, have been proposed to explain ecRNA biogenesis [13, 25, 36]. Exon skipping, as a form of RNA splicing during mRNA biogenesis, may be associated with ecRNA formation. During exon skipping, the downstream exon rotates and leaps one or serveral exons to link the upstream exon, consequently producing a exon-skipped and functional mRNA. Meanwhile, the leaped exons form a lariat precursor containing exons and inrons, finally forming a circRNA after removal of introns [13, 37, 38]. By contrast, the direct backsplicing first generates alternatively spliced RNA and a lariat intermediate regulated by the intron-pairing mechanism. The introns in the lariat are then removed by the canonical splicing process [7, 21, 39–41]. Recent evidence indicates that direct backsplicing, not exon skipping, may be the primary mechanism regulating ecRNA formation [42]. After their biogenesis, ecRNAs must migrate into the cytoplasm to play their regulatory roles. However, the mechanism regulating the migration of mature ecRNAs into the cytoplasm currently remains unclear. The linear counterparts of circRNAs, such as mRNAs or long non-coding RNA (lncRNAs), can penetrate the nuclear membrane through the nuclear pore complex. It was suggested that ecRNA export may be regulated by a mechanism similar to the regulatory mechanism of linear RNA migration [18]. The degradation pathway of circRNAs is another unanswered question. The expression level of circRNA is dynamically modulated by the balance between biogenesis and degradation of circRNAs. circRNAs may be degraded via a mechanism triggered by short interfering RNAs [13]. A recent study found that circRNAs may be cleared by extracellular vesicles or microvesicle release in mammalian cells [43]. However, this conclusion is based on an in vitro study. Whether circRNAs are degraded in vivo by a similar mechanism still needs further elucidation.

In 2013, a novel type of circRNAs consisting of only introns, referred to as ciRNA, was discovered in human cells. It is mainly presented in the nucleus and is involved in the transcriptional regulation of its parental genes [14, 15]. ciRNA biogenesis requires a consensus motif consisting of both a 7 nt GU-rich element near the 5′ splice site and an 11 nt C-rich element near the branchpoint site. This motif may be specifically engaged in ciRNA formation because it is not enriched in regular introns or other types of circRNAs [44]. ciRNA

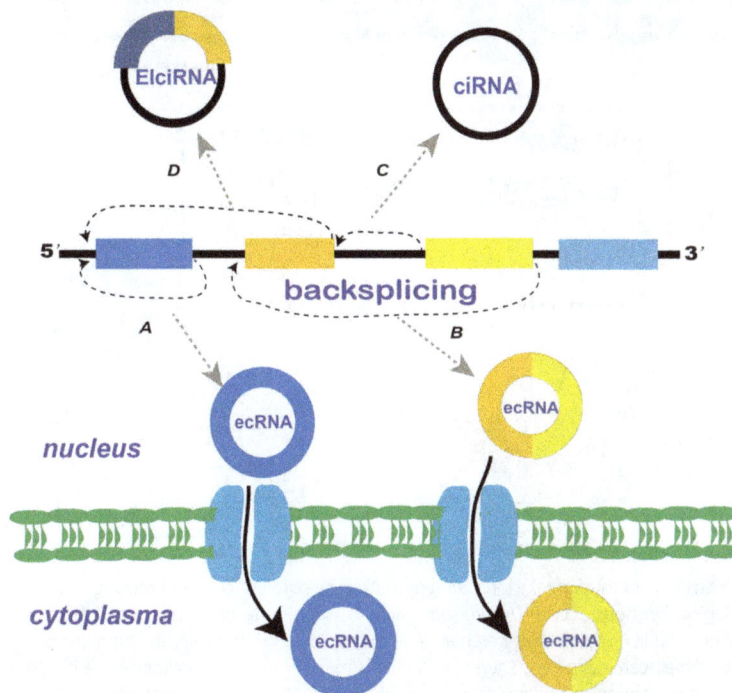

Fig. 1 The biogenesis of circRNAs. In the figure, exons are represented by different coloured rectangles and introns are represented by black lines. Exon-derived circRNA (ecRNA) only consists of exons (a and b). circular intronic RNA (ciRNA) contains only introns (c). In exon–intron circRNA (ElciRNA), an intron is inserted between two exons (d). The pathway through which mature ecRNAs migrate into the cytoplasm remains unclear. In this figure, circRNAs are postulated to pass through the nucleus membrane via a nuclear pore complex

biogenesis is regulated by a eukaryotic spliceosome-mediated splicing mechanism. ciRNAs are circular introns which are circularized at the branchpoint 2′–5′ linkage and degraded from the 3′ end up to the branchpoint. Therefore, ciRNAs are highly stable, due to their resistance to debranching and degradation [15, 45].

Recently, a more interesting EIciRNA in which one intron is inserted between two exons was discovered (illustrated in Fig. 1). Similar to ciRNA, EIciRNAs may also regulate their parental gene transcription in the nucleus [14]. However, the mechanism regulating EIciRNA biogenesis is unclear.

The putative functions of circRNAs

circRNAs are important modulators involved in the transcriptional and post-transcriptional regulation of gene expression. As the linear counterpart of circRNAs,

lncRNAs can fold into complex secondary or higher structures to provide more potential and diversity for both protein and target recognition [46, 47]. Therefore, the functional patterns of lncRNA are highly complicated. On the contrary, the structure of circRNA is circular and lacks complex spatial folding. The functional roles of circRNAs are therefore mainly determined by their base sequence. The putatively functional roles of circRNAs are summarized in Fig. 2.

First, circRNAs can function as a miRNA sponge to regulate the function of miRNAs [19, 27]. Some circRNAs, such as circRNA for miRNA-7 (ciRS-7) or Sry circRNA (circSry), contain some conserved binding sites for miRNAs. Based on the miRNA sponge theory, miRNA, in a form of Argonaute-miRNA complex, can bind to circRNAs. Therefore, circRNAs may function as competitively endogenous RNAs to block the

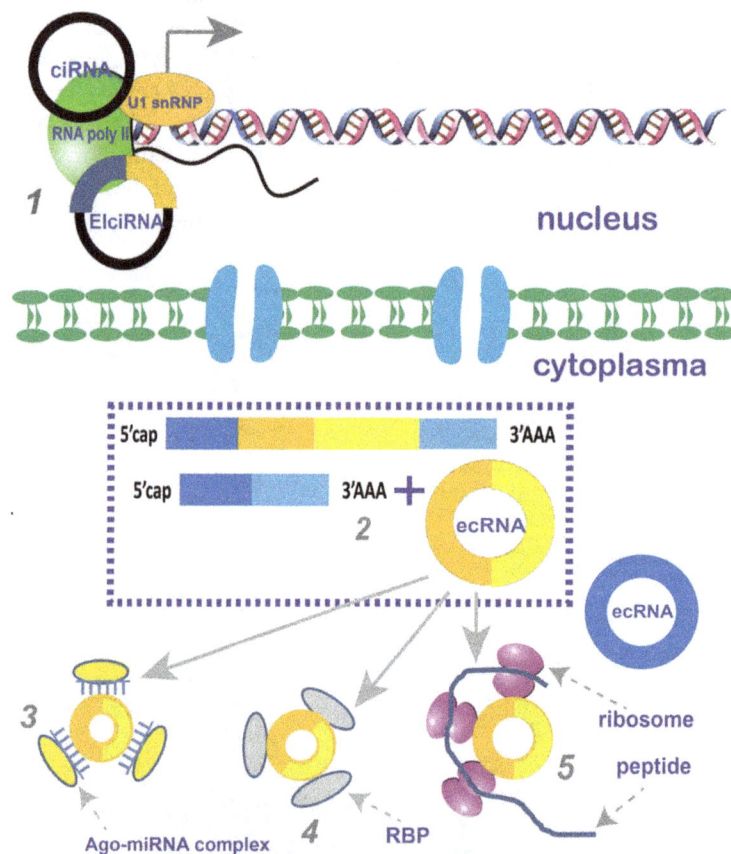

Fig. 2 The putative function of circRNAs. In this figure, exons are represented by different coloured rectangles and introns are represented by black lines. Five potentially biological functions of circRNAs are suggested. 1) To promote transcription of their parental genes: the ciRNAs and EIciRNAs are located in the nucleus and involved in their parental gene expression. 2) mRNA trap: the biogenesis of circRNAs is generally accompanied with transcription of their parental genes. Therefore, circRNAs may competitively influence the biogenesis and processing of mRNA. 3) miRNA sponge: some circRNAs have conserved binding sites for miRNAs. Through competitively binding with miRNAs, these circRNAs can block the binding between miRNAs and their target mRNAs, subsequently prohibiting the repressive effects of miRNAs on the target protein translation. 4) RNA binding protein (RBP) sponge: to regulate the function of RBPs, some circRNAs can interact with RBPs, such as Argonaute (Ago), polymerase II, muscleblind, etc. 5) to encode protein: some circRNAs contain internal ribosome entry site which can bind with ribosomes (shown by two tightly-attached ellipses). Therefore, these circRNAs may have an ability to encode proteins

miRNA-mediated endo-cleavage pathway [45]. Through competitively binding with miRNAs, circRNAs can interfere with the binding procedure between miRNAs and their target mRNAs, consequently weakening the repressive effects of miRNAs on the target protein translation [19, 27]. For instance, ciRS-7 possesses 74 conserved binding sites which can be bound by miR-7. Meanwhile, ciRS-7 can also be bound by Argonaute proteins which can interact with miRNAs [19]. Currently, the coexistence of both ciRS-7 and miR-7 has been affirmed by in vitro microscopy and co-immunoprecipitation experiments [27]. The study of transfecting miR-7 into HeLa cells has revealed that the response of constructed miR-7 targets is more efficient in the cells lacking ciRS-7 expression in comparison with cells expressing ciRS-7 [27]. In addition, miR-7 has shown great potential for applications in cancer therapy [48]. miR-7 can down-regulate some factors associated with cancer signaling pathways, such as epidermal growth factor receptor (EGFR), insulin-receptor substrate-1 (IRS-1), insulin-receptor substrate-2 (IRS-2), rapidly accelerated fibrosarcoma 1 (Raf1), p21-activated kinase 1 (Pak1), activated cdc42 kinase 1 (Ack1), insulinlike growth factor-1 receptor (IGF1R), phosphatidylinositol-4,5-bisphosphate 3-kinase catalytic subunit delta (PIK3CD), and mammalian target of rapamycin (mTOR) [48]. Additionally, E-cadherin can be up-regulated by miR-7, which can target IGF1R [49, 50] and focal adhesion kinase (FAK) [51, 52], causing weakened EMT, reduced anchorage-independent growth, and suppressed metastasis [48]. Therefore, ciRS-7 may play a regulatory role in oncogenesis via its interaction with miR-7.

In a previous study, the overexpression of ciRS-7 resulted in a decrease of the zebrafish midbrain size in zebrafish embryos. Similar phenomena have also been observed after silencing miR-7 via injection of morpholinos to reduce the expression level of miR-7 in zebrafish embryos [19], suggesting that the alteration of ciRS-7 can reversely influence the expression of miR-7. Furthermore, as a natural miRNA sponge for miR-7, ciRS-7 may regulate the expression of miR-7 targeted genes, some of them are known to be associated with Parkinson's disease or Alzheimer's disease [53].

Another example is circSry, which contains 16 conserved binding sites and can act as a miRNA sponge to sequester miR-138 [27]. Wang et al. recently discovered a new circRNA-heart-related circRNA (HRCR) which can function as a sponge to repress the activity of miR-223, subsequently leading to a weakened hypertrophic response [54]. These studies suggest that the miRNA sponge may be an important aspect of circRNA function. However, contradictory findings have also suggested that serving as a miRNA sponge may not be a universal role of circRNAs [12, 42, 45]. In order to test the miRNA sponge roles of circRNAs, Militello et al.

used the list of circRNAs in the circBase database (http:// www.circbase.org) [55] and screened for potential regions which can be bound by Argonaute [56]. Their results indicated that there were approximately 58,063 circRNAs with Argonaute-bound regions among 92,375 circRNAs in the circBase database. The reason why numerous circRNAs possess Argonaute-bound regions may be due to the fact that circRNAs are mainly derived from protein-coding genes which may have Argonaute-binding sites in their sequences [56]. Several highly-expressed circRNAs were selected to verify their miRNA sponge roles using the RNA-binding protein immunoprecipitation- polymerase chain reaction (RIP-PCR) technology. The results, however, were negative which does not support miRNA sponge as a universal function of circRNAs.

Secondly, circRNAs can interact with some RBPs, such as Argonaute [19, 27], RNA polymerase II [15], or MBL [24]. Some circRNAs may act as a RBP sponge to regulate the function of RBPs [19]. In a study carried out by Guo et al., based on the data collected from 20 RBPs in the high-throughput in vivo crosslinking experiment, the cluster densities of circular exons were slightly higher than those of their neighboring exons, possibly due to the fact that RBPs bound with circRNAs cannot be replaced by the translocating ribosome owing to the lack of translating capability in circRNAs [12]. However, in another study, the bioinformatics analysis of 38 RBPs revealed that the density of circRNAs bound with RBPs was lower in comparison with the coding sequence or 3′ untranslated regions (UTRs) of mRNAs [57]. In another study, in order to verify regulatory interactions between circRNAs and RBPs, circScan was adopted to detect backsplicing reads from cross-linking and immunoprecipitation followed by the high-throughput sequencing [58]. The authors screened 1500 crosslinking-immunprecipitation and high-throughput sequencing (CLIP-seq) datasets, identified approximately 12,540 novel bindings between circRNAs and RBPs in the human genome, and 1090 in the mouse genome. Additionally, these results were further confirmed by the RNA immunoprecipitation quantitative PCR (RIP-qPCR) [58]. It is speculated that the circRNAs and RBPs interaction may be engaged in diverse biological processes.

The third potential function of circRNAs is to act as an mRNA trap. Since circRNAs mainly consist of exons which may also be involved in mRNA biogenesis, circRNA formation may compete with the biogenesis of linear mRNA [45, 59]. However, there is evidence against this hypothesis. A typical example of this is the fmn gene. The mutations of the acceptor site in the fourth or fifth exon of the flavin mononucleotide (fmn) gene can cause the removal of corresponding circRNA. However, these mutations cannot influence the splicing efficiency of linear RNAs [59]. Therefore, whether the mRNA trap is merely a byproduct of circRNA biogenesis or an intended product is still unknown.

As newly discovered circRNAs, EIciRNA and ciRNA have been reported to be involved in the transcriptional regulation of their parental genes [14, 15]. EIciRNAs are generally located at the transcriptional site in the nucleus [14]. For example, either circEIF3J or circPAIP2 exists with its corresponding parental genomic loci and the U1 small nuclear ribonucleoprotein particle (U1 snRNP). EIciRNAs promote the transcription of their parental genes in cis with the assistance of the U1 snRNA, which may primarily function via the specific RNA-RNA interaction between U1 snRNA and EIciRNAs. Meanwhile, the down-regulation of EIciRNA expression levels can decrease the expression level of their parental mRNA [14], further suggesting the positive effects of EIciRNAs on the transcription of their parental mRNAs. Similar phenomena are also observed in ciRNAs which have been reported to be involved in the regulation of their parental gene expression [15].

Some circRNAs contain internal ribosome entry sites which can interact with ribosomes, suggesting that they may be translated into proteins [42, 60]. However, earlier works reported that most circRNAs cannot interact with polyribosomes, which leads to the viewpoint that circRNAs translation is less likely [12, 13, 39, 61]. However, as the linear counterparts of circRNAs, lncRNAs encodes some low-conservative peptides, which have been confirmed by ribosome profiling and mass spectrometry [62–64]. Therefore, whether circRNAs can encode proteins still remains a enticing question.

Recently, it was reported that a circRNA with an open reading frame can act as a template to guide protein translation in living cells by the rolling-circle amplification mechanism [65]. More recently, the methylated adenosine, N6-methyladenosine (m^6A), has been reported to promote efficient initiation of protein translation from circRNAs in human cells [66]. Through the polysome profiling, mass spectrometry and computational analysis, the same group also found that the consensus m^6A motifs are enriched in circRNAs, suggesting that they may have translation potential [66]. Similarly, Li et al. also confirmed that some natural circRNAs can interact with cap-independent translation factors including eukaryotic initiation factor 3 and m^6A, suggesting that these circRNAs may have a capability of translating proteins [58]. Based on a recent ribosome footprinting dataset analysis, Pamudurti et al. reported that 37 circRNAs were associated with translating ribosomes. In the same study, it was revealed that a circRNA derived from the muscle-blind locus can be translated into a protein in a cap-independent manner. The produced protein has been

detected in *Drosophila* head extracts by mass spectrometry [67]. Similarly, Legnini et al. also demonstrated that circ-ZNF609, a circRNA specifically regulating the proliferation of myoblasts, can bind to heavy polysomes, which has been confirmed by the sucrose gradient fractionation analysis, finally being translated to a protein in a splicing-dependent and cap-independent manner [68]. Additionally, after treatment with puromycin, circ-ZNF609 in myoblasts shifted to lighter polysomes in a way similarly to that of the corresponding ZNF609 mRNAs, showing the existence of active translation [68]. Another interesting phenomenon is that the presence of poly-adenosine or poly-thymidine in 3′ UTR blocks circRNA translation, which is different from mRNA [25]. Therefore, more and more new evidence is continually emerging to support the protein encoding function of circRNA.

circRNA and reproduction

Despite several sporadic reports about the expression and potential biological functions of circRNAs in reproductive organs, the research regarding the functional roles of circRNAs in this field is still at its infancy. However, these early stage studies shed light for further investigation. The current reports about circRNAs in the reproductive system are summarized in Table 1.

The expression of circRNAs in oocyte and pre-implantation embryo development

Thousands of stable RNAs derived from the introns of the most expressed genes were detected in the cytoplasm and the nucleus of *Xenopus tropicalis* oocytes. These RNAs were named as stable intronic sequence RNAs (sisRNAs) [69, 70]. Approximately 9000 sisRNAs have been identified in the cytoplasm of amphibian oocytes. These RNAs are resistant to the degradation induced by exonucleases and RNase R, due to their lariat structure [70]. Another interesting phenomenon is that the abundance of sisRNAs remained consistent from the germinal vesicle breakdown stage to the blastocyst stage of embryogenesis. Furthermore, the ratio between mRNA and sisRNA did not alter during oocyte and embryo development [70]. The expression pattern of sisRNAs suggests that they may regulate mRNA translation or stability during embryogenesis [70]. However, the functional roles of these sisRNAs in *Xenopus tropicalis* oocytes remain largely unclear. Additionally, Zhang et al. suspected that the biogenesis of sisRNAs may be via a mechanism similar to that of ciRNAs which regulate their parental gene expression [15].

The expression of circRNAs in pre-implantation embryos has only been reported in mice [71] and humans [23] to date. A novel single-cell universal poly (A)-independent RNA sequencing (SUPeR-seq)

Table 1 The recent advances about circRNAs related to reproduction

Species	Sample	Detection methods	Special treatment	Number of circRNAs	References
Xenopus tropicalis	Oocytes	RNA-sequencing	rRNA depletion	About 9000 lariat RNAs	Talhouarne and Gall [70]
Mouse	Embryo	Single-cell universal poly (A)-independent RNA sequencing	none	2891 circRNAs	Fan et al. [71]
Human	Embryo	Single-cell universal poly (A)-independent RNA sequencing	RNase H degradation	10,032 circRNAs from 2974 hosting genes	Dang et al. [23]
Human	Placental tissue	Arraystar circRNA microarray technology	none	301 circRNAs with different expression	Qian et al. [21]
Mouse	Spermatogenic cells	RNA sequencing	RNase R Treatment	15,101 circRNAs in spermatogenic cells	Lin et al. [82]
Human	Testis	RNA sequencing	RNase R Treatment	15,996 circRNAs containing 10,792 new circRNAs	Dong et al. [20]
human	granulosa cells	circRNA microarray technology	RNase R Treatment	57 differentially expressed circRNAs	Cheng et al. [77]

technology has been used for deep sequencing of mouse pre-implantation embryos [71]. A total of 2891 circRNAs derived from 1316 host genes were detected in mouse oocytes and early embryos (from zygotes to blastocysts). Most circRNAs, with a length of less than 2 kb, were derived from internal exons in the same host gene. Moreover, about 91% of circRNAs consist of multiple exons [71]. Different from what has been reported in amphibians [70], the expression pattern of these circRNAs shows a typically developmental stage-specific feature. Additionally, the gene ontology analytical data of the host genes producing these circRNAs revealed that the circRNAs presented in early embryos of mice are potentially responsible for chromosome organization, cell division, and DNA repair [71].

The same group analyzed the number of circRNAs at each embryonic stage. Approximately 2278 circRNAs were expressed in metaphase II mouse oocytes. After fertilization, the circRNA number in zygotes sharply reduced to 1850. At the four-cell embryo stage, the number of circRNA further reduced to only 1422. However, at the morulae stage, the circRNA number increased to 2799 instead. Again, the circRNA number strikingly decreased to only 779 in the blastocyst stage, suggesting the existence of a circRNA degradation mechanism during the morulae-to-blastocyst transition [71]. The fluctuation of circRNA abundance in mouse oocytes and pre-implantation embryos may be associated with their specific roles at different developmental stages.

Using a similar approach, 10,032 circRNAs derived from 2974 host genes were detected in human pre-implantation embryos [23]. Based on the differential expressed gene analysis, 1554 maternal genes and 851 zygotic genes were identified as host genes [23]. The

expression of most circRNAs is developmental stage-specific and dynamically regulated. Many circRNAs are maternally expressed, suggesting their potentially regulatory roles during oogenesis and generation of totipotent zygotes [23].

The circRNAs expressed in human pre-implantation embryos are much more abundant than those presented in mouse embryos, which may be partially due to the increase in intron length during human genome evolution [23]. However, circRNA biogenesis is generally conserved between human and mouse. Among the 1316 circRNA host genes identified in mouse pre-implantation embryos, 835 are also involved in circRNA formation in early human embryos. It was suggested that circRNA host genes in early human embryos may be primarily engaged in the regulation of organelle organization, chromosome organization, cell cycle, and metabolic regulation [23], which is similar to early mouse embryos [71], suggesting that circRNAs may be conserved across species.

The biological function of most detected circRNAs in pre-implantation embryos remains largely unclear. It was suggested that these circRNAs may potentially function as miRNA sponges in the regulation of gene expression during embryo development [72]. An interesting question is why the circRNA number in mouse embryos is significantly less than that in human embryos. Besides some evolutionary factors, it must be noted that there are differences in the technical preparation processes between human [23] and mouse embryo samples [71]. In the study by Dang et al., some human embryos experienced a more complicated process including intracytoplasmic sperm injection, freezing, thawing, and in vitro culture [23], while the mouse embryo samples were freshly isolated [71]. It is unclear if the in vitro manipulation stress triggers more circRNA expression.

Granulosa cells (GCs) play an important role during oocyte maturation and early embryo development [73, 74]. According to some studies, the gene expression patterns of GCs may be used as potential biomarkers to predict oocyte developmental capacity and consequent assistant reproduction results [75, 76]. Recently, Cheng et al. studied the expression pattern of circRNAs in human GCs during maternal aging [77]. The circRNA microarray technology was used to screen the circRNAs expressed in GCs of patients subjected to in vitro fertilization at a young age (less than 30 years) and an older age (more than 38 years). In older women, the expression levels of 46 circRNAs were up regulated. Meanwhile, the expression levels of 11 circRNAs were down regulated. After validation by reverse transcription PCR (RT-PCR) and adjustment of the effects related to gonadotropin treatment, among these differentially expressed circRNAs, the expression level of circRNA_103827 or circRNA_104816 was found to increase with maternal aging. Moreover, a negative correlation existed between the expression level of both circRNAs and the top quality embryo number. The bioinformatics results demonstrated the involvement of both circRNAs in glucose metabolism, mitotic cell cycle, and ovarian steroidogenesis [77]. The results from the receiver operating characteristic curve analysis revealed a higher sensitivity and specificity when circRNA_103827 or circRNA_104816 was used for prediction of live birth. Therefore, the expression patterns of circRNAs in GCs change with aging. Some specific circRNAs, such as circRNA_103827 or circRNA_104816, may be potential biomarkers for prediction of assistant reproduction outcomes [77].

Expression of circRNAs in the testis

Spermatogenesis is a complex and precisely-modulated process which is regulated by many testis- or male germ cell-derived genes [72]. During this process, spermatogonial stem cells experience a series of morphological alterations and finally develop into motile sperm [78]. Previous transcriptome studies primarily focus on mRNAs which can be used as a template for protein translation [79]. However, it must be mentioned that the ratio of protein-coding genes in the transcriptome is largely less than that of ncRNAs. Previous studies have indicated that ncRNAs play an important role during mammalian spermatogenesis [80–83]. For example, piwi-interacting RNAs (piRNAs) present in spermatogonia mainly interact with mRNAs and retrotransposons. However, in spermatocytes and spermatids, piRNAs primarily function in intergenic regions [20]. lncRNA has been reported to be engaged in mammalian spermatogenesis [79]. It has been reported that approximately 3000 human lncRNAs are specifically expressed in testis, suggesting that testis is a natural reservoir of lncRNAs [84].

A recent study confirmed the abundant expression of circRNAs in spermatogenic cells. Approximately 15,101 circRNAs were detected in mouse spermatogenic cells [82]. In terms of cell types, 5573, 5596, 6689, 4677, and 7220 circRNAs were expressed in spermatogonial stem cells, primitive type A spermatogonia, preleptotene spermatocytes, pachytene spermatocytes, and round spermatids, respectively. The circRNAs in round spermatids are higher than those in the other cell types [82]. However, the function of the vast amount of circRNAs in testis remains unknown.

In order to reveal the relationship between exon skipping and circRNA biogenesis, the expression patterns of the cytochrome P-450 2C18 gene in human epidermis and the androgen binding protein (ABP) gene in rat testes were investigated [85]. In human epidermis, besides the common mRNAs derived from nine exons, 2C18 circular transcripts skipping exons are also detected. Similarly, in rat testes, a circRNA composed of exons 6 and 7 of the ABP gene was identified. In this circRNA, the donor splice site of exon 7 is linked with the acceptor splice site of exon 6 [85], suggesting that the biogenesis of circRNAs consisting of various exon combinations may be influenced by the generation of mRNAs skipping the exons presented in the testis [85]. Dong et al. explored the expression profiles of circRNAs in human testes and seminal plasma using a high-throughput sequencing technology [20]. 15,996 circRNAs were discovered in the human testes, in which 10,792 circRNAs were novel. Among the detected circRNAs, 14,033 circRNAs can be mapped to 5928 host genes. Among these host genes, 1017 were newly found to generate circRNAs. Most of the host genes are involved in spermatogenesis, motility, and fertilization. The authors also found that these testis-derived circRNAs stably exist in seminal plasma. Furthermore, the circRNAs in seminal plasma are highly stable at room temperature, which may be due to their binding with proteins in seminal plasma. Therefore, it is suggested that the circRNAs in the seminal plasma may be used as novel noninvasive biomarkers for male fertility [20].

circRNA derived from the Sry gene and sex determination

A study comparing the expression levels of circRNA in brain, liver, heart, lung and testis indicated that circRNA were expressed at high level in testis, only second to that in brain [57], suggesting that circRNAs may have an important role in the testis. A relatively well studied circRNA in the testis is circSry, which is transcribed from the sex-determining region Y (Sry) gene.

In 1990, Sinclair et al. first cloned the Sry gene on the Y chromosome of human sperm [86]. Subsequent studies demonstrated the critically regulatory role of the Sry gene during sex determination [87]. The expression pattern of the Sry gene in mouse testis is developmental stage-dependent [88]. The Sry gene is expressed in the somatic cell lineage of the developing genital ridge between 10.5 and 12.5 days post coitum [87]. During this stage, the Sry gene can be transcribed into a linear mRNA which encodes a protein with a high mobility group (HMG) box. This protein functions as an important transcription factor, regulating sex differentiation during fetal development [89]. On the contrary, in adult testis, the expression of the Sry gene is generally coupled with the first spermatogenesis wave and round spermatid formation. Unlike in the genital ridge, most Sry transcripts in adult testis possess a typically circular structure [88]. It was suggested that long inverted repeats flanking the Sry gene may be responsible for circSry biogenesis [90]. The different transcription pattern of the Sry gene between the genital ridge and adult testis may suggest their specific functions in different developmental stages.

Since circSry possesses an open reading frame and a potential ATG start codon, this circRNA may be capable of protein translation [88]. However, this opinion may be questionable, due to a lack of evidence proving the existence of an interaction between circSry and polysome. Additionally, it is not determined whether circSry can regulate gene expression as a miRNA sponge. In mice, the up-regulation of circSry expression potentially represses the binding of miR-138 with its target mRNAs [27, 36]. According to the report by Hansen et al., biotin-labeled miR-138 has been showed to interact with circSry. Therefore, it is suggested that circSry can function as a miR-138 sponge [27]. However, considering that human circSry has only one miR-138 binding site, the miRNA sponge may be mouse-specific [12, 57]. In addition, the expression pattern of circSry is tissue-specific because circSry cannot be detected in brain, liver, kidney, or spleen [88].

Expression of circRNAs in placenta

The placenta plays an important role during fetal development, including the regulation of fetal metabolism and nutrition, gas and metabolite exchange, and hormone control [21, 91]. Currently, some studies have found that numerous ncRNAs, such as miRNAs [91, 92] or lncRNAs [93], are expressed in placentas. However, there is limited information related to the expression of circRNAs in placentas.

In a recent study carried out by Qian et al., the Arraystar circRNA microarray technology was used to detect differentially expressed circRNAs in placentas of pregnant women with preeclampsia (PE) [21]. Among 301 differentially expressed circRNAs between the PE placental tissues and the healthy tissues, 143 circRNAs were up-regulated and 158 were down-regulated. Many differentially expressed circRNAs, such as hsa_circRNA_101289, hsa_circRNA_101611, or hsa_circRNA_103285, possess miR-17 binding sites, suggesting that these circRNAs may be involved in the functional regulation of miR-17 in human placentas [21]. miR-17, one of the angiogenesis-associated miRNAs in human placentas, has been reported to highly express in PE placentas [94]. It was supposed that the differentially expressed circRNAs, as miRNA sponges, may competitively bind to miR-17, subsequently sequestering miR-17 and leading to the pathogenesis of PE [21]. In another study by Zhang et al., twelve circRNAs were found to be differentially expressed in blood cells of the PE patients as compared to the healthy women via the circRNA microarray analysis. RT-PCR further confirmed that the expression level of the circ_101222 in blood cells of PE patients was significantly higher than that of healthy women. It was suggested that the combination of circ_101222 with plasma protein factor endoglin may be used as a marker for PE [95].

circRNAs as biomarkers in the reproductive system

It was recently reported that the expression abundance of circRNAs in highly proliferating cells is generally lower in comparison with cells with lower proliferating capabilities [96, 97]. The expression level of circRNAs in cancerous tissues is less than the corresponding normal tissues, due to a higher proliferation rate in cancerous cells [96]. In ovarian cancer, the abundance of circRNAs in primary ovarian tumors is significantly different from that in metastasis ovarian lesions [98]. It has been reported that the expression level of ciRS-7, as a miR-7 sponge, was significantly up regulated in tumor samples [96]. miR-7 can regulate various oncogenes like Pak1, which is a kinase generally activated by DNA-damaging factors including radiation or etoposide [99]. Therefore, ciRS-7 may be up regulated in cancerous cells to start DNA repair and inhibit apoptosis during exposure to stress [100]. It will be of interest to study if ciRS-7 may be a biomarker for ovary-related cancers.

Recent studies have indicated that thousands of circRNAs are presented in human peripheral whole blood, suggesting that these blood-derived circRNAs may function as potential biomarkers in an easily available bodily fluid [97]. The new finding is from the group of Zhang et al. in which they discovered that circ_101222 in blood cells may function as a biomarker to diagnose PE [95], suggesting that the reproductive status or disease may be assessed via the measurement of the expression pattern of the circRNAs in the blood.

Many procedures in the field of human assisted reproduction, such as freezing and thawing, in vitro maturation, in vitro fertilization, and in vitro culture, can produce great external stress on gametes or embryos. Therefore, cells must adapt to external stresses by adjusting their gene expression patterns. Since circRNAs are abundantly expressed in gametes and embryos, they may be influenced by these procedures.

A typical example is epidermal growth factor (EGF) which is a growth factor that stimulates cell growth, proliferation, and differentiation. EGF has been used for in vitro maturation of mammalian oocytes. During oocyte meiotic maturation from prophase I to metaphase II, luteinizing hormone stimulates the secretion of EGF, which contributes to cumulus cell expansion and oocyte maturation via its receptor EGFR [101]. EGFR is a target of miR-7, therefore its biogenesis is down regulated by this miRNA [102, 103]. Meanwhile, ciRS-7 can sequester miR-7 and block the functional roles of miR-7. Therefore, ciRS-7 may be engaged in the regulation of EGFR function, further influencing oocyte maturation. Additionally, circRNAs are known to be involved in the regulation of cellular response to external stress, such as redox reactions, heat and cold shock, low temperatures, and salt response [66, 104]. It is thus interesting to study how the assisted reproduction process affects the expression patterns of circRNAs and the significance of these gene alterations.

Conclusions

Although thousands of circRNAs have been detected in ovary, embryo, placenta and testis via high-throughput sequencing technologies, the research on circRNAs in reproductive organs, especially in the ovary, has just begun. The biological functions of these RNAs remain largely unclear. circRNA's putative functions, such as miRNA sponge, RNA binding protein sponge, and mRNA trap, all add novel layers of regulation network to cell function. More excitingly, the recent findings on confirmation of protein coding function of circRNA, and that m^6A-driven translation of circRNAs is potentially a general phenomenon, opens a new array of questions to reproductive physiologists: what are the function of these large group of proteins which are previously unknown? Do they function in a similar manner as those derived from mRNA translation? As most circRNAs are derived from 1 to 2 exon canonical genes, translation of them would likely result in a shorter version of mRNA encoding proteins. Would these group of novel isoforms enhance or interfer with canonical protein function? Answering these questions may reveal a new area of understanding in reproductive physiology.

Abbreviations
ABP: Androgen binding protein; Ack1: Activated cdc42 kinase 1; circMbl: A circRNA derived from the second exon circulation of Mbl pre-mRNA; circRNA: Circular RNA; circSry: A circRNA derived from sex-determined region Y; ciRNA: Circular intronic circRNA; ciRS-7: A circRNA specially bound with miR-7; CLIP-seq: Crosslinking-immunprecipitation and high-throughput sequencing; ecRNA: Exon-derived circRNA; EGF: Epidermal growth factor; EGFR: Epidermal growth factor receptor; ElciRNA: Exon–intron circRNA; EMT: Epithelial-to-mesenchymal transition; FAK: Focal adhesion kinase; fmn: Flavin mononucleotide; GC: Granulosa cell; HMG: High mobility group; HRCR: A heart-related circRNA; IARE: Inverted ALU repeat element; IGF1R: Insulinlike growth factor-1 receptor; IRS-1: Insulin-receptor substrate-1; IRS-2: Insulin-receptor substrate2; lncRNA: Long non-coding RNA; m^6A: N^6-methyladenosine; MBL: Muscleblind; mTOR: Mammalian target of rapamycin; ncRNA: Non-coding RNA; Pak1: p21-activated kinase 1; PE: Preeclampsia; PIK3CD: Phosphatidylinositol-4,5-bisphosphate 3-kinase catalytic subunit delta; piRNA: Piwi-interacting RNA; QKI: Quaking; Raf1: Rapidly accelerated fibrosarcoma 1; RBP: RNA binding protein; RIP-PCR: RNA-binding protein immunoprecipitation- polymerase chain reaction; RIP-qPCR: RNA Immunoprecipitation quantitative PCR; RNase: Ribonuclease; RNA-seq: RNA sequencing; RT-PCR: Reverse transcription PCR; sisRNA: Stable intronic sequence RNA; Sry: Sex-determined region Y; SUPeR-seq: Single-cell universal poly (A)-independent RNA sequencing; U1 snRNP: U1 small nuclear ribonucleoprotein particle; UTR: Untranslated region

Acknowledgements
The authors would apologize to those researchers whose studies could not be cited in this review owing to space limitation. The authors would like to thank Dr. Wei Shen from Qingdao Agricultural University, Bo Pan from University of Guelph for helpful discussion; to Erin Miehe for editing/proof reading of the manuscript.

Funding
This study was funded by the China Scholarship Council (File No. 201508535001) and Natural Sciences and Engineering Research Council of Canada (NSERC).

Authors' contributions
GQ: co-wrote the manuscript; JL: co-wrote, and designed structure of the manuscript. All authors have read and approved the final manuscript.

Competing interests
The authors declare that they have no competing interests.

Author details
[1]Yunnan Animal Science and Veterinary Institute, Jindian, Panlong county, Kunming, Yunnan province 650224, China. [2]Department of Animal Biosciences, University of Guelph, 50 Stone Road East, Building #70, Guelph, ON N1G 2W1, Canada. [3]College of Life Science and Engineering, Foshan University, Foshan, Guangdong province, China.

References
1. Wang KS, Choo QL, Weiner AJ, Ou JH, Najarian C, Thayer RM, Mullenbach GT, Denniston KJ, Gerin JL, Houghton M. Structure, sequence and expression of the hepatitis delta viral genome. Nature. 1986;323:508–13.
2. Rizzetto M, Canese MG, Arico S, Crivelli O, Trepo C, Bonino F, Verme G. Immunofluorescence detection of new antigen-antibody system (delta/anti-delta) associated to hepatitis B virus in liver and in serum of HBsAg carriers. Gut. 1977;18:997–1003.
3. Roossinck MJ, Sleat D, Palukaitis P. Satellite RNAs of plant viruses: structures and biological effects. Microbiol Rev. 1992;56:265–79.
4. Sanger HL, Klotz G, Riesner D, Gross HJ, Kleinschmidt AK. Viroids are single-stranded covalently closed circular RNA molecules existing as

highly base-paired rod-like structures. Proc Natl Acad Sci U S A. 1976;73:3852–6.

5. Coca-Prados M, Hsu MT. Electron microscopic evidence for the circular form of RNA in the cytoplasm of eukaryotic cells. Nature. 1979;280:339–40.

6. Nigro JM, Cho KR, Fearon ER, Kern SE, Ruppert JM, Oliner JD, Kinzler KW, Vogelstein B. Scrambled exons. Cell. 1991;64:607–13.

7. Salzman J, Gawad C, Wang PL, Lacayo N, Brown PO. Circular RNAs are the predominant transcript isoform from hundreds of human genes in diverse cell types. PLoS One. 2012;7:e30733.

8. Barrett SP, Salzman J. Circular RNAs: analysis, expression and potential functions. Development. 2016;143:1838–47.

9. Barrett SP, Wang PL, Salzman J. Circular RNA biogenesis can proceed through an exon-containing lariat precursor. elife. 2015;4:e07540.

10. Schindewolf C, Braun S, Domdey H. In Vitro generation of a circular exon from a linear pre-mRNA transcript. Nucleic Acids Res. 1996;24:1260–6.

11. Starke S, Jost I, Rossbach O, Schneider T, Schreiner S, Hung LH, Bindereif A. Exon circularization requires canonical splice signals. Cell Rep. 2015;10:103–11.

12. Guo JU, Agarwal V, Guo H, Bartel DP. Expanded identification and characterization of mammalian circular RNAs. Genome Biol. 2014;15:409.

13. Jeck WR, Sorrentino JA, Wang K, Slevin MK, Burd CE, Liu J, Marzluff WF, Sharpless NE. Circular RNAs are abundant, conserved, and associated with ALU repeats. RNA. 2013;19:141–57.

14. Li Z, Huang C, Bao C, Chen L, Lin M, Wang X, Zhong G, Yu B, Hu W, Dai L, Zhu P, Chang Z, Wu Q, Zhao Y, Jia Y, Xu P, Liu H, Shan G. Exon–intron circular RNAs regulate transcription in the nucleus. Nat Struct Mol Biol. 2015;22:256–64.

15. Zhang Y, Zhang XO, Chen T, Xiang JF, Yin QF, Xing YH, Zhu S, Yang L, Chen LL. Circular intronic long noncoding RNAs. Mol Cell. 2013;51:792–806.

16. Chen I, Chen CY, Chuang TJ. Biogenesis, identification, and function of exonic circular RNAs. Wiley Interdisciplinary Reviews: RNA. 2015;6:563–79.

17. Salzman J. Circular RNA expression: its potential regulation and function. Trends Genet. 2016;32:309–16.

18. Chen L, Shan G. Circular RNAs remain peculiarly unclear in biogenesis and function. Sci China Life Sci. 2015;58:616–8.

19. Memczak S, Jens M, Elefsinioti A, Torti F, Krueger J, Rybak A, Maier L, Mackowiak SD, Gregersen LH, Munschauer M, Loewer A, Ziebold U, Landthaler M, Kocks C, le Noble F, Rajewsky N. Circular RNAs are a large class of animal RNAs with regulatory potency. Nature. 2013;495:333–8.

20. Dong WW, Li HM, Qing XR, Huang DH, Li HG. Identification and characterization of human testis derived circular RNAs and their existence in seminal plasma. Sci Rep. 2016;6(39080)

21. Qian Y, Lu Y, Rui C, Qian Y, Cai M, Jia R. Potential significance of circular RNA in human placental tissue for patients with preeclampsia. Cell Physiol Biochem. 2016;39:1380–90.

22. Stiefel F, Fischer S, Hackl M, Handrick R, Hesse F, Borth N, Otte K, Grillari J. Noncoding RNAs, post-transcriptional RNA operons and Chinese hamster ovary cells. Pharm Bioprocess. 2015;3:227–47.

23. Dang Y, Yan L, Hu B, Fan X, Ren Y, Li R, Lian Y, Yan J, Li Q, Zhang Y, Li M, Ren X, Huang J, Wu Y, Liu P, Wen L, Zhang C, Huang Y, Tang F, Qiao J. Tracing the expression of circular RNAs in human pre-implantation embryos. Genome Biol. 2016;17(130)

24. Ashwal-Fluss R, Meyer M, Pamudurti NR, Ivanov A, Bartok O, Hanan M, Evantal N, Memczak S, Rajewsky N, Kadener S. circRNA biogenesis competes with pre-mRNA splicing. Mol Cell. 2014;56:55–66.

25. Wang Y, Wang Z. Efficient backsplicing produces translatable circular mRNAs. RNA. 2015;21:172–9.

26. Conn SJ, Pillman KA, Toubia J, Conn VM, Salmanidis M, Phillips CA, Roslan S, Schreiber AW, Gregory PA, Goodall GJ. The RNA binding protein quaking regulates formation of circRNAs. Cell. 2015;160:1125–34.

27. Hansen TB, Jensen TI, Clausen BH, Bramsen JB, Finsen B, Damgaard CK, Kjems J. Natural RNA circles function as efficient microRNA sponges. Nature. 2013;495:384–8.

28. Chen LL, Yang L. Regulation of circRNA biogenesis. RNA Biol. 2015;12:381–8.

29. Ebbesen KK, Hansen TB, Kjems J. Insights into circular RNA biology. RNA Biol. 2017:1–11.

30. De La Mata M, Alonso CR, Kadener S, Fededa JP, Blaustein M, Pelisch F, Cramer P, Bentley D, Kornblihtt AR. A slow RNA polymerase II affects alternative splicing in vivo. Mol Cell. 2003;(2):525–32.

31. Ip JY, Schmidt D, Pan Q, Ramani AK, Fraser AG, Odom DT, Blencowe BJ. Global impact of RNA polymerase II elongation inhibition on alternative splicing regulation. Genome Res. 2011;21:390–401.

32. Khodor YL, Rodriguez J, Abruzzi KC, Tang CHA, Marr MT, Rosbash M. Nascent-seq indicates widespread cotranscriptional pre-mRNA splicing in drosophila. Genes Dev. 2011;(23):2502–12.

33. Ivanov A, Memczak S, Wyler E, Torti F, Porath HT, Orejuela MR, Piechotta M, Levanon EY, Landthaler M, Dieterich C, Rajewsky N. Analysis of intron sequences reveals hallmarks of circular RNA biogenesis in animals. Cell Rep. 2015;10:170–7.

34. Zhang XO, Wang HB, Zhang Y, Lu X, Chen LL, Yang L. Complementary sequence-mediated exon circularization. Cell. 2014;(1):134–47.

35. Vicens Q, Westhof E. Biogenesis of circular RNAs. Cell. 2014;159:13–4.

36. Kulcheski FR, Christoff AP, Margis R. Circular RNAs are miRNA sponges and can be used as a new class of biomarker. J Biotechnol. 2016;238:42–51.

37. Cocquerelle C, Mascrez B, Hetuin D, Bailleul B. Mis-splicing yields circular RNA molecules. FASEB J. 1993;7:155–60.

38. Kelly S, Greenman C, Cook PR, Papantonis A. Exon skipping is correlated with exon circularization. J Mol Biol. 2015;427:2414–7.

39. Salzman J, Chen RE, Olsen MN, Wang PL, Brown PO. Cell-type specific features of circular RNA expression. PLoS Genet. 2013;9:e1003777.

40. Suzuki H, Zuo Y, Wang J, Zhang MQ, Malhotra A, Mayeda A. Characterization of RNase R-digested cellular RNA source that consists of lariat and circular RNAs from pre-mRNA splicing. Nucleic Acids Res. 2006;34:e63.

41. Zaphiropoulos PG. Circular RNAs from transcripts of the rat cytochrome P450 2C24 gene: correlation with exon skipping. Proc Natl Acad Sci USA. 1996;93:6536–41.

42. Jeck WR, Sharpless NE. Detecting and characterizing circular RNAs. Nat Biotechnol. 2014;32:453–61.

43. Lasda E, Parker R. Circular RNAs co-precipitate with extracellular vesicles: a possible mechanism for circRNA clearance. PLoS One. 2016;11:e0148407.

44. Meng X, Li X, Zhang P, Wang J, Zhou Y, Chen M. Circular RNA: an emerging key player in RNA world. Brief Bioinform. 2016:1–11.

45. Shen T, Han M, Wei G, Ni T. An intriguing RNA species—perspectives of circularized RNA. Protein Cell. 2015;6:871–80.

46. Batista PJ, Chang HY. Long noncoding RNAs: cellular address codes in development and disease. Cell. 2013;152:1298–307.

47. Guttman M, Rinn JL. Modular regulatory principles of large non-coding RNAs. Nature. 2012;482:339–46.

48. Li J, Yang J, Zhou P, Le Y, Zhou C, Wang S, Xu D, Lin HK, Gong Z. Circular RNAs in cancer: novel insights into origins, properties, functions and implications. Am J Cancer Res. 2015;5:472–80.

49. Jiang L, Liu X, Chen Z, Jin Y, Heidbreder CE, Kolokythas A, Wang A, Dai Y, Zhou X. MicroRNA-7 targets IGF1R (insulin-like growth factor 1 receptor) in tongue squamous cell carcinoma cells. Biochem J. 2010;432:199–205.

50. Zhao X, Dou W, He L, Liang S, Tie J, Liu C, Li T, Lu Y, Mo P, Shi Y, Wu K, Nie Y, Fan D. MicroRNA-7 functions as an anti-metastatic microRNA in gastric cancer by targeting insulinlike growth factor-1 receptor. Oncogene. 2013;32:1363–72.

51. Kong X, Li G, Yuan Y, He Y, Wu X, Zhang W, Wu Z, Chen T, Wu W, Lobie PE, Zhu T. MicroRNA-7 inhibits epithelial-to-mesenchymal transition and metastasis of breast cancer cells via targeting FAK expression. PLoS One. 2012;7:e41523.

52. Wu DG, Wang YY, Fan LG, Luo H, Han B, Sun LH, Wang XF, Zhang JX, Cao L, Wang XR, You YP, Liu N. MicroRNA-7 regulates glioblastoma cell invasion via targeting focal adhesion kinase expression. Chin Med J (Engl). 2011;124:2616–21.

53. Lu D, Xu AD. Mini review: circular RNAs as potential clinical biomarkers for disorders in the central nervous system. Front Genet. 2016;7(53)

54. Wang K, Long B, Liu F, Wang JX, Liu CY, Zhao B, Zhou LY, Sun T, Wang M, Yu T, Gong Y, Liu J, Dong YH, Li N, Li PF. A circular RNA protects the heart from pathological hypertrophy and heart failure by targeting miR-223. Eur Heart J. 2016;37:2602–11.

55. Glazar P, Papavasileiou P, Rajewsky N. circBase: a database for circular RNAs. RNA. 2014;20:1666–70.

56. Militello G, Weirick T, John D, Döring C, Dimmeler S, Uchida S. Screening and validation of lncRNAs and circRNAs as miRNA sponges. Brief Bioinform. 2016:1–9.

57. You X, Vlatkovic I, Babic A, Will T, Epstein I, Tushev G, Akbalik G, Wang M, Glock C, Quedenau C, Wang X, Hou J, Liu H, Sun W, Sambandan S, Chen T, Schuman EM, Chen W. Neural circular RNAs are derived from synaptic genes and regulated by development and plasticity. Nat Neurosci. 2015;18:603–10.

58. Li B, Zhang XQ, Liu SR, Liu S, Sun WJ, Lin Q, Luo YX, Zhou KR, Zhang CM, Tan YY, Yang JH, Qu LH. Discovering the Interactions between Circular RNAs and RNA-binding Proteins from CLIP-seq Data using circScan. bioRxiv. 2017:115980.

59. Chao CW, Chan DC, Kuo A, Leder P. The mouse formin (Fmn) gene: abundant circular RNA transcripts and gene targeted deletion analysis. Mol Med. 1998;4:614–28.

60. Kos A, Dijkema R, Arnberg AC, van der Meide PH, Schellekens H. The hepatitis delta (δ) virus possesses a circular RNA. Nature. 1986;323:558–60.

61. Granados-Riveron JT, Aquino-Jarquin G. The complexity of the translation ability of circRNAs. Biochim Biophys Acta. 2016;1859:1245–51.

62. Anderson DM, Anderson KM, Chang CL, Makarewich CA, Nelson BR, McAnally JR, Kasaragod P, Shelton JM, Liou J, Bassel-Duby R, Olson EN. A micropeptide encoded by a putative long noncoding RNA regulates muscle performance. Cell. 2015;160:595–606.

63. Bazzini AA, Johnstone TG, Christiano R, Mackowiak SD, Obermayer B, Fleming ES, Vejnar CE, Lee MT, Rajewsky N, Walther TC, Giraldez AJ. Identification of small ORFs in vertebrates using ribosome footprinting and evolutionary conservation. EMBO J. 2014;33:981–93.

64. Ruiz-Orera J, Messeguer X, Subirana JA, Alba MM. Long Non-coding RNAs as a source of new peptides. elife. 2014;3:e03523.

65. Abe N, Matsumoto K, Nishihara M, Nakano Y, Shibata A, Maruyama H, Shuto S, Matsuda A, Yoshida M, Ito Y, Abe H. Rolling circle translation of circular RNA in living human cells. Sci Rep. 2015;5(16435)

66. Yang Y, Fan X, Mao M, Song X, Wu P, Zhang Y, Jin Y, Yang Y, Chen L, Wang Y, Wong CCL, Xiao X, Wang Z. Extensive translation of circular RNAs driven by N6-methyladenosine. Cell Res. 2017;27:626–41.

67. Pamudurti NR, Bartok O, Jens M, Ashwal-Fluss R, Stottmeister C, Ruhe L, Hanan M, Wyler E, Perez-Hernandez D, Ramberger E, Shenzis S, Samson M, Dittmar G, Landthaler M, Chekulaeva M, Rajewsky N, Kadener S. Translation of circRNAs. Mol Cell. 2017;66:9–21.

68. Legnini I, Di Timoteo G, Rossi F, Morlando M, Briganti F, Sthandier O, Fatica A, Santini T, Andronache A, Wade M, Laneve P, Rajewsky N, Bozzoni I. Circ-ZNF609 is a circular RNA that can be translated and functions in myogenesis. Mol Cell. 2017;66:22–37.

69. Gardner EJ, Nizami ZF, Talbot CC, Gall JG. Stable intronic sequence RNA (sisRNA), a new class of noncoding RNA from the oocyte nucleus of Xenopus Tropicalis. Genes Dev. 2012;26:2550–9.

70. Talhouarne GJS, Gall JG. Lariat intronic RNAs in the cytoplasm of Xenopus Tropicalis oocytes. RNA. 2014;20:1476–87.

71. Fan X, Zhang X, Wu X, Guo H, Hu Y, Tang F, Huang Y. Single-cell RNA-seq transcriptome analysis of linear and circular RNAs in mouse preimplantation embryos. Genome Biol. 2015;16(148)

72. Zhang C, Gao L, Xu EY. LncRNA, a new component of expanding RNA-protein regulatory network important for animal sperm development. Semin Cell Dev Biol. 2016;59:110–7.

73. Dumesic DA, Meldrum DR, Katz-Jaffe MG, Krisher RL, Schoolcraft WB. Oocyte environment: follicular fluid and cumulus cells are critical for oocyte health. Fertil Steril. 2015;103:303–16.

74. Moreno JM, Nunez MJ, Quinonero A, Martinez S, de la Orden M, Simon C, Pellicer A, Díaz-García C, Domínguez F. Follicular fluid and mural granulosa cells microRNA profiles vary in in vitro fertilization patients depending on their age and oocyte maturation stage. Fertil Steril. 2015;104:1037–46.

75. Hamel M, Dufort I, Robert C, Gravel C, Leveille MC, Leader A, Sirard MA. Identification of differentially expressed markers in human follicular cells associated with competent oocytes. Hum Reprod. 2008;23:1118–27.

76. Hamel M, Dufort I, Robert C, Leveille MC, Leader A, Sirard MA. Genomic assessment of follicular marker genes as pregnancy predictors for human IVF. Mol Hum Reprod. 2010;16:87–96.

77. Cheng J, Huang J, Yuan S, Zhou S, Yan W, Shen W, Chen Y, Xia X, Luo A, Zhu D, Wang S. Circular RNA expression profiling of human granulosa cells during maternal aging reveals novel transcripts associated with assisted reproductive technology outcomes. PLoS One. 2017;12:e0177888.

78. Griswold MD. Spermatogenesis: The commitment to meiosis. Physiol Rev. 2016;96:1–17.

79. Luk AC, Chan WY, Rennert OM, Lee TL. Long noncoding RNAs in spermatogenesis: insights from recent highthroughput transcriptome studies. Reproduction (Cambridge, England). 2014;147:R131–41.

80. Bettegowda A, Wilkinson MF. Transcription and post-transcriptional regulation of spermatogenesis. Philos Trans R Soc Lond Ser B Biol Sci. 2010;365:1637–51.

81. Chuma S, Nakano T. piRNAe and spermatogenesis in mice. Phil Trans R Soc B. 2013;368:20110338.

82. Lin X, Han M, Cheng L, Chen J, Zhang Z, Shen T, Wang M, Wen B, Ni T, Han C. Expression dynamics, relationships, and transcriptional regulations of diverse transcripts in mouse spermatogenic cells. RNA Biol. 2016;13:1011–24.

83. Yadav RP, Kotaja N. Small RNAs in spermatogenesis. Mol Cell Endocrinol. 2014;382:498–508.

84. Cabili MN, Trapnell C, Goff L, Koziol M, Tazon-Vega B, Regev A, Rinn JL. Integrative annotation of human large intergenic noncoding RNAs reveals global properties and specific subclasses. Gen Dev. 2011;25:1915–27.

85. Zaphiropoulos PG. Exon skipping and circular RNA formation in transcripts of the human cytochrome P-450 2C18 gene in epidermis and of the rat androgen binding protein gene in testis. Mol Cell Biol. 1997;17:2985–93.

86. Sinclair AH, Berta P, Palmer MS, Hawkins JR, Griffiths BL, Smith MJ, Foster JW, Frischauf AM, Lovell-Badge R, Gwdfellow PN. A gene from the human sex-determining region encodes a protein with homology to a conserved DNA-binding motif. Nature. 1990;346:240–4.

87. Koopman P, Gubbay J, Vivian N, Goodfellow P, LovellBadge R. Male development of chromosomally female mice transgenic for Sry. Nature. 1991;357:117–21.

88. Capel B, Swain A, Nicolis S, Hacker A, Walter M, Koopman P, Goodfellow P, Lovell-Badge R. Circular transcripts of the testis-determining gene Sry in adult mouse testis. Cell. 1993;73:1019–30.

89. Harley VR, Jackson D, Hextall P, Hawkins JR, Berkovitz GD, Sockanathan S, Lovell-Badge R, Goodfellow PN. DNA binding activity of recombinant SRY from normal males and XY females. Science. 1992;255:453–8.

90. Dubin RA, Kazmi MA, Ostrer H. Inverted repeated are necessary for circularization of mouse testis Sry transcript. Gene. 1995;167:245–8.

91. Hale BJ, Yang CX, Ross JW. Small RNA regulation of reproductive function. Mol Reprod Dev. 2014;81:148–59.

92. Liang Y, Ridzon D, Wong L, Chen C. Characterization Of microRNA expression profiles in normal human tissues. BMC Genomics. 2017;8:166.

93. Taylor DH, Chu ETJ, Spektor R, Soloway PD. Long non-coding RNA regulation of reproduction and development. Mol Reprod Dev. 2015;82:932–56.

94. Wang W, Feng L, Zhang H, Hachy S, Satohisa S, Laurent LC, Parast M, Zheng J, Chen DB. Preeclampsia up-regulates angiogenesis-associated MicroRNA (i.E., miR-17, −20a, and -20b) that target ephrin-B2 and EPHB4 in human placenta. J Clin Endocrinol Metab. 2012;97:E1051–9.

95. Zhang YG, Yang HL, Long Y, Li WL. Circular RNA in blood corpuscles combined with plasma protein factor for early prediction of pre-eclampsia. BJOG Int J Obstet Gynaecol. 2017;123:2113–8.

96. Bachmayr-Heyda A, Reiner AT, Auer K, Sukhbaatar N, Aust S, Bachleitner-Hofmann T, Mesteri I, Grunt TW, Zeillinger R, Pils D. Correlation of circular RNA abundance with proliferation–exemplified with colorectal and ovarian cancer, idiopathic lung fibrosis, and normal human tissues. Sci Rep. 2015;5(8057)

97. Memczak S, Papavasileiou P, Peters O, Rajewsky N. Identification and characterization of circular RNAs as a new class of putative biomarkers in human blood. PLoS One. 2015;10:e0141214.

98. Ahmed I, Karedath T, Andrews SS, Al-Azwani IK, Mohamoud YA, Querleu D, Rafii A, Malek JA. Altered expression pattern of circular RNAs in primary and metastatic sites of epithelial ovarian carcinoma. Oncotarget. 2016;7:36366.

99. Advani SJ, Camargo MF, Seguin L, Mielgo A, Anand S, Hicks AM, Aguilera J, Franovic A, Weis SM, Cheresh DA. Kinase-independent role for CRAF-driving tumour radioresistance via CHK2. Nat Commun. 2015;6:8154.

100. Fischer JW, AKL L. CircRNAs: A regulator of cellular stress. Crit Rev Biochem Mol Biol. 2017;52:220–33.

101. Jamnongjit M, Gill A, Hammes SR. Epidermal Growth factor receptor signaling is required for normal ovarian steroidogenesis and oocyte maturation. Proc Natl Acad Sci U S A. 2005;102:16257–62.

102. Reddy SD, Ohshiro K, Rayala SK, Kumar R. MicroRNA-7, a homeobox D10 target, inhibits p21-activated kinase 1 and regulates its functions. Cancer Res. 2008;68:8195–200.

103. Webster RJ, Giles KM, Price KJ, Zhang PM, Mattick JS, Leedman PJ. Regulation of epidermal growth factor receptor signaling in human cancer cells by microRNA-7. J Biol Chem. 2009;284:5731–41.

104. Zuo J, Wang Q, Zhu B, Luo Y, Gao L. Deciphering the roles of circRNAs on chilling injury in tomato. Biochem Biophys Res Commun. 2016;479:132–8.

2

Age-dependent difference in impact of fertility preserving surgery on disease-specific survival in women with stage I borderline ovarian tumors

Haiyan Sun[1,2], Xi Chen[1], Tao Zhu[1], Nanfang Liu[1], Aijun Yu[1*] and Shihua Wang[3*]

Abstract

Background: This study was to determine age-specific impact of fertility preserving surgery on disease-specific survival in women with stage I borderline ovarian tumors (BOTs). Patients diagnosed during 1988–2000 were selected from The Surveillance, Epidemiology, and End Results (SEER) database. The age-specific impact of fertility preserving surgery and other risk factors were analyzed in patients with stage I BOTs using Cox proportion hazard regression models. Data from our hospital were collected during 1996–2017 to determine the prevalence of patients who had undergone fertility preserving surgery.

Results: Of a total 6295 patients in the SEER database, this study selected 2946 patients with stage T1 BOTs who underwent fertility preserving or radical surgery. Their median age at diagnosis was 45.0 years and the median follow-up time was 200 months. Fertility preserving surgery was performed in 1000/1751 (57.1%) patients < 50 years and in 1,81/1195 (15.1%) patients ≥50 years. Fertility preserving surgery was significantly associated with worse disease-specific survival only in patients ≥50 years. Increased age, stage T1c and mucinous histology were risk factors for overall patients or patients ≥50 years, but not for < 50 years. Data from our hospital showed that fertility preserving surgery was performed in 53.9 and 12.3%patients < 50 and ≥ 50 years with stage I disease, respectively.

Conclusion: Fertility preserving surgery is safe for women < 50 years with early staged BOTs, but it may decrease disease-specific survival in patients ≥50 years. Conservative surgery is performed at a relatively high rate in patients ≥50 years.

Keywords: Ovarian cancer, Borderline ovarian tumor, Fertility preserving surgery, Survival, Age, Histology, Stage

Background

Borderline ovarian tumors (BOTs) are histologically characterized as atypical epithelial proliferation without the presence of stromal invasion [1]. Serous and mucinous BOTs are the two major histological types [2]. These tumors have a low malignant potential to spread beyond the ovary with peritoneal involvement [1] and have an excellent prognosis [3–5]. This disease accounts for 10–15% of all epithelial ovarian cancers [6]. Compared to invasive epithelial ovarian cancers, BOTs occur more commonly, at an early stage, in women of childbearing ages [7].

The majority of BOTs are managed with surgery alone. Fertility preserving surgery is widely adopted for patients who have early-stage tumor development and a desire for fertility. Current consensus states that fertility preserving surgery is associated with an increased risk of recurrence [8–12]. Data from ours and other groups showed that certain styles of fertility preserving surgery may have a higher risk of recurrence than the others [13–15]. However, fertility preserving surgery was not shown to compromise overall survival in these patients [16–19].

Due to excellent prognosis, many patients with BOTs die due to other diseases. Overall survival is the

* Correspondence: yuaj@zjcc.org.cn; shwang@wakehealth.edu
[1]Department of Gynecologic Oncology, Zhejiang Cancer Hospital, 1 Banshan East Road, Zhejiang 310022, Hangzhou, China
[3]Department of Cancer Biology, Wake Forest School of Medicine, Winston Salem, NC 27157, USA
Full list of author information is available at the end of the article

end-point commonly used in previous studies to determine the impact of fertility preserving surgery; however, this may not accurately reflect the outcome of the surgery. Very few studies have investigated the impact of fertility preserving surgery on disease-specific survival [9]. Fertility preserving surgery has been shown age-dependent differences in its impact on recurrence free survival and other clinical outcomes in patients with BOTs [20]. Using a large population from a publicly available database, the objective of this study was to examine the age-specific impact of fertility preserving surgery on disease-specific survival in women with stage I BOTs.

Methods

The data for this study was obtained from the Surveillance, Epidemiology, and End Results (SEER) database maintained by the National Cancer Institute. This database collects information of cancer patients, which covers approximately 28% of the total US population. The SEER program statistical analysis software package (SEER*Stat version 8.3.4) was used to extract data from SEER18 Regs Research Data + Hurricane Katrina Impacted Louisiana Cases, Nov 2016 Sub (1973–2014 varying) [21]. BOTs in the SEER database between 1988 and 2000 were identified based upon the following histopathology codes: serous 8442–1, 8451–1 and 8462–1; and mucinous 8472–1, 8473–1 [22, 23].

Only patients with stage I BOTs with a record of survival times were included in this study. The status of oophorectomies and hysterectomies were quarried from codes in the site-specific surgery (1983–1997) and RX Summ–Surg Prim Site (1998+) (Additional file 1: Table S1). Fertility preserving surgery refers to preservation of the uterus and at least one side of a functional ovary. This study thus defined the surgery as removal of the tumor or a unilateral oophorectomy without a hysterectomy. Radical surgery was defined as bilateral salpingo-oophorectomy with or without hysterectomy. Women were excluded if they did not receive surgery, their surgical status or survival time was unknown, or other surgical approaches were performed (Additional file 1: Table S1). The flow chart shows the detailed procedure for selecting patients (Additional file 1: Figure S1).

Variables extracted from the database were patients' demographics (age at diagnosis, ethnicities, marital status), surgery information (oophorectomy, hysterectomy, lymphadenectomy), tumor information (size, histology, stage), follow-up time and disease-specific death. Tumor stages were evaluated based on the American Joint Committee on Cancer (AJCC) 3rd staging classification [24].

To understand age-specific prevalence of fertility preserving surgery, women diagnosed with BOTs in Zhejiang Cancer Hospital during the year 1996–2017 were also included in this study. Tumor stages were evaluated based upon of the International Federation of Gynecology and Obstetrics (FIGO) 2014 classification system [25]. Stage T1 defined in AJCC 3rd is the same as stage I in FIGO 2014, except that stage Ic in FIGO 2014 is further divided into Ic1, Ic2 and Ic3 stages. The inclusion and exclusion criteria for these patients has been described previously [15].

Data were analyzed using SAS software V9.3 (SAS Institute, Inc., Cary, NC.). The ordinal/categorical data were examined using the χ^2 test. Univariate or multivariate Cox proportional hazards models were used to determine the impacts of fertility preserving surgery and other risk factors on disease-specific survival. The Kaplan-Meier survival curves were generated and their significant differences were analyzed by log-rank tests. Two-sided P values less than 0.05 were considered statistically significant.

Results

A total of 6295 women with BOTs were initially identified from the SEER database. Based on our inclusion and exclusion criteria, a total of 2946 cases with stage I BOTs were included in this study. The detailed demographic information and pathoclinical features are listed in Table 1. The mean age of these patients was 47.1 ± 17.0 years with a median age of 45.0 years (range 10–96 years). The median follow-up time was 200 months (range 1–323 months). Within this population, 59.4% ($n = 1751$) were < 50 years old and 40.6% ($n = 1195$) were ≥ 50 years. Most patients (85.0%) studied were Caucasian. The majority of BOTs were diagnosed at stage T1a (79.3%). Fertility preserving surgery was performed in 1181 (40.1%) patients. Hysterectomy and recorded lymphadenectomy were performed in 1374 (47.6%) and 341 (11.4%) patients, respectively. At the end of the follow-up year, 70 (2.4%) patients died from this disease.

The characteristics of patients in two age groups (< 50 and ≥ 50 years) are presented in Table 1. Compared to patients < 50 years, patients ≥50 years underwent fertility preserving surgery less frequently (15.1% vs 57.1%, $P < 0.0001$). A higher proportion of them were Caucasian (87.2% vs 83.6%, $P = 0.0049$), underwent hysterectomy (63.7% vs 35.0%, $P < 0.0001$) and lymphadenectomy (14.0% vs 9.6%, $P = 0.0050$). They had a higher rate of disease-specific death (4.5% vs 0.9%, $P < 0.0001$), but a shorter mean follow-up time (163.4 ± 77.8 vs 215.0 ± 59.2 months, $P < 0.0001$).

The features of patients were compared between those who underwent fertility preserving surgery vs. radical surgery. Of the entire population studied, including both age groups, married patients and patients with serous tumors at stage T1b or T1c were less likely to undergo fertility preserving surgery. Patients receiving fertility

Table 1 Demographic and pathoclinical features of BOT patients

Variables		Overall (n = 2946)	< 50 (n = 1751)	≥ 50 (n = 1195)	P value
Age (years)					
	Median (range)	45.0 (10–96)	36.0 (10–49)	64.0 (50–96)	
	Mean ± SD	47.1 ± 17.0	35.3 ± 8.6	64.3 ± 10.2	
Race					
	White	2505 (85.0)	1463 (83.6)	1042 (87.2)	0.0049
	Black	170 (5.8)	102 (5.8)	68 (5.7)	
	Others	271 (9.2)	186 (10.6)	85 (7.1)	
Histology					
	Serous	1646 (55.9)	961 (54.9)	685 (57.3)	0.1905
	Mucinous	1300 (44.1)	790 (45.1)	510 (42.7)	
Marital status					
	Single*	1268 (43.0)	736 (42.0)	532 (44.5)	0.3188
	Married	1560 (53.0)	940 (53.7)	620 (51.9)	
	Unknown	118 (4.0)	75 (4.3)	43 (3.6)	
Lymphadenectomy					
	No	2602 (88.3)	1575 (90.0)	1027 (85.9)	0.0004
	Yes	336 (11.4)	169 (9.6)	167 (14.0)	
	Unknown	8 (0.3)	7 (0.4)	1 (0.1)	
AJCC stage					
	T1a	2337 (79.3)	1407 (80.4)	930 (77.8)	0.0582
	T1b	177 (6.0)	90 (5.1)	87 (7.3)	
	T1c	281 (9.6)	171 (9.8)	110 (9.2)	
	T1x	151 (5.1)	83 (4.7)	68 (5.7)	
Tumor size					
	≤ 5 cm	425 (40.6)	244 (40.3)	181 (40.9)	0.8402
	> 5 cm	622 (59.4)	361 (59.7)	261 (59.1)	
Hysterectomy	No	1572 (53.4)	1138 (65.0)	434 (36.3)	< 0.0001
	Yes	1374 (47.6)	613 (35.0)	761 (63.7)	
Fertility preserving surgery					
	No	1765 (59.9)	751 (42.9)	1014 (84.9)	< 0.0001
	Yes	1181 (40.1)	1000 (57.1)	181 (15.1)	
Laterality					
	Unilateral	1092 (37.1)	646 (36.9)	446 (37.3)	0.9652
	Bilateral	1253 (42.5)	748 (42.7)	505 (42.3)	
	Unknown	601 (20.4)	357 (20.4)	244 (20.4)	
Death	No	2876 (97.6)	1735 (99.1)	1141 (95.5)	< 0.0001
	Yes	70 (2.4)	16 (0.9)	54 (4.5)	
Follow-up time (months)					
	Median (range)	200 (1–323)	217 (1–323)	176 (1–323)	
	Mean ± SD	194.0 ± 72.0	215.0 ± 59.2	163.4 + 77.8	< 0.0001

*including never married, divorced, widowed. Abbreviations: AJCC, American Joint Commission on Cancer; T1x, T1 undefined

preserving surgery were less likely to undergo lymphade-nectomy. Caucasian patients, both in the entire population, as well as in the < 50 age group were less likely to undergo fertility preserving surgery (Table 2).

Results of univariate and multivariate analysis of disease-specific survival in the whole population are presented in Table 3. Increased age (hazard ratio (HR) = 1.06, 95% confidence interval (CI): 1.04–1.08, $P < 0.0001$), stage T1c (vs T1a, HR = 2.42, 95% CI: 1.30–4.48, $P = 0.0051$) were significantly associated with worse disease-specific survival. Without controlling of other confounding factors, fertility preserving surgery (vs radical surgery, HR = 0.52, 95% CI: 0.30–0.88, $P = 0.0142$) was associated with improved disease-specific survival. The survival curves are presented at Additional file 1: Figure S2A and S2B. Multivariate analysis showed that increased age (HR = 1.06, 95% CI: 1.05–1.08, $P < 0.0001$), stage T1b (vs T1a, HR = 2.38, 95% CI: 1.05–5.39, $P = 0.0369$), stage T1c (vs T1a, HR = 3.00, 95% CI: 1.60–5.65, $P = 0.0006$) and mucinous histology (HR = 1.73, 95% CI: 1.06–2.83, $P = 0.0285$) were significantly associated with worse disease-specific survival, whereas fertility preserving

Table 2 Features of patients who underwent fertility preserving surgery (Yes) or radical surgery (No)

Variables		Total (n = 2946)			< 50 (n = 1751)			≥ 50 (n = 1195)		
Fertility preserving surgery		Yes	No	P values	Yes	No	P values	Yes	No	P values
Race										
	White	964 (81.6)	1541 (87.3)	< 0.0001	806 (80.6)	657 (87.5)	< 0.0001	158 (87.3)	884 (87.2)	0.0952
	Black	75 (6.4)	95 (5.4)		60 (6.0)	42 (5.6)		15 (8.3)	53 (5.2)	
	Other	142 (12.0)	129 (7.3)		134 (72.0)	52 (6.9)		8 (4.4)	77 (7.6)	
Marital status										
	Single*	580 (49.1)	688 (39.0)	< 0.0001	487 (48.7)	249 (33.2)	< 0.0001	93 (51.4)	439 (43.3)	0.0220
	Married	555 (35.6)	1005 (56.9)		477 (47.7)	463 (61.6)		78 (43.1)	542 (53.4)	
	Unknown	46 (3.9)	72 (4.1)		36 (3.6)	39 (5.2)		10 (5.5)	33 (3.3)	
Histology										
	Serous	615 (52.1)	1031 (58.4)	0.0007	514 (51.4)	447 (59.5)	0.0007	101 (55.8)	584 (57.6)	0.6533
	Mucinous	566 (47.9)	734 (41.6)		486 (48.6)	304 (40.5)		80 (44.2)	430 (42.4)	
AJCC stage										
	T1a	1000 (84.7)	1337 (75.6)	< 0.0001	850 (85.0)	557 (74.2)	< 0.0001	150 (82.9)	780 (76.9)	0.0008
	T1b	22 (1.9)	155 (8.8)		21 (2.1)	69 (9.2)		1 (0.6)	86 (8.5)	
	T1c	101 (8.6)	180 (10.2)		86 (8.6)	85 (11.3)		15 (8.3)	95 (9.4)	
	T1x	58 (4.9)	93 (5.3)		43 (4.3)	40 (5.3)		15 (8.3)	53 (5.2)	
Hysterectomy										
	No	1181 (100)	391 (22.2)	< 0.0001	100 (100)	138 (18.4)	< 0.0001	181 (100)	253 (25.0)	< 0.0001
	Yes	0 (0)	1374 (77.8)		0 (0)	631 (81.6)		0 (0)	761 (75.0)	
Tumor size										
	<=5	166 (40.3)	259 (40.8)	0.8731	139 (39.8)	105 (41.0)	0.7686	27 (42.9)	154 (40.6)	0.7396
	> 5	246 (59.7)	376 (59.2)		210 (60.2)	151 (59.0)		36 (57.1)	225 (59.4)	
Lymphadenectomy										
	No	1085 (91.9)	1517 (86.0)	< 0.0001	1032 (61.3)	652 (38.7)	0.0001	161 (89.0)	866 (85.4)	0.4254
	Yes	91 (7.8)	245 (13.9)		80 (44.7)	99 (55.3)		20 (11.0)	147 (14.5)	
	Unknown	5 (0.4)	3 (0.2)		5 (71.4)	2 (28.6)		0 (0)	1 (0.1)	
Laterality										
	Unilateral	426 (36.1)	666 (37.7)	0.6573	372 (37.2)	274 (36.5)	0.8792	54 (29.8)	392 (38.7)	0.0679
	Bilateral	510 (43.2)	743 (42.1)		422 (42.2)	326 (43.4)		88 (48.6)	417 (41.1)	
	Unknown	245 (20.7)	356 (20.2)		206 (20.6)	151 (20.1)		39 (21.6)	205 (20.2)	
Death	No	1162 (98.4)	1718 (97.1)	0.0253	994 (99.4)	741 (98.7)	0.1113	168 (92.8)	973 (96.0)	0.0611
	Yes	19 (1.6)	51 (2.9)		6 (0.6)	10 (1.3)		13 (7.2)	41 (4.0)	

*including never married, divorced, widowed. Abbreviations: AJCC, American Joint Commission on Cancer; T1x, T1 undefined

Table 3 Survival analysis of cancer specific survival in the whole population

Variables		Univariate		Multivariate	
		HR (95%CI)	P values	HR (95%CI)	P values
Age		1.06 (1.04–1.08)	< 0.0001	1.06 (1.05–1.08)	< 0.0001
AJCC stage				1	
	T1a	1			
	T1b	2.22 (1.00–4.92)	0.0503	2.38 (1.05–5.39)	0.0369
	T1c	2.42 (1.30–4.48)	0.0051	3.00 (1.60–5.65)	0.0006
	T1x	1.58 (0.63–3.98)	0.3318	1.45 (0.57–3.67)	0.4349
Histology					
	Serous	1		1	
	Mucinous	1.40 (0.88–2.24)	0.1600	1.73 (1.06–2.83)	0.0285
Race					
	White	1			
	Black	0.75 (0.24–2.40)	0.6309		
	Other	0.57 (0.13–1.35)	0.1479		
Marital status					
	Single	1			
	Married	0.82 (0.52–1.32)	0.4191		
Unknown		0	0.9831		
Fertility preserving Surgery					
	No	1			
	Yes	0.52 (0.31–0.88)	0.0142		
Hysterectomy					
	No	1			
	Yes	1.04 (0.65–1.66)	0.8755		
Tumor size					
	<=5	1			
	> 5	1.47 (0.55–3.92)	0.4438		
Lymphadenectomy					
	No	1			
	Yes	0.77 (0.33–1.77)	0.5330		
	Unknown	0	0.9854		
Laterality					
	Unilateral	1			
	Bilateral	1.13 (0.767–1.93)	0.6432		
	Unknown	1.13 (0.59–2.14)	0.7208		

Abbreviations: AJCC, American joint commission on Cancer; T1x, T1 undefined

surgery is not a factor significantly related to disease-specific death.

We further preformed survival analysis for patients in < 50 and ≥ 50 age groups. In patients < 50 years old, only the undefined T1 stage (vs T1a, HR = 5.99, 95% CI: 1.59–22.60, $P = 0.0082$) was significantly associated with poorer disease-specific survival. No other significant risk factors were observed in these patients using univariate analysis. No risk factors were correlated with disease-specific survival using multivariate analysis (Table 4). In patients ≥50 years, univariate analysis showed that increased age (HR = 1.04, 95% CI: 1.01–1.07, $P = 0.0063$), fertility preserving surgery (HR = 2.04, 95% CI: 1.09–3.81, $P = 0.0251$), stage T1c (vs T1a, HR = 2.38, 95% CI: 1.18–4.78, $P = 0.0151$) and hysterectomy (HR = 0.41, 95% CI: 0.24–0.70, $P = 0.0012$) were risk factors significantly associated with disease-specific survival (Table 5). Disease-specific survival curves of the above risk factors are

Table 4 Univariate survival analysis in patients of age < 50 years

Variables		HR (95%CI)	P values
Age		1.04 (0.98–1.11)	0.2070
Race			
	White	1	
	Black	0	0.9908
	Other	1.19 (0. 27–5.25)	0.8173
Marital status			
	Single*	1	
	Married	1.66 (0.58–4.79)	0.3467
	unknown	0	0.9920
Histology	Serous		
	Mucinous	1.20 (0.45–3.19)	0.7200
AJCC stage			
	T1a	1	
	T1b	4.12 (0.87–19.41)	0.0734
	T1c	3.07 (0.81–11.57)	0.0979
	T1x	5.99 (1.59–22.60)	0.0082
Fertility preserving surgery			
	No	1	
	Yes	0.46 (0.17–1.28)	0.1374
Hysterectomy			
	No	1	
	Yes	2.26 (0.84–6.07)	0.1061
Tumor size	≤ 5 cm	1	
	> 5 cm	0.75 (0.110–5.40)	0.7771
Lymphadenectomy	No	1	
	Yes	0	0.9922
	Unknown	0	0.9986
Lymph node number			
	1–10	1	
	> 10	0	0.9911
	Unknown	0	0.9906
Laterality	Unilateral	1	
	Bilateral	150 (0.44–5.12)	0.5183
	Unknown	2.23 (0.60–8.31)	0.2314

*including never married, divorced, widowed. Abbreviations: AJCC, American Joint Commission on Cancer; T1x, T1 undefined

presented at Fig. 1a, b and c. Multivariate analysis showed that the increased age (HR = 1.04, 95% CI: 1.01–1.07, P = 0.0108), fertility preserving surgery (HR = 1.99, 95% CI: 1.059–3.77, P = 0.0253), stage T1c (HR = 2.87, 95% CI: 1.41–5.86, P = 0.0037) and mucinous histology (HR = 1.87, 95% CI: 1.07–3.27, P = 0.0278) were risk factors significantly associated with worse disease-specific survival (Table 5).

Data from our hospital showed that 255 women with BOTs underwent surgery from 1996 to 2017. The median age was 42 years (range 15–87). Among these patients, 108 (42.4%) had serous tumors and 118 (46.3%) had mucinous tumors. A total of 170 (66.7%) cases were stage I, with one case having an unknown age. Fertility preserving surgery was performed in 113 overall (44.3%) patients (Additional file 1: Table S2). The rate of fertility preserving surgery performed in these patients at stage I was further analyzed after dividing them into two age groups (< 50 and ≥ 50 years). Our result showed that 56/104 (53.9%) patients < 50 and 8/65 (12.3%) patients ≥50 underwent fertility preserving surgery. These two groups had other similar pathoclinical features (Table 6).

Discussion

With a sample size of 2946 patients and a median follow-up time of 200 months, this study examined age-specific impact of fertility preserving surgery on disease-specific survival in women with T1 BOTs. The main finding of this study was that fertility preserving surgery was significantly associated with worse disease-specific survival only in patients ≥50 years, but not in overall patients or patients < 50 years. Our results revealed an age-dependent difference in impact of fertility preserving surgery on disease-specific survival in these patients. This finding suggests that while conservative surgery may comprise survival in women ≥50 years, it is safe for patients < 50 years. Future studies with randomized clinical trials are warranted to verify this finding.

Previous studies have consistently shown that fertility preserving surgery may increase the risk of recurrence [11, 14, 15, 26]. Interestingly, the risk of recurrence was higher in younger patients with BOTs [9, 11, 18, 20]. Most of the recurrences showed no malignant transformation and were curable by a single surgery without compromising overall survival [9, 16–18]. Invasive carcinoma diagnosed in recurrences [9, 11, 18, 27–29] is the cause of cancer deaths [30]. A sub-analysis of the Arbeitsgemeinschaft Gynaekologische Onkologie (AGO) ROBOT study evaluated data from a total of 950 patients with BOTs. Their results showed that 66.7% of recurrent diseases were invasive carcinoma in patients ≥40 years, which dramatically contrasted with a recurrence of 12% of invasive carcinomas in patients < 40 years [20]. The increased incidence of invasive recurrent ovarian cancer in older patients may account for the reduced disease-specific survival after fertility preserving surgery.

This study is unable to address the molecular mechanism whereby fertility preserving surgery is associated with reduced disease-specific survival in patients ≥50 years. Akeson et al. [7] reported patients > 60 had significantly more aneuploid tumors. Aneuploidy was

Table 5 Survival analysis in patients ≥ 50 years

Variables		Univariate		Multivariate*	
		HR (95% CI)	P values	HR (95% CI)	P values
Age		1.04 (1.01–1.07)	0.0063	1.04 (1.01–1.07)	0.0108
Fertility preserving surgery					
	No	1		1	
	Yes	2.04(1.09–3.81)	0.0251	1.99 (1.05–3.77)	0.0347
AJCC stage					
	T1a	1		1	
	T1b	1.56 (0.61–3.96)	0.3531	2.30 (0.87–6.09)	0.0931
	T1c	2.38 (1.18–4.78)	0.0151	2.87 (1.41–5.86)	0.0037
	T1x	0.60 (0.14–2.49)	0.4793	0.58 (0.14–2.42)	0.4527
Histology					
	Serous	1		1	
	Mucinous	1.53 (0.90–2.62)	0.1175	1.87 (1.07–3.27)	0.0278
Race					
	White	1			
	Black	1.01 (0.32–3.24)	0.9879		
	Other	0.23 (0.03–1.68)	0.1476		
Marital status					
	Single*	1			
	Married	0.63 (0.37–1.08)	0.0915		
	unknown	N/A	0.9860		
Hysterectomy					
	No	1			
	Yes	0.41 (0.24–0.70)	0.0012		
Size (cm)					
	<=5	1			
	> 5	1.00 (1.00–1.01)	0.3384		
Lymphadenectomy					
	No	1			
	Yes	0.78 (0.33–1.82)	0.5639		
	Unknown	0	0.9888		
Laterality					
	Unilateral				
	Bilateral	1.10 (0.61–1.99)	0.7511		
	Unknown	0.91 (0.42–1.94)	0.7986		

*including never married, divorced, widowed. Abbreviations: AJCC, American Joint Commission on Cancer; T1x, T1 undefined

associated with an increased mortality of patients with BOTs [31]. Furthermore, BRAF, KRAS and other mutations, and ERBB2 overexpression/amplification were frequently observed BOTs [32–34]. It is unknown whether age-related changes in DNA ploidy and gene mutations play a role in increased invasive recurrence in older patients.

It is noted that as high as 15.1% patients ≥ 50 years with stage I BOTs underwent fertility preserving surgery

in this selected population. Reports are still sparse regarding the prevalence of patients undergoing fertility preserving surgery within different age groups. Trillsch et al. reported that fertility preserving surgery was carried out in 53.2% (149/280) of patients < 40 years, 2.8% (19/670) of overall patients ≥40 years with BOTs [20]. It is speculated that a higher rate of conservative surgery was performed in their patients with stage I BOTs. Comparable to the result from the SEER database,

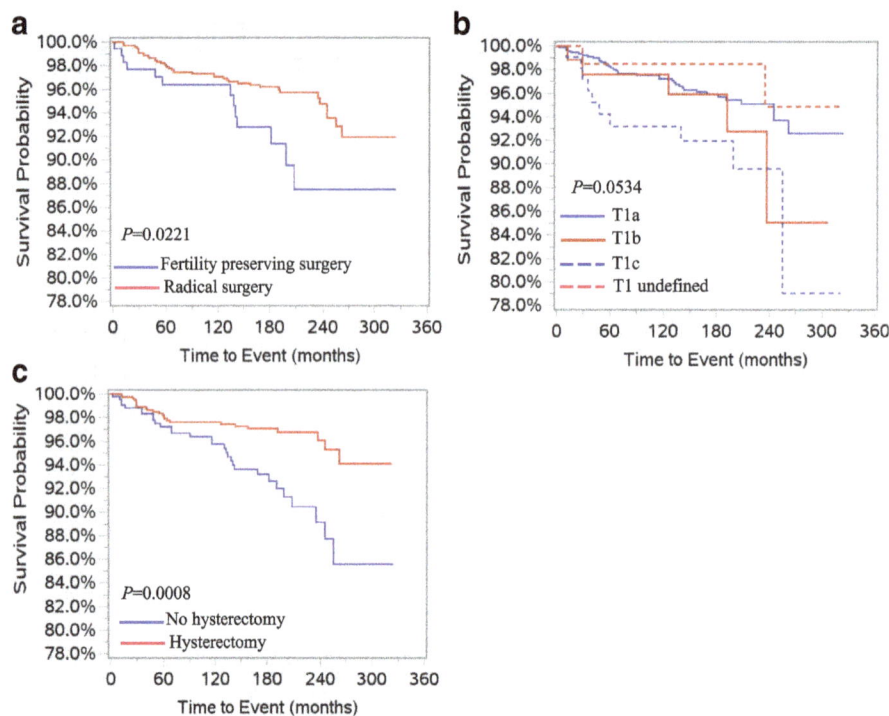

Fig. 1 Kaplan-Meier survival curves for patients ≥50 with stage I borderline ovarian tumors. **a** Fertility preserving surgery vs radical surgery. **b** Sub-stages. **c** Hysterectomy status

data from our hospital showed 12.3% women ≥50 years with stage I disease underwent fertility preserving surgery. Women ≥50 years lose reproductive ability. Preservation of fertility is therefore not the primary objective when adopting conservative surgery in these patients. Conservative surgery brings less postoperative morbidities. Specific reasons older patients undergo conservative surgery remain unknown. Based upon the findings of this study, these patients may need extra attention after conservative surgery.

Our study also identified that increased age, a higher stage (T1c) and mucinous histology were significantly associated with decreased disease-specific survival in overall patients or patients ≥50. Using the same database, a previous study revealed that older age (≥ 50), higher stage and mucinous histology were associated with worse disease-specific survival in patients with stage I BOTs [23]. The tumor stage is a known prognostic factor for patients with BOTs [29]. Our results further revealed that higher stage (T1c) was significantly associated with poorer disease-specific survival in BOT patients at the early stage. Patients with mucinous BOTs were reported to have a worse prognosis compared with to patients with serous BOTs [31, 35]. The worse survival is partially explained by a higher incidence of invasive recurrent carcinoma in patients with mucinous

BOTs. Karlsen et al. [9] found that 6 out of 7 invasive recurrences were patients with mucinous BOTs at FIGO stage I.

An earlier study identified 6017 cases of BOTs from the SEER database. Their results revealed that the lymph node involvement was not significantly associated with disease-specific survival after adjusting with FIGO stages [36]. No impact of lymph node involvement on overall survival in patients with BOT were also observed in other studies [37, 38]. Data from our work and the previous study [23] showed that lymphadenectomy were not a risk factor associated with disease-specific survival.

The use of this database has numerous limitations. Patients were included retrospectively and were not randomly assigned to a treatment. Detailed information of fertility preserving surgery is unavailable. Among patients with stage I disease, 41.6% (2118/5094) were excluded from the study due to unclear surgical information. Many important pathological features of the tumors, such as invasive implants, and micropapillary patterns, are unavailable in these patients. Ovarian cancer related blood biomarkers were not recorded in the SEER database. It is unknown whether there have been recurrences and the types of relapses may have occurred in these patients. The location of harvested lymph nodes are not defined and their numbers are missing in some

Table 6 Pathoclinical features of patients with stage I borderline ovarian tumor from Zhejiang Cancer Hospital

Variables		Age (yeas)		
		< 50	≥50	P values
Fertility preservation surgery				
	No	48 (46.1)	57 (87.7)	< 0.0001
	Yes	56 (53.9)	8 (12.3)	
Histology				
	Serous	43 (41.3)	27 (32.3)	0.9774
	Mucinous	52 (50.0)	39 (60.0)	
	Endometrioid	7 (7.7)	4 (6.1)	
	Clear cells	1 (1.0)	1 (1.5)	
FIGO stage				
	IA	70 (67.3)	42 (64.6)	0.9263
	IB	11 (10.6)	7 (10.8)	
	IC	23 (22.1)	16 (24.6)	
Tumor size (cm)				
	≤5	42 (40.4)	21 (32.3)	0.2908
	> 5	62 (59.6)	44 (67.6)	
Laterality				
	Unilateral	80 (82.7)	49 (76.9)	0.3574
	Bilateral	24 (17.3)	16 (23.1)	
Death				
	No	103 (99.0)	64 (98.5)	0.6938
	Yes	1 (1.0)	1 (1.5)	

patients. Many other limitations using the SEER database have been addressed in a previous study [23].

Use of the SEER database in this study had its strength in its relatively large sample size, long follow-up time, and particularly, relatively large number of disease-specific deaths. Using the same database, the previous study identified 4943 cases with stage T1 BOTs from the same database, and reported a total of 159 (3.2%) deaths in a median follow-up time of 187 months [23]. In contrast, the number of disease-specific deaths reported in previous studies was limited. A cohort included 1143 BOT patients with 1005 (87.9%) patients at FIGO stage I. During a median follow-up time of 49.9 months (range 3.5–99 months), only 7 (0.6%) patients I died of this disease [9]. In another study, a total of 151 patients were recruited. Among them, 87 (64.4%) patients were at FIGO stage I, and 113 patients (74.8%) had follow-up information. After a median follow-up time of 86 (range 0.1–432) months, 7 (6.2%) patients died of this disease [39]. A multi-center study included 457 patients with 390 (85.3%) at stage I. During a mean follow-up of 88.3 months, 9 (2%) patients died of this disease [40]. Leake et al. reported 13 (6.5%) disease-specific deaths in a cohort of 200 patients in a median follow-up time of 120 months [41].

Conclusion

It is safe to perform fertility preserving surgery for women of child-bearing age with stage I BOTs. This surgery may increase the risk of disease-specific death for women of older ages (≥ 50 years). A relatively high proportion of patients (≥ 50 years) receive conservative surgery.

Abbreviations

AJCC: American joint committee on cancer; BOTs: Borderline ovarian tumors; FIGO: International Federation of Gynecology and Obstetrics; SEER: The surveillance, epidemiology, and end results

Acknowledgements
We thank Dr. Kristin Best for her help in manuscript reviewing.

Funding
This research is supported by Zhejiang Natural Science Foundation (LY14H160010).

Authors' contributions

SH, YA and WS conceived the concept. SH, YA and WS analyzed data. SH, CX, LN and ZT participated in data collection and interpretation of results. SH, ZT, YA and WS wrote the manuscript. All authors read and approved the final manuscript.

Competing interests

The authors declare that they have no competing interests.

Author details

[1]Department of Gynecologic Oncology, Zhejiang Cancer Hospital, 1 Banshan East Road, Zhejiang 310022, Hangzhou, China. [2]Department of Gynecology, The First People's Hospital of Aksu, Aksu, China. [3]Department of Cancer Biology, Wake Forest School of Medicine, Winston Salem, NC 27157, USA.

References

1. Serov SF, Scully RE, Sobin LH. Histologic typing of ovarian tumors in international histologic classification of tumors (no. 9). Geneva: World Health Organization; 1973.

2. Seidman JD, Soslow RA, Vang R, Berman JJ, Stoler MH, Sherman ME, et al. Borderline ovarian tumors: diverse contemporary viewpoints on terminology and diagnostic criteria with illustrative images. Hum Pathol. 2004;35:918–33.

3. Benedet JL, Bender H, Jones H 3rd, Ngan HY. Pecorelli S. FIGO staging classifications and clinical practice guidelines in the management of gynecologic cancers. FIGO committee on gynecologic oncology. Int J Gynecol Obstet. 2000;70:209–62.

4. Morice P. Borderline tumours of the ovary and fertility. Eur J Cancer. 2006; 42:149–58.

5. Tinelli R, Tinelli A, Tinelli FG, Cicinelli E, Malvasi A. Conservative surgery for borderline ovarian tumors: a review. Gynecol Oncol. 2006;100:185–91.

6. Skirnisdottir I, Garmo H, Wilander E, Holmberg L. Borderline ovarian tumors in Sweden 1960-2005: trends in incidence and age at diagnosis compared to ovarian cancer. Int J Cancer. 2008;123:1897–901.

7. Akeson M, Zetterqvist BM, Dahllof K, Jakobsen AM, Brannstrom M, Horvath G. Population-based cohort follow-up study of all patients operated for borderline ovarian tumor in western Sweden during an 11-year period. Int J Gynecol Cancer Soc. 2008;18:453–9.

8. Vasconcelos I, de Sousa Mendes M. Conservative surgery in ovarian borderline tumours: a meta-analysis with emphasis on recurrence risk. Eur J Cancer. 2015;51:620–31.

9. Karlsen NMS, Karlsen MA, Hogdall E, Nedergaard L, Christensen IJ, Hogdall C. Relapse and disease specific survival in 1143 Danish women diagnosed with borderline ovarian tumours (BOT). Gynecol Oncol. 2016;142:50–3.

10. Alvarez RM, Vazquez-Vicente D. Fertility sparing treatment in borderline ovarian tumours. Ecancermedicalscience. 2015;9:507.

11. Zanetta G, Rota S, Chiari S, Bonazzi C, Bratina G, Mangioni C. Behavior of borderline tumors with particular interest to persistence, recurrence, and progression to invasive carcinoma: a prospective study. J Clin Oncol Off J Am Soc Clin Oncol. 2001;19:2658–64.

12. Morris RT, Gershenson DM, Silva EG, Follen M, Morris M, Wharton JT. Outcome and reproductive function after conservative surgery for borderline ovarian tumors. Obstet Gynecol. 2000;95:541–7.

13. Suh-Burgmann E. Long-term outcomes following conservative surgery for borderline tumor of the ovary: a large population-based study. Gynecol Oncol. 2006;103:841–7.

14. Chen RF, Li J, Zhu TT, Yu HL, Lu X. Fertility-sparing surgery for young patients with borderline ovarian tumors (BOTs): single institution experience. J Ovarian Res. 2016;9:16.

15. Chen X, Fang C, Zhu T, Zhang P, Yu A, Wang S. Identification of factors that impact recurrence in patients with borderline ovarian tumors. J Ovarian Res. 2017;10:23.

16. Uzan C, Kane A, Rey A, Gouy S, Duvillard P, Morice P. Outcomes after conservative treatment of advanced-stage serous borderline tumors of the ovary. Annals of oncology: official journal of the European society for. Med Oncol. 2010;21:55–60.

17. Fischerova D, Zikan M, Dundr P, Cibula D. Diagnosis, treatment, and follow-up of borderline ovarian tumors. Oncologist. 2012;17:1515–33.

18. Vancraeynest E, Moerman P, Leunen K, Amant F, Neven P, Vergote I, Fertility Preservation I. Safe for serous borderline ovarian tumors. Int J Gynecol Cancer. 2016;26:1399–406.

19. Helpman L, Yaniv A, Beiner ME, Aviel-Ronen S, Perri T, Ben-Baruch G, et al. Fertility preservation in women with borderline ovarian tumors - how does it impact disease outcome? A cohort study. Acta Obstet Gynecol Scand. 2017;96:1300–6.

20. Trillsch F, Mahner S, Woelber L, Vettorazzi E, Reuss A, Ewald-Riegler N, et al. Age-dependent differences in borderline ovarian tumours (BOT) regarding clinical characteristics and outcome: results from a sub-analysis of the Arbeitsgemeinschaft Gynaekologische Onkologie (AGO) ROBOT study. Annals of oncology: official journal of the European society for. Med Oncol. 2014;25:1320–7.

21. Surveillance E, and End Results (SEER) Program. (www.seer.cancer.gov) SEER*Stat Database: Incidence - SEER 18 Regs Research Data + Hurricane Katrina Impacted Louisiana Cases, Nov 2016 Sub (1973–2014 varying) - Linked To County Attributes - Total U.S., 1969–2015 Counties, National Cancer Institute, DCCPS, Surveillance Research Program, Surveillance Systems Branch, released April 2017, based on the November 2016 submission.

22. Sherman ME, Mink PJ, Curtis R, Cote TR, Brooks S, Hartge P, et al. Survival among women with borderline ovarian tumors and ovarian carcinoma: a population-based analysis. Cancer. 2004;100:1045–52.

23. Matsuo K, Machida H, Takiuchi T, Grubbs BH, Roman LD, Sood AK, et al. Role of hysterectomy and lymphadenectomy in the management of early-stage borderline ovarian tumors. Gynecol Oncol. 2017;144:496–502.

24. Beahrs OH, Henson DE, Hutter RVP, Myers MH, editors. AJCC manual for staging of cancer. 3rd ed. Philadelphia: JB Lippincott; 1988. P. 163-8.

25. Prat J, FIGO committee on gynecologic oncology. Staging classification for cancer of the ovary, fallopian tube, and peritoneum. Int J Gynecol Obstet. 2014;124:1–5.

26. Trillsch F, Mahner S, Ruetzel J, Harter P, Ewald-Riegler N, Jaenicke F, et al. Clinical management of borderline ovarian tumors. Expert Rev Anticancer Ther. 2010;10:1115–24.

27. Longacre TA, McKenney JK, Tazelaar HD, Kempson RL, Hendrickson MR. Ovarian serous tumors of low malignant potential (borderline tumors): outcome-based study of 276 patients with long-term (> or =5-year) follow-up. Am J Surg Pathol 2005; 29:707–723.

28. Wong HF, Low JJ, Chua Y, Busmanis I, Tay EH, Ho TH. Ovarian tumors of borderline malignancy: a review of 247 patients from 1991 to 2004. Int J Gynecol Cancer. 2007;17:342–9.

29. du Bois A, Ewald-Riegler N, de Gregorio N, Reuss A, Mahner S, Fotopoulou C, et al. Borderline tumours of the ovary: a cohort study of the Arbeitsgemeinschaft Gynakologische Onkologie (AGO) study group. Eur J Cancer. 2013;49:1905–14.

30. Seong SJ, Kim DH, Kim MK, Song T. Controversies in borderline ovarian tumors. J Gynecol Oncol. 2015;26:343–9.

31. Kaern J, Trope CG, Kristensen GB, Abeler VM. Pettersen EO. DNA ploidy; the most important prognostic factor in patients with borderline tumors of the ovary. Int J Gynecol Cancer. 1993;3:349–58.

32. Malpica A, Wong KK. The molecular pathology of ovarian serous borderline tumors. Ann Oncol. 2016;27(Suppl 1):i16–i9.

33. Anglesio MS, Kommoss S, Tolcher MC, Clarke B, Galletta L, Porter H, et al. Molecular characterization of mucinous ovarian tumours supports a stratified treatment approach with HER2 targeting in 19% of carcinomas. J Pathol. 2013;229:111–20.

34. Mackenzie R, Kommoss S, Winterhoff BJ, Kipp BR, Garcia JJ, Voss J, et al. Targeted deep sequencing of mucinous ovarian tumors reveals multiple overlapping RAS-pathway activating mutations in borderline and cancerous neoplasms. BMC Cancer. 2015;15:415.

35. Levi F, La Vecchia C, Randimbison L, Te VC. Borderline ovarian tumours in Vaud, Switzerland: incidence, survival and second neoplasms. Br J Cancer. 1999;79:4–6.

36. Lesieur B, Kane A, Duvillard P, Gouy S, Pautier P, Lhomme C, et al. Prognostic value of lymph node involvement in ovarian serous borderline tumors. Am J Obstet Gynecol. 2011;204:438 e1–7.

37. McKenney JK, Balzer BL, Longacre TA. Lymph node involvement in ovarian serous tumors of low malignant potential (borderline tumors): pathology, prognosis, and proposed classification. Am J Surg Pathol. 2006;30:614–24.

38. Djordjevic B, Malpica A. Ovarian serous tumors of low malignant potential with nodal low-grade serous carcinoma. Am J Surg Pathol. 2012;36:955–63.

39. Lazarou A, Fotopoulou C, Coumbos A, Sehouli J, Vasiljeva J, Braicu I, et al. Long-term follow-up of borderline ovarian tumors clinical outcome and prognostic factors. Anticancer Res. 2014;34:6725–30.

40. Cusido M, Balaguero L, Hernandez G, Falcon O, Rodriguez-Escudero FJ, Vargas JA, et al. Results of the national survey of borderline ovarian tumors in Spain. Gynecol Oncol. 2007;104:617–22.

41. Leake JF, Currie JL, Rosenshein NB, Woodruff JD. Long-term follow-up of serous ovarian tumors of low malignant potential. Gynecol Oncol. 1992;47:150–8.

3

Retinoic acid enhances germ cell differentiation of mouse skin-derived stem cells

Paul W. Dyce[1*], Neil Tenn[2] and Gerald M. Kidder[2]

Abstract

Background: Retinoic acid (RA) signaling has been identified as a key driver in male and female gamete development. The presence of RA is a critical step in the initiation of meiosis and is required for the production of competent oocytes from primordial germ cells. Meiosis has been identified as a difficult biological process to recapitulate in vitro, when differentiating stem cells to germ cells. We have previously shown that primordial germ cell-like cells, and more advanced oocyte-like cells (OLCs), can be formed by differentiating mouse skin-derived stem cells. However, the OLCs remain unable to function due to what appears to be failure of meiotic initiation. The aim of this study was to determine the effect of RA treatment, during stem cell differentiation to germ cells, particularly on the initiation of meiosis.

Results: Using qPCR we found significant increases in the meiosis markers Stra8 and Sycp3 and a significant reduction in the meiosis inhibitor Nanos2, in the differentiating populations. Furthermore, OLCs from the RA treated group, expressed significantly more of the meiosis regulatory gene Marf1 and the oocyte marker Oct4. At the protein level RA treatment was found to increase the expression of the gap junction protein CX43 and the pluripotency marker OCT4. Moreover, the expression of SYCP3 was significantly upregulated and the localization pattern better matched that of control fetal ovarian cells. RA treatment also improved the structural integrity of the OLCs produced by initiating the expression of all three zona pellucida transcripts (Zp1–3) and improving ZP3 expression levels and localization. Finally, the addition of RA during differentiation led to an almost two-fold increase in the number of OLCs recovered and increased their in vitro growth.

Conclusion: RA is a key driver in the formation of functioning gametes and its addition during stem cell to germ cell differentiation improves OLCs entry into meiosis.

Background

During early embryogenesis mouse primordial germ cells have the potential to either develop to form spermatogonia or begin the process of meiosis and develop into oocytes. In mammals, meiosis onset begins before birth in females, or at the onset of puberty in males. The first evidence of entry into meiosis I can be seen at ~ 13.5 days postcoitum (dpc) in the female fetal mouse [1]. This decision has been shown to be influenced by the presence of retinoic acid (RA) which is produced by mesonephroi during embryogenesis in both sexes [2]. Production of the premeiotic gene stimulated by RA 8 (Stra8) precedes meiosis initiation at ~ 12.5 dpc [2–4]. Conversely, in the male the activity of RA is stopped through the action of the retinoid-degrading enzyme cytochrome P450 26B1 (CYP26B1) [5]. Testicular germ cells do not enter meiosis during fetal development and Stra8 expression is first identified 10 days postpartum, concurrent with the onset of meiosis [6]. In recent years, independent investigations have resulted in RA emerging as a key driver for the entry of both male and female germ cells into meiosis [2, 5, 7–10].

Previous studies have shown that media containing growth factors, including RA, are able to sustain mouse germ cells in the absence of somatic cells and allow them to enter into and progress through meiotic prophase I, in the absence of leukemia inhibitory factor

* Correspondence: pwd0003@auburn.edu
[1]Department of Animal Sciences, College of Agriculture, Auburn University, CASIC Building, 559 Devall Drive, Auburn, AL 36849, USA
Full list of author information is available at the end of the article

(LIF) [2, 11, 12]. Three initial publications demonstrated the induced differentiation of ES cells into oocytes or sperm, though failed to show functioning gametes [13–15]. We have also shown that skin-derived somatic stem cells, from pigs, mice and humans, have the ability to form primordial germ cell-like cells (PGCLCs) and non-functioning oocyte-like cells (OLCs) [16–21]. The OLCs were characterized by their morphology and expression of oocyte markers but have yet to fertilize correctly and function. The failure of OLCs, produced from somatic stem cells, appears to involve a failure to properly initiate and complete meiosis. Recent studies, differentiating ES cells, have included an RA induction phase and resulted in completion of meiosis [22, 23]. ES cells originate from the inner cell mass of developing blastocysts. Therefore, ES cells used for cell therapy are allogenic with the transplanted donor cells not originating from the recipient. This raises the concern of immunogenic response from the host. Moreover, the use of ES cells is impeded by moral, legal, and ethical concerns.

The increased utility provided by the use of somatic stem cells illustrates the necessity for continued investigation of their differentiation capabilities. We hypothesize that the addition of RA during induced differentiation will enhance the ability of skin derived stem cells to develop into OLCs. Therefore, in this study we investigated the use of RA to improve the generation of OLCs from mouse skin-derived somatic stem cells and its ability to improve the induction and progression of meiosis in the OLCs produced.

Methods
Stem cell isolation and culture
All experiments involving animals in the study were conducted according to the Care and Use of Experimental Animals Guidelines of the Canadian Council on Animal Care, and have been approved by the Western University Animal Care and Use Committee. Newborn female transgenic mice [Jackson Lab; 004654; (CBA/CaJ X C57BL/6 J)F2] carrying the Oct4- GFP transgene were euthanized within 24 h of birth and the dorsal skin removed. Skin stem cells were isolated using a protocol by Toma et al. with the following modifications [24]; Skin samples from 4 to 5 pups were grouped and placed in Hank's balanced salt solution (HBSS, Thermo Fisher Scientific) and cut into ~ 1 mm square pieces using dissecting scissors. The samples were then washed 3X using HBSS, and re-suspended in 1 ml of 0.05% trypsin for 40 min. at 37 °C. Following trypsinization, 1 ml of 0.1% DNase (Sigma) was added to the sample and incubated 1 min. at room temperature. Then

9 ml of HBSS was immediately added and the cells pelleted at 500 X G for 5 min. Samples were then washed 1X with HBSS and 2X with DMEM-F12 with antibiotics (Thermo Fisher Scientific). Following the last wash, the samples were mechanically dissociated in 1 ml of DMEM-F12 by pipeting. The partially dissociated samples were then filtered using a 40 μm cell strainer (BD Falcon). This was done by adding 9 ml DMEM-F12 to the dissociated cells and running them through the filter. This was followed by 10–15 ml of DMEM-F12. The resulting filtrate was then pelleted by centrifuging for 5 min. at 500 X G. Each pellet obtained from 4 to 5 pups was then re-suspended in 10 ml stem cell medium (DMEM-F12 with 1 X B27 (Thermo Fisher Scientific), 20 ng/ml epidermal growth factor (EGF, Sigma), and 40 ng/ml basic fibroblast growth factor (Sigma)) and plated on a 10 cm dish (Sarstedt). At ~ 72 h after plating, the skin-derived stem cells grew as suspended spheres, which discriminated them from the rest of the skin cells (attached) in culture. To passage floating cell spheres, medium containing spheres was centrifuged and the pellet was gently dissociated using a large bore pipette. The cells were re-seeded in fresh stem cell medium as above. Cells were passaged every 4–6 days.

Stem cell differentiation
The isolated stem cells at passage two were pelleted at 500 X G and re-suspended in 500 μl of phosphate-buffered saline (PBS). The cells were dissociated to single cells by using vigorous pipetting. The cells were then washed in 9 ml of PBS and counted on a hemocytometer. For the stem cell only group (SC), and ovarian cell only groups, cells were plated at 0.6 X 10^6 cells per well (500 μl) in differentiation medium which consists of TCM199 (no antibiotics, Thermo Fisher Scientific) supplemented with 0.05 IU follicle stimulating hormone (Sioux Biochemical), 0.03 IU luteinizing hormone (Sioux Biochemical), 3 mg/ml bovine serum albumin (BSA, Sigma), 5 μl/ml ITS (Life Technologies), 0.23 mM sodium pyruvate (Life Technologies), 1 mg/ml Fetuin (Sigma), and 1 ng/ml EGF (Sigma). Cells were cultured at 37 °C for 12 days, changing half the medium every 2 days. Spent medium was centrifuged and the pelleted cells returned to the culture dish. A 10 mM RA stock solution was prepared by diluting the RA in dimethyl sulfoxide (DMSO, Sigma). During the differentiations, at the beginning of day 4, cultures were treated with either 10 μm RA or treated with the same concentration of dimethyl sulfoxide (DMSO, vehicle only control) for 24 h. At the end of the 12 days of

differentiation, the aggregates were trypsinized and large cells collected using a stereoscope and mouth pipette.

Western blot

For immunoblotting, protein from differentiated cells and adult ovary samples were isolated using radio-immunoprecipitation assay (RIPA) lysis buffer with complete mini protease inhibitors (Roche) added fresh prior to use. 30 µg of protein (as determined using a BSA protein assay kit, Pierce) were mixed with 5X reducing sample buffer, boiled for 5 min, and electrophoresed under reducing conditions on 12% polyacrylamide gels. Protein was transferred using an iBlot (Thermo Fisher Scientific) onto nitrocellulose membranes. Membranes were incubated for 2 h in 5% non-fat dry milk blocking buffer at room temperature, followed by an overnight incubation at 4 °C in primary antibody (HSP70 1:5000; Chemicon, CX43 1:10000; Sigma, OCT4 1:300; Santa Cruz Biotech). After a 1 h incubation with anti-mouse IgG (alexa 680; 1:10000; Thermo Fisher Scientific) or goat anti-rabbit (Alexa 488; 1/1000; Thermo Fisher Scientific) at room temperature, expression was detected following three washes, using the LI-COR Odyssey fluorescent scanner. Blots were incubated in 1X strip buffer (re-blot plus mild, Millipore) at room temperature for 15 min and re-blocked 1 h between antibody staining. All blots were stripped, blocked, and re-probed between antibodies.

RNA isolation and RT-PCR

RNA was isolated using the RNeasy Mini Kit (Qiagen) according to the manufacturer's protocol. RT-PCR on differentiated cultures was performed as previously described [20]. Briefly, RT-PCR on groups of 15 OLCs or oocytes was performed by freezing cells in 7 µl of lysis buffer containing 14 U of porcine RNase inhibitor (Amersham) and 5 mM DTT (Thermo Fisher Scientific) at −80 °C until use. Cells were then lysed by boiling for 1 min and vortexing for 2 min (repeated for a total of 3X), and then stored on ice. Samples were then DNase treated by adding 1 µl 10X DNase buffer and 1 µl amplification grade DNase (Thermo Fisher Scientific) and incubating 15 min. at room temperature. 1 µl EDTA (25 mM) was then added and the samples were incubated for 10 min. at 65 °C. RT was then performed by adding 0.5 µl H_2O, 5 µl 5X buffer, 1.25 µl of random hexamer primers, 6.25 µl 2 mM dNTPs, and 1 µl MMLV reverse transcriptase to the sample. The samples were incubated at 25 °C for 10 min., 37 °C for 50 min., and 70 °C for 15 min. Real-Time PCR was carried out on a Smart Cycler (Cepheid) by using the QuantiTect SYBR green PCR kit (Qiagen): 2.5 µl, for cell populations, and 3.1 µl for groups of 15 cells, of DNase treated cDNA

(from a 25 µl RT reaction) was added to 12.5 µl of SYBR green mix and 0.3 µM each of forward and reverse primers (final volume 25 µl). The housekeeping gene hypoxanthine guanine phosphoribosyl transferase (Hprt) was used to calculate the relative transcript levels of target genes using the ΔΔCT method. Product sizes were confirmed on a 1% agarose gel. The identities of the products were confirmed by sequencing.

Immunofluorescence

Cells were washed twice with PBS and fixed in 4% para-formaldehyde in PBS for 20 min. Cells were then washed three times in PBS with 0.1% Tween 20 and incubated for 10 min, and then for 20 min in PBS with 1% Triton-X-100. Next, cells were blocked for 2 h in PBS with 5% BSA, and 0.05% Triton-X-100 (PBS-B, blocking solution), followed by an incubation with primary antibody, 1:400 anti-ZP3 (Sigma) or 1:300 anti OCT4 (Santa Cruz Biotech) for 2 h at 37 °C, or overnight at 4 °C. Cells were then washed in blocking solution (PBS with 5% BSA and 0.05% Triton X 100), and incubated with 1:1000 PE-conjugated goat anti-rabbit IgG or 1:500 FITC-conjugated rat anti-mouse IgG for 1 h at room temperature. This was followed with a blocking solution wash and incubation with 4′-6-diamidino-2-phenylindole (DAPI) for 1 min, followed by washing three times with PBS-B. Cells were mounted using fluorescent mount medium (DakoCytomation) and viewed using an Olympus BX-UCB microscope and MetaMorph analysis software (Universal Imaging Corporation).

Chromosome spreading and SYCP3 staining

At day 6 cells from the RA treated or control differentiations were trypsinized (Thermo Fisher Scientific) for 3 min at 37 °C, washed once in DMEM H21 (Life Technologies) with 10% fetal calf serum (FCS, Life Technologies) and then resuspended in 0.5 ml PBS. Thirty µl of the suspension was then placed on a slide and incubated for 5 min at room temperature to attach the cells to the slide surface. To spread the cells, 90 µl of 3% sucrose was gently added to the slide which was then held for 20 to 30 min at room temperature. Fixative was prepared as 2% paraformaldehyde with 2 µl of 10% sodium dodecyl sulfate (SDS, Life Technologies) per ml. The pH was adjusted to between 9 and 11 by adding 10 µl NaOH (1 N) per 8 ml of fixative followed by 3 rinses in PBS block with tween (PBT), each for 10 min at room temperature. PBT was made by adding 0.15 g BSA and 100 µl Tween20 to 100 ml PBS. The primary antibody against synaptonemal complex protein 3 (SYCP3, 1/100) was then added and the slides were incubated in humidity chambers overnight at 4 °C. Prior to adding anti-rabbit FITC (1/500; Abcam), the slides were washed three times with PBT for 10 min in each wash. The slides were then incubated for 2 h at room temperature, then washed twice with PBT for 10 min at room temperature. Slides were stained with Hoechst (Life Technologies) for 7 min, washed once in PBT, and then mounted using fluorescent mounting medium (Dako, S3023). Slides were viewed using an Olympus BX-UCB microscope and MetaMorph analysis software (Universal Imaging Corporation).

Statistical analysis
Experiments were repeated at least three times and the data were analyzed using a t-test (on comparison of germ cell marker expression levels between OLC and the oocyte groups) or ANOVA, followed by the Tukey test. Results were considered significant at $P < 0.05$.

Results
Treatment of differentiations with RA results in altered expression of meiosis markers
Initially, in order to determine the induction of meiosis we compared transcript levels of the meiosis marker genes Stra8 and Sycp3. We found the expression of Stra8 was significantly higher, at 11.63 ± 7.64 fold, following RA treatment ($p < 0.01$, Fig. 1a). Similarly, the expression of Sycp3 was significantly increased 1.65 ± 0.42 fold higher than the vehicle only control ($p < 0.05$, Fig. 1b). Finally, we compared the expression of the gene encoding the meiosis inhibitor NANOS2 and found significantly less was present following the treatment with RA ($p < 0.05$). The RA treated groups expression decreased to 0.32 ± 0.08 fold the level of that in the vehicle only control, 0.90 ± 0.25 fold ($p < 0.05$, Fig. 1c).

Treatment with RA results in increased expression of Marf1, Oct4, and Sycp3 genes in OLCs
We next set out to test the expression of oocyte specific markers in OLCs produced from RA treated and vehicle only controls. Groups of 10 OLCs produced either with or without RA treatment were compared using qRT-PCR. The expression of the gene encoding meiosis regulator and mRNA stability factor 1 (MARF1) was found to be lower than in natural oocytes in our control differentiations. The treatment with RA resulted in the expression of Marf1 significantly increasing to higher levels than the untreated control and the natural oocyte control ($p < 0.05$, Fig. 2a). Conversely, the expression of the pluripotent marker gene Oct4, in our control OLCs, was found to be significantly lower than in our oocyte controls ($p < 0.05$, Fig. 2b). OLCs produced following RA treatment expressed significantly higher Oct4 mRNA, not significantly different from that of control oocytes ($p > 0.05$, Fig. 2b). Finally, we tested the expression of the meiosis marker gene Sycp3. We did not see a significant difference in the expression of Sycp3 in either our treated or untreated OLCs nor in the control oocytes ($p > 0.05$, Fig. 2c).

Treatment with RA results in increased CX43 and OCT4 expression
The requirement of cellular cooperation between granulosa and the oocyte, through the presence of connexin 43 (CX43) based gap junctions, for the correct development of oocytes has been well defined (for review see [25]). Therefore, we were interested in investigating the effect of RA on the expression of CX43 and the oocyte marker octamer-binding transcription factor 4 (OCT4). We compared the expression of OCT4 and CX43 at the protein level using Western blotting. The expression of OCT4 was significantly higher in the RA treated differentiations when compared to the vehicle only control ($p < 0.05$, Fig. 3a and b). Similarly, the expression of the gap junction protein CX43 was found to be significantly higher following treatment with RA when compared to the control untreated differentiations ($p < 0.01$, Fig. 3a and b).

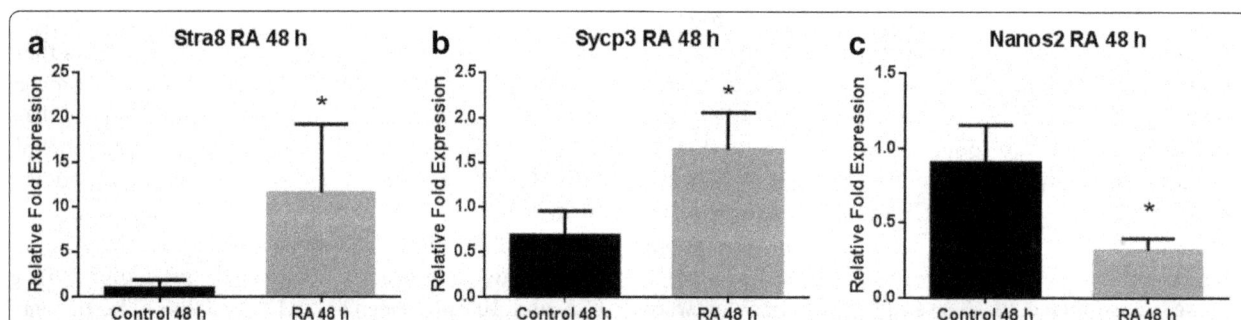

Fig. 1 RT real-time PCR analysis of meiosis related gene expression in differentiation cultures exposed to RA or vehicle only for 48 h. **a** The expression of Stra8 was significantly higher (11.63 ± 7.64 fold) following exposure to 10 μm RA when compared to the vehicle only control. **b** Similarly, the expression of Sycp3 was significantly higher (1.65 ± 0.42 fold) following exposure to 10 μm RA when compared to the vehicle only control. Conversely, the expression of the meiosis inhibitor gene Nanos2 was significantly lower, 0.32 ± 0.08 fold when compared to the vehicle only contol. * denotes significant difference $p < 0.05$ using a t-test.

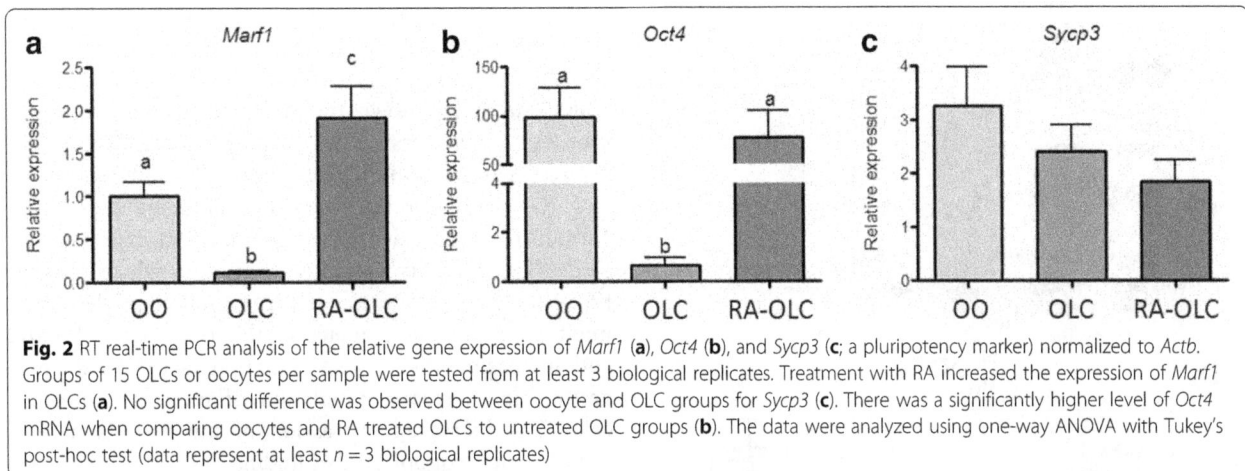

Fig. 2 RT real-time PCR analysis of the relative gene expression of *Marf1* (**a**), *Oct4* (**b**), and *Sycp3* (**c**; a pluripotency marker) normalized to *Actb*. Groups of 15 OLCs or oocytes per sample were tested from at least 3 biological replicates. Treatment with RA increased the expression of *Marf1* in OLCs (**a**). No significant difference was observed between oocyte and OLC groups for *Sycp3* (**c**). There was a significantly higher level of *Oct4* mRNA when comparing oocytes and RA treated OLCs to untreated OLC groups (**b**). The data were analyzed using one-way ANOVA with Tukey's post-hoc test (data represent at least $n = 3$ biological replicates)

The localization of SYCP3 is improved following treatment with RA

In order to determine if the PGCLCs were entering meiosis we utilized Western blotting to detect the expression level of the synaptonemal complex protein SYCP3. The overall expression of SYCP3 was found to be significantly higher following treatment with RA when compared to the undifferentiated or differentiated cells exposed to vehicle only ($p < 0.05$, Fig. 4a). We next utilized immunofluorescent staining for SYCP3 in chromosomal spreads to determine the localization. The majority of cells stained in the control culture had cytoplasmic SYCP3 staining (Fig. 4b). This was contrasted dramatically by stained control female fetal gonad spreads which had the phenotypically characteristic synapsed staining pattern of SYCP3. Following treatment with RA the SYCP3 staining more resembled the positive control staining with SYCP3 at least partially synapsed with the DNA.

RA treatment improved the formation of the zona pellucida

In our earlier work we found that the OLCs are much more fragile than natural oocytes [17–20]. We have previously shown that this may potentially be due to the failure of OLCs to produce ZP1 and ZP2, components of the zona pellucida [19]. We utilized RT-PCR to determine if the treatment of the differentiations with RA improved the expression of the genes *Figla*, *Zp1*, *Zp2*, and *Zp3*. We found that the treatment of the differentiations with RA resulted in the expression of all four transcripts while the control differentiation failed to express *Zp1* and *Zp2* (Fig. 5a). Moreover, while the protein expression of ZP3 was membrane localized in both OLCs from untreated and RA treated differentiations, the expression was more intense and continuous in the OLCs from RA

treated cultures (Fig. 5c). It is important to note that the ZP membrane, while improved with the RA treatment, remains not as strong in the OLCs (unpublished results).

RA treatment improves the efficiency of OLC generation from skin derived stem cells

We next compared the number of OLCs generated per 10^6 starting cells. RA treatment was found to increase the number of OLCs from 8.17 ± 2.22 in the control differentiations to 18.39 ± 1.58 per 10^6 cells ($p < 0.01$, Fig. 6a). Recovered oocytes were measured and found to be on average significantly larger in the RA treated group (49.25 ± 11.66 µm, $p < 0.01$) when compared to the untreated control OLCs (68.75 ± 5.94 µm, Fig. 6b).

Discussion

Currently, many stem cell types have been demonstrated to have the potential to form germ cells in vitro (for review see [26]). However, there have been very few examples of the germ cells produced successfully initiating and completing meiosis, indicating a lack of competency for efficiently producing gametes from stem cells in vitro. The ability to produce functioning gametes from stem cells will provide a closed system in which to study germ cell formation and development.

Retinoic acid, the biologically active form of vitamin A, was initially identified as a requirement through nutritional studies (for review see [27]). Recent investigations have shown that RA is involved in meiosis initiation and is an important regulator of many organ systems during development (for review see [28]). We reasoned that for the successful production of a female gamete the presence of RA would be required to properly enter the meiotic process. Therefore, we initially treated our differentiations with RA while monitoring the expression level of genes critical for meiosis. We found the early meiosis marker *Stra8* and the later

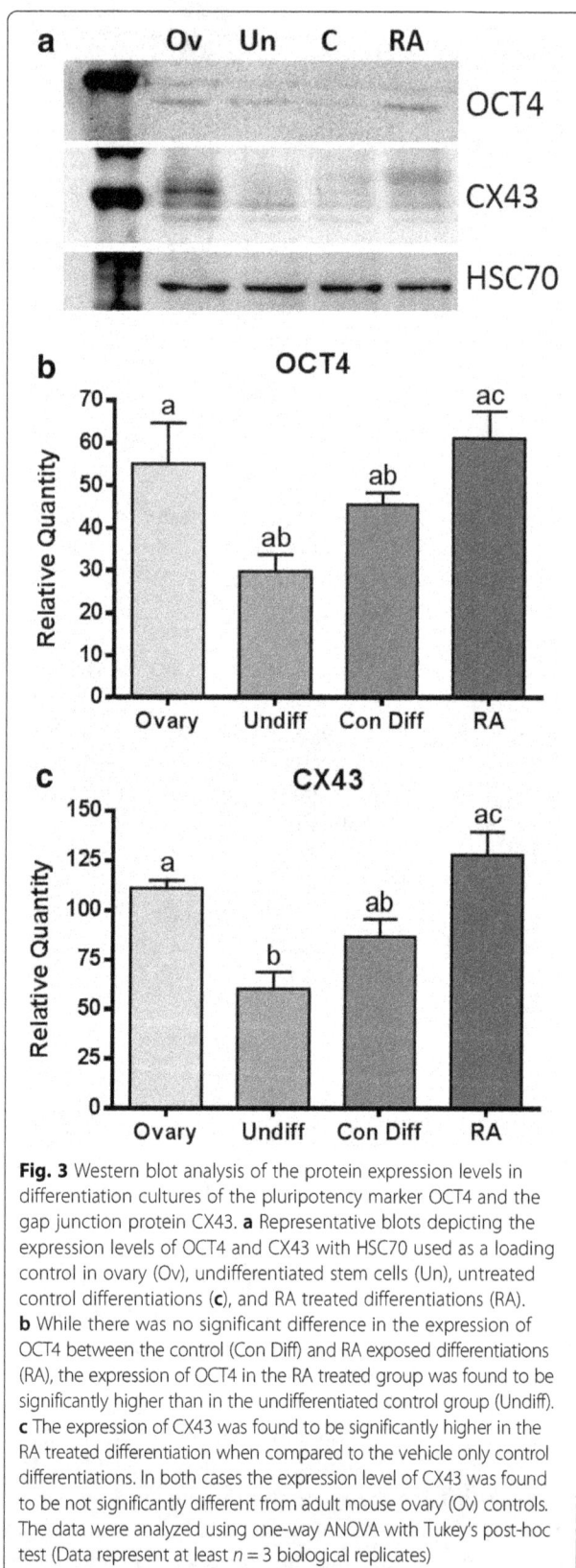

Fig. 3 Western blot analysis of the protein expression levels in differentiation cultures of the pluripotency marker OCT4 and the gap junction protein CX43. **a** Representative blots depicting the expression levels of OCT4 and CX43 with HSC70 used as a loading control in ovary (Ov), undifferentiated stem cells (Un), untreated control differentiations (**c**), and RA treated differentiations (RA). **b** While there was no significant difference in the expression of OCT4 between the control (Con Diff) and RA exposed differentiations (RA), the expression of OCT4 in the RA treated group was found to be significantly higher than in the undifferentiated control group (Undiff). **c** The expression of CX43 was found to be significantly higher in the RA treated differentiation when compared to the vehicle only control differentiations. In both cases the expression level of CX43 was found to be not significantly different from adult mouse ovary (Ov) controls. The data were analyzed using one-way ANOVA with Tukey's post-hoc test (Data represent at least $n = 3$ biological replicates)

meiosis marker *Sycp3* were both significantly upregulated following the RA treatment. We next wanted to test the expression of the RNA-binding protein *Nanos2*, which has been shown to inhibit meiosis entry in the mouse by suppressing the expression of *Stra8* [29]. Interestingly, we found treatment of the differentiations with RA resulted in significantly decreased expression of *Nanos2* that coincided with the increased expression of *Stra8* (Fig. 1). This suggested that, as a whole population, the differentiations were responding to RA treatment by removing a meiosis inhibiting factor *Nanos2* and increasing the meiosis initiation factor *Stra8*, suggesting an increased population of meiosis competent cells. The increased expression of the meiosis marker *Sycp3* further supported this finding.

We next compared the expression of oocyte markers specifically in the OLCs. To do this we took groups of 15 RA treated and untreated OLCs and compared them to groups of 10 natural mouse oocytes. We initially tested the expression levels of *Marf1*, a recently identified marker important for controlling meiosis and the maintenance of genomic integrity [30, 31]. The mutation of *Marf1* results in large scale alterations to gene expression and a failure of meiosis in oocytes [30]. *Marf1* was found to be expressed at a significantly lower level in our untreated, control differentiation produced, OLCs when compared to natural oocytes (Fig. 2a). OLCs produced following RA treatment had significantly higher *Marf1* expression than untreated OLCs and natural OLCs (Fig. 2a). Further study will be required to determine if a higher expression of *Marf1* leads to issues with progression through meiosis. Similarly, *Oct4* expression was found to be significantly lower in the untreated OLCs when compared to natural oocytes (Fig. 2b). The RA treated OLCs had a similar expression level of *Oct4* compared to natural oocytes (Fig. 2b). Interestingly, the expression of *Sycp3* was not found to be significantly different between the three groups (Fig. 2c) at the mRNA level. In order to investigate this further, we next compared the expression level and localization of SYCP3 in the untreated and RA treated differentiations. We utilized mouse fetal ovaries as a positive control. Comparing the protein level of SYCP3 in our treated, untreated, and undifferentiated stem cell populations we found the treatment with RA led to significantly higher SYCP3 expression (Fig. 3a). Due to the role of SYCP3 in forming the synaptonemal complex during meiosis it was important to specifically look at how SYCP3 was interacting with the chromosomes. Therefore, following chromosome spreads and immunolocalization of SYCP3 we found the expected phenotype in our fetal ovary controls of synapsed chromosomes labelling positive (Fig. 4b). In our control untreated differentiations positive staining was seen largely as cytoplasmic, suggesting

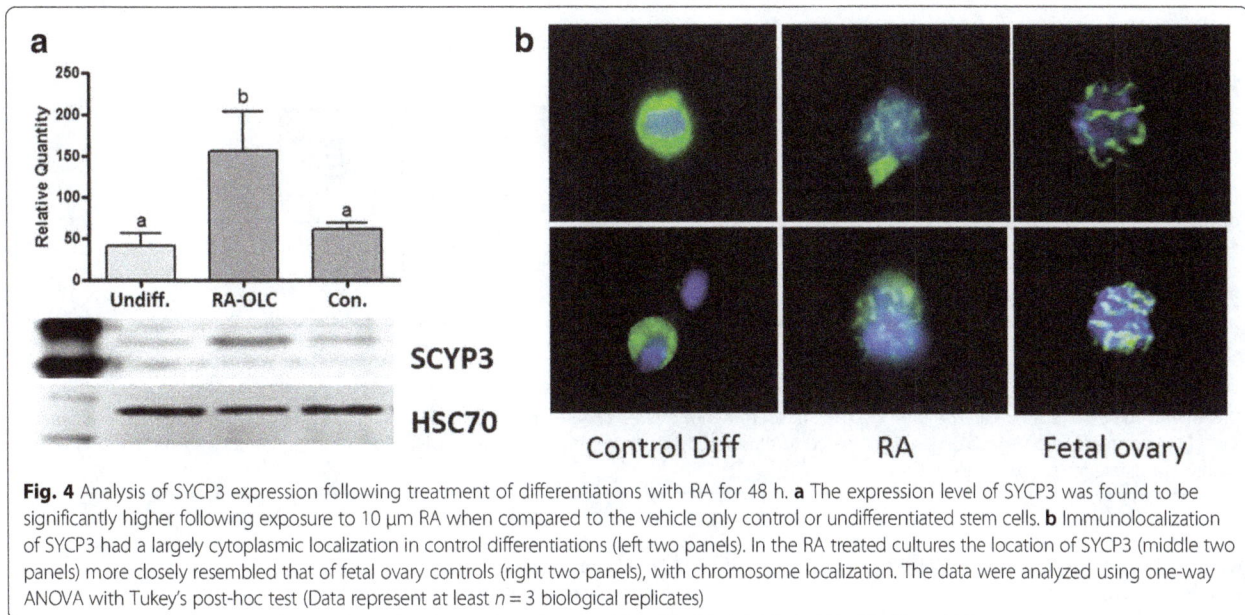

Fig. 4 Analysis of SYCP3 expression following treatment of differentiations with RA for 48 h. **a** The expression level of SYCP3 was found to be significantly higher following exposure to 10 μm RA when compared to the vehicle only control or undifferentiated stem cells. **b** Immunolocalization of SYCP3 had a largely cytoplasmic localization in control differentiations (left two panels). In the RA treated cultures the location of SYCP3 (middle two panels) more closely resembled that of fetal ovary controls (right two panels), with chromosome localization. The data were analyzed using one-way ANOVA with Tukey's post-hoc test (Data represent at least $n = 3$ biological replicates)

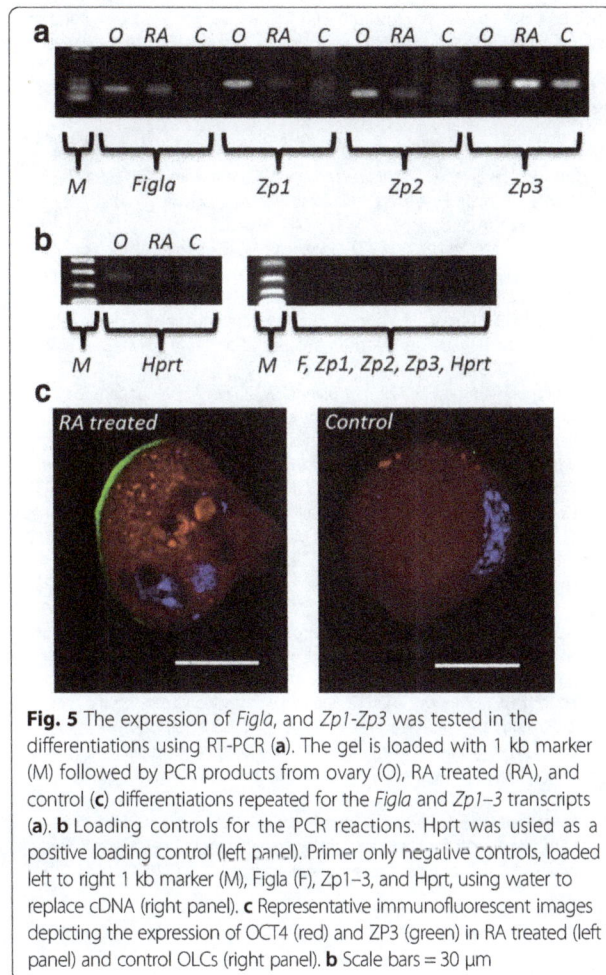

Fig. 5 The expression of *Figla*, and *Zp1-Zp3* was tested in the differentiations using RT-PCR (**a**). The gel is loaded with 1 kb marker (M) followed by PCR products from ovary (O), RA treated (RA), and control (**c**) differentiations repeated for the *Figla* and *Zp1–3* transcripts (**a**). **b** Loading controls for the PCR reactions. Hprt was used as a positive loading control (left panel). Primer only negative controls, loaded left to right 1 kb marker (M), Figla (F), Zp1–3, and Hprt, using water to replace cDNA (right panel). **c** Representative immunofluorescent images depicting the expression of OCT4 (red) and ZP3 (green) in RA treated (left panel) and control OLCs (right panel). **b** Scale bars = 30 μm

a dysregulation in SYCP3 chromosome loading (Fig. 4b). Interestingly, the treatment with RA resulted in a phenotype more consistent with our fetal ovary control cells (Fig. 4b). Following RA treatment SYCP3 was localized on the chromosomes and not in the cytoplasm, though it is unclear if the chromosomes are fully synapsed. This suggests that RA treatment is improving the transition into meiosis of the OLCs.

During the production of OLCs we noticed that the RA treated OLCs had a thicker zona pellucida-like membrane and were less fragile. Previously we have determined that OLCs only expressed *ZP3* and not *Zp1* and *Zp2* [19]. Therefore, we tested the expression of *Zp1–3* in the differentiations following treatment with RA. We found the expression of factor in the germline alpha *(Figla)* in the untreated and RA treated differentiations as well as in the ovary control (Fig. 5a). FIGLA has been shown to be required for the expression of the ZP genes [32]. While the expression of all three *Zp* transcripts were found following RA treatment and in the ovary control, again *Zp1* and *Zp2* failed to be expressed in our control differentiations (Fig. 5a). We next compared the localization of ZP3 in the untreated and RA treated OLCs (Fig. 5c). ZP3 stained more intensely in the RA treated OLCs and appeared to be more membrane localized and continuous, when compared to the control OLCs (Fig. 5c). This likely explains the less fragile OLCs produced in the RA treated differentiation. It is of note to mention that the majority of the OLCs did not show 100 % continuous ZP3 staining and remained more fragile when being handled when compared to natural oocytes (Fig. 5c). Suggesting the RA treatment does not completely correct ZP

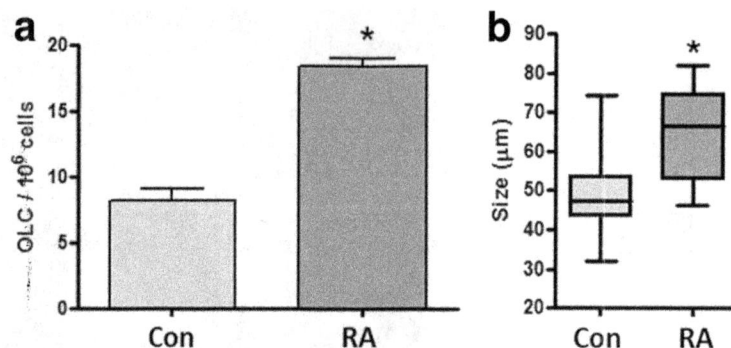

Fig. 6 Analysis of OLC production and growth efficiency. **a** The number of OLCs was determined from starting cell numbers with or without RA treatment. There were significantly more OLCs produced in the RA treated cultures. **b** Over the 6 day differentiation, OLC in the RA treated (left panel)) group reached a larger size when compared to those recovered from the vehicle only control differentiation (right panel). * denotes significant difference $p < 0.05$ using a t-test.

membrane issues and potentially prohibiting full functionality in the OLCs.

Finally, we wanted to determine if the treatment of the differentiations resulted in improved OLC production efficiency and growth. While the system remains relatively inefficient, the production of OLCs following RA treatment more than doubled compared to the untreated controls, 18.39 ± 1.58 OLCs per million starting cells compared to 8.17 ± 2.22 OLCs per million starting cells (Fig. 6a). Moreover, the OLCs displayed better growth characteristics following RA treatment, reaching a significantly greater size (Fig. 6a).

Conclusions

Overall, we have demonstrated that RA can improve the differentiation of skin-derived stem cells into OLCs. It improved the meiotic progress and overall efficiency of the system. Further research will be required to determine if RA treatment improves the functional competency of somatic derived OLCs produced in vitro.

Acknowledgements
The authors thank Kevin Barr for providing expert technical assistance.

Funding
The authors thank Auburn University, the Alabama Agricultural Experiment Station, and the Canadian Institutes of Health Research for funding.

Authors' contributions
PWD and GMK provided funding. PWD and GMK designed the experiments. PWD collected and analyzed the results except for Fig. 2. NT performed the qPCR experiments for preparation of Fig. 2. All authors read and approved the final manuscript.

Competing interests
The authors declare that they have no competing interests.

Author details
[1]Department of Animal Sciences, College of Agriculture, Auburn University, CASIC Building, 559 Devall Drive, Auburn, AL 36849, USA. [2]Department of Physiology and Pharmacology, The University of Western Ontario and Children's Health Research Institute, 800 Commissioners Road East, London, ON N6C 2V5, Canada.

References
1. Speed RM. Meiosis in the foetal mouse ovary. I. An analysis at the light microscope level using surface-spreading. Chromosoma. 1982;85:427–37.
2. Bowles J, Knight D, Smith C, Wilhelm D. Retinoid signaling determines germ cell fate in mice. Science. 2006;312(5773):596–600.
3. Baltus AE, Menke DB, Hu Y-CC, Goodheart ML, Carpenter AE, de Rooij DG, Page DC. In germ cells of mouse embryonic ovaries, the decision to enter meiosis precedes premeiotic DNA replication. Nat Genet. 2006;38:1430–4.
4. Menke DB, Koubova J, Page DC. Sexual differentiation of germ cells in XX mouse gonads occurs in an anterior-to-posterior wave. Dev Biol. 2003;262:303–12.
5. White JA, Ramshaw H, Taimi M, Stangle W, Zhang A, Everingham S, Creighton S, Tam SP, Jones G, Petkovich M. Identification of the human cytochrome P450, P450RA1-2, which is predominantly expressed in the adult cerebellum and is responsible for all-trans-retinoic acid metabolism. Proc Natl Acad Sci. 2000;97:6403–8.
6. Zhou Q, Li Y, Nie R, Friel P, Mitchell D, Evanoff RM, Pouchnik D, Banasik B, McCarrey JR, Small C, Griswold MD. Expression of stimulated by retinoic acid gene 8 (Stra8) and maturation of murine gonocytes and spermatogonia induced by retinoic acid in vitro. Biol Reprod. 2008;78:537–45.
7. Adams IR, McLaren A. Sexually dimorphic development of mouse primordial germ cells: switching from oogenesis to spermatogenesis. Development. 2002;129(5):1155–64.
8. Koubova J, Menke DB, Zhou Q. Retinoic acid regulates sex-specific timing of meiotic initiation in mice. Proc Natl Acad Sci. 2006;103(8):2474–9.
9. Li H, Clagett-Dame M. Vitamin a deficiency blocks the initiation of meiosis of germ cells in the developing rat ovary in vivo. Biol Reprod. 2009;81(5):996–1001.
10. Raverdeau M, Gely-Pernot A, Féret B. Retinoic acid induces Sertoli cell paracrine signals for spermatogonia differentiation but cell autonomously drives spermatocyte meiosis. Proc Natl Acad Sci. 2012;109(41):16582–7.

11. Farini D, Scaldaferri ML, Iona S, Sala LG. Growth factors sustain primordial germ cell survival, proliferation and entering into meiosis in the absence of somatic cells. Dev Biol. 2005;285(1):49–56.

12. Koshimizu U, Watanabe M, Nakatsuji N. Retinoic acid is a potent growth activator of mouse primordial germ cells in vitro. Dev Biol. 1995;168(2):683–5.

13. Hübner K, Fuhrmann G, Christenson LK, Kehler J, Reinbold R, De La Fuente R, Wood J, Strauss JF, Boiani M, Schöler HR. Derivation of oocytes from mouse embryonic stem cells. Science. 2003;300:1251–6.

14. Geijsen N, Horoschak M, Kim K, Gribnau J, Eggan K, Daley GQ. Derivation of embryonic germ cells and male gametes from embryonic stem cells. Nature. 2004;427:148–54.

15. Toyooka Y, Tsunekawa N, Akasu R, Noce T. Embryonic stem cells can form germ cells in vitro. Proc Natl Acad Sci U S A. 2003;100:11457–62.

16. Linher K, Dyce P, Li J. Primordial germ cell-like cells differentiated in vitro from skin-derived stem cells. PLoS One. 2009;4(12):e8263.

17. Dyce PW, Wen L, Li J. In vitro germline potential of stem cells derived from fetal porcine skin. Nat Cell Biol. 2006;8:384–90.

18. Dyce PW. Differentiation of newborn mouse skin derived stem cells into germ-like cells in vitro. J Vis Exp. 2013;77:e50486.

19. Dyce PW, Liu J, Tayade C, Kidder GM, Betts DH, Li J. In vitro and in vivo germ line potential of stem cells derived from newborn mouse skin. PLoS One. 2011;6(5):e20339.

20. Dyce PW, Shen W, Huynh E, Shao H, Villagómez DA, Kidder GM, King WA, Li J. Analysis of oocyte-like cells differentiated from porcine fetal skin-derived stem cells. Stem Cells Dev. 2011;20:809–19.

21. Ge W, Ma H-GG, Cheng S-FF, Sun Y-CC, Sun L-LL, Sun X-FF, Li L, Dyce P, Li J, Shi Q-HH, Shen W. Differentiation of early germ cells from human skin-derived stem cells without exogenous gene integration. Sci Rep. 2015;5:13822.

22. Nayernia K, Nolte J, Michelmann HW, Lee JH. In vitro-differentiated embryonic stem cells give rise to male gametes that can generate offspring mice. Dev Cell. 2006;11(1):125–32.

23. Zhou Q, Wang M, Yuan Y, Wang X, Fu R, Wan H, Xie M, Liu M, Guo X, Zheng Y, Feng G, Shi Q, Zhao X-YY, Sha J, Zhou Q. Complete meiosis from embryonic stem cell-derived germ cells in vitro. Cell Stem Cell. 2016;18:330–40.

24. Toma J, Akhavan M, Fernandes K, Barnabé-Heider F, Sadikot A, Kaplan D, Miller F. Isolation of multipotent adult stem cells from the dermis of mammalian skin. Nat Cell Biol. 2001;3:778–84.

25. Winterhager E, Kidder GM. Gap junction connexins in female reproductive organs: implications for women's reproductive health. Hum Reprod Update. 2015;21(3):340–52.

26. Ge W, Cheng SF, Dyce PW, De Felici M, Shen W. Skin-derived stem cells as a source of primordial germ cell-and oocyte-like cells. Cell Death Dis. 2016; 7(11):e2471.

27. Semba RD (2012). On the "discovery" of vitamin a. Annals of nutrition and metabolism.

28. Rhinn M, Dollé P. Retinoic acid signalling during development. Development. 2012;139(5):843–58.

29. Suzuki A, Saga Y. Nanos2 suppresses meiosis and promotes male germ cell differentiation. Genes Dev. 2008;22:430–5.

30. Su Q, Sugiura S, Pendola C, Handel S, Eppig. MARF1 regulates essential Oogenic processes in mice. Science. 2012;335:14961499.

31. Su Y-Q, Sun F, Handel M, Schimenti J, Eppig J. Meiosis arrest female 1 (MARF1) has nuage-like function in mammalian oocytes. Proc Natl Acad Sci. 2012;109:18653–60.

32. Liang L, Soyal SM, Dean J. FIGalpha, a germ cell specific transcription factor involved in the coordinate expression of the zona pellucida genes. Development. 1997;124(24):4939–47.

Deregulation of the spindle assembly checkpoint is associated with paclitaxel resistance in ovarian cancer

Taryne Chong[1], Amila Sarac[1], Cindy Q. Yao[2], Linda Liao[1], Nicola Lyttle[1], Paul C. Boutros[2,3,4], John M. S. Bartlett[1,5,6] and Melanie Spears[1,5*]

Abstract

Background: Ovarian cancer is the leading gynecologic cancer diagnosed in North America and because related symptoms are not disease specific, this often leads to late detection, an advanced disease state, and the need for chemotherapy. Ovarian cancer is frequently sensitive to chemotherapy at diagnosis but rapid development of drug resistance leads to disease progression and ultimately death in the majority of patients.

Results: We have generated paclitaxel resistant ovarian cell lines from their corresponding native cell lines to determine driver mechanisms of drug resistance using gene expression arrays. These paclitaxel resistant ovarian cells demonstrate: (1) Increased IC_{50} for paclitaxel and docetaxel (10 to 75-fold) and cross-resistance to anthracyclines (2) Reduced cell apoptosis in the presence of paclitaxel (3) Gene depletion involving mitotic regulators BUB1 mitotic checkpoint serine/threonine kinase, cyclin BI (CCNB1), centromere protein E (CENPE), and centromere protein F (CENPF), and (4) Functional data validating gene depletion among mitotic regulators.

Conclusions: We have generated model systems to explore drug resistance in ovarian cancer, which have revealed a key pathway related to the spindle assembly checkpoint underlying paclitaxel resistance in ovarian cell lines.

Keywords: Spindle assembly checkpoint, Ovarian cancer, Paclitaxel, Mitotic checkpoint serine/threonine kinase (BUB1), centromere protein E (CENPE), Centromere protein F (CENPF), Cyclin B1 (CCNB1)

Background

Each year approximately 158,000 women die of ovarian cancer worldwide [1]. Ovarian cancer is the most common gynecological cancer diagnosed in North America and has one of the lowest survival rates among all cancers [2]. Symptoms are not disease specific and often overlap with other common gastrointestinal and gynecological conditions, which can result in late detection, an advanced disease state, and the need for chemotherapy [2–4]. Roughly 70% of ovarian cancers are sensitive to chemotherapy treatment at diagnosis, but rapid development of drug resistance and the inability to halt metastasis leads to treatment failure and disease progression when detected at later stages [4–6]. Paclitaxel is a frontline therapy used to treat advanced ovarian cancer, and in many instances, paclitaxel is combined with platinum based therapeutic drugs, such as carboplatin to improve overall survival [4, 7]. Paclitaxel inhibits cell replication by stabilizing microtubule assembly, thereby promoting mitotic arrest at the spindle assembly checkpoint [8–10]. Previous evidence points to numerous components of the spindle assembly checkpoint and mitotic regulation playing a major role in several cancers [11, 12]. We have generated isogenic paclitaxel resistant cell lines from their corresponding native cell lines which reflect the 3 most common ovarian histologic subtypes, these include serous, clear cell and endometrioid subtypes [2]. These pre-clinical models were used to observe cytotoxicity, cell cycle modulation and changes in gene expression to examine the mechanisms driving drug resistance. Lastly, through gene expression profiling we have demonstrated disruption of the spindle assembly

* Correspondence: Melanie.Spears@oicr.on.ca
[1]Diagnostic Development, Ontario Institute for Cancer Research, MaRS Centre, 661 University Avenue, Suite 510, Toronto, Ontario M5G 0A3, Canada
[5]Department of Laboratory Medicine and Pathobiology, University of Toronto, 27 King's College Circle, Toronto, Ontario M5S 1A1, Canada
Full list of author information is available at the end of the article

checkpoint in the paclitaxel resistant cell lines, indicating a potential therapeutic pathway.

Methods

Cell lines and cell culture

Human ovarian cancer cell lines TOV21G (representing clear cell ovarian carcinoma) and TOV112D (representing endometrioid adenocarcinoma) were purchased from American Type Culture Collection (Manassas, VA). The human ovarian epithelial-serous cell line COV504 was purchased from Sigma Aldrich (St. Louis, MO). The identity of each cell line was validated prior to use by short tandem repeat genotyping at The Centre for Applied Genomics at The Hospital for Sick Children (Toronto, ON). All cell lines were cultured in Dulbecco's modified eagles' medium (DMEM) supplemented with 2 mM glutamine and 10% heat inactivated fetal bovine serum (FBS) from Life Technologies (Carlsbad, CA) and maintained at 37°C in a 5% CO_2 atmosphere. The following chemotherapeutic drugs: paclitaxel, docetaxel, doxorubicin, epirubicin and carboplatin were purchased from Sigma Aldrich (St. Louis, MO), dissolved in dimethyl sulfoxide (DMSO) from Sigma Aldrich (St. Louis, MO) and supplemented in complete media at increasing concentrations. Cells were exposed to an incremental dose escalation of paclitaxel (2 nM) for approximately 2 passages, up to a final concentration of 25 nM, once paclitaxel resistance was achieved.

Cell viability and cytotoxicity assays

IC_{50} values were determined using the CCK-8 assay from Dojindo Molecular Technologies (Rockville, MD). Briefly, all cell suspensions were plated in 100 μl per well across a 96-well plate, allowed to grow for 24 hours and incubated at 37°C in a humidified 5% CO_2 atmosphere. Following a 24 hour incubation, cells were treated with complete DMEM with 10% FBS and supplemented with or without increasing concentrations of drugs (0, 0.3, 1, 3, 10, 30, 100, 1000 or 3000 nM) in DMSO. After 72 hours of exposure to varying drug concentrations, 10 μl of the CCK-8 assay reagent was added to 90 μl DMEM and the cells were incubated for an additional 4 hours at 37°C in a 5% CO_2 atmosphere. The absorbance of each sample was measured using a microplate reader at 450 nm from BioRad (Hercules, CA). Negative controls were prepared using cell-free complete DMEM containing the CCK-8 reagent.

Annexin V staining

Cultured cells were treated with or without paclitaxel for 24 hours prior to collection. According to the manufacturer's protocol from eBioscience (San Diego, CA); cells were washed once in 1X phosphate buffered saline (PBS) and 1X Binding Buffer from eBioscience, then resuspended in 1X Binding Buffer. Following the addition of 5 μl fluorochrome-conjugated Annexin V staining solution to 100 μl cell suspension, cells were incubated in the dark for 15 minutes at room temperature and evaluated for apoptosis on a flow cytometer from Becton Dickinson (San Jose, CA). Negative controls included cells with vehicle (DMSO) stained for Annexin V and cells without staining.

Cell cycle analysis

Cell cycle distribution was evaluated by using propidium iodide staining and the BD FACSCanto II system (San Jose, CA). Cells were arrested in G1/S phase by employing a double thymidine block (2 mM) from Sigma Aldrich (St. Louis, MO). The following day, the reaction was halted by replacing media with fresh thymidine containing media and cells were collected at varying time points thereafter. Once the cell pellets were collected, they were washed with 1X PBS (pH 7.2) from Life Technologies (Carlsbad, CA) and fixed with ice cold 80% ethanol from Commercial Alcohols (Tiverton, ON). We used 0.1 mg/ml propidium iodide and 2 mg/ml RNase A purchased from Sigma Aldrich (St. Louis, MO) which were added to each sample prior to incubation in the dark for 30 minutes. The cell cycle data were collected using the BD FACSCanto II system and analyzed using FlowJo software (San Jose, CA).

Microarray sample submission

Illumina Human HT-12-V4 Bead Chips were used for the whole genome microarray analysis by the University Health Network (UHN) Microarray Centre in Toronto, Canada. Total RNA was extracted with the RNeasy Mini kit from Qiagen (Toronto, ON) and used for profiling gene expression changes.

Gene expression analysis

Summary-level data from GenomeStudio (defaulted to have no normalization or background correction) were loaded into the R statistical environment (v3.0.2) using the lumi package (v2.12.0) from BioConductor [13]. The remaining samples were transformed using variance-stabilizing transformation (VST) and normalized using robust spline normalization. Samples from the same cell lines (native and drug resistant) were pre-processed together to avoid confounding effects from normalizing multiple cell lines together. Following pre-processing, we used general linear-modeling to identify genes that are differentially expressed in drug resistant cell lines relative to native cell line controls. The gene expression levels across all cell lines were determined using a per-gene linear model that assessed both basal levels and drug resistance-induced effects. Coefficients were fitted to terms representing each effect and the standard errors of the coefficients were adjusted using an empirical

Bayes moderation of the standard error [14]. To test if each coefficient was statistically different from zero, we applied model-based t-tests, followed by a false discovery rate (FDR) adjustment for multiple testing [15]. Genes were deemed to be significant if their adjusted p-values were less than or equal to 0.05. All statistical analyses were performed using the limma package (v3.16.8) within the R statistical environment (v3.0.2). Genes showing significant differential gene expression levels between the resistant and native samples across all types of cell lines were loaded into the Cytoscape Reactome Functional Interaction (FI) plugin in Cytoscape (v3.0.2). Symbols were loaded as a gene set with the 2013 version of the FI network. FI network was constructed with FI annotations and linker genes. Spectral clustering and Pathway Enrichment were computed for each module using the Reactome FI plugin functions and the pathways exhibiting FDR < 0.05 were considered enriched.

Immunoblot analysis

Cell lysates were normalized using the BCA Protein Assay Kit by Pierce and equivalent amounts of total protein were separated by electrophoresis on 4-20% BioRad Mini Protean TGX Precast Gels (Hercules, CA). Gels were transferred to nitrocellulose membranes and incubated with rabbit anti-cyclin B1 (1:1000 dilution) from Cell Signaling (Danvers, MA), mouse anti-BubR1 (1:1000 dilution) from BD Transduction Laboratories (San Jose, CA), rabbit anti-CENPE (1:2000 dilution) from Sigma (Oakville, ON), and rabbit anti-CENPF (1:1000 dilution) from Novus Biologicals (Oakville, ON) antibodies. The visualization of blots was performed using the ChemiDoc Imaging System and accompanying Image Lab software from BioRad (Hercules, CA). The membranes were stripped and re-probed for β-actin (1:10,000 dilution) from Proteintech Group (Rosemont, IL) which served as a loading control.

Results

Increased resistance to paclitaxel, docetaxel and anthracyclines in human ovarian cancer cells

To study chemotherapeutic resistance in ovarian cancer cells, we established three paclitaxel resistant cell lines by incremental and continuous exposure to paclitaxel, up to a final concentration of 25 nM. We observed marked increases in IC_{50} values for both paclitaxel and docetaxel (up to 75 fold) in all 3 cell lines representing three different histologic subtypes (Table 1). In addition, we observed distinct cross-resistance to anthracyclines, including epirubicin and doxorubicin (typically 3-10 fold) across all 3 cell line pairs (Table 1). Carboplatin is currently a standard treatment option, and we show cross-resistance to carboplatin in the TOV112D cell line,

which may indicate improved clinical benefit in the endometrioid ovarian subtype (Table 1).

Reduced cell apoptosis in paclitaxel resistant human ovarian cancer cells

During exposure of native and resistant cell lines to increasing concentrations of paclitaxel, we demonstrated that paclitaxel resistant cell lines exhibited reduced cell apoptosis relative to their native counterparts, following exposure to 25 and 1000 nM paclitaxel treatment (Table 2). For example, the percentage of apoptotic cells in the native TOV21G ovarian cells was 59% versus 14% in the resistant cells, following the addition of 25 nM paclitaxel. This result was equally marked in the TOV112D ovarian cells where 63% of native cells were apoptotic versus 4% in the resistant cell line. Lastly, a similar trend was observed in the COV504 ovarian cells where 26% of the native cells were apoptotic compared to 10% of the resistant ovarian cells in the presence of 25 nM paclitaxel. The treatment of resistant ovarian cell lines with 25 nM paclitaxel clearly resulted in reduced cell apoptosis across all subtypes observed.

Paclitaxel resistant human ovarian cells overcome G2/M arrest

We monitored cell cycle progression in both the native and resistant ovarian cell lines (±) 25 nM paclitaxel and we found that the resistant cell lines were able to overcome paclitaxel induced G2/M arrest and progress through the cell cycle. At 12 hours, paclitaxel treatment of the native TOV21G, TOV112D and COV504 cells caused a G2/M block and a failure to progress to the G0/G1 phase (Fig. 1). Specifically, the G2/M population of TOV112D native cells increased considerably from 26% to 55% upon exposure to paclitaxel, indicating mitotic arrest in G2/M, compared with a minimal change of 29% to 36% in the TOV112D resistant cells. The increase in cell accumulation at the G2/M phase was accompanied by a decrease of cell population in the G1 phase for the native cells. Similar results were observed in the COV504 resistant cell line, whereby the G1 population changed minimally from 35% to 36% following paclitaxel treatment. These results verify that paclitaxel inhibits cell growth by inducing a block at G2/M phase in several subtypes of ovarian cancer cells, however this effect is more apparent in the native cell lines rather than the resistant cell lines, and overcoming G2/M arrest is a potential process linked to paclitaxel resistance.

Gene expression analysis in paclitaxel resistant human ovarian cancer cells

The effect of paclitaxel resistance across several subtypes was examined and a number of statistically significant alterations in gene expression levels (q ≤ 0.05) were observed between the native and paclitaxel resistant cells

Table 1 The half maximal inhibitory concentration (IC_{50}) in human ovarian cancer cells

	Paclitaxel (nM)	Docetaxel (nM)	Epirubicin (nM)	Doxorubicin (nM)	Carboplatin (uM)
TOV21G N	1.31 ± 0.75	0.17 ± 4.43	6.30 ± 1.90	0.02 ± 1.01	17.99 ± 1.27
TOV21G R	44.64 ± 15.41 (34)	10.73 ± 1.28 (63)	20.06 ± 1.48 (3)	9.90 ± 1.72 (495)	0.59 ± 4.64
TOV112D N	1.49 ± 1.40	0.86 ± 1.50	9.60 ± 1.10	11.19 ± 1.11	80.81 ± 1.08
TOV112D R	28.26 ± 1.06 (19)	13.91 ± 1.11 (16)	34.78 ± 1.10 (3.6)	30.16 ± 1.09 (3)	140.0 ± 1.45 (2)
COV504 N	1.91 ± 1.85	0.30 ± 3.37	31.56 ± 1.48	47.58 ± 1.81	103.68 ± 1.14
COV504 R	75.51 ± 27.44 (40)	23.08 ± 1.25 (77)	290.33 ± 2.20 (9)	250.58 ± 2.50 (5)	35.16 ± 1.35

The IC_{50} in both native (N) and drug resistant (R) ovarian cancer cell lines were determined by incremental and continuous exposure to drug. Drug resistance is clearly defined in all subtypes and most evident in the epithelial serous cell line, represented by COV504 for both taxanes and anthracyclines (± standard deviation, average of 3 independent experiments). The resistance factor is shown in parentheses and highlights drug resistance (resistant IC_{50}/native IC_{50}) for each cell line pair

(Fig. 2). These changes in gene expression include 49 deregulated genes across the ovarian histologic subtypes. Among the differentially expressed genes were a number of key regulators that maintain the mitotic spindle checkpoint. Specifically, we determined that 21 genes were found depleted when compared to the native cell lines (Additional file 1: Table S1), and many of these genes were associated with cell cycle regulation and the mitotic checkpoint, and include the following: Aurora kinase A (AURKA), abnormal spindle microtubule assembly (ASPM), BUB1, CCNB1, CENPE, and CENPF and NIMA-related kinase 2 (NEK2). Alternatively, gene enrichment patterns were observed in several functions controlling structural scaffolding and development and apoptotic control; these genes include BCL2/adenovirus E1B 19 kDa interacting protein 3 (BNIP3), sprouty

homolog 2 (SPRY2), and the WW domain binding protein 5 (WBP5). Overall, several genes governing G2/M transition were found depleted and to ultimately affect mitotic function, corresponding to acquired paclitaxel resistance in ovarian cell lines.

Pathway analysis in paclitaxel resistant human ovarian cancer cells

We explored pathway analysis and observed several gene alterations between resistant cells and their respective native cell lines (q ≤ 0.05) (Fig. 3). The majority of gene nodes display gene depletion and include the following candidate genes: AURKA, ASPM, NEK2, BUB1, CCNB1, CENPE and CENPF. Reactome network analysis revealed significant pathways and genes associated with mitotic regulation, and these include: (1) mitotic pro metaphase (2) mitotic metaphase and anaphase (3) mitotic G2-G2/M phase and (4) APC/C-mediated degradation of cell cycle proteins (Table 3). An additional pathway linked to the spindle checkpoint control involves ubiquitin conjugating enzyme E2C (UBE2C) which was found depleted across the ovarian subtypes. Cell cycle progression was shown to be modified by UBE2C which can affect the degradation of cyclin B1 required for mitotic exit [16].

Validation of reduced protein expression in paclitaxel resistant human ovarian cancer cells

Immunoblotting of ovarian cancer cells revealed a decrease in spindle assembly checkpoint proteins in the paclitaxel resistant cells (Fig. 4). Specifically, there was a marked decrease in both BUB1-related protein (BubR1) and cyclin B1 protein expression in the paclitaxel resistant cells versus the corresponding natives. Our results support previous work illustrating lower expression of BubR1 and cyclin B1 in paclitaxel resistant ovarian cells OVCAR-3 and SKOV-3 versus their corresponding native cells, thus validating our functional data [8]. Furthermore, a significant decrease in CENPE and CENPF protein expression was observed in the paclitaxel resistant cells versus the corresponding native cells (Fig. 4).

Table 2 Percentages of apoptotic ovarian cells following the absence or presence of paclitaxel

	DMSO	Paclitaxel (25nM)	Paclitaxel (1000 nM)
TOV21G N	6.00	58.60	63.00
	(±0.38)	(±4.50)	(±2.80)
TOV21G R	11.20	13.60[1]	56.70
	(±5.50)	(±1.10)	(±30.70)
TOV112D N	1.80	63.20	82.00
	(±0.18)	(±0.50)	(±0.25)
TOV112D R	2.00	3.70[2]	69.00
	(±0.27)	(±0.57)	(±0.87)
COV504 N	7.40	25.70	49.60
	(±4.40)	(±6.70)	(±25.30)
COV504 R	8.40	10.00[3]	29.60
	(±4.40)	(±1.80)	(±6.20)

Annexin V staining was used to determine the early detection of apoptotic cells and after 72 hours, apoptosis is evident in both native (N) and paclitaxel resistant (R) cell lines, in all three subtypes TOV21G, TOV112D and COV504. Both the native and resistant cell lines were exposed to increasing concentrations of paclitaxel; all three paclitaxel resistant cell lines exhibited reduced apoptotic induction when exposed to 25 and 1000 nM paclitaxel treatment (± standard deviation, average of 3 independent experiments). [1](p < 0.01) [2](p < 0.04) [3](p < 0.05) versus corresponding native groups

Fig. 1 (See legend on next page.)

(See figure on previous page.)
Fig. 1 Cell cycle distributions in native and paclitaxel resistant cell lines (**a**) TOV21G, (**b**) TOV112D and (**c**) COV504. Using a double thymidine block, native and paclitaxel resistant cells were synchronized and incubated in the presence of DMSO or 25 nM paclitaxel. Cells were collected at 12 hours and the cell cycle distributions within the cell population were analysed by flow cytometry. The cellular response of 3 cell lines was consistent whereby the resistant ovarian cancer cells treated with paclitaxel were able to overcome paclitaxel induced G2/M arrest and progressed through the cell cycle. The percentages shown represent a single experiment; 3 independent experiments were conducted for each cell line

Clinical tumour samples and kaplan-meier survival curve analysis

The Cancer Genome Atlas (TCGA) is a large scale database containing human cancer genomics data [17, 18]. We have analyzed our candidate genes using the TCGA clinical database and web based tool cBio Cancer Genomics Portal (http://www.cbioportal.org/), which was developed for mining cancer genome sequencing data [17, 18]. We have evaluated the mRNA expression of primary serous ovarian tumour samples via Agilent microarray to validate the impact of candidate genes BUB1, CCNB1, CENPE and CENPF on overall survival. Using Kaplan-Meier survival curve analysis, we have found that overall survival of 489 patients was significantly less ($p < 0.02$) when the candidate genes were deregulated (Fig. 5). Moreover, patient prognosis with altered expression was significantly poorer than those with unaltered mRNA expression.

Discussion

Our study revealed gene depletion across a number of molecular components involved in the spindle assembly checkpoint and mitotic regulation, including BUB1, CCNB1, CENPE and CENPF in paclitaxel resistant ovarian cancer cell lines. We found molecular pathways involving mitotic regulation, mitotic pro metaphase, mitotic anaphase and mitotic G2-G2/M phase showing significant depletion. Using the TCGA clinical database, we have shown that altered expression of candidate genes in patients with serous ovarian cancer contributes to significantly poorer survival status in patients. Taken together, we have found evidence of a deregulated spindle assembly checkpoint with significant alteration in mitotic regulators linked to the acquisition of paclitaxel resistance across ovarian subtypes. Several chemotherapeutic agents, such as paclitaxel, target the spindle assembly checkpoint which affects mitotic progression and arrest, thus emphasizing

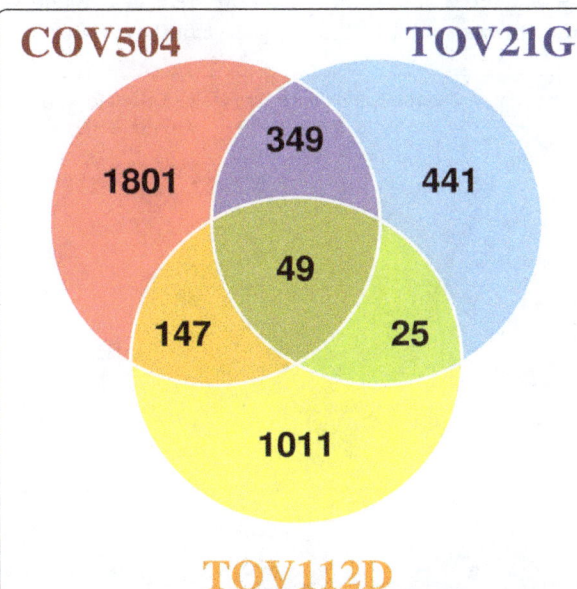

Fig. 2 Venn diagram showing overlapping genes between the paclitaxel resistant cell lines. Paclitaxel resistant cell lines TOV21G, TOV112D and COV504 were differentially expressed across multiple histologic subtypes (q ≤ 0.05). The changes in mRNA abundance include an overlap of 49 significant genes highlighting both enrichment and depletion of genes across human ovarian cell lines

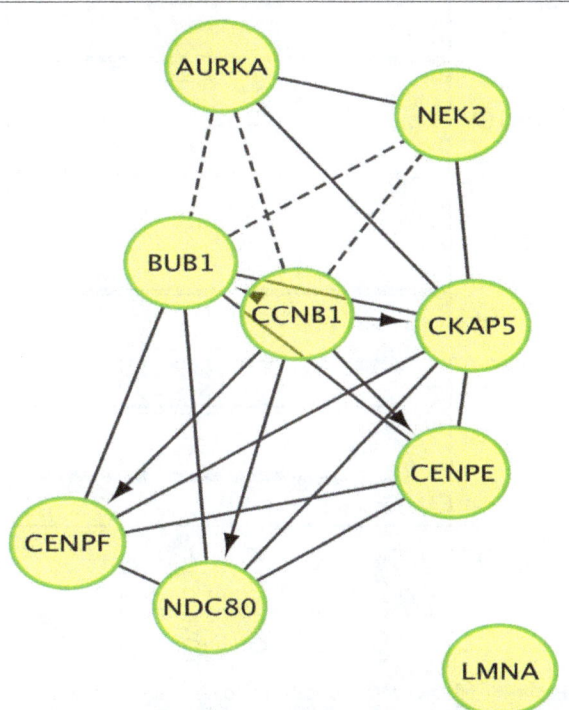

Fig. 3 Pathway analysis illustrating differential gene expression and association between gene nodes. The gene nodes display gene depletion (q ≤ 0.05) and include the following candidate genes: BUB1, CCNB1, CENPE and CENPF. The arrows with blunt ends denote negative regulation and sets with overlapping content are connected by a line of long dashes. The arrows represent positive regulation

Table 3 Reactome network analysis revealing significant association with mitotic regulation

Associated Pathway	Genes	FDR
mitotic pro metaphase	CCNB1, CKAP5, BUB1, CENPF, CENPE, NDC80	FDR ≤ 3.33 x 10^{-4}
mitotic metaphase and anaphase	CKAP5, LMNA, BUB1, CENPF, CENPE, NDC80, UBE2C, PSME1	FDR ≤ 1.00 x 10^{-3}
mitotic G2-G2/M phase	CCNB1, CKAP5, NEK2, CENPF, AURKA	FDR ≤ 1.00 x 10^{-3}
APC/C-mediated degradation of cell cycle proteins	AURKA, UBE2C, CCNB1, PSME1	FDR ≤ 4.80 x 10^{-3}

Reactome network analysis revealed pathways associated with mitotic regulation. These networks predominantly involve spindle assembly checkpoint, centromere-kinetochore complex and cell cycle regulation

the importance of the mitotic spindle and associated genes as a therapeutic target [19–21].

Cyclin B1 and cyclin dependent kinases (cdks) are associated with mitosis and cell cycle regulation [8, 22]. Our gene expression data reveal significant depletion of cyclin B1 across all three resistant ovarian subtypes. Our findings are consistent with recent data showing reduced cyclin B1 protein expression in two additional paclitaxel resistant ovarian cell lines, OVCAR-3 and SKOV-3 versus their respective parental cell lines [8, 19]. Furthermore, a functional decrease in cyclin B1 protein expression was observed in conjunction with reduced CDK1 (cdc2) expression in human ovarian cisplatin resistant A2780 cells [22]. Since cyclin B1 is a marker specific for the G2/M phase, the decrease in cyclin B1 is associated with the deregulation and weakening of the G2/M phase of the cell cycle [19]. Therefore, a functional loss of cyclin B1 can be attributed to the destabilization of the spindle checkpoint, thus emphasizing the role of cyclin B1 on cell cycle dynamics and the regulatory mechanisms associated with paclitaxel resistance.

Cell cycle progression is tightly orchestrated and many of the spindle assembly checkpoint genes associated with regulation, including BUB1 and BUBR1 are conserved throughout evolution [19, 23]. BUB1 is a molecular component of the spindle checkpoint and required for proper checkpoint signalling and deletions of BUB1 or BUBR1 were detected in several cancers [12, 24]. Previously, mitotic checkpoint defects and the inactivation of the BUB1 gene have been implicated in human colorectal cancer cells [12, 25]. These colorectal cell lines with loss of altered checkpoint function were also found to show chromosomal instability [12]. Consistent with this

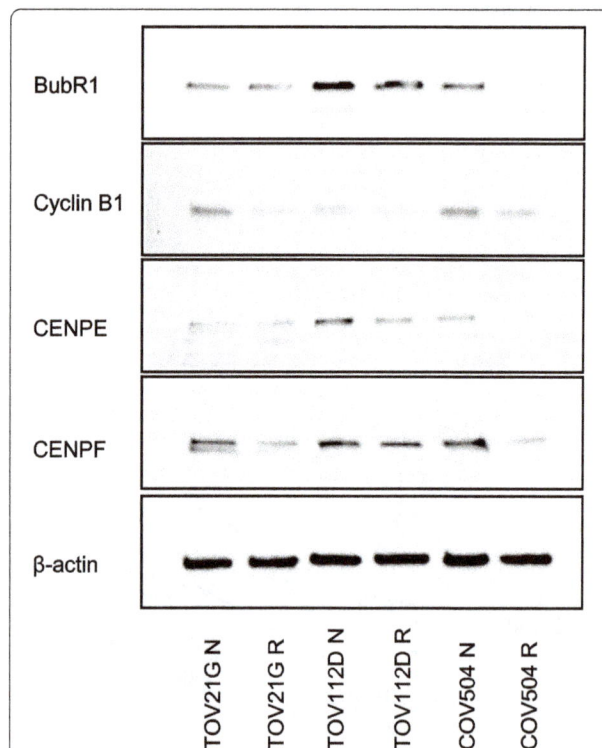

Fig. 4 The effect of paclitaxel resistance on key regulators of the mitotic spindle checkpoint. Immunoblot analysis of cell cycle proteins BubR1, cyclin B1, CENPE and CENPF isolated from native and resistant cell lines. Individual lanes contained 20-50 µg of total protein; each gel was normalized. The proteins were resolved on 4-20% Mini Protean TGX Precast Gels, transferred to nitrocellulose membranes and probed using antibodies specific for BubR1, cyclin B1, CENPE and CENPF proteins. β-actin served as a loading control. The immunoblots represent a single experiment; 3 independent experiments were conducted

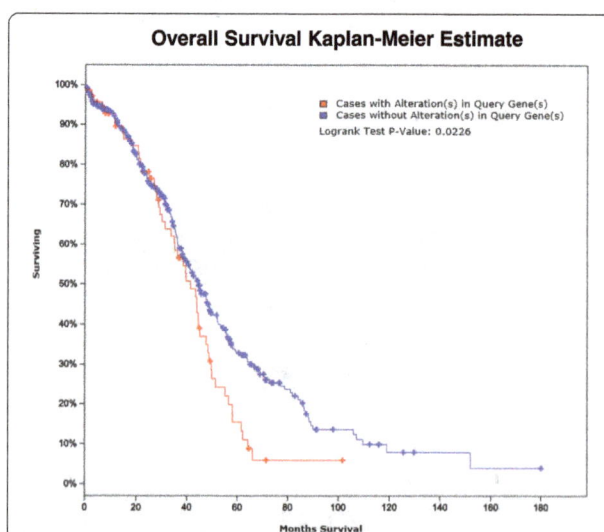

Fig. 5 Kaplan-Meier survival curve analysis in primary serous ovarian tumours. Kaplan-Meier survival analysis comparing the mRNA status with overall survival in 489 primary serous ovarian tumour samples. Z-Scores of mRNA expression of candidate genes were downloaded using cBioPortal. Survival status was significantly poorer in patients with altered expression of all 4 candidate genes ($p < 0.02$)

finding, one study examining a subset of human colorectal tumours revealed a statistically significant association of low BUB1 and BUBR1 mRNA expression with increased metastasis, and a higher recurrence rate [26]. A corresponding observation found BubR1 protein expression was considerably reduced in polyploid cells, and in 31.3% (21/67) of the human colon adenocarcinoma examined [27]. Collectively, these results illustrate that deregulation of the spindle assembly checkpoint is associated with the lack of BUB1 gene function and this deficiency is associated with paclitaxel resistance.

Kinetochore motor proteins CENPE and CENPF are required for proper microtubule attachment and regulation of the spindle checkpoint [23, 28]. Our results reveal significant depletion of CENPE and CENPF mRNA levels across the ovarian subtypes when compared to native cells. In support of our findings, recent evidence shows CENPF siRNA knockdown resulting in cisplatin resistance in a variant small cell lung carcinoma and a non-small cell lung adenocarcinoma [29]. Similar observations reveal depletion of CENPE resulting in unstable kinetochore-microtubule capture and chromosomal instability [30]. Furthermore, evidence illustrated reduced CENPE mRNA expression found in a human hepatocellular carcinoma (HepG2) versus a normal liver cell line (LO2); the results were further validated using western blot analysis and quantitative real-time PCR [31]. In vitro immunofluorescence staining demonstrated that CENPE is co-localized with BUBR1 at kinetochores [28]. The direct interaction between the centromere-kinetochore complex and BUBR1, along with spindle microtubules is believed to modulate mitotic checkpoint signaling events and thus highlights the interaction of kinetochores, spindle checkpoint control and mitotic progression [24].

Conclusions

We have generated model systems to explore drug resistance in ovarian cancer, which reveal a defective spindle assembly checkpoint associated with acquired paclitaxel resistance. Our results demonstrate that depletion of spindle checkpoint related genes BUB1, CCNB1, CENPE and CENPF during paclitaxel resistance correlates with significant disruption to the cell cycle, which can lead to the suppression of paclitaxel induced cell death. Specifically, multiple cancers exhibit gene down regulation involving CCNB1 and BUB1, highlighting the relationship between a disrupted spindle assembly checkpoint and tumour formation. Since paclitaxel is an effective microtubule drug and exerts apoptotic effect through the regulation of the spindle assembly checkpoint, restoration of gene function to spindle checkpoint related genes would seem an effective target for minimizing cancer progression.

Abbreviations

ASPM: Asp abnormal spindle homolog, microcephaly associated (Drosophila); AURKA: Aurora kinase A; BCA: Bicinchoninic acid assay; BNIP3: BCL2/adenovirus E1B 19 kDa interacting protein 3; BUB1: Mitotic checkpoint serine/threonine kinase; BUBR1: BUB1 related protein; CCNB1: Cyclin B1; CDK: Cyclin dependent kinase; CENPE: Centromere protein E; CENPF: Centromere protein F; CKAP5: Cytoskeleton associated protein 5; LMNA: Lamin A/C; NDC80: Kinetochore complex component; NEK2: NIMA-related kinase 2; PSME1: Proteasome activator subunit 1; SPRY2: Sprouty homolog 2; UBE2C: Ubiquitin conjugating enzyme E2C; WBP5: WW domain binding protein 5

Acknowledgements

We thank Nazleen Lobo for her exceptional technical skills and contributions to the manuscript.

Funding

TC, AS, CQY, LL, NL, PCB, JMSB and MS were supported by funding from OICR. We thank the government of Ontario for funding, which is provided through the Ontario Ministry of Research, Innovation and Science.

Authors' contributions

TC performed experimental procedures, data analysis, experimental design and drafted the manuscript; AS performed experimental procedures and data analysis; CQY data analysis; LL performed experimental procedures and data analysis; NL performed experimental procedures and data analysis; PCB data analysis; JMSB experimental design; MS coordination and experimental design. All authors read and approved the final manuscript.

Competing interests

The authors declare that they have no competing interests.

Author details

[1]Diagnostic Development, Ontario Institute for Cancer Research, MaRS Centre, 661 University Avenue, Suite 510, Toronto, Ontario M5G 0A3, Canada. [2]Informatics Program, Ontario Institute for Cancer Research, MaRS Centre, 661 University Avenue, Suite 510, Toronto, Ontario M5G 0A3, Canada. [3]Department of Medical Biophysics, University of Toronto, 101 College Street, Room 15-701, Toronto, Ontario M5G 1L7, Canada. [4]Department of Pharmacology and Toxicology, University of Toronto, 1 King's College Circle, Room 4207, Toronto, Ontario M5S 1A8, Canada. [5]Department of Laboratory Medicine and Pathobiology, University of Toronto, 27 King's College Circle, Toronto, Ontario M5S 1A1, Canada. [6]Biomarkers and Companion Diagnostics, Edinburgh Cancer Research Centre, Crewe Road South, Edinburgh EH4 2XR, UK.

References

1. Fitzmaurice C, Dicker D, Pain A, Hamavid H, Moradi-Lakeh M, et al. The Global Burden of Cancer. J Am Med Assoc Oncol. 2015;1(4):505–27.
2. Bowtell D. The genesis and evolution of high-grade serous ovarian cancer. Nat Rev Cancer. 2010;10:803 8.
3. Berns E, Bowtell D. The changing view of high-grade serous ovarian cancer. Cancer Res. 2012;72(11):2701–4.
4. Bast R Jr. Molecular approaches to personalizing management of ovarian cancer. Ann Oncol. 2011;22(Suppl 8):viii5–viii15.
5. Tagawa T, Morgan R, Yen Y, et al. Ovarian cancer: Opportunity for targeted therapy. J Oncol. 2012;2012:1–9.

6. Swanton C, Marani M, Pardo O, Warne P, Kelly F, Sahai E, et al. Regulators of mitotic arrest and ceramide metabolism are determinants of sensitivity to paclitaxel and other chemotherapeutic drugs. Cancer Cell. 2007;11:498–512.

7. Yap T, Carden C, Kaye S. Beyond chemotherapy: targeted therapies in ovarian cancer. Nature Reviews Cancer. 2009;9:167–81.

8. Wang X, Wu E, Wu J, et al. An antimitotic and antivascular agent BPR0L075 overcomes multidrug resistance and induces mitotic catastrophe in paclitaxel-resistant ovarian cancer cells. PLoS One. 2013;8:1–12.

9. Bharadwaj R, Yu H. The spindle checkpoint, aneuploidy, and cancer. Oncogene. 2004;23:2016–27.

10. Rowinsky E, Donehower R. Paclitaxel (taxol). N Engl J Med. 1995;332:1004–14.

11. Hartwell L, Kastan M. Cell cycle control and cancer. Science. 1994;266:1821–8.

12. Cahill D, Lengauer C, Yu J, et al. Mutations of mitotic checkpoint genes in human cancers. Nature. 1998;392:300–3.

13. Du P, Kibbe W, Lin S. lumi: a pipeline for processing Illumina microarray. Bioinformatics. 2008;24:1547–8.

14. Smyth GK. Linear models and empirical bayes methods for assessing differential expression in microarray experiments. Stat Appl Genet Mol Biol. 2004;3:Article 3.

15. Storey JD, Tibshirani R. Statistical significance for genomewide studies. Proc Natl Acad Sci U S A. 2003;100:9440–5.

16. Gene [Internet]. National Library of Medicine (US). National Center for Biotechnology Information. 2004-2017. Available from: https://www.ncbi.nlm.nih.gov/gene/

17. Cerami E, Gao J, Dogrusoz U, et al. The cBio Cancer Genomics Portal: An Open Platform for Exploring Multidimensional Cancer Genomics Data. Cancer Discov. 2012;5:401–4.

18. Gao J, Aksoy B, Dogrusoz U, et al. Integrative Analysis of Complex Cancer Genomics and Clinical Profiles Using the cBioPortal. Sci Signal. 2013;6(269):pl1.

19. Fu Y, Ye D, Chen H, et al. Weakened spindle checkpoint with reduced BubR1 expression in paclitaxel-resistant ovarian carcinoma cell line SKOV3-TR30. Gynecol Oncol. 2007;105:66–73.

20. Sudo T, Nitta M, Saya H, et al. Dependence of Paclitaxel Sensitivity on a Functional Spindle Assembly Checkpoint. Cancer Res. 2004;64:2502–8.

21. Rath O, Kozielski F. Kinesins and Cancer. Nat Rev Cancer. 2012;12:527–39.

22. Wang XL, Zhao J, Ding H, et al. Antiproliferative effect of ß-elemene in chemoresistant ovarian carcinoma cells is mediated through arrest of the cell cycle at the G2-M phase. Cell Mol Life Sci. 2005;62:894–904.

23. Chan GK, Jablonski SA, Sudakin V, et al. Human BUBR1 is a mitotic checkpoint kinase that monitors CENP-E functions at kinetochores and binds the cyclosome/APC. The Journal of Cell Biology. 1999;146:941–54.

24. Lopes C, Sunkel C. The spindle checkpoint: From normal cell division to tumorigenesis. Arch Med Res. 2003;34:155–65.

25. Ohshima K, Haraoka S, Yoshioka S, et al. Mutation analysis of mitotic checkpoint genes (hBUB1 and hBUBR1) and microsatellite instability in adult T-cell leukemia/lymphoma. Cancer Letters. 2000;158:141–50.

26. Shichiri M, Yoshinaga K, Hisatomi H, et al. Genetic and epigenetic inactivation of mitotic checkpoint genes hBUB1 and hBUBR1 and their relationship to survival. Cancer Research. 2002;62:13–7.

27. Shin H-J, Baek K-H, Jeon A-H, et al. Dual roles of human BubR1, a mitotic checkpoint kinase, in the monitoring of chromosomal instability. Cancer Cell. 2003;4:483–97.

28. Mao Y, Abrieu A, Cleveland D. Activating and silencing the mitotic checkpoint through CENP-E-dependent activation/inactivation of BubR1. Cell. 2003;114:87–98.

29. Fridley B, Abo R, Tan X-L, et al. Integrative gene set analysis: Application to platinum pharmacogenomics. OMICS A Journal of Integrative Biology. 2014;18:34–41.

30. Putkey F, Cramer T, Morphew M, et al. Unstable kinetochore-microtubule capture and chromosomal instability following deletion of CENP-E. Dev Cell. 2002;3:351–65.

31. Liu Z, Ling K, Wu X, et al. Reduced expression of cenp-e in human hepatocellular carcinoma. J Exp Clin Cancer Res. 2009;28:156–63.

5

Consanguineous familial study revealed biallelic *FIGLA* mutation associated with premature ovarian insufficiency

Beili Chen[1†], Lin Li[2†], Jing Wang[3], Tengyan Li[4], Hong Pan[4], Beihong Liu[4], Yiran Zhou[1], Yunxia Cao[1,5,6*] and Binbin Wang[1,4,7*]

Abstract

Background: To dissect the genetic alteration in two sisters with premature ovarian insufficiency (POI) from a consanguineous family.

Methods: Whole-exome sequencing technology was used in the POI proband, bioinformatics analysis was carried out to identify the potential genetic cause in this pedigree. Sanger sequencing analyses were performed to validate the segregation of the variant within the pedigree. In silico analysis was also used to predict the effect and pathogenicity of the variant.

Results: Whole-exome sequencing analysis identified novel and rare homozygous mutation associated with POI, namely mutation in *FIGLA* (c.2 T > C, start codon shift). This homozygous mutation was also harbored by the proband's sister with POI and was segregated within the consanguineous pedigree. The mutation in the start codon of the *FIGLA* gene alters the open reading frame, leading to a *FIGLA* knock-out like phenotype.

Conclusions: Biallelic mutations in *FIGLA* may be the cause of POI. This study will aid researchers and clinicians in genetic counseling of POI and provides new insights into understanding the mode of genetic inheritance of *FIGLA* mutations in POI pathology.

Keywords: Premature ovarian insufficiency, FIGLA, Whole-exome sequencing

Background

Premature ovarian insufficiency (POI) is a severe disorder of ovarian dysfunction and is characterized as decreased ovarian reserve and increased follicle-stimulating hormone (FSH) level. The aetiology is complex, among which the genetic alteration is one of the causes of POI and includes X chromosomal abnormalities, balanced translocations, and fragile X mental retardation 1 (*FMR1*) premutations and single gene defects [1]. Although several single gene variants have been associated with POI in recent decades [1], only a few have been proven to cause POI, e.g., *FSHR, BMP15, NOBOX, MCM8, MCM9, STAG3, HFM1, MSH4*, and *MSH5* [2]. Recently, we and another groups suggested that some genes and mutations cause POI in an autosomal recessive mode of inheritance rather than previous suggested heterozygous manner [3–6]. Together, these findings have expanded our knowledge on POI and helped distinguish causative mutations and risk alleles for POI.

In recent years, whole-exome sequencing (WES) technology has become a powerful tool for elucidating the genetic causes of familial POI, especially in consanguineous pedigrees [2]. In this study, we used WES to identify a novel mutation for POI in a consanguineous family. Our study is the first to report that mutations in *FIGLA* cause POI in a recessive manner. Our findings will aid researchers and clinicians to understand genetic causes for POI and help patients by genetic counseling.

* Correspondence: caoyunxia_profr@126.com; wbbahu@163.com
†Beili Chen and Lin Li contributed equally to this work.
[1]Department of Obstetrics and Gynecology, Reproductive Medicine Center, The First Affiliated Hospital of Anhui Medical University, Meishan Road, Shushan, Hefei 230022, China
Full list of author information is available at the end of the article

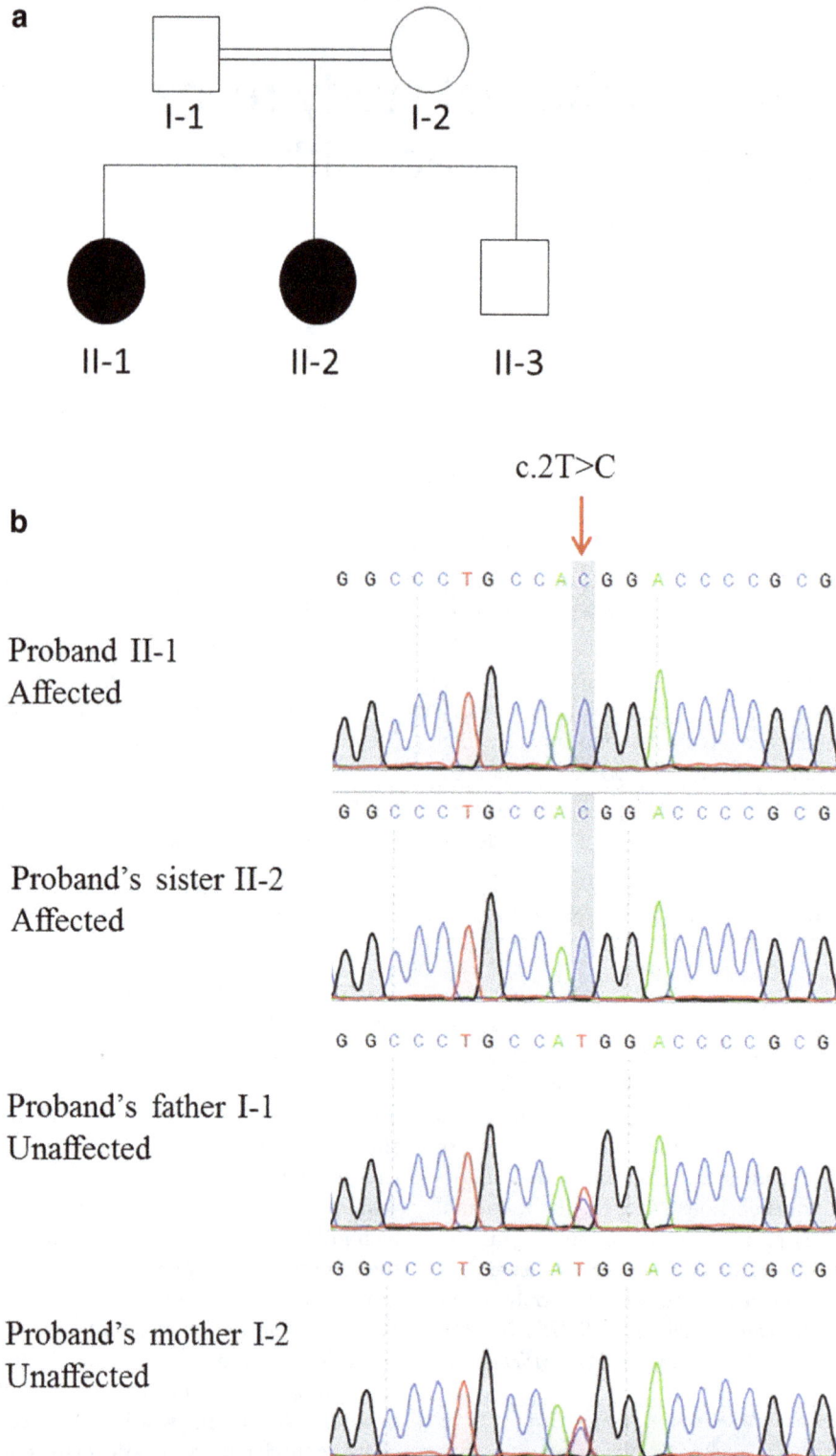

Fig. 1 Pedigree and genetic analysis of the patients in family 1. (**a**) Two POI patients in a Chinese consanguineous pedigree. The black circle indicates the affected family members. (**b**) Sanger sequencing validation of the mutation in family members. Red arrow indicates the mutation site

Table 1 In silico analysis of the *FIGLA* mutation

Gene	Mutation	Amino acid change	Consanguinity	Zygosity	Mutation Taster[a]	SNPs&GO[b]	FATHMM-MKL[c]	ExAC (total)[d]	ExAC (East Asian)[e]	gnomAD (total)[f]
FIGLA	c.2 T > C	Start ATG shift	Yes	Homozygous	Disease causing (1)	Neutral (0.157)	Damaging (0.8119)	0	0	0

[a]Mutation Taster (http://www.mutationtaster.org/). The probability value is the probability of the prediction, i.e., a value close to 1 indicates a high 'security' of the prediction

[b]SNPs&GO (http://snps.biofold.org/snps-and-go/). Disease probability (if > 0.5 mutation is predicted Disease)

[c]FATHMM-MKL (http://fathmm.biocompute.org.uk/fathmmMKL.htm). Values above 0.5 are predicted to be deleterious, while those below 0.5 are predicted to be neutral or benign

[d]Frequency of variations in total of ExAC database.

[e]Frequency of variations in East Asian population of ExAC database

[f]Frequency of variation in total of gnomAD (genome Aggregation Database, a big database containing 123,136 exome sequences and 15,496 whole-genome sequences)

Methods

Patients

Two sisters with POI were recruited from The First Affiliated Hospital of Anhui Medical University. Their parents were consanguineous marriage. POI was diagnosed if the patients had amenorrhea for at least 4 months under the age of 40 and two consecutive follicle stimulating hormone (FSH) measurements > 25 IU/L taken 4 weeks apart [7]. None of the patients showed any of the following: karyotypic abnormality, auto-immune disorder, history of radiotherapy and chemotherapy, or pelvic surgery. Before the patients came to our hospital, they had been on hormone replacement therapy. This study was approved by the Ethics Committee of Anhui Medical University. Written informed consent was obtained from all participants, and peripheral blood (5 mL) was subsequently collected from each participant.

WES and sanger sequencing validation

WES was performed as previously described [8]. WES was carried out on the proband. The sequencing raw reads were 32,530,181, and the raw depth (×) was 161. 44. Sanger sequencing was performed using gene-specific primers. Firstly, the PCR product containing the *FIGLA*'s mutation site was amplified using the specific primers as follow, 5'-GCGAGAAAGAGGGCAACG-3' for forward primer, and 5'-TGGTGGTAGAGCAGG GAAGG-3' for reverse primer.

Bioinformatic analysis of the sequence variant

Three online prediction tools were used in this study to predict the pathogenicity of the variant. For Mutation Taster (http://www.mutationtaster.org/), the probability value is the probability of the prediction, i.e., a value close to 1 indicates a high 'security' of the prediction. For SNPs&GO (http://snps.biofold.org/snps-and-go/), if the value was more than 0.5, the mutation is predicted as Disease. For FATHMM-MKL (http://fathmm.biocompute.org. uk/fathmmMKL.htm), values above 0.5 are predicted to be damaging, while those below 0.5 are predicted to be neutral or benign. The allele frequency was evaluated by searching

the human exome-seq or whole genome-seq databases such as Exome Aggregation Consortium (ExAC, http://exac.broadinstitute.org/) and genome Aggregation Database (gnomAD, http://gnomad.broadinstitute.org/). ExAC contained 60,706 unrelated individuals' exome sequencing data, and gnomAD is a big database containing 123,136 exome sequences and 15,496 whole-genome sequences.

Results

Clinical features of the family

Both the proband (II-1, Fig. 1a) and her younger (II-2) were diagnosed as POI with primary amenorrhea. The proband's father and mother were in a consanguineous marriage. The proband's paternal grandfather and maternal grandmother were siblings. The proband was 31 years old when diagnosed with POI in 2011. Her height was 172 cm and weight was 75 kg. Hormone levels of the proband were as follows: FSH, 36.81 IU/L; luteinizing hormone (LH), 10.2 IU/L; testosterone (T), 1.47 nmol/L; estradiol (E2), 122 pmol/L; prolactin (PRL), 8.8 ng/mL; and anti-Müllerian hormone (AMH), 0.05 ng/mL. The proband's ovaries were not detected by transvaginal color Doppler ultrasound examination. The hormone levels of the proband's sister were as follows: FSH, 54. 49 IU/L; LH, 16.29 IU/L; T, 0.43 nmol/L; E2, 14 pmol/L; and PRL, 10.46 ng/mL. The proband's mother (I-2) underwent menopause at the age of 53. The proband's brother (II-3) was fertile and had twin daughters.

Whole-exome sequencing analysis

To identify the genetic cause for POI in these two sisters, we first set an analysis pipeline. Each patient underwent WES, with sequence reads aligned and variants called, as previously described [8]. Pedigree analysis suggested a recessive mode of inheritance. Likely causative mutations were identified after filtering polymorphisms with allele frequencies > 1% in Exome Aggregation Consortium (ExAC), Genome Aggregation Database (gnomAD), 1000 Genomes and dbSNP databases. A list of genes harboring homozygous variants was further filtered by the functional impact of the mutation, e.g., conservation and functional prediction. Gene relevance for

a

original gDNA sequence snippet	CTGCCATGGACCCCGCGCCCGGCGTCC
altered gDNA sequence snippet	CTGCCACGGACCCCGCGCCCGGCGTCC
original cDNA sequence snippet	CTGCCATGGACCCCGCGCCCGGCGTCC
altered cDNA sequence snippet	CTGCCACGGACCCCGCGCCCGGCGTCC
wildtype AA sequence	MDPAPGVLDP RAAPPALLGT PQAEVLEDVL REQFGPLPQL AAVCRLKRLP SGGYSSTENL QLVLERRRVA NAKERERIKN LNRGFARLKA LVPFLPQSRK PSKVDILKGA TEYIQVLSDL LEGAKDSKKQ DPDEQSYSNN SSESHTSSAR QLSRNITQHI SCAFGLKNEE EGPWADGGSG EPAHACRHSV MSTTEIISPT RSLDRFPEVE LLSHRLPQV*
mutated AA sequence	MSRAIVTTVL NHIHPRQDSC QETSPNISAV LSA*

b

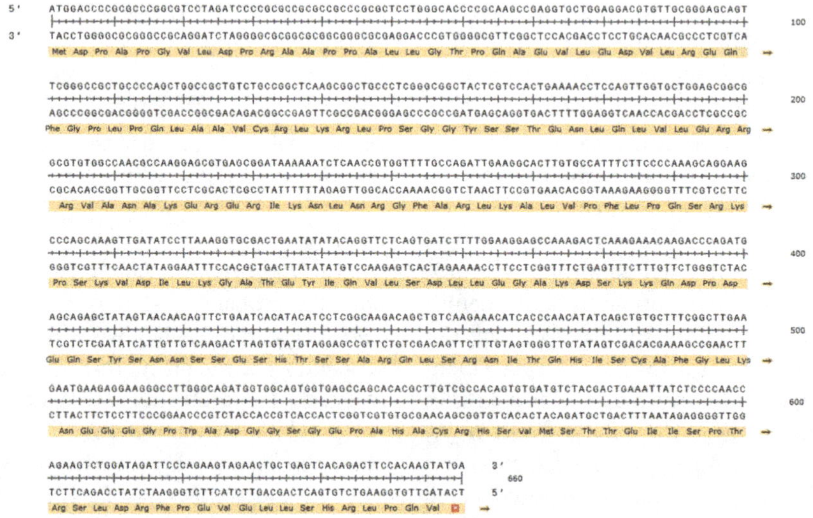

c

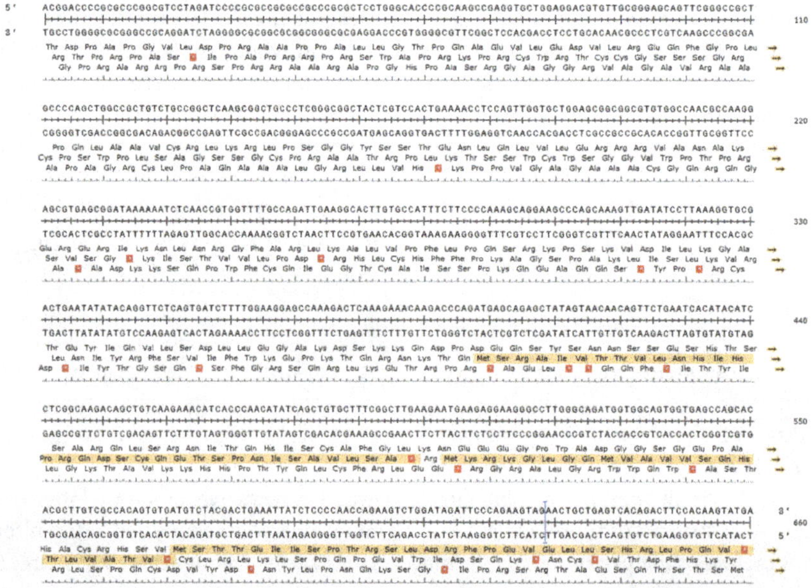

Fig. 2 (See legend on next page.)

(See figure on previous page.)

Fig. 2 (**a**) In silico analysis of the alternative start site and potential resulting protein. The MutationTaster online prediction tool (http://www.mutationtaster.org/) was used in the current analysis. The predicted results for c.2 T > C showed that the start ATG shifted, the Kozak consensus sequence changed, and the entire protein amino acid sequence frameshifted and was changed. The green box indicates the wild-type amino acid sequence, while the red box indicates the mutated amino acid sequence. (**b**) and (**c**) The wild-type (**b**) and mutated (**c**) sequences of FIGLA. The light grown indicate the putative translated protein sequences

ovarian function was also assessed using gene expression data (Human Protein Atlas, http://www.proteinatlas.org/) and mouse model phenotype data (Mouse Genome Informatics, http://www.informatics.jax.org/).

According to pipeline and several filtering steps after WES, only the *FIGLA* (folliculogenesis specific bHLH transcription factor) gene and its homozygous mutation, NM_001004311:exon1:c.2 T > C, was identified in the proband. This homozygous mutation was also harbored by the proband's sister and was segregated within the pedigree (Fig. 1b). *FIGLA* has been shown to be specifically expressed in human ovary [9, 10] and was reported to be associated with POI by haploinsufficiency effect [11]. However, our finding did not support the haploinsufficiency effect of *FIGLA* causing POI.

Bioinformatics analysis of the mutation

In silico analysis by four online prediction tools suggested that the c.2 T > C mutation was a pathogenic mutation (Table 1). The c.2 T > C mutation lost the start codon and therefore the open reading frame of *FIGLA* was altered (Fig. 2a, b and c). The c.2 T > C mutation was absent in the ExAC, gnomAD, 1000G and dbSNP databases, indicating the extremely rarity of this mutation.

Discussion

Here we report that a novel homozygous mutation in *FIGLA* is associated with POI in one consanguineous pedigree.

FIGLA encodes a basic helix-loop-helix transcription factor that regulates primordial follicle formation [12, 13]. FIGLA is specifically expressed in human and mouse ovaries [9, 10, 14]. *Figla* knockout mice cannot form primordial follicles, leading to oocyte loss and female sterility [13]. FIGLA transcriptionally activates oocyte-related genes, such as *ZP1*, *ZP2* and *ZP3* [10, 13], and represses sperm-associated genes during postnatal oogenesis [15].

A previous study found that *FIGLA* haploinsufficiency may be associated with premature ovarian failure [11]. The study found a heterozygous p.G6 fs*66 mutation in a patient with secondary amenorrhea at 36 years of age, and a heterozygous p.140delN mutation in a patient with secondary amenorrhea at 27 years of age [11]. The p.G6 fs*66 mutation creates *FIGLA* haploinsufficiency, because the truncated protein only shares five amino acids with the wild-type protein [11]. The p.140delN mutation disrupts FIGLA binding to TCF3 [11], however no

dominant negative effect of p.140delN was observed in that study. So that study did not prove the cause and effect of the variants. While our findings indicate a novel underlying mechanism based on two facts: one is that, the patient's mother, who is heterozygous for the mutation, was neither a POI patient nor had the phenotype of premature menopause; another is that, the c.2 T > C mutation abolishes the start codon, leading to an alternative open reading frame. The two facts above indicated that loss of function in one *FIGLA* allele can not cause POI. Therefore, our consanguineous pedigree analysis suggests that recessive inheritance of the *FIGLA* mutation is implicated in POI pathogenesis. However, our study did not oppose the previous finding, as the patient with homozygous mutation in our study was primary amenorrhea while the patient with heterozygous mutation in the previous study was secondary amenorrhea. Based on the current results and those of previous studies, we hypothesized that *FIGLA* haploinsufficiency may cause a milder POI than the *FIGLA* homozygous allele mutations.

Conclusions

Taken together, our study demonstrates biallelic *FIGLA* mutation causing POI with primary amenorrhea. This study will aid researchers and clinicians in genetic counseling of POI and provides new insight into understanding the mode of genetic inheritance of certain genes and POI.

Acknowledgments

We thank Rachel James, Ph.D., from Edanz Group (www.edanzediting.com/ac) for editing a draft of this manuscript.

Funding

Research funding was provided by the National Natural Science Foundation of China (81701405) and the National Research Institute for Family Planning (2017GJZ05).

Authors' contributions

Beili Chen carried out the clinical sample collection and clinical diagnosis. Lin Li provided the manuscript preforming and carried out experiments preforming. Jing Wang and Hong Pan carried out the manuscript revision and the data analysis. Tengyan Li, Beihong Liu and Yiran Zhou participated in the experiments preforming. Yunxia Cao and Binbin Wang conceived the study. All authors read and approved the final manuscript.

Author details

[1]Department of Obstetrics and Gynecology, Reproductive Medicine Center, The First Affiliated Hospital of Anhui Medical University, Meishan Road, Shushan, Hefei 230022, China. [2]Central Laboratory, Beijing Obstetrics and Gynecology Hospital, Capital Medical University, Chaoyang, Beijing 100026, China. [3]Department of Medical Genetics and Developmental Biology, School of Basic Medical Sciences, Capital Medical University, No. 10 Xitoutiao, Youanmenwai, Fengtai, Beijing 100069, China. [4]Center for Genetics, National Research Institute for Family Planning, 12 Dahuisi Road, Haidian, Beijing 100081, China. [5]Institute of Reproductive Genetics, Anhui Medical University, Meishan Road, Shushan, Hefei 230032, China. [6]Anhui Provincial Engineering Technology Research Center for Biopreservation and Artificial Organs, Meishan Road, Shushan, Hefei 230027, China. [7]Key Laboratory of Family planning and Reproductive Genetics, National Health and Family Planning Commission, Heb Research institute For Family Planning, Beijing 050071, People's Republic of China.

References

1. Qin Y, Jiao X, Simpson JL, Chen ZJ. Genetics of primary ovarian insufficiency: new developments and opportunities. Hum Reprod Update. 2015; 21:787–808.
2. Laissue P. The molecular complexity of primary ovarian insufficiency aetiology and the use of massively parallel sequencing. Mol Cell Endocrinol. 2017;
3. Li L, Wang BB, Zhang W, Chen BL, Luo MN, Wang J, Wang X, Cao YX, Kee K. A homozygous NOBOX truncating variant causes defective transcriptional activation and leads to primary ovarian insufficiency. Hum Reprod. 2017;32:248–55.
4. Mayer A, Fouquet B, Pugeat M, Misrahi M. BMP15 "knockout-like" effect in familial premature ovarian insufficiency with persistent ovarian reserve. Clin Genet. 2017;92:208–12.
5. Franca MM, Funari MFA, Nishi MY, Narcizo AM, Domenice S, Costa EMF, Lerario AM, Mendonca BB. Identification of the first homozygous 1-bp deletion in GDF9 gene leading to primary ovarian insufficiency by using targeted massively parallel sequencing. Clin Genet. 2017;
6. Franca MM, Funari MFA, Lerario AM, Nishi MY, Pita CC, Fontenele EGP, Mendonca BB. A novel homozygous 1-bp deletion in the NOBOX gene in two Brazilian sisters with primary ovarian failure. Endocrine. 2017;58:442–7.
7. Webber L, Davies M, Anderson R, Bartlett J, Braat D, Cartwright B, Cifkova R, de Muinck K-SS, Hogervorst E, Janse F, et al. ESHRE guideline: management of women with premature ovarian insufficiency. Hum Reprod. 2016;31:926–37.
8. Wang B, Li L, Zhu Y, Zhang W, Wang X, Chen B, Li T, Pan H, Wang J, Kee K, Cao Y. Sequence variants of KHDRBS1 as high penetrance susceptibility risks for primary ovarian insufficiency by mis-regulating mRNA alternative splicing. Hum Reprod. 2017;32:2138–46.
9. Huntriss J, Gosden R, Hinkins M, Oliver B, Miller D, Rutherford AJ, Picton HM. Isolation, characterization and expression of the human factor in the germline alpha (FIGLA) gene in ovarian follicles and oocytes. Mol Hum Reprod. 2002;8:1087–95.
10. Bayne RA, Martins Da Silva SJ, Anderson RA. Increased expression of the FIGLA transcription factor is associated with primordial follicle formation in the human fetal ovary. Mol Hum Reprod. 2004;10:373–81.
11. Zhao H, Chen ZJ, Qin YY, Shi YH, Wang S, Choi Y, Simpson JL, Rajkovic A. Transcription factor FIGLA is mutated in patients with premature ovarian failure. Am J Hum Genet. 2008;82:1342–8.
12. Pangas SA, Rajkovic A. Transcriptional regulation of early oogenesis: in search of masters. Hum Reprod Update. 2006;12:65–76.
13. Soyal SM, Amleh A, Dean J. FIGalpha, a germ cell-specific transcription factor required for ovarian follicle formation. Development. 2000;127:4645–54.
14. Liang L, Soyal SM, Dean J. FIGalpha, a germ cell specific transcription factor involved in the coordinate expression of the zona pellucida genes. Development. 1997;124:4939–47.
15. Hu W, Gauthier L, Baibakov B, Jimenez-Movilla M, Dean J. FIGLA, a basic helix-loop-helix transcription factor, balances sexually dimorphic gene expression in postnatal oocytes. Mol Cell Biol. 2010;30:3661–71.

6

The molecular mechanism of ovarian granulosa cell tumors

Jiaheng Li[1], Riqiang Bao[1], Shiwei Peng[2] and Chunping Zhang[3*]

Abstract

Over these years, more and more sex cord-stromal tumors have been reported. Granulosa cell tumor (GCT) is a rare tumor in ovaries, accounts for 2% to 5% of ovarian cancers. The main different feature of GCTs from other ovarian cancers is that GCTs can lead to abnormally secreted hormones (estrogen, inhibin and Müllerian inhibiting substance). The GCT is divided into two categories according to the age of patients, namely AGCT (adult granulosa cell tumor) and JGCT (Juvenile granulosa cell tumor). AGCT patients accounts for 95%. Although the pathogenesis is not clear, FOXL2 (Forkhead box L2) mutation was considered as the most critical factor in AGCT development. The current treatment is dominated by surgery. Target therapy remains in the adjuvant therapy stage, such as hormone therapy. During these years, other pathogenic factors were also explored, such as PI3K/AKT (phosphatidylinositol-3-kinase; serine/threonine kinase), TGF-β (Transforming growth factor beta) signaling pathway, Notch signaling pathway, GATA4 and VEGF (vascular endothelial growth factor). These factors and signaling pathway play important roles in GCT cell proliferation, apoptosis, or angiogenesis. The purpose of this review is to summarize the possible pathogenic factors and signaling pathways, which may shed lights on developing potential therapeutic targets for GCT.

Keywords: GCT, FOXL2, PI3K/AKT signaling, TGF-β signaling, Notch signaling

Background

Granulosa cell tumor (GCT) is the most common sex cord-stromal tumor that stem from granulosa cells. GCT accounts for 2% to 5% of all ovarian cancers and can be divided into two subtypes according to the differences of the age of patients, clinical and histopathologic features [1]. About 95% of GCT belong to the adult granulosa cell tumors (AGCTs), and others are juvenile granulosa cell tumors (JGCTs). JGCT only occurs in people who are younger than 30 years old with the features of hypoestrogenism and abnormal abdominal mass [2, 3]. Clinical features of AGCT include abnormal uterine bleeding in postmenopausal patients and menometrorrhagia in youngers. Some reports also indicated that patients were with stopping ovulating symptom [4]. The incidence of GCT is around 0.47 to 1.6 per 100,000. The main risk factors of GCT include nulliparity, fatness, oral contraceptives and family cancer history. From the cancer databases in Finland, Iceland, Norway and Sweden, the GCT onset showed scattered feature. There was no increasing trend over the 60 years [5]. Abnormal cell cycle is related to the occurrence and development of cancers. The recent studies provided powerful evidences that fork head box protein L2 (FOXL2), PI3K/AKT signaling pathway, TGF-β signaling pathway, Notch signaling pathway and etc. were involved in granulosa cell tumor through influencing cell proliferation and apoptosis [6–10].

In the development of GCT, a variety of cell signaling pathways, such as TGF-β, Notch and PI3K/AKT, are involved. In fact, these signal pathways are not isolated, but make up a complex network and contribute to the formation and development of GCT. FOXL2 is the most important mutant gene in GCT formation. Studies showed that FOXL2 is involved in the TGF-β pathway. For example, FOXL2 mutation has negative effect on SMAD3 (drosophila mothers against decapentaplegic protein) activation by interacting with BMPs, follistatin and activin A [11]. FOXO1/3 (forkhead box O1/3) also inhibited SMAD3 [12]. The interaction between Notch signaling and PI3K/AKT were also proved [13]. In the following sections, we will summarize the influence of different cell signaling network on GCT.

* Correspondence: zhangcp81@163.com
[3]Department of Cell Biology, School of Medicine, Nanchang University, Nanchang, Jiangxi 330006, People's Republic of China
Full list of author information is available at the end of the article

FOXL2

Forkhead transcription factor 2 (FOXL2) is a transcription factor. The gene is 2.7 kb long and encodes 376 amino acids, which locates at human chromosome 3q23. The sequence of FOXL2 is highly conserved. It is mainly expressed in ovarian granulosa cell and pituitarium. FOXL2 is the first confirmed autosomal gene that maintains normal function of ovary, and it is also a marker of sexual selection and development. FOXL2 knockout mouse model showed sex reversal [14]. Further studies showed that FOXL2 regulated the ovarian granulosa cell proliferation, follicle development and ovarian hormones synthesis [14].

In 2009, a breakthrough of AGCT, using the whole-transcriptome paired-end RNA sequencing, showed that a somatic missense mutation (402C»G) occurred in four different AGCT samples at C134W (amino acid position 134) [15]. From the published results, the mutation exists in more than 97% of AGCT, and it is rarely detected in other ovarian cancer [16]. Some reports showed that the expression of FOXL2 was also downregulated in aggressive JGCT [17, 18]. These studies make FOXL2 as one possible pathognomonic defining feature. The mechanism of mutant FOXL2 in GCT was also widely explored. Some studies showed that prominent serine 33 (S33) phosphorylation of FOXL2, which is induced by GSK3β, was detected in C134W mutation. The phosphorylation modification of FOXL2 contributes to the growths of GCTs [19, 20]. The growth of GCT was proportional to the S33 phosphorylation status, and GSK3β inhibitor might serve as an effective intervention for GCT therapy [19].

Some studies examined the transcriptional targets of mutant FOXL2. Wile-type FOXL2 plays a key role in inhibiting granulosa cell proliferation and promoting apoptosis [21]. However, mutant FOXL2 downregulated the INHA, one of a proliferative signaling ligand [22]. Death signaling mediators, TNF-R1 (Tumor necrosis factor receptor 1) and FAS, were also decreased [23]. Caspase 8, BID and BAK determine the FOXL2 depended granulosa cell apoptotic pathway, but mutant FOXL2 was unable to elicit the apoptotic signaling responses [24]. In addition, mutant FOXL2 has been shown to reduce GnRH receptor expression, thus conferring resistance to GnRH-induced cell apoptosis [25]. Follistatin is mainly expressed in granulosa cells of developing follicles and it binds to activin A to block activin A-stimulated granulosa cells proliferation [26]. Mutant FOXL2 suppresses follistatin expression and leads to increased cells proliferation and tumor formation [6, 11]. Furthermore, FOXL2 mutation also leads to TGF-β signaling pathway deregulation [23].

More and more clinical data show that FOXL2 mutation is the main factor in AGCT So, understanding the FOXL2 regulation mechanism is instrumental to develop new prevention and therapy methods.

Notch signaling pathway

Notch signaling is highly conserved in evolution, which plays critical role in organisms' development. In mammalian, there are four Notch receptors, Notch1 to 4, There are three domains in Notch receptors, including functional extracellular (NECD), transmembrane (TM) and intracellular (NICD). Five Notch ligands, Jagged-1, Jagged-2, Delta-like-1 (DLL1), Delta-like-3 (DLL3) and Delta-like-4 (DLL4) had been identified [27, 28]. Both the Notch ligands and the receptors are transmembrane proteins. When ligands bind receptors, Notch receptors become susceptible to proteolytic cleavage mediated by secretase complex, which releases the intracellular domain of Notch. NICD enters nucleus and forms a complex with recombination signal binding protein-Jk, which contains a DNA binding domain. The complex regulates Myc, P21, HES family, Cyclin D3 and other Notch target genes. The deregulation of Notch signaling has been proved to be related to several cancers [27]. Studies showed that DLL4, Jagged-1, Notch1 and Notch4 were highly expressed in KGN cells (FOXL2-mutated granulosa tumor cell line), compared with granulosa-lutein cells. DAPT, an inhibitor of γ-secretase, was used to treat KGN cells and the inhibition of Notch system lead to lower proliferation and viability, as well as estradiol and progesterone secretion of KGN cells [13, 29]. Several apoptotic parameters such as BAX, BCLXs, PARP and caspase eight cleavages were increased after DAPT treatment. The interaction of Notch signaling and PI3K/AKT signaling were also been proved in the process. AKT phosphorylation was decreased and PTEN (phosphatase and tensin homolog deleted on chromosome ten) protein was increased after Notch signaling inhibition [13]. More studies are needed to demonstrate that Notch signaling would be potential therapeutic targets for AGCT.

TGF-β signaling pathway

TGF-β super family is composed of 30 different growth and differential factors, including TGF-βs, activin, inhibin and BMPs (bone morphogenic proteins) [30]. TGF-β related signaling pathway plays critical roles in regulating stem cell cycle, organ development and immune cells through regulating cell proliferation, differentiation, and death [31]. SMAD proteins are general signaling pathway mediated proteins in TGFβ signaling network [32]. When the signaling pathway is abnormally activated, it may lead to diseases.

Activin and inhibin

Inhibin and activin are two hydrophilic non-steroid substances and are mainly synthesized by pituitary cells and ovarian granulosa cells. They have two α and β subunits. α and β subunits are encoded by different genes respectively.

The β subunit consists of five different types of homologous compositions, βA, βB, βC, βD and βE. βA and βB units can form three kinds of activins linked by a disulfide bond, including activin A (βA-βA), B (βB-βB) and C(βA-βB) [33]. Inhibins were composed of Inhibin βA, βB units shared with activins, and a unique α-subunit (INHA), inhibin A (α-βA) and inhibin B (α-βB) [34]. Activins function via combining with activin-type 1 receptors and activin-type 2 receptors. The complex can activate SMAD2/3 through phosphorylation [35]. While inhibins carry out their biological role by antagonizing activin pathway [36].

Inhibin was first defined in 1932 [37]. As one gonadal hormone, Inhibin played important role in regulating folliculogenesis, steroidogenesis and FSH production [34]. Inhibin was also defined as a critical negative regulator of gonadal stromal cell proliferation and was identified to have tumour-suppressor activity [38]. Inhibin-α can inhibit granulosa cell proliferation and promotes apoptosis [39]. High expression of inhibin-α subunit exists in most human gonadal cancers. Loss of inhibin-α can lead to more aggressive GCT by using INHA knockout mice [38, 40–42]. As to the two subtypes of inhibin, studies showed that almost all the GCT patients had higher level of inhibin B, and over synthesized inhibin A was also detected in some cases [43]. Lower inhibin sensitive is also related to GCT development and tumor metastasis. Betaglycan or p120 was identified as inhibin receptors, which is associated with the type II or type I activin receptor subunits (ActR), respectively [44]. Studies showed that only p120 was especially high in GCT patients [44]. Not only in GCT, but also other types of ovarian tumor, abnormal elevated inhibin had been proved [43].

Activins have critical functions in genital system. Activin synthesized by pituitary gonadotrophic cells decreases the activation of luteotropic and promotes the expression of follicle stimulating hormone receptors, so it enhances the follicle development [45]. Activin binds to type II receptors, and then recruits and phosphorylates of type I receptor ALK4, which phosphorylates both SMAD2 and SMAD3 proteins. GCT cells show high inhibinβA subunit expression level and the proliferation rate was positively correlated with a high activin A to inhibin A ratio, suggesting that the tumor cells stimulated their growth through an activin A autocrine signaling pathway [46]. In GCT patients, abnormal activin receptors may lead to failure of granulosa cell apoptosis [26]. There are controversies about GCT markers. Early studies suggested that inhibin B and activin A were elevated in GCT patients. But recently it has also been suggested that inhibin B is more specific than activin A [47, 48]. In fact, activin still does not have the significance of large-scale application in the diagnosis and prognosis of GCT. The healthy activin levels are also increased significantly in postmenopausal women and ovarian cancer patients. The relationship between GCT and elevated inhibin is still unclear. The clinical application of inhibin as a tumor marker remains controversial. However, the clinical data and available studies suggest that the inhibin test may be used as part of a GCT screening and be used for disease prognosis [49, 50].

BMPs

Bone morphogenetic proteins (BMPs) are a group of at least 20 growth factors. They were firstly found in ostosis as induction proteins [51]. BMPs are multi-functional growth factors and have been implicated in a variety of functions. BMPs induce the formation of both cartilage and bone. BMPs also play a role in a number of non-osteogenic developmental processes, such as epidermal induction, inhibition of limb bud and myogenesis [52, 53]. BMPs can inhibit the growth of normal cells and human colon, prostate and breast cancer cell lines when the BMP signal components are complete. In addition, the BMP pathway was inactivated in 70% of colorectal cancers. The lack of two BMP type I receptors, Bmpr1a and Bmpr1b in the ovarian granulosa cells of mice were involved in the development of GCT [54]. The expression of Myc, cyclin D2 and cyclinE2 was highly increased in BMPR1a and BMPR1b double knockout mice, which result in the promotion of granulosa cell tumor proliferation [55]. BR-SMADs represented SMAD1/5/9 signal via interacting with BMP receptors. The study showed GCT development in BR-SMADs conditional knock out mice [56]. The studies in KGN cell line confirmed that FSH increased the expression of BMP type 1 receptors (BMPR1A/B) and BMP type 2 receptors (BMPR2). BMP6/7 induced phosphorylation of SMAD1/5/8. What' more, FSH also promoted SMAD1/5 expression, while it reduced the inhibitory SMAD, SMAD6/7 expression [57].

As the upstream ligand for BMPR, BMP-2 is proved to be greatly associated with follicle formation. BMP7 was highly expressed in granulosa cell. Studies proved that BMP7 induced a rise rate in DNA synthesis and proliferation in granulosa cells [58, 59]. Studies showed that BMP15 was involved in polycystic ovary syndrome (PCOS). BMP15/SMAD1 may regulate granulosa cell apoptosis, which expression were significantly decreased in PCOS [60]. However, the relationship between BMPs and GCT is still unclear.

AMH

AMH is a regulator in sexual differentiation and it was also considered as an inhibitor in ovary cancer development. Normal granulosa cells and GCT both synthesize AMH. In human GCT, there was a controversy of high serum but low tissue AMH level. But it had been confirmed that serum AMH levels were positively correlate with the GCT size [61–63]. It can be speculated that AMH in the tumor microenvironment was lower than normal level [61]. AMH participates in the BMP signaling pathway to inhibit GCT formation, and lower expression of AMH reduced the activation of BMP signaling components. In addition, Extrinsic AMH reduced the number of KGN cells and primary GCT cells. It was proved that overexpression of AMH induced an increased activation of caspase-3 and subsequent apoptosis [64].

SMAD

SMADs are intracellular proteins, which occupy critical position in transducing TGF-β signaling from the receptors on cell surface to nucleus. According to the structures, SMADs divided in to three sub-families, R-SMAD (receptor-regulated type), Co-SMAD (common-mediator type) and I-SMAD (inhibitory type) [65]. In follicle development, many studies have showed these factors have co-operative functions.

SMAD 4 is the common mediator, is also a well-known tumor suppressor in human [66]. However, no ovarian tumors develop in SMAD4$^{loxp/loxp}$ AMHR2 Cre mice. The deletion of SMAD4 significantly disturbed the reproduction ability of mice. The lack of SMAD4 also promoted luteinization [67]. SMAD4 is necessary for FSH synthesis. Studies also indicated that SMAD4 played its role with FOXL2. When SMAD4 and FOXL2 were double deleted, FSH synthesis was almost stopped and females were sterile. The phenotype is similar to Fshb-knockout mice [68]. In ovulation period, SMAD4 was necessary in ERK1/2 activation [69]. During ovary development, the expression of SMAD4 was increased with the growth. SMAD4 silencing can increase the expression of CDK1 and CCNB2, suggesting that SMAD4 can also regulate cell cycle [70, 71].

Conditional deletion of SMAD1 and SMAD5 in ovarian granulose cells causes metastatic granulose cell tumors (GCTs) in female mice and phenocopies human juvenile GCTs (JGCTs) [54]. SMAD1/4/5 triple knockout mice showed increased survival rate and smaller tumor size, means that SMAD4 regulated signaling pathway may be a cancer promotor.

Both SMAD2 and SMAD3 are considered as important factors in ovarian development and functions. The ability of fecundity was reduced in the SMAD3-type (SMAD3-/-) mice, which also showed poor granulosa proliferation [72]. The TGF β-SMAD2/3 pathway is active in JGCTs. TGF-β may play as a promoting factor in JGCT, because the related signaling pathway can inhibit cell apoptosis [73]. Growing GCT cells expressed high levels of nuclear SMAD3 [46]. In KGN cell line, when NFκB expression is inhibited, the SMAD3 expression is also reduced, while SMAD3 is been proved overexpressed

in AGCT [74]. SMAD3 interacted with FOXL2 and GATA4 modulated cell viability and apoptosis in ovarian granulosa cell tumour cells through regulating the expression of CCND2 [7, 75].

SMADs are critical regulation proteins in TGF-β family and they are significant in TGF-β signaling dynamic accommodation between cell plasma and nucleus. But the complete process is not clear now. The future study need to concentrate on the co-regulation among different SMADs and other regulating factors in GCT.

PI3K/AKT signaling pathway

It has been demonstrated that activation of AKT pathway via PI3K is highly related to tumorigenesis. In ovarian cancers, AKT signaling blocks cell apoptosis through inhibiting FOXO1 and Bcl-2 proteins transcription [76, 77]. Forkhead box O1/O3, are the O class of the forkhead family. FOXO1 locates at chromosome 13, while FOXO3 locates at chromosome 6. In normal condition, FOXOs combine with the promotor of P27KIP1. P27 (Cyclin-dependent kinase inhibitor 1B) is an inhibitor in cell cycle. Once FOXOs were phosphorylated by AKT, the transcription of p27 would be influenced and lead to abnormal cell proliferation. [78]. Evidences showed FOXO1a influenced p27 nuclear localization and inhibited granulosa cell proliferation [79]. TRAIL has the effect of high efficiency and rapid induction of apoptosis of tumor cells and virus infected cells, but not normal cells [80]. FOXOs can also regulate TRAIL [81]. The knockdown of TRAIL obviously reduced the apoptosis induced by FOXO3 [82]. FOXO1/3 double knock out mice have high risk in getting GCT [83].

PTEN is one negative regulator of PI3K signaling and its mutation is very common in human cancers. PTEN is an important tumour suppresser. Studies indicated that lower PTEN expression levels was related to cancer development [84]. The expression of PTEN in ovarian cancer was negatively correlated with clinical stage, diferentiation and VEGF expression. The overall survival of PTEN-positive patients was significantly longer than that of negative expression [85]. The depletion of PTEN and FOXO1/3 has a synergistic effect in GCT development, but the single knockout PTEN mice rarely developed to GCT [83]. In ovaries, PTEN mutation leaded to over-phosphorylation of AKT. In addition, FOXOs can promote PTEN transcription, suggesting that there exists a negative feedback among them [81, 86]. In addition, uncontrolled PI3K activity within oocytes irreversibly transforms granulosa cells into GC tumors through perturbed local cell communication [46]. Lague et al. provided powerful evidence for the role of the dysregulation of the PI3K/AKT pathway in the pathogenesis of GCTs by means of a Pten$^{flox/flox}$, Amhr$^{cre/+}$ mouse model. Activation of WNT/CTNNB1 signaling causes late-onset GCT development. However, activation of both the PI3K/AKT and WNT/CTNNB1 pathways in the granulosa cell. Had 100% penetrance and extremely rapid growth and the ability to spread [87].

Others
GATA4

GATA4 belongs to the GATA family of zinc finger transcription factors. In human, it locates at 8p23.1. The current study indicated that GATA4 played key role in embryogenesis and cardiac development. GATA4 mutations can lead to heart disease due to abnormal fold or other embryogenic failure in heart. Based on statistics of clinical GCT samples, overexpression of GATA-4 is associated with higher recurrence and more aggressive of GCT [63]. Evidences show GATA4 can regulate GCT cell apoptosis and proliferation by activating Bcl-2 and cyclin D2, respectively [88, 89]. Overexpressing GATA4 protects GCTs from TRAIL-induced apoptosis in KGN cells [90]. In other species, like dogs, GATA-4 is also the GCT markers [91]. In

previous sections, we introduced the role of SMAD3 and FOXOL2. Studies showed that FOXL2, GATA4, and SMAD3 expression patterns overlap in the fetal and adult ovary. The three factors co-operatively modulate the cell viability and apoptosis in ovarian granulosa cell tumour cells through regulating the expression of CCND2 [7].

VEGF

Vascular endothelial growth factor played important role in cancer development, as a cell factor that mainly regulates vasculogenesis. VEGF and its receptors were hugely expressed in GCTs [92, 93]. In anti-VEGF therapy, some case reports showed that bevacizumab was benefited to recurrent GCT patients [93]. VEGFR1 normally be considered as a decoy receptor and it showed unobvious phosphorylation when combined with VEGF [94]. VEGFR2, was usually seen as the main mediator of VEGF [95]. The expression levels of VEGFR2 were higher in GCT patients, while VEGF1 expression levels showed no increase trendy [93].

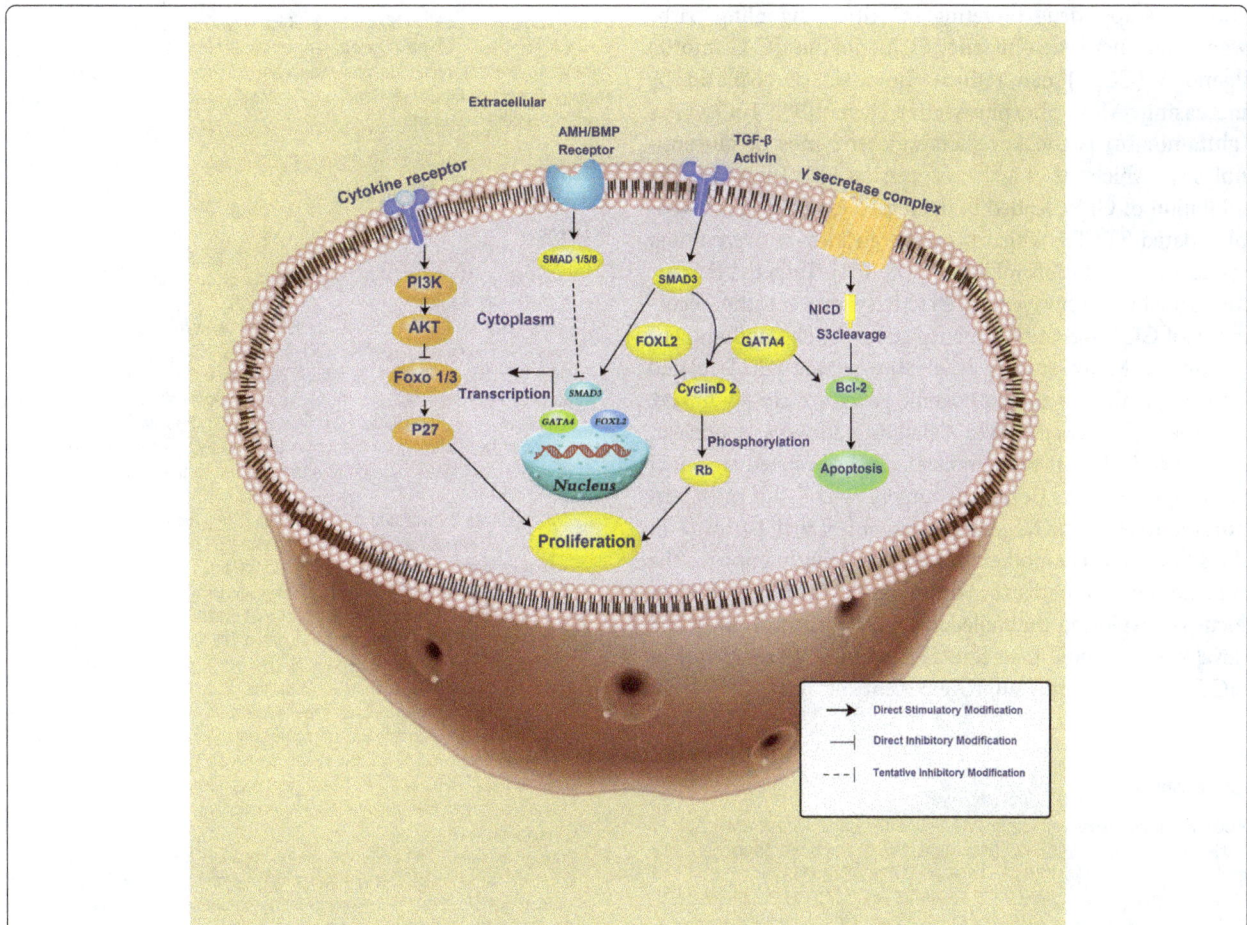

Fig. 1 Schematic representation of the cell signaling pathways in GCT development. PI3K, phosphatidylinositol-3-kinase; AKT, serine/threonine kinase; FOXO 1/3, forkhead box O1/3; AMH, anti-Mullerian hormone; BMP, bone morphogenetic protein; SMAD, drosophila mothers against decapentaplegic protein; FOXL2, forkhead transcription factor 2; Rb, retinoblastoma protein; Bcl-2, B-cell lymphoma 2

Conclusion

GCT incidence of ovarian cancer accounts for about 2% to 5%, while the prognosis is usually better. Five-year survival rate is up to 90%. High recurrent rate is the most critical factor for GCT death. At present, the most important problem lies in the early diagnosis and prevention of recurrence. FOXL2 mutation is the main cause of GCT, while other factors also contributed to it, such as GATA4, SMAD, VEGF, PI3K/AKT, AMH and TGF-β. The \treatment for GCT includes surgery, radiotherapy, chemotherapy and hormone therapy. Studies showed that hormones play a critical role in the pathogenesis and treatment of GCT, especially in some ineffective cases for radiotherapy and chemotherapy. However, the serious adverse effects were followed. New treatment strategies need to be explored. The employment of anti-VEGFA antibody in mouse model successfully slowed the tumor development through inhibiting the tumor cell proliferation [96]. Other studies also demonstrated anti-VEGF (or VEGFR) had conspicuous function in inhibiting GCT development [97, 98]. As for chemotherapy, drug targeting in critical signaling pathways can increase efficiency. Chemokine (C-C motif) ligand 5 (CCL5) can reduce the toxic of cisplatin by increasing AKT phosphorylation level [99, 100]. GLS (glutaminase) is the key metabolic enzymes of glutaminolysis, which is highly expression in tumors. The inhibition of GLS1 leaded to decreased expression of phosphorylated STAT3, which provided an idea in overcoming the resistance of PI3K inhibitor [100, 101]. Targeted therapy for signaling pathways can effectively prevent the recurrence of GCT and reduce the resistance of chemotherapeutic drugs. Many studies have shown that GCT-related signaling pathways and pathogenic genes are closely linked, and the link between these signaling pathways is unclear. As shown in Fig. 1, we summarized these related signaling pathways network. Certainly, surgery is still the most important treatment. Targeting drugs for signal pathway in the subsequent chemotherapy can significantly improve the survival rate of patients. Future research should further focus on exploring the molecular mechanisms of GCT and developing targeted medicines. Prevention of recurrence of GCT will significantly improve patient survival.

Abbreviations

AGCT: Adult granulosa cell tumor; AKT: Serine/threonine kinase; AMH: Anti-Mullerian hormone; Bcl-2: B-cell lymphoma 2; BMP: Bone morphogenetic protein; DLL1: Delta-like-1; DLL3: Delta-like-3; DLL4: Delta-like-4; FOXL2: Forkhead box L2; FOXO 1/3: Forkhead box O1/3; GCT: Granulosa cell tumor; GLS: Glutaminase; INHA: Inhibin α-subunit; JGCT: Juvenile granulosa cell tumor; PI3K: Phosphatidylinositol-3-kinase; PTEN: Phosphatase and tensin homolog deleted on chromosome ten; Rb: Retinoblastoma protein; SMAD: Drosophila mothers against decapentaplegic protein; TGF-β: Transforming growth factor beta; VEGF: Vascular endothelial growth factor

Acknowledgements

Not applicable.

Funding

This study was supported by National Natural Science Foundation of China (81601242) and Natural Science Foundation of Jiangxi province (20161BAB215199).

Authors' contributions

JL executed and drafted the manuscript, RB and SP made critical discussion about the study. CZ designed the study. All authors read and approved the final manuscript.

Competing interests

The authors declare that they have no competing interests.

Author details

[1]Joint programme of Nanchang University and Queen Mary University of London, Nanchang, China. [2]Department of Gynecology and Obstetrics, Jiangxi Provincial People's Hospital, Nanchang, China. [3]Department of Cell Biology, School of Medicine, Nanchang University, Nanchang, Jiangxi 330006, People's Republic of China.

References

1. Schumer ST, Cannistra SA. Granulosa cell tumor of the ovary. J Clin Oncol. 2003;21:1180–9.
2. Rao AC, Kishore M, Monappa V. Juvenile Granulosa cell tumour: anaplastic variant with omental deposits. J Clin Diagn Res. 2016;10:ED01–3.
3. Kalfa N, Philibert P, Patte C, Thibaud E, Pienkowski C, Ecochard A, Boizet-Bonhoure B, Fellous M, Sultan C. Juvenile granulosa-cell tumor: clinical and molecular expression. Gynecol Obstet Fertil. 2009;37:33–44.
4. Obendorf DL. Pathology of the female reproductive tract in the koala, Phascolarctos Cinereus (Goldfuss), from Victoria, Australia. J Wildl Dis. 1981; 17:587–92.
5. Bryk S, Pukkala E, Martinsen JI, Unkila-Kallio L, Tryggvadottir L, Sparen P, Kjaerheim K, Weiderpass E, Riska A. Incidence and occupational variation of ovarian granulosa cell tumours in Finland, Iceland, Norway and Sweden during 1953-2012: a longitudinal cohort study. BJOG. 2017;124:143–9.
6. Leung DT, Fuller PJ, Chu S. Impact of FOXL2 mutations on signaling in ovarian granulosa cell tumors. Int J Biochem Cell Biol. 2016;72:51–4.
7. Anttonen M, Pihlajoki M, Andersson N, Georges A, L'Hote D, Vattulainen S, Farkkila A, Unkila-Kallio L, Veitia RA, Heikinheimo M. FOXL2, GATA4, and SMAD3 co-operatively modulate gene expression, cell viability and apoptosis in ovarian granulosa cell tumor cells. PLoS One. 2014;9:e85545.
8. Farkkila A, Andersson N, Butzow R, Leminen A, Heikinheimo M, Anttonen M, Unkila-Kallio L. HER2 and GATA4 are new prognostic factors for early-stage ovarian granulosa cell tumor-a long-term follow-up study. Cancer Med. 2014;3:526–36.
9. Hua G, He C, Lv X, Fan L, Wang C, Remmenga SW, Rodabaugh KJ, Yang L, Lele SM, Yang P, et al. The four and a half LIM domains 2 (FHL2) regulates ovarian granulosa cell tumor progression via controlling AKT1 transcription. Cell Death Dis. 2016;7:e2297.
10. Chang HM, Cheng JC, Taylor E, Leung PC. Oocyte-derived BMP15 but not GDF9 down-regulates connexin43 expression and decreases gap junction intercellular communication activity in immortalized human granulosa cells. Mol Hum Reprod. 2014;20:373–83.

11. McTavish KJ, Nonis D, Hoang YD, Shimasaki S. Granulosa cell tumor mutant FOXL2C134W suppresses GDF-9 and activin A-induced follistatin transcription in primary granulosa cells. Mol Cell Endocrinol. 2013;372:57–64.

12. Wang XW, Yu Y, Gu L. Dehydroabietic acid reverses TNF-alpha-induced the activation of FOXO1 and suppression of TGF-beta1/Smad signaling in human adult dermal fibroblasts. Int J Clin Exp Pathol. 2014;7:8616–26.

13. Irusta G, Pazos MC, Abramovich D, De Zuniga I, Parborell F, Tesone M. Effects of an inhibitor of the gamma-secretase complex on proliferation and apoptotic parameters in a FOXL2-mutated granulosa tumor cell line (KGN). Biol Reprod. 2013;89:9.

14. Schmidt D, Ovitt CE, Anlag K, Fehsenfeld S, Gredsted L, Treier AC, Treier M. The murine winged-helix transcription factor Foxl2 is required for granulosa cell differentiation and ovary maintenance. Development. 2004;131:933–42.

15. Shah SP, Kobel M, Senz J, Morin RD, Clarke BA, Wiegand KC, Leung G, Zayed A, Mehl E, Kalloger SE, et al. Mutation of FOXL2 in granulosa-cell tumors of the ovary. N Engl J Med. 2009;360:2719–29.

16. Suh DS, Oh HK, Kim JH, Park S, Shin E, Lee K, Kim YH, Bae J. Identification and validation of differential Phosphorylation sites of the nuclear FOXL2 protein as potential novel biomarkers for adult-type Granulosa cell tumors. J Proteome Res. 2015;14:2446–56.

17. Benayoun BA, Kalfa N, Sultan C, Veitia RA. The forkhead factor FOXL2: a novel tumor suppressor? Biochim Biophys Acta. 2010;1805:1–5.

18. Kalfa N, Philibert P, Patte C, Ecochard A, Duvillard P, Baldet P, Jaubert F, Fellous M, Sultan C. Extinction of FOXL2 expression in aggressive ovarian granulosa cell tumors in children. Fertil Steril. 2007;87:896–901.

19. Kim JH, Kim YH, Kim HM, Park HO, Ha NC, Kim TH, Park M, Lee K, Bae J. FOXL2 posttranslational modifications mediated by GSK3beta determine the growth of granulosa cell tumours. Nat Commun. 2014;5:2936.

20. Benayoun BA, Caburet S, Dipietromaria A, Georges A, D'Haene B, Pandaranayaka PJ, L'Hote D, Todeschini AL, Krishnaswamy S, Fellous M, et al. Functional exploration of the adult ovarian granulosa cell tumor-associated somatic FOXL2 mutation p.Cys134Trp (c.402C>G). PLoS One. 2010;5:e8789.

21. Farkkila A, Haltia UM, Tapper J, McConechy MK, Huntsman DG, Heikinheimo M. Pathogenesis and treatment of adult-type granulosa cell tumor of the ovary. Ann Med. 2017;49:435–47.

22. Rosario R, Araki H, Print CG, Shelling AN. The transcriptional targets of mutant FOXL2 in granulosa cell tumours. PLoS One. 2012;7:e46270.

23. Rosario R, Cohen PA, Shelling AN. The role of FOXL2 in the pathogenesis of adult ovarian granulosa cell tumours. Gynecol Oncol. 2014;133:382–7.

24. Kim JH, Yoon S, Park M, Park HO, Ko JJ, Lee K, Bae J. Differential apoptotic activities of wild-type FOXL2 and the adult-type granulosa cell tumor-associated mutant FOXL2 (C134W). Oncogene. 2011;30:1653–63.

25. Cheng JC, Klausen C, Leung PC. Overexpression of wild-type but not C134W mutant FOXL2 enhances GnRH-induced cell apoptosis by increasing GnRH receptor expression in human granulosa cell tumors. PLoS One. 2013;8: e55099.

26. Cheng JC, Chang HM, Qiu X, Fang L, Leung PC. FOXL2-induced follistatin attenuates activin A-stimulated cell proliferation in human granulosa cell tumors. Biochem Biophys Res Commun. 2014;443:537–42.

27. Ranganathan P, Weaver KL, Capobianco AJ. Notch signalling in solid tumours: a little bit of everything but not all the time. Nat Rev Cancer. 2011; 11:338–51.

28. Masek J, Andersson ER. The developmental biology of genetic notch disorders. Development. 2017;144:1743–63.

29. Terauchi KJ, Shigeta Y, Iguchi T, Sato T. Role of notch signaling in granulosa cell proliferation and polyovular follicle induction during folliculogenesis in mouse ovary. Cell Tissue Res. 2016;365:197–208.

30. Budi EH, Duan D, Derynck R. Transforming growth factor-beta receptors and Smads: regulatory complexity and functional versatility. Trends Cell Biol. 2017;27:658–62.

31. Massague J. TGFbeta signalling in context. Nat Rev Mol Cell Biol. 2012;13: 616–30.

32. Pangas SA. Bone morphogenetic protein signaling transcription factor (SMAD) function in granulosa cells. Mol Cell Endocrinol. 2012;356:40–7.

33. Thompson TB, Cook RW, Chapman SC, Jardetzky TS, Woodruff TK. Beta A versus beta B: is it merely a matter of expression? Mol Cell Endocrinol. 2004;225:9–17.

34. Makanji Y, Zhu J, Mishra R, Holmquist C, Wong WP, Schwartz NB, Mayo KE, Woodruff TK. Inhibin at 90: from discovery to clinical application, a historical review. Endocr Rev. 2014;35:747–94.

35. Ethier JF, Findlay JK. Roles of activin and its signal transduction mechanisms in reproductive tissues. Reproduction. 2001;121:667–75.

36. Looyenga BD, Wiater E, Vale W, Hammer GD. Inhibin-A antagonizes TGFbeta2 signaling by down-regulating cell surface expression of the TGFbeta coreceptor betaglycan. Mol Endocrinol. 2010;24:608–20.

37. McCullagh DR. Dual endocrine activity of the testes. Science. 1932;76:19–20.

38. Matzuk MM, Finegold MJ, Su JG, Hsueh AJ, Bradley A. Alpha-inhibin is a tumour-suppressor gene with gonadal specificity in mice. Nature. 1992;360:313–9.

39. Kadariya I, Wang J, ur Rehman Z, Ali H, Riaz H, He J, Bhattarai D, Liu JJ, Zhang SJ. RNAi-mediated knockdown of inhibin alpha subunit increased apoptosis in granulosa cells and decreased fertility in mice. J Steroid Biochem Mol Biol. 2015;152:161–70.

40. Suresh PS, Rajan T, Tsutsumi R. New targets for old hormones: inhibins clinical role revisited. Endocr J. 2011;58:223–35.

41. Myers M, Middlebrook BS, Matzuk MM, Pangas SA. Loss of inhibin alpha uncouples oocyte-granulosa cell dynamics and disrupts postnatal folliculogenesis. Dev Biol. 2009;334:458–67.

42. Bilandzic M, Chu S, Farnworth PG, Harrison C, Nicholls P, Wang Y, Escalona RM, Fuller PJ, Findlay JK, Stenvers KL. Loss of betaglycan contributes to the malignant properties of human granulosa tumor cells. Mol Endocrinol. 2009; 23:539–48.

43. Burger HG, Fuller PJ, Chu S, Mamers P, Drummond A, Susil B, Neva P, Robertson DM. The inhibins and ovarian cancer. Mol Cell Endocrinol. 2001; 180:145–8.

44. Fuller PJ, Zumpe ET, Chu S, Mamers P, Burger HG. Inhibin-activin receptor subunit gene expression in ovarian tumors. J Clin Endocrinol Metab. 2002; 87:1395–401.

45. Oktem O, Akin N, Bildik G, Yakin K, Alper E, Balaban B, Urman B. FSH stimulation promotes progesterone synthesis and output from human granulosa cells without luteinization. Hum Reprod. 2017;32:643–52.

46. Kim SY, Ebbert K, Cordeiro MH, Romero MM, Whelan KA, Suarez AA, Woodruff TK, Kurita T. Constitutive activation of PI3K in oocyte induces ovarian Granulosa cell tumors. Cancer Res. 2016;76:3851–61.

47. Robertson DM, Cahir N, Burger HG, Mamers P, Groome N. Inhibin forms in serum from postmenopausal women with ovarian cancers. Clin Endocrinol. 1999;50:381–6.

48. Vihko KK, Blauer M, Puistola U, Tuohimaa P. Activin B in patients with granulosa cell tumors: serum levels in comparison to inhibin. Acta Obstet Gynecol Scand. 2003;82:570–4.

49. Geerts I, Vergote I, Neven P, Billen J. The role of inhibins B and antimullerian hormone for diagnosis and follow-up of granulosa cell tumors. Int J Gynecol Cancer. 2009;19:847–55.

50. Robertson DM, Stephenson T, Pruysers E, Burger HG, McCloud P, Tsigos A, Groome N, Mamers P, McNeilage J, Jobling T, Healy D. Inhibins/activins as diagnostic markers for ovarian cancer. Mol Cell Endocrinol. 2002;191:97–103.

51. ten Dijke P, Fu J, Schaap P, Roelen BA. Signal transduction of bone morphogenetic proteins in osteoblast differentiation. J Bone Joint Surg Am. 2003;85-A(Suppl 3):34–8.

52. Reddi AH, Reddi A. Bone morphogenetic proteins (BMPs): from morphogens to metabologens. Cytokine Growth Factor Rev. 2009;20:341–2.

53. Kouroukis T, Meyer R, Benger A, Marcellus D, Foley R, Browman G. An evaluation of age-related differences in quality of life preferences in patients with non-Hodgkin's lymphoma. Leuk Lymphoma. 2004;45:2471–6.

54. Tripurani SK, Cook RW, Eldin KW, Pangas SA. BMP-specific SMADs function as novel repressors of PDGFA and modulate its expression in ovarian granulosa cells and tumors. Oncogene. 2013;32:3877–85.

55. Edson MA, Nalam RL, Clementi C, Franco HL, Demayo FJ, Lyons KM, Pangas SA, Matzuk MM. Granulosa cell-expressed BMPR1A and BMPR1B have unique functions in regulating fertility but act redundantly to suppress ovarian tumor development. Mol Endocrinol. 2010;24:1251–66.

56. Van Nieuwenhuysen E, Lambrechts S, Lambrechts D, Leunen K, Amant F, Vergote I. Genetic changes in nonepithelial ovarian cancer. Expert Rev Anticancer Ther. 2013;13:871–82.

57. Miyoshi T, Otsuka F, Suzuki J, Takeda M, Inagaki K, Kano Y, Otani H, Mimura Y, Ogura T, Makino H. Mutual regulation of follicle-stimulating hormone signaling and bone morphogenetic protein system in human granulosa cells. Biol Reprod. 2006;74:1073–82.

58. Shimasaki S, Zachow RJ, Li D, Kim H, Iemura S, Ueno N, Sampath K, Chang RJ, Erickson GF. A functional bone morphogenetic protein system in the ovary. Proc Natl Acad Sci U S A. 1999;96:7282–7.

59. Lee WS, Otsuka F, Moore RK, Shimasaki S. Effect of bone morphogenetic protein-7 on folliculogenesis and ovulation in the rat. Biol Reprod. 2001;65:994–9.

60. Cui X, Jing X, Wu X, Bi X, Liu J, Long Z, Zhang X, Zhang D, Jia H, Su D, Huo K. Abnormal expression levels of BMP15/Smad1 are associated with granulosa cell apoptosis in patients with polycystic ovary syndrome. Mol Med Rep. 2017;16:8231–6.

61. Chang HL, Pahlavan N, Halpern EF, MacLaughlin DT. Serum Mullerian inhibiting substance/anti-Mullerian hormone levels in patients with adult granulosa cell tumors directly correlate with aggregate tumor mass as determined by pathology or radiology. Gynecol Oncol. 2009;114:57–60.

62. Weenen C, Laven JS, Von Bergh AR, Cranfield M, Groome NP, Visser JA, Kramer P, Fauser BC, Themmen AP. Anti-Mullerian hormone expression pattern in the human ovary: potential implications for initial and cyclic follicle recruitment. Mol Hum Reprod. 2004;10:77–83.

63. Anttonen M, Unkila-Kallio L, Leminen A, Butzow R, Heikinheimo M. High GATA-4 expression associates with aggressive behavior, whereas low anti-Mullerian hormone expression associates with growth potential of ovarian granulosa cell tumors. J Clin Endocrinol Metab. 2005;90:6529–35.

64. Anttonen M, Farkkila A, Tauriala H, Kauppinen M, Maclaughlin DT, Unkila-Kallio L, Butzow R, Heikinheimo M. Anti-Mullerian hormone inhibits growth of AMH type II receptor-positive human ovarian granulosa cell tumor cells by activating apoptosis. Lab Investig. 2011;91:1605–14.

65. Li Q. Inhibitory SMADs: potential regulators of ovarian function. Biol Reprod. 2015;92:50.

66. Hahn SA, Schutte M, Hoque AT, Moskaluk CA, da Costa LT, Rozenblum E, Weinstein CL, Fischer A, Yeo CJ, Hruban RH, Kern SE. DPC4, a candidate tumor suppressor gene at human chromosome 18q21.1. Science. 1996;271:350–3.

67. Pangas SA, Li X, Robertson EJ, Matzuk MM. Premature luteinization and cumulus cell defects in ovarian-specific Smad4 knockout mice. Mol Endocrinol. 2006;20:1406–22.

68. Fortin J, Boehm U, Deng CX, Treier M, Bernard DJ. Follicle-stimulating hormone synthesis and fertility depend on SMAD4 and FOXL2. FASEB J. 2014;28:3396–410.

69. Yu C, Zhang YL, Fan HY. Selective Smad4 knockout in ovarian preovulatory follicles results in multiple defects in ovulation. Mol Endocrinol. 2013;27:966–78.

70. Zhang L, Du X, Wei S, Li D, Li Q. A comprehensive transcriptomic view on the role of SMAD4 gene by RNAi-mediated knockdown in porcine follicular granulosa cells. Reproduction. 2016;152:81–9.

71. Miao ZL, Wang ZN, Cheng LQ, Zhang Y. Expression of Smad4 during rat ovarian development. Di Yi Jun Yi Da Xue Xue Bao. 2005;25:127–31.

72. Coutts SM, Childs AJ, Fulton N, Collins C, Bayne RA, McNeilly AS, Anderson RA. Activin signals via SMAD2/3 between germ and somatic cells in the human fetal ovary and regulates kit ligand expression. Dev Biol. 2008;314:189–99.

73. Mansouri-Attia N, Tripurani SK, Gokul N, Piard H, Anderson ML, Eldin K, Pangas SA. TGFbeta signaling promotes juvenile granulosa cell tumorigenesis by suppressing apoptosis. Mol Endocrinol. 2014;28:1887–98.

74. Bilandzic M, Chu S, Wang Y, Tan HL, Fuller PJ, Findlay JK, Stenvers KL. Betaglycan alters NFkappaB-TGFbeta2 cross talk to reduce survival of human granulosa tumor cells. Mol Endocrinol. 2013;27:466–79.

75. Mancari R, Portuesi R, Colombo N. Adult granulosa cell tumours of the ovary. Curr Opin Oncol. 2014;26:536–41.

76. Fuller PJ, Leung D, Chu S. Genetics and genomics of ovarian sex cord-stromal tumors. Clin Genet. 2017;91:285–91.

77. Manning BD, Cantley LC. AKT/PKB signaling: navigating downstream. Cell. 2007;129:1261–74.

78. Polyak K, Lee MH, Erdjument-Bromage H, Koff A, Roberts JM, Tempst P, Massague J. Cloning of p27Kip1, a cyclin-dependent kinase inhibitor and a potential mediator of extracellular antimitogenic signals. Cell. 1994;78:59–66.

79. Cunningham MA, Zhu Q, Hammond JM. FoxO1a can alter cell cycle progression by regulating the nuclear localization of p27kip in granulosa cells. Mol Endocrinol. 2004;18:1756–67.

80. von Karstedt S, Montinaro A, Walczak H. Exploring the TRAILs less travelled: TRAIL in cancer biology and therapy. Nat Rev Cancer. 2017;17:352–66.

81. Zhang X, Tang N, Hadden TJ, Rishi AK. Akt, FoxO and regulation of apoptosis. Biochim Biophys Acta. 2011;1813:1978–86.

82. Ausserlechner MJ, Salvador C, Deutschmann A, Bodner M, Viola G, Bortolozzi R, Basso G, Hagenbuchner J, Obexer P. Therapy-resistant acute lymphoblastic leukemia (ALL) cells inactivate FOXO3 to escape apoptosis induction by TRAIL and Noxa. Oncotarget. 2013;4:995–1007.

83. Liu Z, Ren YA, Pangas SA, Adams J, Zhou W, Castrillon DH, Wilhelm D, Richards JS. FOXO1/3 and PTEN depletion in Granulosa cells promotes ovarian Granulosa cell tumor development. Mol Endocrinol. 2015;29:1006–24.

84. Brandmaier A, Hou SQ, Shen WH. Cell cycle control by PTEN. J Mol Biol. 2017;429:2265–77.

85. Shen W, Li HL, Liu L, Cheng JX. Expression levels of PTEN, HIF-1alpha, and VEGF as prognostic factors in ovarian cancer. Eur Rev Med Pharmacol Sci. 2017;21:2596–603.

86. Verhagen PC, van Duijn PW, Hermans KG, Looijenga LH, van Gurp RJ, Stoop H, van der Kwast TH, Trapman J. The PTEN gene in locally progressive prostate cancer is preferentially inactivated by bi-allelic gene deletion. J Pathol. 2006;208:699–707.

87. Lague MN, Paquet M, Fan HY, Kaartinen MJ, Chu S, Jamin SP, Behringer RR, Fuller PJ, Mitchell A, Dore M, et al. Synergistic effects of Pten loss and WNT/CTNNB1 signaling pathway activation in ovarian granulosa cell tumor development and progression. Carcinogenesis. 2008;29:2062–72.

88. Kyronlahti A, Ramo M, Tamminen M, Unkila-Kallio L, Butzow R, Leminen A, Nemer M, Rahman N, Huhtaniemi I, Heikinheimo M, Anttonen M. GATA-4 regulates Bcl-2 expression in ovarian granulosa cell tumors. Endocrinology. 2008;149:5635–42.

89. Virgone C, Cecchetto G, Ferrari A, Bisogno G, Donofrio V, Boldrini R, Collini P, Dall'Igna P, Alaggio R. GATA-4 and FOG-2 expression in pediatric ovarian sex cord-stromal tumors replicates embryonal gonadal phenotype: results from the TREP project. PLoS One. 2012;7:e45914.

90. Kyronlahti A, Kauppinen M, Lind E, Unkila-Kallio L, Butzow R, Klefstrom J, Wilson DB, Anttonen M, Heikinheimo M. GATA4 protects granulosa cell tumors from TRAIL-induced apoptosis. Endocr Relat Cancer. 2010;17:709–17.

91. Durkes A, Garner M, Juan-Salles C, Ramos-Vara J. Immunohistochemical characterization of nonhuman primate ovarian sex cord-stromal tumors. Vet Pathol. 2012;49:834–8.

92. Farkkila A, Pihlajoki M, Tauriala H, Butzow R, Leminen A, Unkila-Kallio L, Heikinheimo M, Anttonen M. Serum vascular endothelial growth factor a (VEGF) is elevated in patients with ovarian granulosa cell tumor (GCT), and VEGF inhibition by bevacizumab induces apoptosis in GCT in vitro. J Clin Endocrinol Metab. 2011;96:E1973–81.

93. Farkkila A, Anttonen M, Pociuviene J, Leminen A, Butzow R, Heikinheimo M, Unkila-Kallio L. Vascular endothelial growth factor (VEGF) and its receptor VEGFR-2 are highly expressed in ovarian granulosa cell tumors. Eur J Endocrinol. 2011;164:115–22.

94. Roskoski R Jr. Vascular endothelial growth factor (VEGF) and VEGF receptor inhibitors in the treatment of renal cell carcinomas. Pharmacol Res. 2017;120:116–32.

95. Karasic TB, Rosen MA, O'Dwyer PJ. Antiangiogenic tyrosine kinase inhibitors in colorectal cancer: is there a path to making them more effective? Cancer Chemother Pharmacol. 2017;80:661–71.

96. Tsoi M, Lague MN, Boyer A, Paquet M, Nadeau ME, Boerboom D. Anti-VEGFA therapy reduces tumor growth and extends survival in a Murine model of ovarian Granulosa cell tumor. Transl Oncol. 2013;6:226–33.

97. Schmidt M, Kammerer U, Segerer S, Cramer A, Kohrenhagen N, Dietl J, Voelker HU. Glucose metabolism and angiogenesis in granulosa cell tumors of the ovary: activation of Akt, expression of M2PK, TKTL1 and VEGF. Eur J Obstet Gynecol Reprod Biol. 2008;139:72–8.

98. Tao X, Sood AK, Deavers MT, Schmeler KM, Nick AM, Coleman RL, Milojevic L, Gershenson DM, Brown J. Anti-angiogenesis therapy with bevacizumab for patients with ovarian granulosa cell tumors. Gynecol Oncol. 2009;114:431–6.

99. Zhou B, Sun C, Li N, Shan W, Lu H, Guo L, Guo E, Xia M, Weng D, Meng L, et al. Cisplatin-induced CCL5 secretion from CAFs promotes cisplatin-resistance in ovarian cancer via regulation of the STAT3 and PI3K/Akt signaling pathways. Int J Oncol. 2016;48:2087–97.

100. Zhang X, Huang X, Fang C, Li Q, Cui J, Sun J, Li L. miR-124 regulates the expression of BACE1 in the hippocampus under chronic cerebral hypoperfusion. Mol Neurobiol. 2017;54:2498–506.

101. Guo L, Zhou B, Liu Z, Xu Y, Lu H, Xia M, Guo E, Shan W, Chen G, Wang C. Blockage of glutaminolysis enhances the sensitivity of ovarian cancer cells to PI3K/mTOR inhibition involvement of STAT3 signaling. Tumour Biol. 2016;37:11007–15.

7

Endometriosis does not confer improved prognosis in ovarian clear cell carcinoma

Ting Zhao[†], Yu Shao[†], Yan Liu, Xiao Wang, Luyao Guan and Yuan Lu[*]

Abstract

Background: Considered as the precursor lesion of a subset of ovarian clear cell carcinoma (OCCC), the prognostic role of endometriosis in OCCC patients remains controversial. This study aimed to investigate the prognostic role of coexisting endometriosis in the survival of patients with OCCC, and also sought to identify other prognostic factors.

Results: A total of 125 patients were diagnosed with OCCC during the study period. Of these, 55 (44.0%) patients had coexisting endometriosis. Patients with endometriosis were younger ($p = 0.030$), had smaller tumor diameter ($p = 0.005$) and lower preoperative CA125 levels ($p = 0.005$). More patients with endometriosis had International Federation of Gynecology and Obstetrics (FIGO) stage I disease (83.6% vs. 51.4%, $p = 0.000$) and exhibited sensitivity to platinum-based regimen (89.6% vs. 66.7%, $p = 0.003$). Univariate and multivariate analysis revealed that coexisting endometriosis was not a predictor of 5-year overall survival (OS) or progression-free survival (PFS) of OCCC patients. For OS, chemosensitivity was the only useful prognostic factor (Hazards ratio (HR) 109.33, 95% Confidence Interval (CI) 23.46–511.51; $p = 0.000$). For PFS, the useful prognostic factors were ascites (HR 2.78, 95% CI 1.21–6.47; $p = 0.016$), FIGO stage (HR 1.61, 95% CI 1.04–2.49; $p = 0.033$), and chemosensitivity (HR 101.60, 95% CI 29.45–350.49; $p = 0.000$). Moreover, higher FIGO stage was the only risk factor for resistance to platinum-based chemotherapy (Exp (B) = 0.292, 95% CI 0.123–0.693; $p = 0.005$).

Conclusions: In this study, coexisting endometriosis was not a prognostic factor for the survival of OCCC patients. The most important predictor of both 5-year OS and PFS was chemosensitivity to platinum-based regimen, which decreased significantly with increase in FIGO stage.

Keywords: Clear cell carcinoma, Chemosensitivity, Endometriosis, Ovarian cancer, Survival

Background

Ovarian clear cell carcinoma (OCCC) is the second most common histological subtype of epithelial ovarian carcinoma (EOC) after high-grade serous carcinoma (HGSC) and accounts for > 10% of EOC [1, 2]. OCCC typically presents as a large unilateral pelvic mass and is frequently diagnosed at an early stage [3]. Unlike HGSC, this subtype of EOC is typically insensitive to conventional platinum-based chemotherapy [4]. As a result, it has a poorer prognosis as compared to that of HGSC of comparable stage [5]. In the absence of alternative chemotherapy regimens, treatment of patients with OCCC represents a clinical challenge [4].

Endometriosis is a common gynecological condition that affects 5–20% of premenopausal women [6]. It is a benign condition that exhibits some characteristics of malignant disease such as tissue invasion and distant spread [7]. In 1925, Sampon first described a case of endometriosis that transformed to ovarian carcinoma [8]. Subsequently, a consistent body of evidence has addressed the relationship between endometriosis and certain EOC subtypes. A pooled analysis published in *Lancet* showed that self-reported endometriosis was associated with a significantly increased risk of OCCC [Odds ratio (OR) 3.05, 95% Confidence Interval (CI) 2.43–3.84)], ovarian endometrioid carcinoma (OEC) (OR 2.04, 95% CI 1.67–2.48), and low-grade serous

* Correspondence: yuanlu@fudan.edu.cn
[†]Ting Zhao and Yu Shao contributed equally to this work.
Department of Gynecology, Obstetrics and Gynecology Hospital of Fudan University, 419 Fangxie Road, Shanghai 200011, China

carcinoma (OR 2.11, 95% CI 1.39–3.20) [9]. Histopathology studies have also provided compelling evidence that endometriosis is a precursor lesion for OCCC and OEC [3].

It was suggested that OCCC is distinct disease entity from other endometriosis-associated ovarian tumors (EAOCs) with a distinct gene expression profile. As reported by a number of researchers, hepatocyte nuclear factor 1β (HNF-1β) was exclusively expressed in almost all OCCC cases, but not in other EOCs including OEC [10–12]. Positive expression of HNF-1β was detected in 61.1% of ovarian endometriod cysts [13]. It was subsequently extrapolated that OCCC arises from HNF-1β positive epithelial cells while OEC arises from HNF-1β negative epithelial cells of endometriosis [13].

Theoretically, only a subset of OCCC is derived from endometriosis [9]. Yet controversy still remains regarding the prognostic role of endometriosis in OCCC patients [14]. So far, most of the studies that have investigated the prognostic role of endometriosis in the context of EAOC have included multiple histological types, while OCCC only consisted a small subgroup of the subjects [14]. Some studies precluded other subtypes but included OCCC mixed with other histological types such as serous carcinoma [15]. Owing to heterogeneity with respect to histological subtypes of EAOCs, the results of these studies should be interpreted with caution. Only a few studies have focused exclusively on pure OCCC. Of these, 3 studies reported series of 47 [16], 55 [17] and 84 [3] patients, respectively. The sample size in these studies was limited and the last study spanned over a period of 27 years, during which time considerable changes in adjuvant therapies took place. The other studies also did not reach a consensus about the prognostic role of endometriosis [2, 18, 19]. The purpose of the present study was to investigate whether concomitant endometriosis affects the survival of patients with pure OCCC and to identify other prognostic factors in these patients.

Methods

This was a retrospective study approved by the ethics committee of the OB/GYN Hospital of Fudan University. The inclusion criteria were: [1] patients who underwent primary surgery in the hospital between January 1995 and December 2014; [2] histological diagnosis of pure OCCC. The exclusion criteria were: [1] patients with mixed histological subtypes such as OCCC with high-grade serous carcinoma or endometrioid carcinoma; [2] patients with concurrent genital or extra-genital primary malignancy.

A total of 135 patients were diagnosed with ovarian clear cell carcinoma in the study period. All the patients received primary surgery in our institute and none of

them had concurrent primary malignancies of other organs. Of these, there were 10 patients diagnosed with mixed types according to the pathological reports (Fig. 1). Finally 125 patients were included in this study and were divided into two groups based on the presence or absence of endometriosis. OCCC with endometriosis was defined as endometriosis involving the same or the contralateral ovary or the pelvic peritoneum of the same patient. All the histological slides were independently reviewed by two pathologists.

A comprehensive review of the medical records was performed. Data pertaining to the following variables were obtained: age at diagnosis; personal medical history; reproductive history; preoperative level of CA125; ultrasonography findings; surgery details; adjuvant chemotherapy; date of disease progression or death; and status of the patient at the most recent follow-up. Comprehensive surgical staging was defined according to International Federation of Gynecology and Obstetrics (FIGO) guidelines (version 2015) for ovarian cancer. Satisfactory debulking surgery was defined as residual lesion ≤1 cm. Platinum-sensitivity was defined as relapse occurring ≥6 months after the completion of last regimen or lack of recurrence. Platinum-resistance was defined as relapse occurring within 6 months of the completion of last regimen.

The expressions of tumor suppressor gene protein p53, cell proliferation index Ki-67, estrogen receptor (ER) and progesterone receptor (PR) were evaluated using standard immunoperoxidase technique. The immunoreactivity was determined by counting the positively stained nuclei in at least 100 cells of the tumor tissue samples. Ki-67 immunoreactivity was expressed as a percentage. ER, PR, and p53 expressions were scored semiquantitatively as 0 (< 5% positive cells in $10 \times$ HPF), 1 (5–25%), 2 (25–50%), 3 (51–75%), or 4 (75–100%).

Statistical analysis was performed using SPSS software (version 16.0, Chicago, IL, USA). All data are expressed as mean ± standard deviation (SD). Between-group differences with respect to continuous variables were assessed by t-test or Mann-Whitney test, as appropriate. The Pearson Chi-square test or Fisher's exact test was used to assess differences with respect to categorical variables. Spearman's correlation analysis was used to assess the correlation between variables. Variables with $p < 0.05$ were included in the logistic regression model. Overall survival (OS) and progression-free survival (PFS) was calculated from the date of primary surgery to death and recurrence, respectively, or the last disease-free visit. Survival analysis was performed using Kaplan-Meier model. Variables associated with p values < 0.1 in univariate analyses were included in the Cox regression model to account for the confounding factors. All p values reported are two-tailed and a $p < 0.05$ was considered significant.

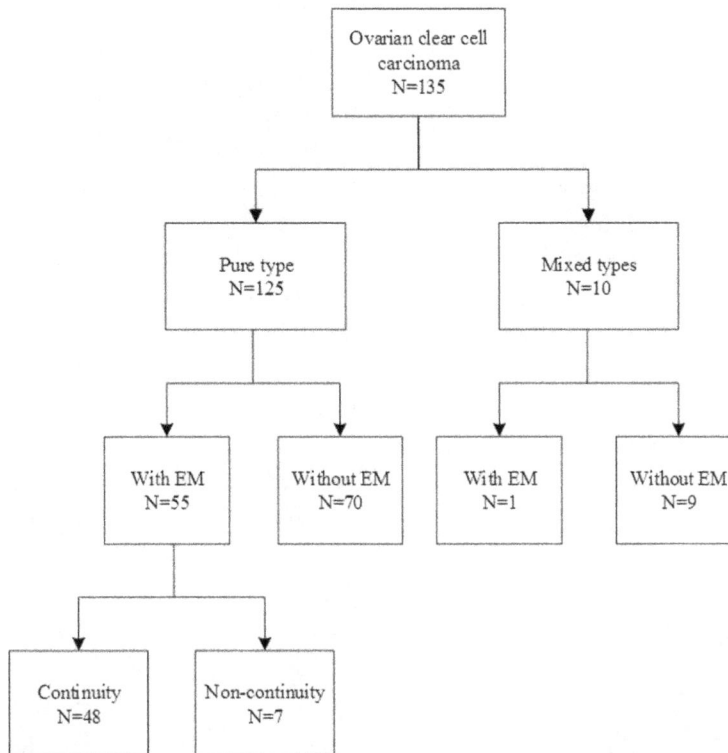

Fig. 1 An overview of the subject of this study. A total of 135 cases were diagnosed with ovarian clear cell carcinoma in the study period. Finally 125 cases were included in the analysis and 10 cases were excluded for mixed subtypes. There were 55 cases with endometriosis while 70 cases without. Of the 55 patients, continuity of clear cell carcinoma from endometriosis was detected in 48 cases. EM: endometriosis. Continuity: continuity of clear cell carcinoma from endometriosis.

Results

Characteristics of the study population

A total of 125 patients treated during the 19-year study period qualified the inclusion and exclusion criteria. Mean age at the time of diagnosis was 51.6 ± 7.8 years (range, 31–75). Mean tumor diameter was 11.3 ± 4.6 cm (range, 2.3–25.2) (Table 1). Over a median follow-up period of 28.9 months (range, 3.2–93.9 months), 5 patients (4.0%) were lost to follow-up. Twenty-four disease-specific deaths were observed. The 5-year OS and PFS for the entire study cohort was 78.7 and 74.5%, respectively. In total, 82 (65.6%), 12 (9.6%), 28 (22.4%), and 3 (2.4%) patients were diagnosed with FIGO stage I, II, III, and IV, respectively. Most patients with FIGO stage I and IIA disease received comprehensive staging surgery including total hysterectomy, salpingo-oophorectomy, pelvic lymphadnectomy, and omentum resection; however, 3, 2, and 1 patient with FIGO stage I disease only received hysterectomy and salpingo-oophorectomy, salpingo-oophorectomy, and ovarian cystectomy, respectively. All patients with FIGO stage IIB disease or higher received debulking surgery. The 5-year OS of patients with FIGO stage I, II, III and IV was 89.9, 80.2, 45.5, and 33.3%, respectively ($p = 0.000$). The corresponding 5-year PFS was 88.8, 55.6, 22.4, and 33.3%, respectively ($p = 0.000$) (Fig. 2). There were 122 patients who received platinum-based chemotherapy regimen after surgery while 3 patients with FIGO stage I disease did not receive chemotherapy. Of these, 119 patients received TP or TC regimen (paclitaxel taxol 135 mg/m^2 and carboplatin AUC (area under the curve) = 5, or cisplatin 75 mg/m^2); 1 patient with FIGO stage I received PAC regimen (cisplatin, doxorubicin, and cyclophosphamide); 1 patient with FIGO stage IIIC disease received PEFC regimen (carboplatin, etoposide, fluorouracil, and cyclophosphamide); and 1 patient with FIGO stage IV disease received TVP regimen (paclitaxel taxol, etoposide, and cisplatin). Most (96.2%, 76/79) patients with FIGO stage I disease received ≥4 courses and most (95.3%, 41/43) patients with FIGO stage II disease or higher received ≥6 courses of regimen. For 11 out of the 122 patients, the status pertaining to chemosensitivity could not be verified due to the following reasons: [1] loss of follow-up for 5 patients (4 patients with FIGO stage I and 1 patient with FIGO stage III); [2] Until the cut-off date for the present study the follow-up time was not long enough to assess the

Table 1 Clinicopathological features of patients with ovarian clear cell carcinoma

Characteristics	All ($N = 125$)	NEM ($N = 70$)	EM ($N = 55$)	p value
Age (years)	51.6 ± 7.8	52.9 ± 8.5	49.9 ± 6.4	0.030
Parity	0.9 ± 0.5	1.0 ± 0.5	0.8 ± 0.5	0.040
Nulliparous (%)	20 (16.1%) ($n = 124$)	8 (11.6%) ($n = 69$)	12 (21.8%) ($n = 55$)	0.145
Tumor size (cm)	11.3 ± 4.6 ($n = 118$)	12.3 ± 5.0 ($n = 66$)	9.9 ± 3.7 ($n = 52$)	0.005
Serum CA 125 (U/mL)	295.0 ± 934.7	433.5 ± 1188.2	94.7 ± 198.4	0.005
Normal (%)	40 (34.8%)	20 (29.4%)	20 (42.6%)	0.167
Elevated (%)	75 (65.2%) ($n = 115$)	48 (70.6%) ($n = 68$)	27 (57.4%) ($n = 47$)	
Laterality (%)				0.045
Left	61 (48.8%)	32 (45.7%)	29 (52.7%)	
Right	52 (41.6%)	28 (40.0%)	24 (43.6%)	
Both	12 (9.6%)	10 (14.3%)	2 (3.6%)	
FIGO stage (%)				0.000
I	82 (65.6%)	36 (51.4%)	46 (83.6%)	
II	12 (9.6%)	7 (10.0%)	5 (9.1%)	
III	28 (22.4%)	24 (34.3%)	4 (7.3%)	
IV	3 (2.4%)	3 (4.3%)	0 (0%)	
Surgical method (%)				0.070
Laparoscopy	21 (16.8%)	8 (11.4%)	13 (23.6%)	
Laparotomy	104 (83.2%)	62 (88.6%)	42 (76.4%)	
Comprehensive staging (%)				0.829
Yes	114 (91.2%)	63 (90.0%)	51 (92.7%)	
No	11 (8.8%)	7 (10.0%)	4 (7.3%)	
Ascites (%)	48 (38.4%)	37 (52.9%)	11 (20%)	0.000
Ascites positivity (%)	20 (41.7%)	18 (48.6%)	2 (18.2%)	0.147
Lymph nodes status (%)				0.031
Positive	12 (10.6%)	10 (16.9%)	2 (1.8%)	
Negative	101 (89.4%) ($n = 113$)	49 (83.1%) ($n = 59$)	52 (96.3%) ($n = 54$)	
Residual lesion (%)	120 (96.0%)	66 (94.3%)	54 (98.2%)	0.520
0	113 (90.4%)	60 (85.7%)	53 (96.4%)	
≤1 cm	7 (5.6%)	6 (8.6%)	1 (1.8%)	
>1 cm	5 (4.0%)	4 (5.7%)	1 (1.8%)	
Cycles of chemotherapy	6.3 ± 1.8	6.4 ± 1.9	6.1 ± 1.6	0.382
Chemosensitivity (%)				0.003
Sensitive	85 (76.6%)	42 (66.7%)	43 (89.6%)	
Resistant	26 (23.4%) ($n = 111$)	21 (33.3%) ($n = 63$)	5 (10.4%) ($n = 48$)	

EM endometriosis, *NEM* without endometriosis

status of 6 patients (all with FIGO stage I disease). Among the other patients, 76.6% (85/111) patients were sensitive to platinum-based chemotherapy. Specifically, 91.4% (74/81) of patients with FIGO stage I or II disease exhibited chemosensitivity; for patients with advanced disease (FIGO stage III and IV), the response rate was 36.7% (11/30).

Of the study population, 55 (44.0%) patients with endometriosis were assigned to EM group; 70 patients (56.0%) with no evidence of endometriosis were assigned to NEM group.

Comparison of clinical and pathological features between the two groups

The clinical parameters of the two groups are shown in Table 1. Compared to NEM group, patients in the EM group were younger (49.9 ± 6.4 vs.52.9 ± 8.5 years, $p = 0.030$), gave fewer births (0.8 ± 0.5 vs.1.0 ± 0.5, $p = 0.040$),

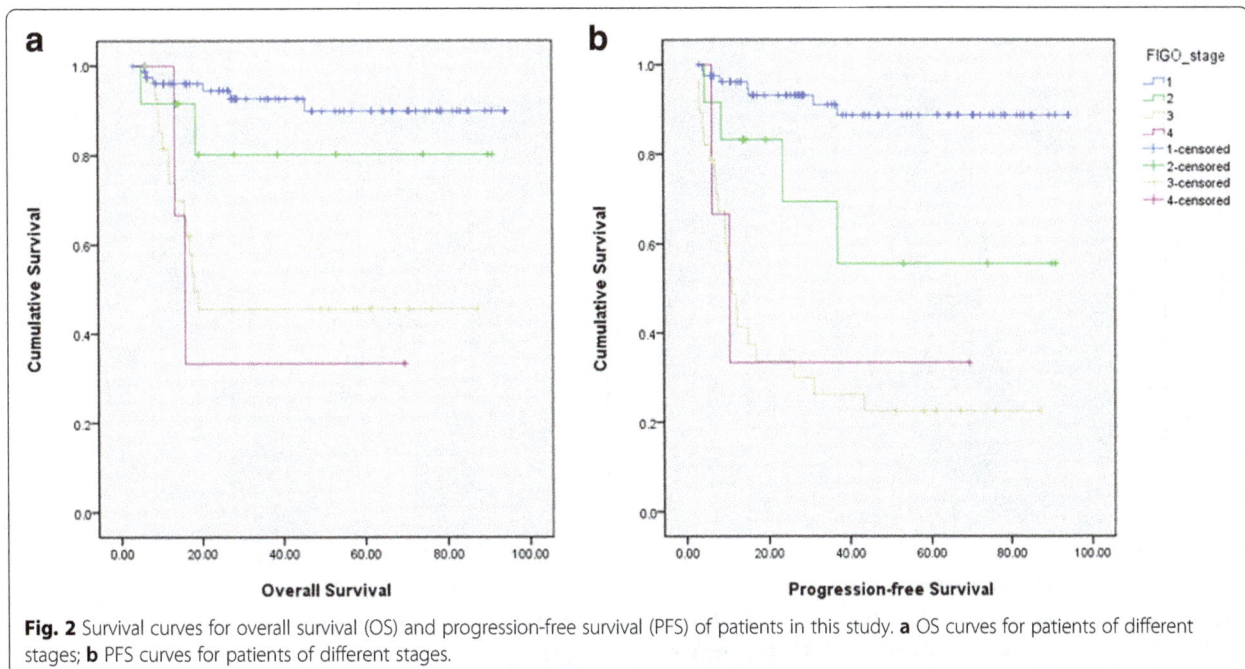

Fig. 2 Survival curves for overall survival (OS) and progression-free survival (PFS) of patients in this study. **a** OS curves for patients of different stages; **b** PFS curves for patients of different stages.

and had smaller tumor diameter (9.9 ± 3.7 vs. 12.3 ± 5.0 cm, $p = 0.005$), and lower preoperative CA125 levels (94.7 ± 198.4 vs. 433.5 ± 1188.2 U/ml, $p = 0.005$). More patients in the EM group had FIGO stage I disease (83.6% vs. 51.4%, $p = 0.000$). On the contrary, a lower proportion of patients in the EM group showed bilateral involvement (3.6% vs. 14.3%, $p = 0.045$), lymph node involvement (1.8% vs. 16.9%, $p = 0.031$), or ascites (20.0% vs. 52.9%, $p = 0.000$). A significantly greater proportion of patients in the EM group were sensitive to platinum-based regimen (89.6% vs. 66.7%, $p = 0.003$).

No significant between-group difference was observed with respect to the proportion of patients who underwent laparotomy, the ratio of patients who received satisfactory debulking surgery and chemotherapy cycles. Immunoreactivity of ER, PR, p53, and Ki-67 was also comparable between the two groups (Table 2).

Comparison of survival outcomes between the two groups

As estimated from Kaplan-Meier survival curves, both the 5-year OS and PFS in the EM group were better

Table 2 Immunohistochemical staining intensity of ER, PR, p53, and Ki-67 in ovarian clear cell carcinoma patients

Index	NEM	EM	p value[a]
ER	0.50 ± 1.00	0.56 ± 0.91	0.478
PR	0.21 ± 0.51	0.12 ± 0.44	0.207
p53	0.93 ± 0.97	0.77 ± 0.61	0.769
Ki-67	32.54 ± 24.15	32.35 ± 19.30	0.662

EM endometriosis, *NEM* without endometriosis
[a]Mann-Whitney test

than that in the NEM group (OS: 89.4% vs. 67.7%, $p = 0.013$) (PFS: 87.9% vs. 53.3%, $p = 0.001$) (Fig. 3).

As some features such as age, FIGO stage, and preoperative CA125 level were different between the two groups, Cox regression model was used to account for the influence of these factors. No significant between-group difference with respect to survival was observed after controlling for these confounding factors ($p > 0.05$).

Of the 55 patients from EM group, there were 48 cases had endometriosis in direct continuity from the OCCC lesion, and seven cases not (Fig. 1). We also compared the survival outcomes between them. They were comparable in 5-year OS (92.7% vs. 71.4%, $p = 0.083$) but significant difference of 5-year PFS (93.4% vs. 53.6%, $p = 0.004$) was observed. However, after controlling for confounding factors such as FIGO stage, no significant difference with respect to PFS was observed in Cox regression model ($p = 0.607$).

Predictors of survival in univariate and multivariate survival analysis

We performed the *log*-rank test using $p < 0.1$ as a criteria to identify predictors of survival. The potential prognostic factors for PFS were: presence of endometriosis, preoperative CA125 level, bilateralism, tumor diameter, size of residual lesion, ascites, lymph node positivity, FIGO stage, number of chemotherapy cycles, and chemosensitivity. The potential prognostic factors for OS were: presence of endometriosis, bilateralism, comprehensive staging, size of residual lesion, ascites, lymph node positivity, FIGO stage, and chemosensitivity.

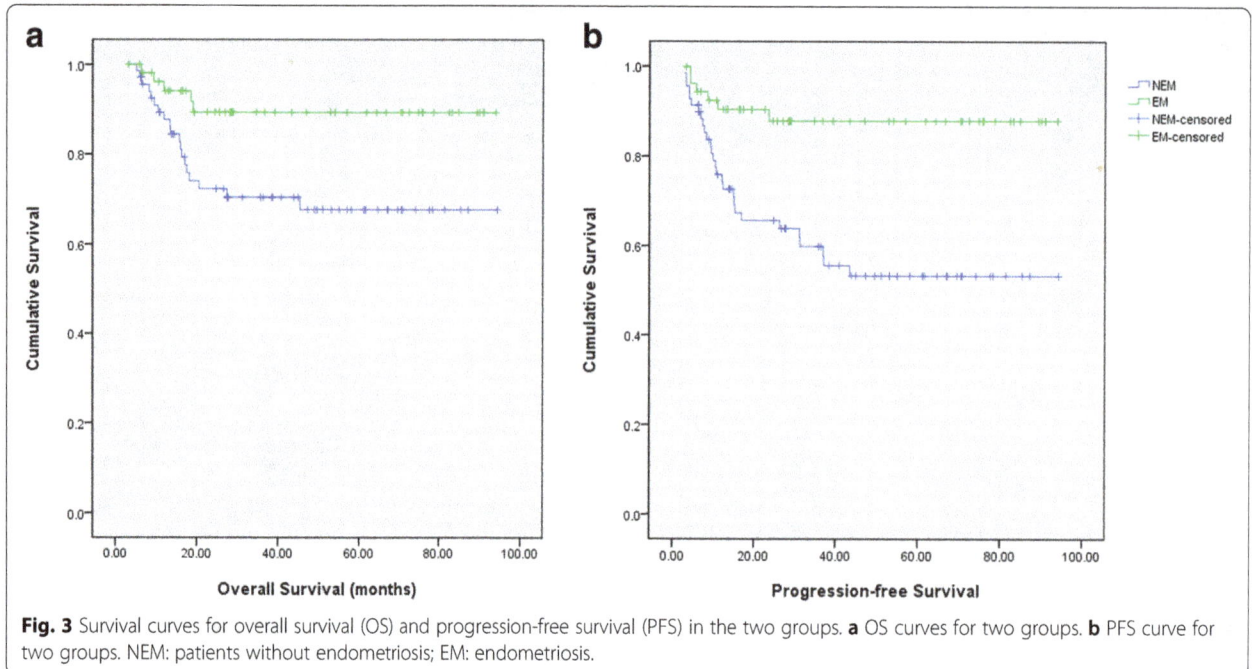

Fig. 3 Survival curves for overall survival (OS) and progression-free survival (PFS) in the two groups. **a** OS curves for two groups. **b** PFS curve for two groups. NEM: patients without endometriosis; EM: endometriosis.

After recalculation in Cox regression model, the useful prognostic factors for PFS were ascites (Hazards ratio (HR) 2.78, 95% CI1.21–6.47; $p = 0.016$), FIGO stage (HR 1.61, 95% CI1.04–2.49; $p = 0.033$), and chemosensitivity (HR 101.60, 95% CI29.45–350.49; $p = 0.000$). For OS, chemosensitivity was the only useful prognostic factor (HR 109.33, 95% CI23.46–511.51; $p = 0.000$) (Table 3).

Factors related to chemosensitivity in the logistic regression model

As chemosensitivity was the most important prognostic factor for both OS and PFS of patients with OCCC, further analysis was performed to identify covariates of chemosensitivity. Spearman's correlation analysis showed that preoperative CA125 level, ascites, size of residual lesion, lymph node positivity, FIGO stage, and presence of endometriosis were associated with chemosensitivity ($p < 0.05$). However, after entering into logistic regression equation, only FIGO stage was significantly associated with chemosensitivity (Exp (B) = 0.292, 95% CI0.123–0.693; $p = 0.005$) (Table 4).

Discussion

Pathological evidence of the synchronous presence of endometriosis and OCCC has been consistently reported [20]. A review of 15 published reports concluded that 39.2% of patients with OCCC had coexisting endometriosis [21]. In the present study, this percentage was 44.0% (55/125), which is comparable to the reported figure. The histological characteristics of OCCC include large cuboidal, hobnailed or flattened epithelial cells containing abundant clear cytoplasm lining the tubules and cysts, and exhibiting a solid/tubular or glandular growth pattern [22]. The hobnail cells present a very strong morphological resemblance to endometrial Arias-Stella cells [23].

The mechanism by which endometriosis develops into OCCC remains largely unknown. It was suggested that OCCC develops in a step-wise fashion from endometriosis through metaplastic, hyperplastic, and atypical endometriosis [24]. Atypical endometriosis is characterized by epithelial cells showing nuclear enlargement, crowding, slight hyperchromasia, and possible chromocentres/nucleoli architectural abnormalities [25]. It was reported that OCCC-associated endometriosis already harbors aberrant gene expression, such as altered expressions of *eEF1A2*, *PTCH2*, *PPP1R14B*, and *XRCC5*, which may not be found in endometriosis tissue in the absence of cancer [26]. Shared gene alterations such as *PTEN*, *PIK3CA* or *ARID1A* mutation were documented between ovarian cancers and adjacent normal-appearance endometriosis, which suggests that these gene mutations represent early events in the carcinogenic pathway before the appearance of the atypical precancerous lesions [27–29]. Moreover, HNF-1β expression is significantly increased and ER expression is significantly down-regulated in primary OCCC lesions as compared to that in matched endometriosis, which suggests that the changes in these proteins were relatively late carcinogenic events [26]. The product of *H3K27me3* gene sets and one of its target proteins, WT1, were found enriched in neighboring endometriosis, but silenced in OCCC lesion, which suggests that epigenetic reprogramming transformed the endometriotic cells to a pluripotent stage as OCCC [26].

Table 3 Prognostic factors for progression-free survival (PFS) and overall survival (OS) of ovarian clear cell carcinoma patients

Variables	5 year-PFS %	p value[a]	p value[b]	HR (95%CI)	5 year-OS %	p value[a]	p value[b]	HR (95%CI)
Endometriosis		0.001	0.295			0.013	0.677	
With	87.9				89.4			
Without	53.3				67.7			
Age (years)		0.628				0.550		
< 60	72.0				79.6			
≥60	47.8				69.6			
CA-125 (U/mL)		0.001	0.620			0.142		
< 200	76.6				80.0			
≥200	38.4				64.4			
Parity		0.342				0.382		
0	70.8				89.5			
≥1	53.6				75.9			
Laterality		0.034	0.093			0.028	0.360	
Unilateral	70.1				79.3			
Bilateral	46.7				56.2			
Tumor diameter		0.084	0.662			0.236		
< 10	77.7				83.4			
≥10	59.8				70.0			
Comprehensive staging		0.348				0.070	0.441	
Yes	68.6				79.0			
No	58.9				56.2			
Residual lesion		0.000	0.126			0.001	0.731	
Yes	72.8				82.6			
No	25.0				33.3			
Ascites		0.000	0.016			0.001	0.052	
Yes	45.9			2.78 (1.21–6.47)	60.8			
No	82.0				87.6			
Lymph nodes status		0.000	0.324			0.012	0.395	
Positive	33.3				58.3			
Negative	76.0				85.6			
FIGO stage		0.000	0.033	1.61 (1.04–2.49)		0.000	0.874	
I	88.8				89.9			
II	55.6				80.2			
III	22.4				45.5			
IV	33.3				33.3			
Chemotherapy cycles		0.050	0.290			0.421		
≥6	72.5				78.4			
> 6	49.9				69.5			
Chemosensitivity		0.000	0.000	101.60 (29.45–350.49)		0.000	0.000	109.55
Sensitive	87.3				96.5			(23.46–511.51)
Resistant	0				9.2			

[a]log-rank test; [b] Cox-proportional hazards model

Table 4 Risk factors for chemosensitivity to platinum-based regimen of ovarian clear cell carcinoma patients

Variables	p value[a]	Correlation Coefficent	p value[b]	Exp (B) (95% CI)
Age	0.995			
Tumor diameter	0.396			
CA125 value	0.028	−0.216	0.887	
Number of live birth	0.448			
Ascites	0.004	−0.267	0.673	
Residual lesion	0.000	−0.348	0.467	
Lymph nodes positivity	0.002	−0.306	0.858	
FIGO stage	0.000	−0.546	0.005	0.292 (0.123–0.693)
Bilaterality	0.060			
Endometriosis	0.003	0.279	0.671	
ER	0.579			
PR	0.191			
p53	0.990			
Ki67	0.681			

[a]Spearman's correlation test; [b]Logistic regression model

Compared to NEM group, patients in the EM group presented favorable characteristics such as younger age and earlier stage, which is consistent with previously reported results [7, 30]. This is likely attributable to the typical symptoms of endometriosis which may facilitate earlier attendance to the clinics [7, 30]. Moreover, in advanced stage malignancies the tumor might have masked the deriving tissue of origin; this may have contributed to the lower frequency of detection of endometriosis [31].

Some studies have suggested that OCCC patients with concomitant endometriosis have a better prognosis than that of patients without endometriosis [31]. However, other studies have found no difference in survival after adjusting for stage and age [7, 32, 33]. A meta-analysis of evidence from 10 cohort studies also concluded that endometriosis is not a prognostic factor for the survival of OCCC patients [34]. A study conducted in Korea found that only in FIGO stage I patients was endometriosis an independent prognostic factor [19]. However, studies conducted in China found no prognostic role of endometriosis in OCCC patients [2], even when the tumor was confined to FIGO stage I [18]. In the present study, either, endometriosis was not found to be a prognostic factor in OCCC patients. These results collectively suggest that endometriosis may not affect the progression after the onset of ovarian cancer [7]. Moreover, there was no difference with respect to key molecular characteristics such as the expressions of p53, Ki-67, ER and PR between the two groups, which also suggests homogeneity across the two groups.

In the present study, the most important prognostic factor for survival was the sensitivity to platinum-based chemotherapy. With a HR of 109.55 (95% CI 23.46–

511.51) for 5-year OS and 101.60 (95% CI 29.45–350.49) for PFS, it is reasonable to conclude that chemosensitivity to platinum-based chemotherapy was a key determinant of the survival of OCCC patients. For 5-year OS, chemosensitivity was the only prognostic factor while FIGO stage was not. However, FIGO stage was the only risk factor for chemosensitivity in the logistic regression equation. Specifically, the higher the FIGO stage, the more the resistance to platinum-based chemotherapy. Patients affected by localized (FIGO stage I and II) OCCC exhibited a response rate of 91.4% to platinum-based chemotherapy while their counterparts with advanced disease (FIGO stage III and IV) exhibited a response rate of only 36.7%. The prognosis of patients with FIGO stage I and II OCCC was reported to be comparable to that of serous adenocarcinoma, while the prognosis of patients with FIGO stage III and IV disease was much poorer compared to that of serous adenocarcinoma [4, 35, 36]. The reported median survival time for patients with advanced disease was only 12.7–23.0 months [23, 37, 38]. It is generally recognized that the poor survival of patients with advanced stage disease is largely due to the insensitivity to conventional platinum-based chemotherapy [39]. The mechanism of resistance includes decreased drug efflux, increased drug inactivation, and increased DNA repair activity [39]. These results indicate that platinum-based chemotherapy may not be the optimum treatment regimen for patients with advanced OCCC. However, the National Comprehensive Cancer Network (NCCN) guidelines (version 2016) still recommend treatment of OCCC with platinum-based chemotherapy. New molecular targets have been identified and experimented with in the past decades such as mitogen-activated protein kinase kinase (MAPK), phosphatidylinositol 3′-kinase (PI3K) signaling pathway [40], and epidermal growth-factor receptor (EGFR) [41]. However, no definite consensus has been reached about the efficacy of the above strategies.

Conclusions

Although this work has limitations inherent to retrospective studies, to the best of our knowledge, this is the largest study to compare patients diagnosed with OCCC with and without concomitant endometriosis. The two groups in this study were heterogeneous in many aspects such as age and FIGO stage. However, the prognosis was not different after controlling for confounding factors. The most important prognostic factor for the survival of OCCC patients was the chemosensitivity to platinum-based chemotherapy, which showed an inverse correlation with FIGO stage. This study calls for further research to unravel the mechanism of development of chemoresistance and underlines the need to develop novel therapeutic strategies for patients with advanced stage OCCC.

Abbreviations

AUC: Area under the curve; CI: Confidence interval; EAOCs: Endometriosis-associated ovarian tumors; EGFR: Epidermal growth-factor receptor; EOC: Epithelial ovarian carcinoma; ER: Estrogen receptor; FIGO: International Federation of Gynecology and Obstetrics; HGSC: High-grade serous carcinoma; HNF-1β: Hepatocyte nuclear factor 1β; HR: Hazards ratio; MAPK: Mitogen-activated protein kinase kinase; NCCN: National Comprehensive Cancer Network; OCCC: Ovarian clear cell carcinoma; OEC: Ovarian endometrioid carcinoma; OS: Overall survival; OR: Odds ratio; PFS: Progression-free survival; PI3K: Phosphatidylinositol 3'-kinase; PR: Progesterone receptor; SD: Standard deviation

Acknowledgements

We thank the members of the Department of Pathology of Obstetrics and Gynecology Hospital of Fudan University for their help with the pathological reviews in this study.

Funding

This study was supported by grants from Shanghai Municipal Commission of Health and Family Planning (Y.L.) (grant 201540224).

Authors' contributions

YL is the corresponding author contributed to the intellectual planning of the project and to revise the paper. TZ analyzed the data and wrote the manuscript. YL, XW and LG collected data from medical records and did telephone interview of the patients. All authors read and approved the final manuscript.

Competing interests

The authors declare that they have no competing interests.

References

1. Kobel M, Kalloger SE, Huntsman DG, Santos JL, Swenerton KD, Seidman JD, et al. Differences in tumor type in low-stage versus high-stage ovarian carcinomas. Int J Gynecol Pathol. 2010;29:203–11.
2. Ye S, Yang J, You Y, Cao D, Bai H, Lang J, et al. Comparative study of ovarian clear cell carcinoma with and without endometriosis in People's Republic of China. Fertil Steril. 2014;102:1656–62.
3. Orezzoli JP, Russell AH, Oliva E, Del Carmen MG, Eichhorn J, Fuller AF. Prognostic implication of endometriosis in clear cell carcinoma of the ovary. Gynecol Oncol. 2008;110:336–44.
4. Sugiyama T, Kamura T, Kigawa J, Terakawa N, Kikuchi Y, Kita T, et al. Clinical characteristics of clear cell carcinoma of the ovary: a distinct histologic type with poor prognosis and resistance to platinum-based chemotherapy. Cancer. 2000;88:2584–9.
5. Chan JK, Teoh D, JM H, JY Shin KO, Kapp DS. Do clear cell ovarian carcinomas have poorer prognosis compared to other epithelial cell types? A study of 1411 clear cell ovarian cancers. Gynecol Oncol. 2008;109:370–6.
6. Bulun SE. Endometriosis. N Engl J Med. 2009;360:268–79.
7. Kim HS, Kim TH, Chung HH, Song YS. Risk and prognosis of ovarian cancer in women with endometriosis: a meta-analysis. Br J Cancer. 2014;110:1878–90.
8. Sampson J. Endometrial carcinoma of the ovary arising in endometrial tissue in that organ. Arch Surg. 1925;10:1–72.
9. Pearce CL, Templeman C, MA Rossing A, Lee AM. Near, PM Webb et al. association between endometriosis and risk of histological subtypes of ovarian cancer: a pooled analysis of case-control studies. Lancet Oncol. 2012;13:385–94.
10. Tsuchiya A, Sakamoto M, Yasuda J, Chuma M, Ohta T, Ohki M, et al. Expression profiling in ovarian clear cell carcinoma: identification of hepatocyte nuclear factor-1 beta as a molecular marker and a possible molecular target for therapy of ovarian clear cell carcinoma. Am J Pathol. 2003;163:2503–12.
11. Kato N, Sasou S, Motoyama T. Expression of hepatocyte nuclear factor-1beta (HNF-1beta) in clear cell tumors and endometriosis of the ovary. Mod Pathol. 2006;19:83–9.
12. Yamamoto S, Tsuda H, Aida S, Shimazaki H, Tamai S, Matsubara O. Immunohistochemical detection of hepatocyte nuclear factor 1beta in ovarian and endometrial clear-cell adenocarcinomas and nonneoplastic endometrium. Hum Pathol. 2007;38:1074–80.
13. Kajihara H, Yamada Y, Shigetomi H, Higashiura Y, Kobayashi H. The dichotomy in the histogenesis of endometriosis-associated ovarian cancer: clear cell-type versus endometrioid-type adenocarcinoma. Int J Gynecol Pathol. 2012;31:304–12.
14. Scarfone G, Bergamini A, Noli S, Villa A, Cipriani S, Taccagni G, et al. Characteristics of clear cell ovarian cancer arising from endometriosis: a two center cohort study. Gynecol Oncol. 2014;133:480–4.
15. Schnack TH, Hogdall E, Thomsen LN, Hogdall C. Demographic, clinical, and prognostic factors of ovarian clear cell adenocarcinomas according to endometriosis status. Int J Gynecol Cancer. 2017;27:1804–12.
16. Komiyama S, Aoki D, Tominaga E, Susumu N, Udagawa Y, Nozawa S. Prognosis of Japanese patients with ovarian clear cell carcinoma associated with pelvic endometriosis: clinicopathologic evaluation. Gynecol Oncol. 1999;72:342–6.
17. Noli S, Cipriani S, Scarfone G, Villa A, Grossi E, Monti E, et al. Long term survival of ovarian endometriosis associated clear cell and endometrioid ovarian cancers. Int J Gynecol Cancer. 2013;23:244–8.
18. Bai H, Cao D, Yuan F, Sha G, Yang J, Chen J, et al. Prognostic value of endometriosis in patients with stage I ovarian clear cell carcinoma: experiences at three academic institutions. Gynecol Oncol. 2016;143:526–31.
19. Park JY, Kim DY, Suh DS, Kim JH, Kim YM, Kim YT, et al. Significance of ovarian endometriosis on the prognosis of ovarian clear cell carcinoma. Int J Gynecol Cancer. 2018;28:11–8.
20. Vigano P, Somigliana E, Parazzini F, Vercellini P. Bias versus causality: interpreting recent evidence of association between endometriosis and ovarian cancer. Fertil Steril. 2007;88:588–93.
21. Yoshikawa H, Jimbo H, Okada S, Matsumoto K, Onda T, Yasugi T, et al. Prevalence of endometriosis in ovarian cancer. Gynecol Obstet Investig. 2000;50(Suppl 1):11–7.
22. Scully RE. Recent progress in ovarian cancer. Hum Pathol. 1970;1:73–98.
23. Aure JC, Hoeg K, Kolstad P. Clinical and histologic studies of ovarian carcinoma. Long-term follow-up of 990 cases. Obstet Gynecol. 1971;37:1–9.
24. Prefumo F, Todeschini F, Fulcheri E, Venturini PL. Epithelial abnormalities in cystic ovarian endometriosis. Gynecol Oncol. 2002;84:280–4.

25. King CM, Barbara C, Prentice A, Brenton JD, Charnock-Jones DS. Models of endometriosis and their utility in studying progression to ovarian clear cell carcinoma. J Pathol. 2016;238:185–96.

26. Worley MJ Jr, Liu S, Hua Y, Kwok JS, Samuel A, Hou L, et al. Molecular changes in endometriosis-associated ovarian clear cell carcinoma. Eur J Cancer. 2015;51:1831–42.

27. Sato N, Tsunoda H, Nishida M, Morishita Y, Takimoto Y, Kubo T, et al. Loss of heterozygosity on 10q23.3 and mutation of the tumor suppressor gene PTEN in benign endometrial cyst of the ovary: possible sequence progression from benign endometrial cyst to endometrioid carcinoma and clear cell carcinoma of the ovary. Cancer Res. 2000;60:7052–6.

28. Wiegand KC, Shah SP, Al-Agha OM, Zhao Y, Tse K, Zeng T, et al. ARID1A mutations in endometriosis-associated ovarian carcinomas. N Engl J Med. 2010;363:1532–43.

29. Yamamoto S, Tsuda H, Takano M, Tamai S, Matsubara O. Loss of ARID1A protein expression occurs as an early event in ovarian clear-cell carcinoma development and frequently coexists with PIK3CA mutations. Mod Pathol. 2012;25:615–24.

30. Wang S, Qiu L, Lang JH, Shen K, Yang JX, Huang HF, et al. Clinical analysis of ovarian epithelial carcinoma with coexisting pelvic endometriosis. Am J Obstet Gynecol. 2013;208(413):e1–5.

31. Somigliana E, Vigano P, Parazzini F, Stoppelli S, Giambattista E, Vercellini P. Association between endometriosis and cancer: a comprehensive review and a critical analysis of clinical and epidemiological evidence. Gynecol Oncol. 2006;101:331–41.

32. Erzen M, Rakar S, Klancnik B, Syrjanen K. Endometriosis-associated ovarian carcinoma (EAOC): an entity distinct from other ovarian carcinomas as suggested by a nested case-control study. Gynecol Oncol. 2001;83:100–8.

33. Mangili G, Bergamini A, Taccagni G, Gentile C, Panina P, Vigano P, et al. Unraveling the two entities of endometrioid ovarian cancer: a single center clinical experience. Gynecol Oncol. 2012;126:403–7.

34. Kim HS, Kim MA, Lee M, Suh DH, Kim K, No JH, et al. Effect of endometriosis on the prognosis of ovarian clear cell carcinoma: a two-center cohort study and meta-analysis. Ann Surg Oncol. 2015;22:2738–45.

35. Goff BA, Sainz de la Cuesta R, Muntz HG, Fleischhacker D, Ek M, Rice LW, et al. Clear cell carcinoma of the ovary: a distinct histologic type with poor prognosis and resistance to platinum-based chemotherapy in stage III disease. Gynecol Oncol. 1996;60:412–7.

36. Mizuno M, Kikkawa F, Shibata K, Kajiyama H, Ino K, Kawai M, et al. Long-term follow-up and prognostic factor analysis in clear cell adenocarcinoma of the ovary. J Surg Oncol. 2006;94:138–43.

37. Behbakht K, Randall TC, Benjamin I, Morgan MA, King S, Rubin SC. Clinical characteristics of clear cell carcinoma of the ovary. Gynecol Oncol. 1998;70:255–8.

38. Itamochi H, Kigawa J, Sugiyama T, Kikuchi Y, Suzuki M, Terakawa N. Low proliferation activity may be associated with chemoresistance in clear cell carcinoma of the ovary. Obstet Gynecol. 2002;100:281–7.

39. Itamochi H, Kigawa J, Terakawa N. Mechanisms of chemoresistance and poor prognosis in ovarian clear cell carcinoma. Cancer Sci. 2008;99:653–8.

40. Kawaguchi W, Itamochi H, Kigawa J, Kanamori Y, Oishi T, Shimada M, et al. Simultaneous inhibition of the mitogen-activated protein kinase kinase and phosphatidylinositol 3′-kinase pathways enhances sensitivity to paclitaxel in ovarian carcinoma. Cancer Sci. 2007;98:2002–8.

41. Fujimura M, Hidaka T, Saito S. Selective inhibition of the epidermal growth factor receptor by ZD1839 decreases the growth and invasion of ovarian clear cell adenocarcinoma cells. Clin Cancer Res. 2002;8:2448–54.

8

Role of BMI1 in epithelial ovarian cancer: investigated via the CRISPR/Cas9 system and RNA sequencing

Qianying Zhao[1,2], Qiuhong Qian[1,3], Dongyan Cao[1], Jiaxin Yang[1], Ting Gui[1*] and Keng Shen[1*]

Abstract

Background: B-cell-specific Moloney murine leukemia virus integration site 1 (BMI1) might be an appropriate biomarker in the management of epithelial ovarian cancer (EOC). However, the biological role of BMI1 and its relevant molecular mechanism needs further elaboration. Clustered regularly interspaced short palindromic repeats (CRISPR)/Cas9 system is an excellent genome-editing tool and is scarcely used in EOC studies.

Methods: We first applied CRISPR/Cas9 technique to silence BMI1 in EOC cells; thereafter we accomplished various in vivo and in vitro experiments to detect biological behaviors of ovarian cancer cells, including MTT, flow cytometry, Transwell, real-time polymerase chain reaction and western blotting assays, etc.; eventually, we used RNA sequencing to reveal the underlying molecular traits driven by BMI1 in EOC.

Results: We successfully shut off the expression of BMI1 in EOC cells using CRISPR/Cas9 system, providing an ideal cellular model for investigations of target gene. Silencing BMI1 could reduce cell growth and metastasis, promote cell apoptosis, and enhance the platinum sensitivity of EOC cells. BMI1 might alter extracellular matrix structure and angiogenesis of tumor cells through regulating Focal adhesion and PI3K/AKT pathways.

Conclusion: BMI1 is a potential biomarker in EOC management, especially for tumor progression and chemo-resistance. Molecular traits, including BMI1 and core genes in Focal adhesion and PI3K/AKT pathways, might be alternatives as therapeutic targets for EOC.

Keywords: B-cell-specific Moloney murine leukemia virus integration site 1 (BMI1), Clustered regularly interspaced short palindromic repeats (CRISPR)/Cas9, Epithelial ovarian cancer (EOC), Focal adhesion pathway, PI3K/AKT pathway

Background

Epithelial ovarian cancer (EOC) is the leading cause of mortality among gynecologic cancers, and the majority of patients are diagnosed in advanced stages [1, 2]. Approximately, 70% of the patients would relapse even if they have received optimal cytoreductive surgery (CRS) combined with standard platinum-based chemotherapy. The 5-year survival rate for advanced-stage patients is very low [3]. It has been a major research focus and challenge to search for appropriate tumor markers and effective therapeutic targets because the etiology of EOC is largely unknown and the tumors present heterogeneity in multiple dimensions.

As a core member of Polycomb group proteins (PcG), B-cell-specific Moloney murine leukemia virus integration site 1 (BMI1) plays an important role in epigenetics, participates in important cellular events and is identified as aberrantly expressed in various human cancers [4–11]. In our previous study, we also found significant over-expression of BMI1 in metastatic lymph nodes and recurrent tumors compared to primary ovarian carcinomas. In addition, intensive expression of BMI1 in metastatic and recurrent tumors was an independent prognostic factor for survival and relapse, respectively [12]. However, the biological functions and related mechanism of BMI1 in EOC lack elaboration.

Among a variety of genome-editing techniques, the clustered regularly interspaced short palindromic repeats,

* Correspondence: gt_greating@sina.com; shenkeng.pumc@hotmail.com
[1]Department of Obstetrics and Gynecology, Peking Union Medical College Hospital, Chinese Academy of Medical Sciences and Peking Union Medical College, No.1 Shuaifuyuan, Dongcheng District, Beijing, China
Full list of author information is available at the end of the article

(CRISPR)/Cas9 system has enormous prospects in tumor genesis and progression researches. The technique is highly effective at thoroughly shutting off gene expression with ~ 20 bp guide RNAs (gRNAs) [13, 14], by which can establish ideal cellular models for functional investigation. To date, studies involving the CRISPR/Cas9 technique in ovarian cancer studies are still scarce.

Therefore, we 1) explored the feasibility of the CRISPR/Cas9 system as a genome editing tool to construct BMI1 knock-out EOC cell models, 2) investigated the changes in biological behaviors after silencing BMI1 using in vitro and in vivo experiments, and 3) identified the differences in mRNA profiles between wild-type and BMI1 knock-out EOC cells using transcriptome sequencing technique in order to reveal the potential molecular mechanism. 4) revealed the potential of BMI1 serving as a biomarker in EOC management with basic research evidences.

Methods
Knocking out BMI1 in EOC cell lines using CRISPR/Cas9 technique
Cell culture
The ovarian cancer cell line SKOV3 was obtained from Institute of Basic Medical Sciences Chinese Academy of

Medical Sciences & School of Basic Medicine, Peking Union Medical College. The SKOV3 cells were cultured in McCOY' 5A medium (Macgene; Beijing, CN), supplemented with 10% fetal bovine serum (FBS, HyClone; Logan, UT, US), 100 U/ml penicillin (Solarbio; Beijing, CN), and 100 μg/ml streptomycin (Solarbio; Beijing, CN).

CRISPR/Cas9 vector construction and transfection
Specific gRNAs (Table 1) were designed using http://crispr.mit.edu/, and they were subsequently connected to linear pX330-BbsI vectors. To enhance editing efficiency, two gRNAs were synthesized targeting distinct domains of BMI1. Successively, two expression vectors (pX330-Cas9-gRNA1 and pX330-Cas9-gRNA2) were established, and co-transfected SKOV3 simultaneously with pLLexp-puro plasmid. Then, we used puromycin (1 μg/ml) to screen out those cells which have not been successfully transfected. Eventually, we cultured the viable cells surviving drug-sifting in 96-well plates using limited dilution method and amplified all the single-cell derived sub-clones.

Validation of BMI1 knock-out
Genomic DNA was extracted from each sub-clone for polymerase chain reaction (PCR) and Sanger sequencing

Table 1 Sequences of gRNAs and primers

Name	Sequences (5'- > 3')		PAM/ Length
	Forward	Reverse	
CRISPR gRNAs for BMI1			
gRNA1	CACCGAACGTGTATTGTTCGTT	AAACGGTAACGAACAATACACGTTC	ACC
gRNA2	CACCGTGGTCTGGTCTTGTGAAC	AAACAGTTCACAAGACCAGACCAC	TGG
Primers for PCR			
BMI1[a]	TTGATGCCACAACCATAATAGAAT CTAACACCAATGATTTATCCACTC	AATTACAAACAAGGAATTTCAACA	494 bp 194 bp
Primers for real-time PCR			
Caspase3	GAAATTGTGGAATTGATGCGTGA	CTACAACGATCCCCTCTGAAAAA	166 bp
Bcl-2	CTAAGGGTATGAAGGACCTGTA	CTCTGGAATCTAAAGGTCGT	111 bp
COL1A1	GTGCGATGACGTGATCTGTGA	CGGTGGTTTCTTGGTCGGT	119 bp
COL4A1	GGACTACCTGGAACAAAAGGG	GCCAAGTATCTCACCTGGATCA	240 bp
TNC	TCCCAGTGTTCGGTGGATCT	TTGATGCGATGTGTGAAGACA	131 bp
LAMA3	TGCTCAACTACCGTTCTGCC	TCCAGTTCTTTTGCGCTTTGT	181 bp
ITGA7	CAGCGAGTGGACCAGATCC	CCAAAGAGGAGGTAGTGGCTATC	203 bp
ITGB4	CTCCACCGAGTCAGCCTTC	CGGGTAGTCCTGTGTCCTGTA	133 bp
AKT3	AATGGACAGAAGCTATCCAGGC	TGATGGGTTGTAGAGGCATCC	130 bp
CREB5	AAAGACTGCCCAATAACAGCC	AAGCTGGGACAGGACTAGCA	88 bp
PIK3CA	GAAACAAGACGACTTTGTGACCT	CTTCACGGTTGCCTACTGGT	76 bp
PIK3CD	AGCCGGAAGACTACACGCT	GGTCAGGTGAGGGGTCAAC	122 bp
BIRC3	TTTCCGTGGCTCTTATTCAAACT	GCACAGTGGTAGGAACTTCTCAT	96 bp
GAPDH	ACAACTTTGGTATCGTGGAAGG	GCCATCACGCCACAGTTTC	101 bp

[a]Longer fragments obtained by the first BMI1 primer is more suitable for subsequent Sanger sequencing, whereas the second primer is better for revealing fragments shortening after silencing BMI1 on Agarose gel

of the targeted fragments. PCR primers are listed in Table 1. Protein was subsequently extracted from sub-clones with shortened nucleic acid sequences for western blotting. All validated BMI1 knock-out clones were then amplified and stored.

Comparison of biological behaviors using in vitro and in vivo experiments

MTT assays

Cell viability was detected using MTT assays. Twenty microliters of MTT reagent (5 mg/ml) was added to each well (96-well plate) and incubated for 4 h and then terminated by adding 100 μl dimethylsulfoxide (DMSO) and incubating at 37 °C in the dark for 10 min. Cell proliferation was assessed by measuring the absorbance at 570 nm and 630 nm wavelength (Optical density, $OD_{570-630nm}$). Growth curves were drawn with doubling time calculated for each group by consecutive MTT assays for seven days.

Flow cytometry (FCM)

The cell pattern of each sub-clone was detected using C6 FCM (BD Biosciences; New Jersey, US). Briefly, cell pre-treatment comprised cold-ethanol fixation for 2 h and propidium iodide (PI, Keygene; Wageningen, the Netherlands) staining for 30 min in the dark. Modfit software (Verity; Maine, US) was used for analysis. Similarly, apoptosis could be compared by FCM after Annexin V-fluorescein isothiocyanate (FITC) and PI staining.

Transwell migration and invasion assays

The cell migration assay was performed using a Transwell chamber (BD Falcon™, San Jose, CA). These chambers were inserted into 24-well cell culture plates. Wild-type SKOV3 cells and BMI1 knock-out clones in 200 μl serum-free culture solution were added to the upper chambers. Ten percent FBS-containing McCOY' 5A medium was added into the lower chambers to serve as the chemo-attractant. For invasion assays upper chambers were pre-coated with Matrigel (BD BioCoat™, BD Biosciences, San Jose, CA). After incubation for 24 h, the medium, the gel and uncrossed cells in the upper chambers were removed, while the migrated/invaded cells at the lower side of the membranes were fixed with paraformaldehyde (4%) and stained with crystal violet. Pictures were taken at 200X magnification, and cell numbers from five random microscopic fields were counted for statistical comparison.

Real-time PCR and western blotting

Expression levels of marker proteins in apoptosis were compared between wild-type and BMI1 knock-out cells by real-time PCR and western blotting. Primers and antibodies are listed in Tables 1 and 2, respectively.

Table 2 Antibodies

Name	Corporation	Dilution ratio
BMI1	Cell signaling	1:1000
Caspase3	Abcam	1:1000
Bcl-2	Abcam	1:500
COL1A1	Abcam	1:1000
COL4A1	Bioworld	1:500
TNC	Abcam	1:2000
LAMA3	Abcam	1:2000
ITGA7	Bioworld	1:500
ITGB4	Abcam	1:2000
AKT3	Proteintech	1:500
CREB5	Proteintech	1:500
PIK3CA	Abcam	1:1000
PIK3CD	Abcam	1:500
BIRC3	Abcam	1:1000
β-Tubulin	Bioworld	1:3000
β-Actin	Cell signaling	1:1000

Total RNA was isolated using Trizol reagent (Invitrogen; California, US). For quantitative analysis, mRNA levels of target sequences were compared: RNA was first retro-transcribed with random primers using Trans-Script First-Strand cDNA Synthesis Kit (TransGen; Beijing, CN), and then real-time PCR was carried out using TransStart Tip Green qPCR SuperMix (TransGen; Beijing, CN) with specific primers. The comparative Ct method was used to calculate the relative abundance of mRNA compared to GAPDH expression.

Harvested EOC cells were washed in phosphate buffer (PBS) and lysed in ice-cold cell lysis buffer with freshly added 0.01% protease inhibitor and then incubated on ice for 15 min. Cell debris was discarded after ultrasonic breaking and centrifugation at 14000 rpm for 10 min at 4 °C. Afterwards, the supernatant was run on a sodium-dodecyl sulphate (SDS)-PAGE gel, transferred to a poly-vinylidene fluoride (PVDF) membrane, hybridized with specific antibodies, and developed using electrochemilu-minescence (ECL) methodology.

Chemotherapeutic response

MTT assays were also used to estimate the cells' sensitivity to cisplatin, carboplatin and paclitaxel (National Institutes for Food and Drug Control; CN). Each anti-neoplastic medicine was diluted at gradient concentrations and added to 96-well plates (6 wells per group per concentration). After incubation at 37 °C for 48 h, MTT assays were performed as previously described. With OD_{570nm} and OD_{630nm} detected, the growth inhibition ratio was calculated under each concentration for each group (Formula 1). Afterwards, the drug concentration at which 50% of the cells were prevented from proliferating was obtained using GraphPad Prism 5.0 software (California, US).

$$\left(1 - \frac{\text{Test well } OD_{570\text{-}630nm} - \text{Blank well } OD_{570\text{-}630nm}}{\text{Lowest Concentration well } OD_{570\text{-}630nm} - \text{Blank well } OD_{570\text{-}630nm}}\right) \times 100\%$$

Growth inhibition rate =

Xenografted tumor experiments

Female nude mice (BALB/c) were purchased from Beijing Vital River Laboratory Animal Technology Corporation (Beijing, CN). All mice were housed and fed under specific pathogen-free conditions in an institution approved by the Beijing Laboratory Animal Research Center. All studies were approved and supervised by Peking Union Medical College Hospital. All mice used were 5 weeks old when the experiments initiated. Six mice were assigned per group. Cells cultivated from different groups (2×10^7 cells) were injected subcutaneously. To compare the ability of tumor formation in vivo, the transplanted tumors were checked and dimensioned every 2 days. Feeding was stopped at the same time for each group after 10 weeks. Tumor formation rate and average tumor size (Length×Width^2 × 0.5) were calculated and compared.

Investigation of underlying molecular mechanism using RNA sequencing

Total RNA was extracted from wild-type SKOV3 and BMI1 knock-out clones, and transcriptome libraries were subsequently constructed using a KAPA stranded mRNA-Seq Kit (KAPA Biosystems; Massachusetts, US). High-throughput sequencing was accomplished on a Hiseq2000 platform (Illumina; California, US). Bioinformatics analyses included estimation of gene-expression amount, clustering, GO (Gene ontology) and KEGG (Kyoto Encyclopedia of Genes and Genome). Differential gene-expression profiles were validated by real-time quantitative PCR and western blotting; corresponding primers and antibodies are listed in Tables 1 and 2. Eventually, potential pathways involving BMI1 in tumor genesis and progression were proposed.

Statistical analysis

Biological behaviors and transcriptome profiles were compared between wild-type and BMI1 knock-out EOC cells. Each experiment was performed in triplicate assays and repeated at least three times. All values were expressed as the means ± SD (standard deviation). Statistical significance was determined using two-sided Student's t test or Fish's exact test, and a value of $P < 0.05$ was considered significant. Statistical analyses were performed using Statistical Package for the Social Sciences 20.0 (IBM; New York, US).

Results

Knock-out BMI1 in EOC cells using CRISPR/Cas9 system

Specific gRNAs were inserted into pX330-Cas9 vectors as shown in Fig. 1 with a success rate of 100%. After transfection and drug sifting, we obtained 23 single-cell derived BMI1 knock-out clones after limited-dilution culture. Figure 1 also depicts the validation results of target-gene editing: Agarose electrophoresis results revealed PCR products from the treated group had shortened nucleic acid sequences (9/23, Fig. 1b); target fragments of these sub-clones were confirmed deleted by Sanger sequencing (9/9); and western blotting experiments further verified that all nine sub-clones completely lack expression of BMI1 protein (Fig. 1c).

Silencing BMI1 suppressed cell proliferation, migration and invasion of EOC cells

Growth curves showed that BMI1 knocking out reduced cell proliferation straight from the second through the seventh day, compared to the wild-type SKOV3 (Fig. 2a). The doubling times for BMI1 knock-out and wild-type clones were 2.10 ± 0.7 d and 5.62 ± 1.57 d, respectively ($P < 0.05$). BMI1 silencing also led to cell pattern alteration, as the proportion of EOC cells in S phase significantly decreased (23.7% vs. 12.2%, Fig. 2b). Cell invasiveness assessed using Matrigel-coated Transwell chambers presented a significant inhibition (Fig. 2c). Figure 2d shows reduced migration of SKOV3 cells transfected with CRISPR/Cas9-gRNAs. The numbers of migrated/invaded cells in either group are listed in Table 3. In addition, in vivo experiments (Fig. 2e) revealed that 1) tumor formation rate of subcutaneous inoculation reduced from 100% to 50% after BMI1 silencing and 2) the average xenografted tumor size was dramatically smaller in the BMI1 knock-out group (5.3 mm^3) than in the wild-type group (1986.7 mm^3).

BMI1 knock-out promoted apoptosis of EOC cells

We next examined the effect of BMI1 knocking out on cell apoptosis. First, FCM detected a higher apoptosis rate in BMI1 knock-out EOC cells than in the untreated group ($3.3 \pm 0.2\%$ vs. $1.9 \pm 0.2\%$, $P < 0.05$). Established markers of apoptosis include caspases. Therefore, we determined the expression of caspase 3 cleavages in control and BMI1-gRNAs-transfected EOC cells. An increase of active caspase 3 was observed in BMI1 knock-out cells (Fig. 2f). Bcl-2 suppresses apoptosis in a variety of cell systems, including functioning in a feedback loop system with caspases. We detected a remarkable reduction of Bcl-2 expression after knocking-out BMI1, indicating an ongoing apoptotic process (Fig. 2f, Additional file 1: Figure S1).

Silencing BMI1 enhanced platinum sensitivity of EOC cells

We tested whether BMI1 silencing would affect chemotherapeutic responses of EOC cells. After drawing cell

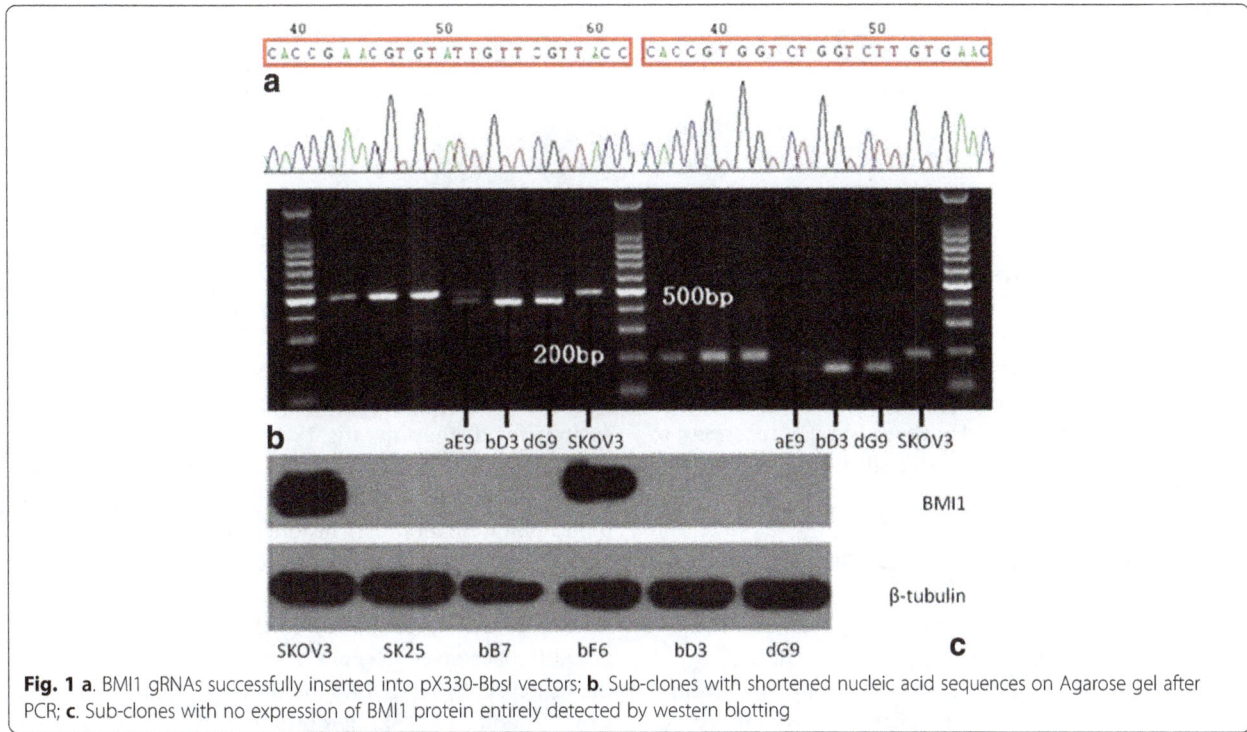

Fig. 1 a. BMI1 gRNAs successfully inserted into pX330-BbsI vectors; **b**. Sub-clones with shortened nucleic acid sequences on Agarose gel after PCR; **c**. Sub-clones with no expression of BMI1 protein entirely detected by western blotting

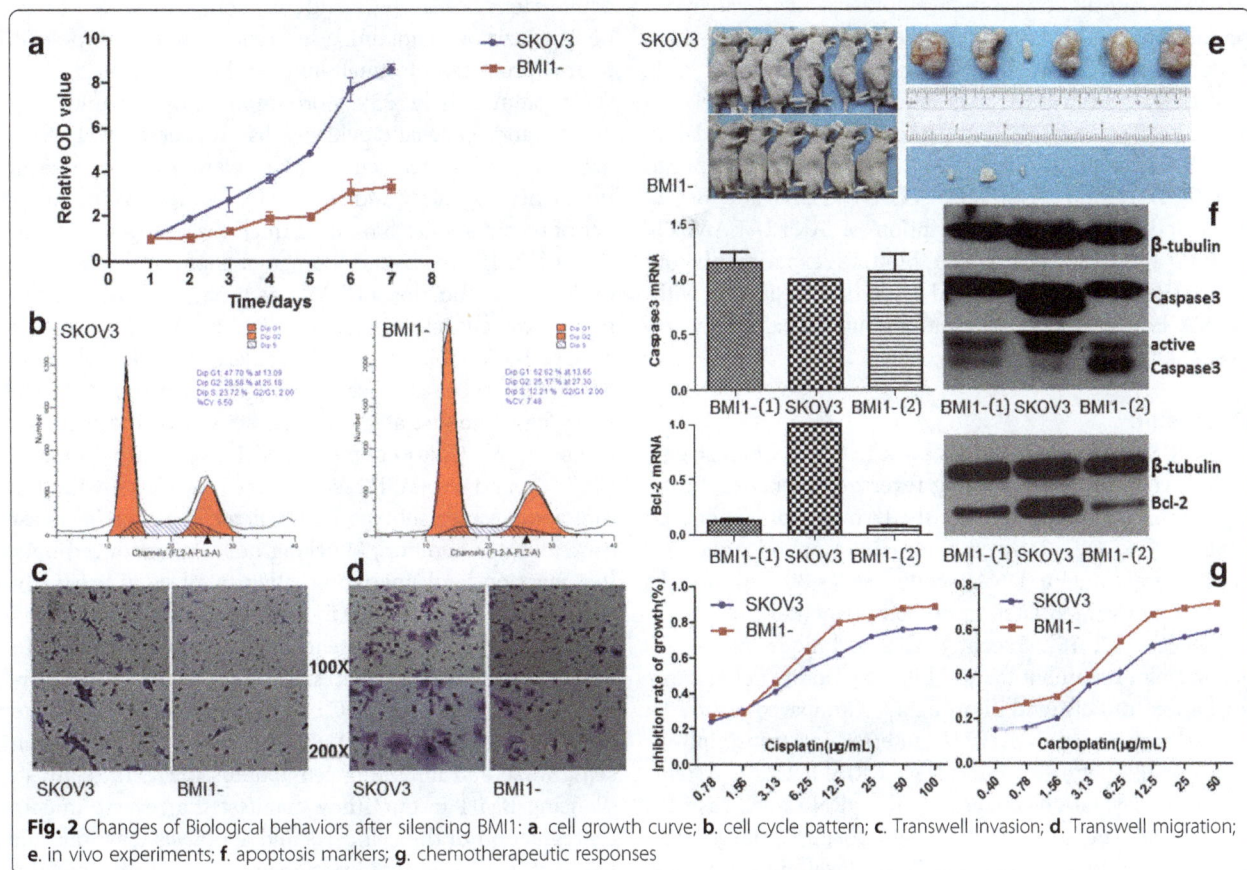

Fig. 2 Changes of Biological behaviors after silencing BMI1: **a**. cell growth curve; **b**. cell cycle pattern; **c**. Transwell invasion; **d**. Transwell migration; **e**. in vivo experiments; **f**. apoptosis markers; **g**. chemotherapeutic responses

Table 3 Results of Transwell experiments and IC50 for anti-neoplastic drugs

Group	Cell numbers (median ± SD)		IC50 (µg/ml)		
	Invasion	Migration	Cisplatin	Carboplatin	Paclitaxel
Wild-type SKOV3	9.2 ± 0.4	27.8 ± 3.2	5.9	14.5	16.6
BMI1 knock-out clone	4.2 ± 1.1	11.0 ± 0.7	3.4	5.2	13.6
P value	< 0.05	< 0.05	< 0.05	< 0.05	> 0.05

growth inhibition curves under gradient drug concentrations (Fig. 2g), IC50s of either sub-clone to cisplatin, carboplatin and paclitaxel were calculated (Table 3). The data demonstrated that BMI1 knock-out sensitized EOC cells to platinum medications ($P < 0.05$), including both cisplatin and carboplatin. However, similar reactions to paclitaxel were observed in BMI1-silenced and untreated cells ($P > 0.05$).

BMI1 modulated focal adhesion and PI3K/AKT pathways in EOC cells

Total RNA extracted from either group was qualified for RNA sequencing, revealing appropriate $OD_{260nm/280nm}$ values (1.8–2.0) and abundances (≥5.0 µg per group). Raw reads were filtered and aligned to reference sequences. With GO analyses, we demonstrated that the majority of differentially expressed genes after BMI1 silencing participated in extracellular matrix (ECM) construction and blood vessel development. KEGG analyses revealed that BMI1 might alter the biological behaviors of EOC cells by modulating the focal adhesion and PI3K/AKT pathways. Expressions levels of related markers at both mRNA and protein levels were validated (Fig. 3): shutting-off BMI1 down-regulated transcription of COL1A1, COL4A1, TNC, ITGA7, ITGB4 and Bcl-2, while it up-regulated transcription of AKT3, LAMA3, CREB5 and BIRC3. Western blotting experiments on translational aspects showed results consistent with mRNA levels, except for additional under-expression of PIK3CA protein.

Discussion

The CRISPR technique traces back to 1987, when scientists discovered corresponding reverse sequences following certain DNA fragments at the terminus of a bacterial genome [15, 16]. Between these short palindromic repeats were random DNA sequences (~ 30 bp), which were demonstrated later to be complementary to phage sequences [17, 18]. Recently, this technique has been generating excitement for its ability to modify genetic information rapidly and thoroughly. Compared to traditional techniques (e.g. RNA interfering, transcription activator-like effector nuclease), CRISPR/Cas9 system possesses several advantages: 1) the gRNAs are easy to design and stable in double-chain form; 2) target sequences are directly cut on DNA level, inducing an entire shut-off of gene expression; 3) multiple genes could be edited simultaneously, and DNA sequences could be knock-in as well as knock-out [13, 14]. We have successfully applied the CRISPR/Cas9 system and established a stable EOC cell model with BMI1 silenced entirely for further investigations.

BMI1 protein is one component of the polycomb repressive complex 1 (PRC1), which catalyzes lysine 119 mono-ubiquitination of histone H2A (H2AK119Ub1). H2AK119Ub1 is thought to contribute to gene silencing through the induction of chromatin compaction and inhibition of transcriptional elongation [19–21]. BMI1 has a broad impact on a diversity of cellular events: it controls the cell cycle by regulating the tumor suppressor proteins p16[INK4a] and p14[ARF] [22]; it promotes cell proliferation by suppressing the p16[INK4a]/retinoblastoma and/or the p14[ARF]/MDM2/p53 pathways [10]; it bypasses senescence and immortalizes cells by inducing telomerase activity in adult stem cells [9]; and it contributes to tissue homeostasis by maintaining self-renewal of hematopoietic, neural, prostate, intestinal, lung epithelial and bronchoalveolar stem cells [5, 23]. More importantly, accumulating genetic and epigenetic evidence has revealed BMI1, serving as a cancer stem cell marker, plays a crucial role in tumor heterogeneity and relapse [6, 24]. A growing number of recent studies have confirmed the oncogenic activation of BMI1 in diverse human malignancies and have explored the function of BMI1 as a pathway regulator in both stem cells and cancer cells [25, 26]. We discovered a remarkable inhibition of cell proliferation from silencing BMI1, with more EOC cells staying in G1 phase. A recent study has demonstrated that the activity of the estrogen receptor α (ERα)-coupled BMI1 signature impacts p16[INK4a] and cyclin D1 status and correlates with the tumor molecular subtype and biologic behavior in breast cancer [9]. In addition, knocking out BMI1 reduced both the invasion and migration abilities of EOC cells. In accordance, other studies found that BMI1 was involved in inducing epithelial mesenchymal transition, leading to tumor invasion and metastasis [26]. Moreover, overexpression of BMI1 in EOC cells was found to up-regulate the expression of cyclin D1, CDK4 and Bcl-2, promoting cell growth and inhibiting cell apoptosis [27]. In contrast, silencing BMI1 in our study manifested a reverse impact on regulation of the cell cycle and apoptosis. Last but not the least, we found that knocking out BMI1 enhanced the

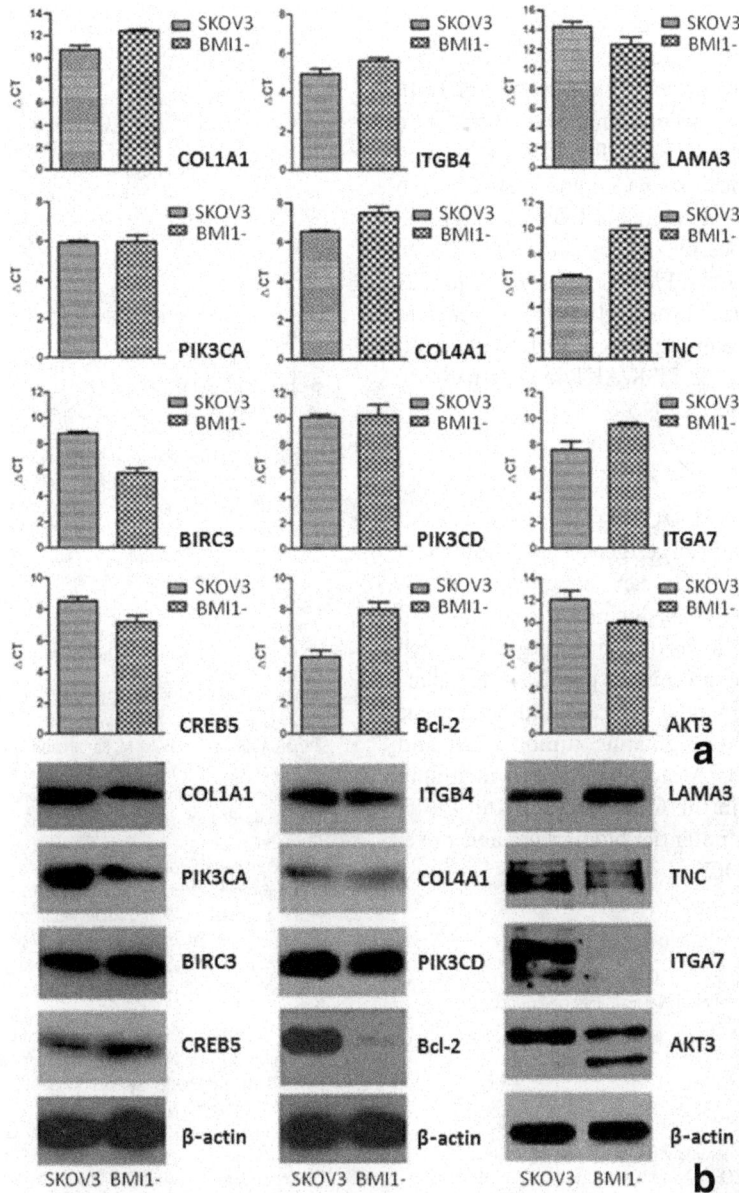

Fig. 3 Validation of RNA sequencing results by **a**. RT-PCR; **b**. western blotting

platinum sensitivity of EOC cells. Similarly, Wang et al. revealed that down-regulating BMI1 increased the amount of reactive oxygen species, stimulated the DNA damage repair pathway, and eventually promoted the cisplatin-induced apoptosis [28]. Altogether, these evidences might shed light upon the most vexing conundrum in EOC management: chemo-resistance.

The CRISPR/Cas9 technique has provided an excellent cell model for analysis of one single variable: BMI1. We further investigated the most relevant genes using RNA sequencing. Most genes differentially expressed after silencing BMI1 were engaged in tissue development, ECM organization and blood vessel development, which might alter the microenvironment and angiogenesis of tumors, and then lead to transformation of malignant phenotypes: decrease in COL1A1 and COL4A1 might redress the reconstruction disorder of ECM [29, 30]; regulation of TNC and LAMA could increase tissue tension, reduce invasion and prevent migration of ovarian cancer cells [31, 32]. However, the clinical significance of these biomarkers in EOC management still needs validation because of controversial results from different studies. Furthermore, KEGG analyses revealed that the focal adhesion and PI3K/AKT pathways were involved after silencing BMI1. Aberrant expression of focal adhesion kinase (FAK) was related to the uncontrolled proliferation, suppressed apoptosis, invasion, angiogenesis and immune-depression of tumor cells [33]. One meta-analysis demonstrated that up-regulation of FAK indicated shorter overall survival in a variety of human cancers with a pooled hazards ratio of 1.815 and site specificity [34]. A growing number of studies have proved the activation of the PI3K/AKT/mTOR pathway in EOC [35–38], although the Cancer Genome Atlas research detected a low mutational rate (< 5%) of PI3KCA, AKT and PTEN in high-grade serous ovarian carcinomas (HsOCs) [39]. Other research found that PI3K genes were frequently mutated in non-HsOCs, which were relatively insensitive to platinum [38]. Another promising thing is that diverse anti-neoplastic drugs targeting the PI3K/AKT/mTOR pathway are under clinical investigations [39, 40].

Conclusions

It is feasible to use the CRISPR/Cas9 system to construct ideal EOC cell models with target gene expression thoroughly shut off. Silencing BMI1 can change various biological behaviors of EOC cells, including reducing cell proliferation, migration, invasion, and promoting cell death; BMI1 might be a promising predictor for platinum sensitivity. BMI1 may accelerate tumor genesis and metastasis through dysregulating tumor ECM and blood vessel assemblies. Molecular traits, including BMI1 and crucial genes in the focal adhesion and PI3K/AKT pathways, might be potential biomarkers and novel therapeutic targets for EOC.

Funding

This study was supported by the National Natural Science Foundation of China (No 81402140 and No 81372780).

Authors' contributions

Conceptualization: ZQ, GT, SK; Formal analysis: ZQ, QQ, GT; Funding acquisition: GT, SK; Investigation: ZQ, QQ; Methodology: ZQ, QQ; Project administration: GT, SK; Resources: ZQ, QQ, CD, YJ, GT, SK; Software: ZQ, QQ; Supervision: CD, YJ, SK; Validation: ZQ, CD, YJ, GT; Writing - original draft: ZQ; Writing - review & editing: GT, CD, YJ, SK. All authors read and approved the final manuscript.

Competing interests

The authors declare that they have no competing interests.

Author details

[1]Department of Obstetrics and Gynecology, Peking Union Medical College Hospital, Chinese Academy of Medical Sciences and Peking Union Medical College, No.1 Shuaifuyuan, Dongcheng District, Beijing, China. [2]Department of Gynecology and Obstetrics, West China Second University Hospital, Sichuan University, Key Laboratory of Birth Defects and Related Diseases of Women and Children (Sichuan University), Ministry of Education, Chengdu, China. [3]Department of Obstetrics and Gynecology, Qilu Hospital of Shandong University, Shandong, China.

References

1. Tangjitgamol S, Manusirivithaya S, Laopaiboon M, Lumbiganon P. Interval debulking surgery for advanced epithelial ovarian cancer: a Cochrane systematic review. Gynecol Oncol. 2009;112(1):257–64.
2. Torre LA, Bray F, Siegel RL, Ferlay J, Lortet-Tieulent J, Jemal A. Global cancer statistics, 2012. CA Cancer J Clin. 2015;65(2):87–108.
3. Tanda ET, Budroni M, Cesaraccio R, Palmieri G, Palomba G, Capobianco G, et al. Epidemiology of ovarian cancer in North Sardinia, Italy, during the period 1992-2010. Eur J Gynaecol Oncol. 2015;36(1):69–72.
4. Bracken AP, Kleine-Kohlbrecher D, Dietrich N, Pasini D, Gargiulo G, Beekman C, et al. The Polycomb group proteins bind throughout the INK4A-ARF locus and are disassociated in senescent cells. Genes Dev. 2007;21(5):525–30.
5. Siddique HR, Saleem M. Role of BMI1, a stem cell factor, in cancer recurrence and chemoresistance: preclinical and clinical evidences. Stem Cells. 2012;30(3):372–8.
6. Song LB, Zeng MS, Liao WT, Zhang L, Mo HY, Liu WL, Set a. Bmi-1 is a novel molecular marker of nasopharyngeal carcinoma progression and immortalizes primary human nasopharyngeal epithelial cells. Cancer Res. 2006;66(12):6225–32.
7. Huber GF, Albinger-Hegyi A, Soltermann A, Roessle M, Graf N, Haerle SK, et al. Expression patterns of Bmi-1 and p16 significantly correlate with overall, disease-specific, and recurrence-free survival in oropharyngeal squamous cell carcinoma. Cancer. 2011;117(20):4659–70.
8. Crea F, Duhagon Serrat MA, Hurt EM, Thomas SB, Danesi R, Farrar WL. BMI1 silencing enhances docetaxel activity and impairs antioxidant response in prostate cancer. Int J Cancer. 2011;128(8):1946–54.
9. Wang H, Liu H, Li X, Zhao J, Zhang H, Mao J, et al. Estrogen receptor α-coupled Bmi1 regulation pathway in breast cancer and its clinical implications. BMC Cancer. 2014;14:122.
10. Park IK, Morrison SJ, Clarke MF. Bmi1, stem cells, and senescence regulation. Clin Invest. 2004;113(2):175–9.
11. Engelsen IB, Mannelqvist M, Stefansson IM, Carter SL, Beroukhim R, Øyan AM, et al. Low BMI-1 expression is associated with an activated BMI-1-driven signature, vascular invasion, and hormone receptor loss in endometrial carcinoma. Br J Cancer. 2008;98(10):1662–9.
12. Gui T, Bai H, Zeng J, Zhong Z, Cao D, Cui Q, et al. Tumor heterogeneity in the recurrence of epithelial ovarian cancer demonstrated by polycomb group proteins. Onco Targets Ther. 2014;7:1705–16.
13. Hsu PD, Lander ES, Zhang F. Development and applications of CRISPR-Cas9 for genome engineering. Cell. 2014;157(6):1262–78.
14. Cho SW, Kim S, Kim JM, Kim JS. Targeted genome engineering in human cells with the Cas9 RNA-guided endonuclease. Nat Biotechnol. 2013;31(3):230–2.
15. Ishino Y, Shinagawa H, Makino K, Amemura M, Nakata A. Nucleotide sequence of the iap gene, responsible for alkaline phosphatase isozyme conversion in Escherichia coli, and identification of the gene product. J Bacteriol. 1987;169(12):5429–33.
16. Mojica FJ, Díez-Villaseñor C, Soria E, Juez G. Biological significance of a family of regularly spaced repeats in the genomes of archaea, Bacteria and mitochondria. Mol Microbiol. 2000;36(1):244–6.
17. Pennisi E. The CRISPR craze. Science. 2013;341(6148):833–6.
18. Barrangou R, Fremaux C, Deveau H, Richards M, Boyaval P, Moineau S, et al. CRISPR provides acquired resistance against viruses in prokaryotes. Science. 2007;315(5819):1709–12.
19. Morey L, Helin K. Polycomb group protein-mediated repression of transcription. Trends Biochem Sci. 2010;35(6):323–32.
20. Francis NJ, Kingston RE, Woodcock CL. Chromatin compaction by a polycomb group protein complex. Science. 2004;306(5701):1574–7.
21. Zhou W, Zhu P, Wang J, Pascual G, Ohgi KA, Lozach J, et al. Histone H2A monoubiquitination represses transcription by inhibiting RNA polymerase II transcriptional elongation. Mol Cell. 2008;29(1):69–80.
22. Abd El hafez A, El-Hadaad HA. Immunohistochemical expression and prognostic relevance of Bmi-1, a stem cell factor, in epithelial ovarian cancer. Ann Diagn Pathol. 2014;18(2):58–62.
23. Molofsky AV, He S, Bydon M, Morrison SJ, Pardal R. Bmi-1 promotes neural stem cell self-renewal and neural development but not mouse growth and survival by repressing the p16Ink4a and p19Arf senescence pathways. Genes Dev. 2005;19(12):1432–7.
24. Allegra E, Trapasso S, Pisani D, Puzzo L. The role of BMI1 as a biomarker of cancer stem cells in head and neck cancer: a review. Oncology. 2014;86(4):199–205.

25. Bhattacharya R, Nicoloso M, Arvizo R, Wang E, Cortez A, Rossi S, et al. MiR-15a and MiR-16 control Bmi-1 expression in ovarian cancer. Cancer Res. 2009;69(23):9090–5.

26. Koren A, Rijavec M, Kern I, Sodja E, Korosec P, Cufer T. BMI1, ALDH1A1, and CD133 transcripts connect epithelial-mesenchymal transition to Cancer stem cells in lung carcinoma. Stem Cells Int. 2016;2016:9714315.

27. Kim BR, Kwon Y, Rho SB. BMI-1 interacts with sMEK1 and inactivates sMEK1-induced apoptotic cell death. Oncol Rep. 2017;37(1):579–86.

28. Wang E, Bhattacharyya S, Szabolcs A, Rodriguez-Aguayo C, Jennings NB, Lopez-Berestein G, et al. Enhancing chemotherapy response with Bmi-1 silencing in ovarian cancer. PLoS One. 2011;6(3):e17918.

29. Wilson KE, Bartlett JM, Miller EP, Smyth JF, Mullen P, Miller WR, et al. Regulation and function of the extracellular matrix protein tenascin-C in ovarian cancer cell lines. Br J Cancer. 1999;80(5–6):685–92.

30. Campo E, Merino MJ, Tavassoli FA, Charonis AS, Stetler-Stevenson WG, Liotta LA. Evaluation of basement membrane components and the 72 kDa type IV collagenase in serous tumors of the ovary. Am J Surg Pathol. 1992;16(5):500–7.

31. Byers LJ, Osborne JL, Carson LF, Carter JR, Haney AF, Weinberg JB, et al. Increased levels of laminin in ascitic fluid of patients with ovarian cancer. Cancer Lett. 1995;88(1):67–72.

32. Didem T, Faruk T, Senem K, Derya D, Murat S, Murat G, et al. Clinical significance of serum tenascin-c levels in epithelial ovarian cancer. Tumour Biol. 2014;35(7):6777–82.

33. Sulzmaier FJ, Jean C, Schlaepfer DD. FAK in cancer: mechanistic findings and clinical applications. Nat Rev Cancer. 2014;14(9):598–610.

34. de Graeff P, Crijns AP, de Jong S, Boezen M, Post WJ, de Vries EG, et al. Modest effect of p53, EGFR and HER-2/neu on prognosis in epithelial ovarian cancer: a meta-analysis. Br J Cancer. 2009;101(1):149–59.

35. Levine DA, Bogomolniy F, Yee CJ, Lash A, Barakat RR, Borgen PI, et al. Frequent mutation of the PIK3CA gene in ovarian and breast cancers. Clin Cancer Res. 2005;11(8):2875–8.

36. Bai H, Li H, Li W, Gui T, Yang J, Cao D, et al. The PI3K/AKT/mTOR pathway is a potential predictor of distinct invasive and migratory capacities in human ovarian cancer cell lines. Oncotarget. 2015;6(28):25520–32.

37. Carpten JD, Faber AL, Horn C, Donoho GP, Briggs SL, Robbins CM, et al. A transforming mutation in the pleckstrin homology domain of AKT1 in cancer. Nature. 2007;448(7152):439–44.

38. Kuo KT, Mao TL, Jones S, Veras E, Ayhan A, Wang TL, et al. Frequent activating mutations of PIK3CA in ovarian clear cell carcinoma. Am J Pathol. 2009;174(5):1597–601. 6

39. Verhaak RG, Tamayo P, Yang JY, Hubbard D, Zhang H, Creighton CJ, et al. Cancer genome atlas research network. Prognostically relevant gene signatures of high-grade serous ovarian carcinoma. J Clin Invest. 2013;123(1):517–25.

40. Engelman JA, Chen L, Tan X, Crosby K, Guimaraes AR, Upadhyay R, et al. Effective use of PI3K and MEK inhibitors to treat mutant Kras G12D and PIK3CA H1047R murine lung cancers. Nat Med. 2008;14(12):1351–6.

9

Wounding promotes ovarian cancer progression and decreases efficacy of cisplatin in a syngeneic mouse model

Yooyoung Lee[1,2,3], Alexandra Kollara[2], Taymaa May[1,3†] and Theodore J. Brown[2,3*†] (iD)

Abstract

Background: Primary cytoreductive surgery followed by adjuvant chemotherapy is the standard treatment for advanced epithelial ovarian cancer. The average interval between surgery and chemotherapy initiation is approximately 4-weeks at most centers; however, since surgery may accelerate residual tumor growth, a shorter interval may be more beneficial.

Methods: The murine ID8 cell model of ovarian cancer was used to examine the efficacy of cisplatin treatment administered perioperatively or 7 days after surgical wounding. Luciferase-expressing cells ID8 cells were injected intraperitoneally (i.p.) into female C57/Bl6 mice. Fourteen days post-injection, animals received an abdominal incision or anesthesia alone and received i.p. cisplatin either on the surgical day or 7 days later, or received no chemotherapy. Additional animals received cisplatin 28 days after wounding for comparison.

Results: Abdominal tumor mass increased 2.5-fold in wounded vs. unwounded animals as determined by bioluminescent in vivo tumor imaging. Cisplatin administered on the day of wounding decreased tumor burden by 50%, as compared to 90% in unwounded animals. Cisplatin on day 7 or day 28 decreased tumor burden by 80 and 37% respectively.

Conclusions: Surgical wounding increases ovarian tumor mass and decreases perioperative cisplatin efficacy in this animal model. Administration of cisplatin 1 week after surgery was more effective than cisplatin administered perioperatively or 4 weeks after surgery.

Keywords: Ovarian cancer, ID8 cells, Wound healing, Cisplatin, Mouse, Chemoresistance

Background

Advanced epithelial ovarian cancer has a poor prognosis with a 5-year survival rate of less than 40% [1]. Standard treatment consists of a combination of maximal cytoreductive surgery followed by adjuvant chemotherapy to eliminate residual macroscopic or microscopic disease [2, 3]. Despite this approach, disease recurs in more than 70% of patients, underscoring the inability of this treatment strategy to cure the disease. Ovarian cancer patients who achieve microscopic as compared to macroscopic residual disease at primary surgical cytoreduction have a significantly longer overall survival [4]. Thus, a key therapeutic goal is to optimize chemotherapy efficacy to maximize residual tumor elimination.

Ovarian cancer patients generally begin adjuvant chemotherapy 3–5 weeks after primary cytoreductive surgery [5], although there is no consensus regarding the optimal postoperative waiting period. Delayed initiation of chemotherapy could negatively impact survival since factors released during wound healing can act to promote proliferation of residual tumor cells [6, 7]. A case series of 8 patients with testicular cancer found dramatic exacerbation of residual disease after cytoreductive surgery [8]. Similarly, work by Retsky and colleagues [9] indicated that surgery may reawaken dormant breast cancer cells. A tumor-promoting effect of surgery is

* Correspondence: brown@lunenfeld.ca

†Taymaa May and Theodore J. Brown contributed equally to this work.
2Lunenfeld-Tanenbaum Research Institute at Sinai Health Systems, Mt. Sinai Hospital, 60 Murray Street, 6-10016-3, Toronto, ON M5T 3L9, Canada
3Department of Obstetrics and Gynecology, University of Toronto, Toronto, ON, Canada
Full list of author information is available at the end of the article

further supported by studies using animal models of breast and colorectal cancers, where incomplete or non-curative surgery was performed to determine the impact on residual disease. In these models, surgery increased proliferation of residual tumor cells and accelerated tumor growth [10, 11].

Administration of chemotherapy near the time of surgery may mitigate surgery-induced increased tumor growth since actively dividing cells are most susceptible to chemotherapeutic agents. Reducing the interval between surgery and initiation of adjuvant chemotherapy associates with better survival in patients with early breast [12] and colorectal cancer [13]. In a post-trial ad hoc analysis of Gynecologic Oncology protocol 218, which investigated the time from surgery to initiation of chemotherapy in advanced ovarian carcinoma, Tewari et al. [5] found earlier initiation of chemotherapy (time intervals less than 25 days) was associated with improved overall survival in those patients with microscopic residual disease. Importantly, a study with cyclophosphamide in a subcutaneous mouse mammary tumor model indicates that perioperative administration of chemotherapy is most effective in decreasing residual tumor growth after cytoreductive surgery [14]. Surprisingly, studies addressing the interval from primary surgery to adjuvant chemotherapy in animal models of ovarian cancer have not been reported.

In the present study, we used the widely accepted ID8 animal model of ovarian cancer to determine if surgical abdominal wounding impacts peritoneal dissemination of tumor expansion and the efficacy of cisplatin administered at either the time of surgical wounding or 1 week later. These cells were derived by Roby and coworkers [15] from mouse ovarian surface epithelial cells that had spontaneously transformed in repeated passage tissue culture. Advantages to this model include its recapitulation of high-grade serous ovarian cancer [16], the most commonly diagnosed epithelial ovarian cancer histotype, and the ability to use non-immunocompromised syngeneic C57Bl6 mice. In this model, cells were injected intraperitoneally (i.p.) at a level to reflect a clinical situation of microscopic residual disease following cytoreductive surgery.

Methods
Cell culture
ID8-luciferase expressing cells were generated by stably co-transfecting ID8 cells (obtained from Dr. Jim Petrik, University of Guelph, Guelph, ON, Canada) with pCMV-hyPBase (Trust Sanger Institute, Cambridge, UK) [17] and the PB-CAG-Luciferase-IRES-eGFP-pA vector (provided by Dr. Andras Nagy, Lunenfeld-Tanenbaum Research Institute, Toronto, ON, Canada), in 1:3 ratio using lipofectamine 2000 (Invitrogen, Burlington, ON,

Canada). Cells were grown in RPMI 1640 medium without phenol red, supplemented with 5% heat-inactivated normal fetal bovine serum, 100 units/mL penicillin and 100 μg/mL streptomycin (Invitrogen) in a humidified chamber with 5% CO_2 at 37°C. Transfected cells were clonally selected in medium supplemented with 1 μg/ml puromycin (Invitrogen) and were initially screened for luciferase activity using a Luciferase Assay System (Promega) and a GloMAX microplate luminometer (Promega, Madison, WI, USA).

Animals
C57/Bl6 female mice 6–8 weeks of age were obtained from Charles River Laboratories (Sherbrooke, QC, Canada) and group-housed under standard conditions in accordance with the guidelines of the Canadian Council on Animal Care. Mice were maintained on a 12–12 h light-dark schedule and were provided food and water ad libitum. All animal procedures were approved by the University of Toronto Animal Care and Use Committee.

ID8-Luc 11 cells (5×10^6 cells in 0.2 ml phosphate-buffered saline; PBS) were injected intraperitoneally (i.p.) to mimic peritoneal dissemination. Surgical wounding simulating a laparotomy was performed under isoflurane anesthesia (Baxter, Deerfield, IL, USA) and consisted of a single 1.5 cm midventral abdominal incision through the skin and musculature and gentle exploration of the intra-peritoneal cavity. The abdominal wall was closed with absorbable sutures. Control animals were subjected to anesthesia without surgical wounding. Cisplatin (Sigma, St. Louis, MO, USA) was dissolved in PBS (1.4 mg/ml) and administered i.p. as a single dose (14 mg/kg) [18] immediately after surgery, or 7 or 28 days after surgery. Animals were evaluated daily for tumor growth, ascites accumulation, and postoperative complications including wound problems. Animals were weighed and given health assessments at least every other day. Animals were euthanized by CO_2 inhalation followed by cervical dislocation 12 weeks after tumor cell inoculation or upon evidence of excessive ascites formation, 20% weight gain or loss, signs of debilitation, or wound ulceration.

In vivo bioluminescent imaging
Bioluminescent imaging was performed on an IVIS Spectrum In Vivo Imaging System (Perkin Elmer, Rodgau, Germany). As recommended by the manufacturer, the auto-exposure setting was used to automatically set the exposure time, f/stop and binning to keep the signal within an optimal range for quantification and to avoid overexposure during image acquisition. Auto-exposure sensitivity settings used for the snapshot image were adjusted to obtain a minimal target count of 3000.

Luminescence was measured as total flux (photons per second (P/S)).

Two highly expressing clones (ID8–11 and ID8–15) were subjected to bioluminescent imaging to select the best clone for in vivo study. Cells were seeded in 100 μl medium at varying concentrations into 96-well black culture plates. An equal amount of in vivo glow solution (D-Luciferin, Promega) was added just prior to imaging. Images were acquired with a 12.8 cm width field of view, 2×2 binning factor, and an exposure time of 1 s.

For in vivo imaging of dissemination of tumor cells, animals were anesthetized with 1.5–2.5% isoflurane inhalation, maintained throughout the imaging procedure. Animals received 150 mg D-luciferin/kg body weight i.p. at a concentration of 15 mg/L, 8 min prior to imaging. Images were acquired with a 12.8 cm field of view, 4×4 binning factor, and an exposure time ranging from 0.5–1 s.

Serum collection

Blood was collected via cardiac puncture just prior to necropsy and centrifuged for 10 min at 500 g. Serum from each group of animals were pooled and filtered through a 0.22-μm syringe filter (Millipore, Burlington, MA, USA) and stored at − 80 °C.

XTT dye-reduction assay

ID8 or ID8 luciferase-expressing cells (ID8–11 and ID8–15) were seeded into 96-well plates at 2.0×10^3 cells per well. Cisplatin was added 24 h after seeding and cell number was determined by XTT dye-reduction assay. Briefly, 50 μl of XTT (Invitrogen) solution (1 mg/ml) were added to each well. Following incubation for 3 h in a humidified 5% CO_2 atmosphere at 37 °C, reduced XTT was measured spectrophotometrically at 492 nm using a microtiter plate reader.

To determine the impact of serum on cell growth, ID8 cells were seeded into 96-well plates at 2.0×10^3 cells per well. Culture medium was replaced 24 h after seeding with fresh medium supplemented to 10% (vol/vol) with mouse serum. Cells were incubated in the presence or absence of 10 μM cisplatin for 72 h. Cell number was determined by XTT dye reduction as described.

Statistical analysis

Data are expressed as mean ± SEM and were analyzed by one-way ANOVA followed by a Fisher LSD Multiple Comparison Test using Prism v7 (Graphpad Software, La Jolla, CA, USA). A natural log transformation was applied to the datasets if Bartlett's test indicated unequal variances. Survival outcome is presented as Kaplan-Meier survival curves and was analyzed using the Log-Rank (Mantel-Cox) Test. Data on ascites development were compared using a Chi-square analysis. Data were considered statistically significant at $p < 0.05$.

Results

ID8 cells were transfected with a constitutively active luciferase expression vector to enable noninvasive longitudinal assessment of tumor burden in vivo. Transfected cells were clonally selected and screened for luciferase activity. Out of 15 clones screened, ID8-L11 and ID8-L15, were found to express high levels of luciferase activity (Additional file 1: Table S1) and robust growth. Luciferase activity assays and bioluminescent imaging of these two sublines in vitro indicated a linear relationship between luciferase activity and cell number (Fig. 1a and b). Parental ID8 cells were growth inhibited in culture by 25 or 50 μM cisplatin (Fig. 1c), with both cell sublines exhibiting similar sensitivity to these doses and to 10 μM cisplatin (Fig. 1d and e). ID8-L11 cells produced a stronger bioluminescence signal than ID8-L15 cells, imparting a greater sensitivity for detection while maintaining a dose-dependent response to cisplatin; therefore, these cells were selected for further study.

The ability to detect ID8-L11 cells in vivo was tested in a preliminary study. C57/Bl6 mice were injected i.p. with 5×10^6 cells 13 days prior to imaging. On day 14, mice were anesthetized and subjected to surgical wounding (abdominal incision; $n = 6$) or left unwounded ($n = 6$). Half of the animals in each group were treated with i.p. cisplatin and animals were sacrificed 4 days later following cardiac puncture (Fig. 2a). Bioluminescence was not detectable in control mice not injected with ID8-L11 cells ($n = 3$) whereas all mice injected with the cells exhibited abdominal luminescence consistent with the presence of luciferase-expressing cells (Fig. 2b). Neither macroscopic tumor formation nor ascites were detected at the time of necropsy in any of the animals (Fig. 2c), indicating that this model is representative of microscopic residual disease following primary cytoreductive surgery.

To determine if factors released into the serum as a result of wounding affect the growth of cancer cells in vitro, ID8 cells were cultured with medium supplemented to 10% with pooled sera obtained from the four treatment groups, in either the presence or absence of 25 μM cisplatin. No difference in cell viability or response to cisplatin was apparent due to exposure to sera from the different treatment groups (Fig. 2d; $p > 0.05$).

To determine the impact of surgical wounding on disease progression and sensitivity to cisplatin, 72 mice were injected with ID8-L11 cells and imaged 13 days later. Two mice died prior to imaging and two mice had no detectable tumor cells. The remaining animals were stratified to the amount of disease present in pretreatment imaging and were assigned to seven treatment groups: Group S = surgery alone; Group S + C_0 = surgery

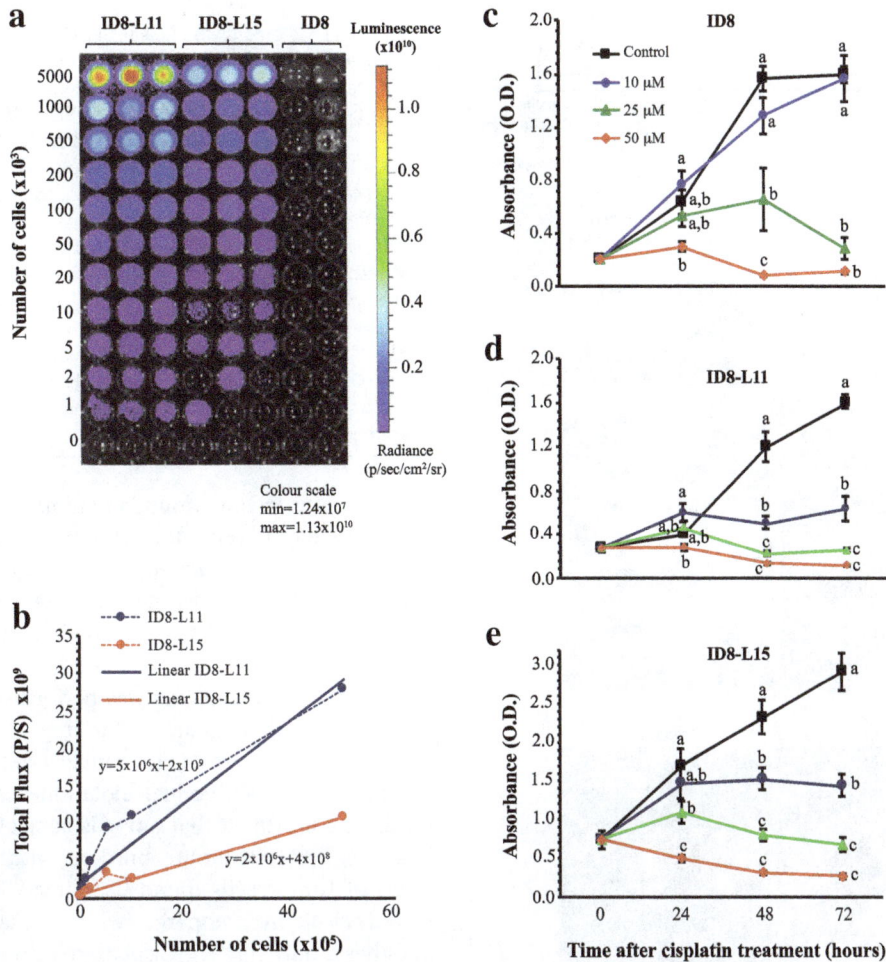

Fig. 1 Bioluminescent luciferase activity and sensitivity to cisplatin of ID8-L11 and ID8-L15 cells in vitro. **a** Concentration-dependent bioluminesence imaging of both cell sublines compared to non-luciferase expressing parental ID8 cells. Different concentrations of cells were added to a 96-well tissue culture plate and imaged on an IVIS Spectrum In Vivo Imaging System. **b** Graphical representation of the quantitation of images shown in Panel A (dashed lines). Solid lines indicate a linear fitting of the data. **c-e** Response of cells to cisplatin. Parental ID8 (**c**), ID8-L11 (**d**), or ID8-L15 (**e**) cells were seeded into 96 well plates. One day later, cells were treated with 0, 10, 25, or 50 μM cisplatin and relative cell viability was determined by a XTT dye-reduction assay. Points represent the mean ± SEM of 8 determinations. Within each time point, points with different letters are statistically different from one another as determined by ANOVA followed by SNK multiple comparison test ($p < 0.05$)

plus cisplatin on the same day; Group S + C$_7$ = surgery plus cisplatin on post-operative day (POD) 7; Group S + C$_{28}$ = surgery plus cisplatin on POD 28; Group A = anesthesia alone; Group A + C$_0$ = anesthesia plus cisplatin on the same day; Group A + C$_7$ = surgery plus cisplatin on POD 7. Animals were reimaged 21 or 35 days after wounding or control (anesthesia only) treatment (Fig. 3a). Several mice died during or within 3 days of surgery/anesthesia or were euthanized because of superficial wound dehiscence (Fig. 3b). As a result, 61 mice were imaged at all three time points and were further followed for indications of significant ascites (moribund), excessive weight gain or loss, or debilitation (cachexia, hunched back with tremor, increased respiratory frequency), which were taken as a surrogate for death. The

study was terminated 13 weeks after tumor cell injection.

There were no differences between groups in overall change in body weight during the study duration (Fig. 4a, $p = 0.8271$). Animals assigned to anesthesia alone appeared to have the greatest incidence of ascites development (Fig. 4b); however, chi-square analysis indicated the differences in ascites occurrences between treatment groups was not statistically significant ($p = 0.160$).

There was a statistically significant overall impact of treatment group on survival ($p = 0.0012$). In general, lower survival was observed for mice that received anesthesia alone or surgery combined with perioperative cisplatin. Highest survival was observed for animals that received cisplatin on day 7, regardless of surgical

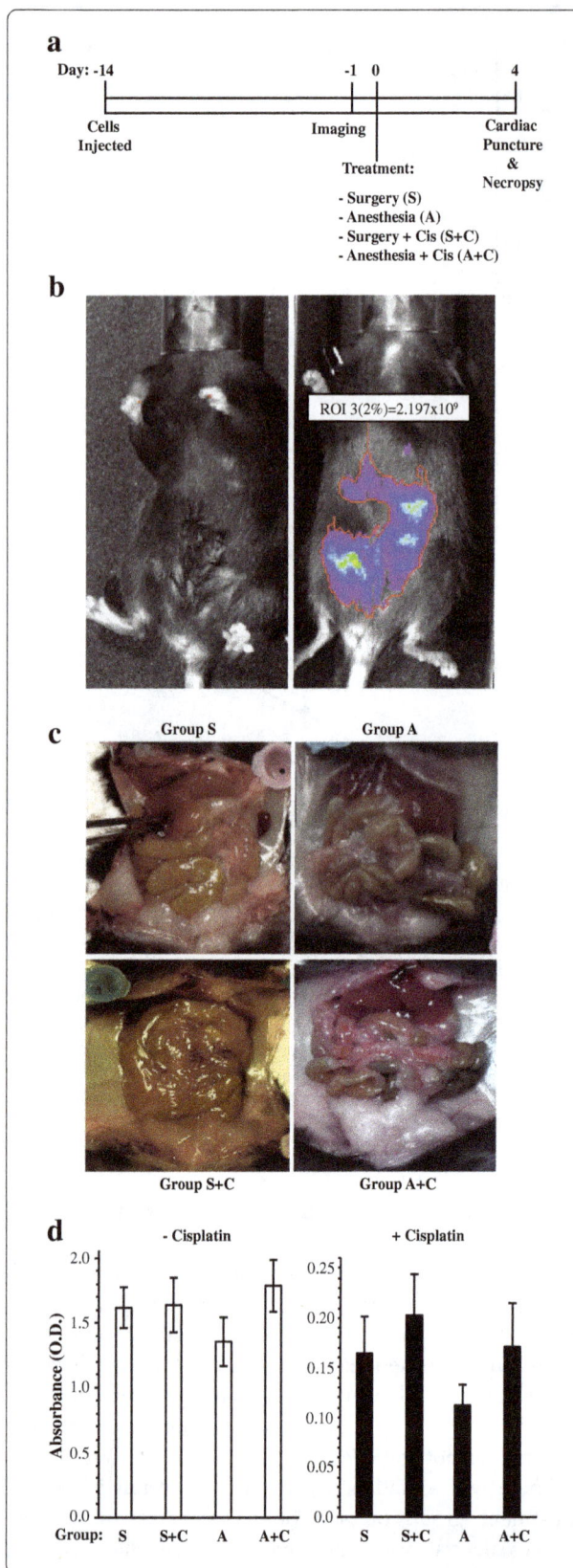

Fig. 2 In vivo imaging of ID8-L11 cells and effect of serum from wounded mice on growth of parental ID8 cells. **a** Schematic of the treatment paradigm used in the preliminary study. **b** Representative bioluminescence images of a mouse not injected with ID8-L11 cells (left) and a mouse injected with 5 million ID8-L11 cells i.p. 13 days earlier (right). **c** Representative images of the abdominal viscera of mice in each of the four treatment groups at time of necropsy. No evidence of macroscopic seeding was found. **d** Serum from mice of the different treatment groups did not impact the growth of parental ID8 cells in vitro. Cells were grown in medium supplemented to 10% with serum pooled from within the four treatment groups in the presence or absence of 25 µM cisplatin. XTT dye reduction assay was performed 72 h after initiation of treatment. Bars represent the mean ± SEM of 8 replicates. Two-way ANOVA performed on natural log-transformed data indicated a statistically significant effect of cisplatin but no statistically significant effect of serum from the different treatment groups or interaction

wounding, or in non-wounded animals that received cisplatin on day 0 (Fig. 4c). Multiple comparison testing using a Bonferroni-corrected statistical threshold indicated that cisplatin treatment resulted in improved survival in non-wounded animals but not in wounded animals.

Bioluminesence imaging was performed on day 21 and 35 after wounding to assess the impact of treatment on tumor burden. Representative images are shown in Fig. 5. Quantitation of abdominal bioluminescence determined on day 21 indicated that animals subjected to wounding had the greatest tumor burden, with 2.5-fold higher levels of tumor cells found in animals that had not received cisplatin compared with animals subjected to anesthesia only (Fig. 6). Cisplatin treatment administered on either the perioperative day or on day 7 reduced tumor burden in both wounded and non-wounded animals, with lower levels achieved in non-wounded animals. Cisplatin administered on the same day as wounding decreased the collective peritoneal tumor mass by approximately 50%, which was 18-fold more than the tumor mass measured in non-wounded animals treated with cisplatin at the same time. Cisplatin treatment in non-wounded animals reduced tumor burden by more than 90%. Administration of cisplatin 1 week after wounding was more effective, resulting in a reduction of tumor mass by approximately 80%, which was not statistically different from the tumor mass measured in non-wounded animals treated with cisplatin at the same time. Cisplatin treatment in non-wounded animals at this time reduced tumor burden by a similar percentage, approximately 89%. Importantly, the levels of bioluminescence measured in wounded animals treated with cisplatin on either day were not statistically different from levels measured in non-wounded animals that had not received cisplatin, indicating that perioperative cisplatin mitigated the tumor promoting effects of wounding.

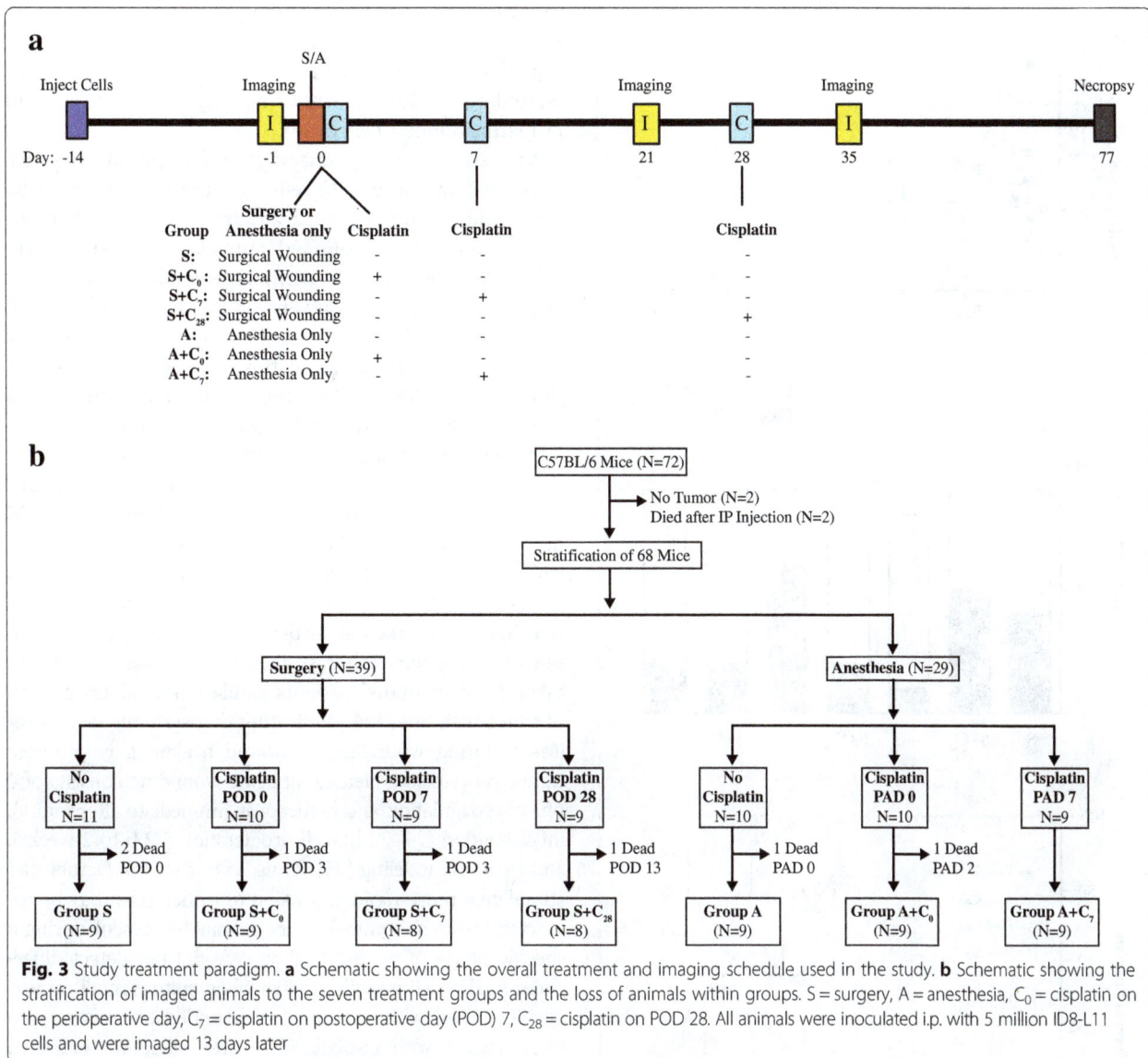

Fig. 3 Study treatment paradigm. **a** Schematic showing the overall treatment and imaging schedule used in the study. **b** Schematic showing the stratification of imaged animals to the seven treatment groups and the loss of animals within groups. S = surgery, A = anesthesia, C_0 = cisplatin on the perioperative day, C_7 = cisplatin on postoperative day (POD) 7, C_{28} = cisplatin on POD 28. All animals were inoculated i.p. with 5 million ID8-L11 cells and were imaged 13 days later

While the primary objective of the study was to compare perioperative cisplatin to cisplatin administered on day 7 following wounding, an additional group of wounded animals treated with cisplatin on day 28 was included as a comparator to reflect the current average waiting period to initiate adjuvant chemotherapy [19]. As determined by imaging performed 1 week later (day 35), wounded mice receiving chemotherapy on day 28 had 73% of the amount of tumor mass as untreated wounded mice (Fig. 6). This decrease was not statistically significant. At this imaging time point, wounded animals not treated with cisplatin showed highest levels of tumor burden; however, this level was not statistically different from that measured in untreated non-wounded animals. Of wounded animals, those treated with cisplatin on day 7, but not on the perioperative day, exhibited reduced tumor burden compared to untreated wounded animals. In contrast, cisplatin administered to non-wounded animals during the perioperative period or on day 7 effectively reduced tumor burden.

Discussion

Using the ID8 syngeneic ovarian cancer mouse model, we report that surgical wounding increased growth of tumor cells within the peritoneal cavity, as determined by quantitation of bioluminescence 3 weeks later. While cisplatin decreased tumor burden, its efficacy was affected by surgical wounding and timing of chemotherapy. Cisplatin administered on the day as wounding decreased collective peritoneal tumor mass by only 50%, whereas more than a 90% reduction was measured in non-wounded animals. Administration of cisplatin 1 week after wounding appeared more effective, resulting in a reduction of tumor mass by 80%. These results

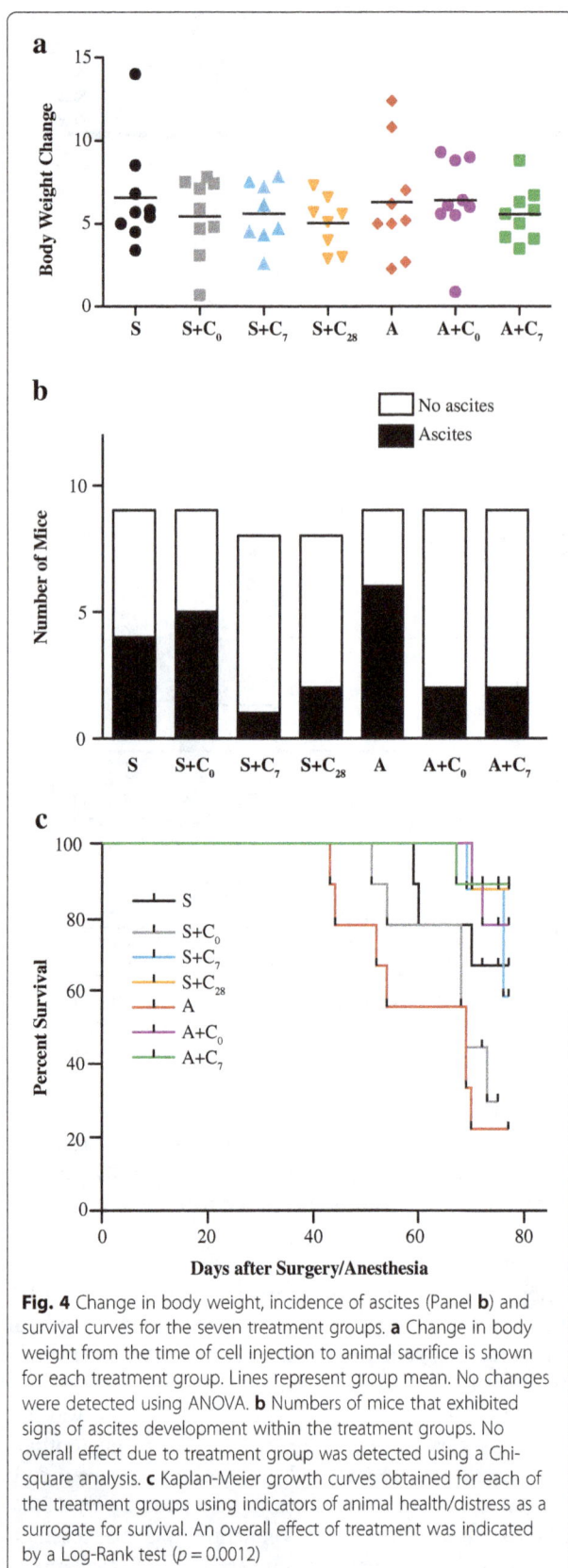

Fig. 4 Change in body weight, incidence of ascites (Panel **b**) and survival curves for the seven treatment groups. **a** Change in body weight from the time of cell injection to animal sacrifice is shown for each treatment group. Lines represent group mean. No changes were detected using ANOVA. **b** Numbers of mice that exhibited signs of ascites development within the treatment groups. No overall effect due to treatment group was detected using a Chi-square analysis. **c** Kaplan-Meier growth curves obtained for each of the treatment groups using indicators of animal health/distress as a surrogate for survival. An overall effect of treatment was indicated by a Log-Rank test ($p = 0.0012$)

indicate that surgical wounding negatively impacts the efficacy of perioperatively delivered cisplatin, suggesting that systemic factors released at the time of wounding or during wound healing protect cells from cisplatin-induced cell death.

As determined by imaging performed on day 35, chemotherapy on day 28 reduced tumor burden by 27%, which did not differ statistically from the level of tumor cells measured in wounded animals that had not received chemotherapy. In contrast, wounded mice treated with cisplatin perioperatively or on day 7 had 65 and 19%, respectively, of the tumor mass measured in untreated wounded animals at this time point. Our results thus support the assertion that earlier administration of cisplatin following surgery is more efficacious.

Studies have indicated that surgical wounding promotes the growth and metastasis of solid tumors [20, 21]. Ramolu et al. [22] found that fluid taken from wounds 24 or 48 h after breast surgery stimulated the growth of MCF-7 and HCC1937 cancer cells, but not non-malignant MCF-10A cells, in vitro. While this and a similar study [23] have been taken as evidence to explain recurrence at the operative site, other studies have shown that serum taken from wounded patients similarly stimulates growth of cancer cell lines [24], indicating that systemic factors released during wounding or wound healing may promote tumor progression. Healing of acute wounding consists of 4 phases: coagulation and hemostasis (immediate after injury), inflammation (24–72 h), cell proliferation (72 h to 2 weeks), and tissue remodeling [25]. Thus, in our model, factors that stimulate a more rapid expansion of tumor cells may be restricted to the abdominal cavity or may be present during a specific phase of wound healing. We did not detect differences in ID8 cell growth in vitro when culture medium was supplemented with serum from wounded animals or animals treated with cisplatin. However, since we collected serum samples 4 days after wounding, it remains possible that differences might be seen with serum collected nearer the time of wounding.

A key finding of our study, that perioperative cisplatin efficacy was inhibited by wounding, was unexpected. Surgical wounding has been reported to activate quiescent tumor cells [26]. The mitotic activity of residual cancer cells increases within 1 day of surgery [27] and remains elevated for 1–2 weeks [26]. Since actively dividing cells are more susceptible to cisplatin [28], we hypothesized that the perioperative environment would maximize cisplatin effects. Moreover, an animal study performed more than 30 years ago by Fisher et al. [14] with transplanted mouse syngeneic mammary cancer cells indicated that preoperative or perioperative cyclophosphamide treatment was more effective than treatment administered 3 days later. In fact, a delay of treatment for 1 week was least effective.

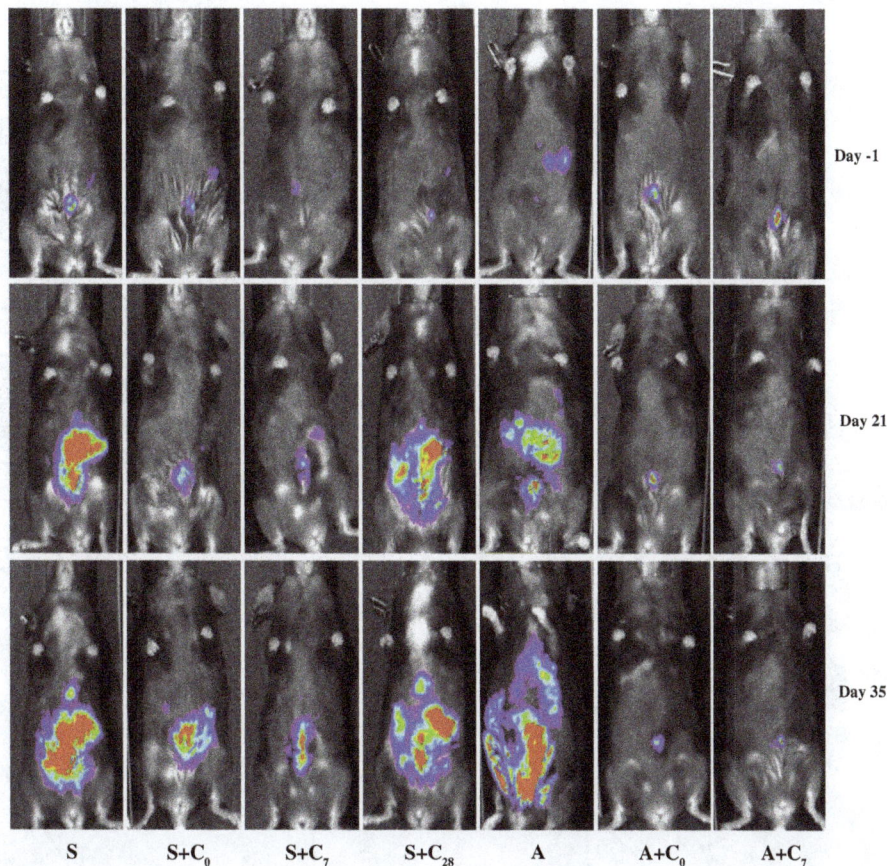

Fig. 5 Representative bioluminescence images obtained for the seven treatment groups at each of the three imaging sessions

Aside from the chemotherapy and cell line used, key differences in the design of these two studies could contribute to the discrepancy in findings. The model used by Fisher et al. [14] consisted of subcutaneously injecting tumor cells into both hind legs of mice. Surgery, consisting of amputating the leg inoculated with the greater number of cells (the primary tumor), increased tumor growth in the remaining leg. The macroscopic amount of residual disease remaining at the time of surgery, its subcutaneous location, and the extent of surgery differed from the microscopic i.p. disease and incision-wounding modeled in our study. Interestingly, a recent animal study reported that expression of survivin in residual tumor tissues, taken as a surrogate marker of chemoresistance, began increasing within 6 h of surgery, peaked at post-operative day 2, and decreased to baseline levels by post-operative day 7 [29]. This suggested chemoresistance pattern during the immediate post-operative period is consistent with our finding of impaired cisplatin activity perioperatively vs. 7 days later.

An alternative interpretation of our data is that perioperative cisplatin mitigates the impact of surgical wounding on residual tumor expansion. The level of tumor burden in wounded animals treated with

perioperative cisplatin was equivalent to untreated non-wounded animals at both imaging sessions. This has important clinical implications as there is growing interest in the use of hyperthermic intraperitoneal chemotherapy (HIPEC) in ovarian cancer. HIPEC is typically administered intraoperatively at the time of cytoreductive surgery and enables direct administration of a high volume of systemic therapy with a homogenous distribution at the nadir of residual disease. In select patients with colorectal carcinoma and peritoneal carcinomatosis, perioperative i.p. chemotherapy enhanced the overall median survival, particularly for patients in which surgery resulted in microscopic residual disease [30]. Although a recent randomized clinical trial showed no benefit of HIPEC on survival in patients with advanced ovarian cancer [31], they noted a trend favoring HIPEC in patients that had received neoadjuvant chemotherapy. This has since been demonstrated in a recent report by van Driel et al. [32], who showed increased progression-free and overall survival of stage III ovarian cancer patients randomized to receive interval cytoreductive surgery with HIPEC vs. interval cytoreductive surgery alone. Further studies examining the

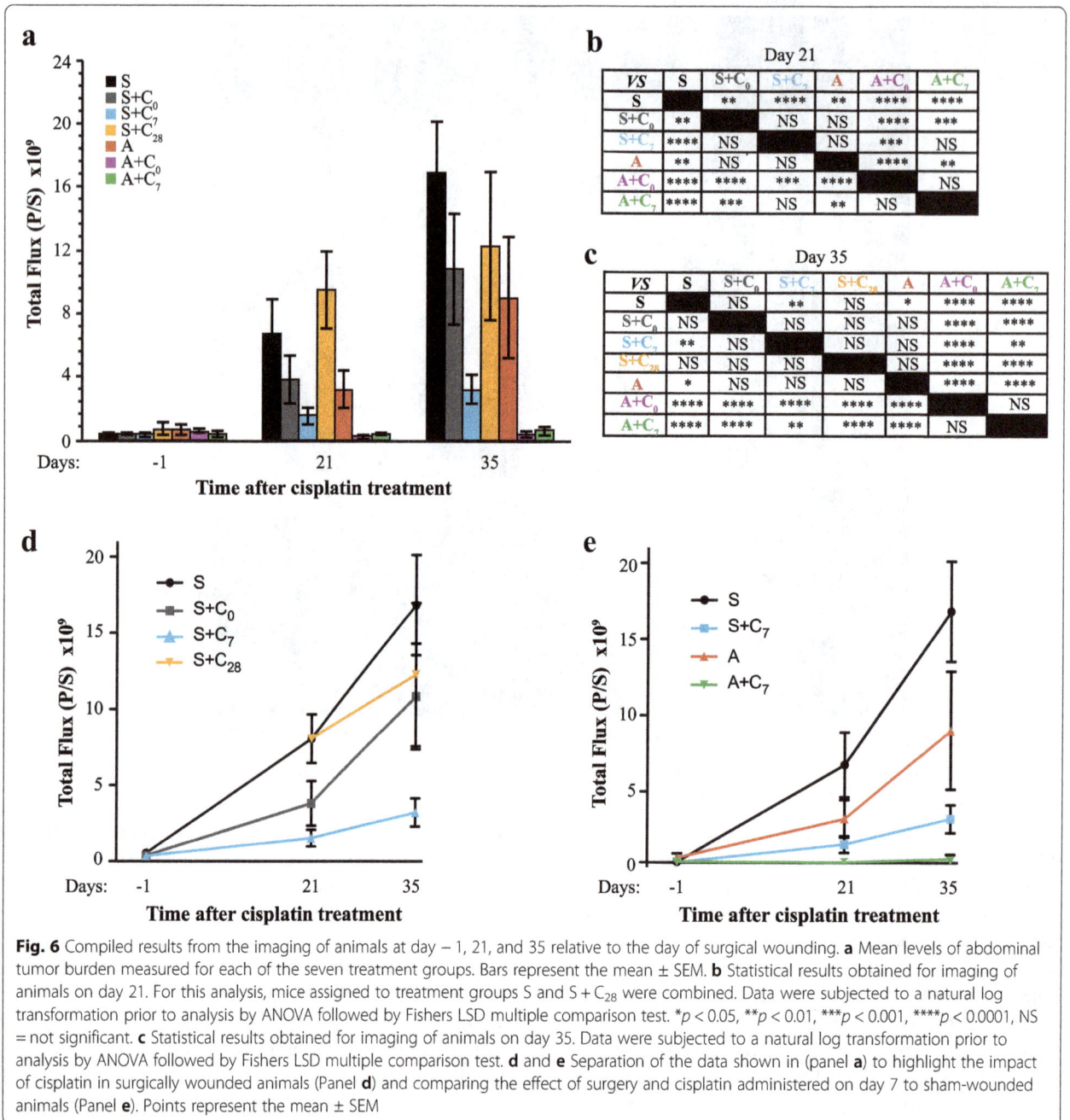

Fig. 6 Compiled results from the imaging of animals at day − 1, 21, and 35 relative to the day of surgical wounding. **a** Mean levels of abdominal tumor burden measured for each of the seven treatment groups. Bars represent the mean ± SEM. **b** Statistical results obtained for imaging of animals on day 21. For this analysis, mice assigned to treatment groups S and $S + C_{28}$ were combined. Data were subjected to a natural log transformation prior to analysis by ANOVA followed by Fishers LSD multiple comparison test. $*p < 0.05$, $**p < 0.01$, $***p < 0.001$, $****p < 0.0001$, NS = not significant. **c** Statistical results obtained for imaging of animals on day 35. Data were subjected to a natural log transformation prior to analysis by ANOVA followed by Fishers LSD multiple comparison test. **d** and **e** Separation of the data shown in (panel **a**) to highlight the impact of cisplatin in surgically wounded animals (Panel **d**) and comparing the effect of surgery and cisplatin administered on day 7 to sham-wounded animals (Panel **e**). Points represent the mean ± SEM

impact of surgical wounding and efficacy of i.p. chemotherapy in a model of neoadjuvant chemotherapy are warranted.

A possible mechanism underlying surgery-driven accelerated residual tumor growth may be an increase in the level of angiogenic cytokines during the perioperative period. For example, perioperative levels of systemic proangiogenic cytokines such as vascular endothelial growth factor (VEGF), basic fibroblast growth factor (bFGF) and transforming growth factor beta (TGF-β) are increased in blood samples drawn from breast, lung, and gastric cancer patients during the perioperative period [33–35]. VEGF levels were also found to be increased in wound fluid collected during the perioperative period [23, 24]. Other factors released during wound healing that have been implicated in promoting tumor growth and metastases include epidermal growth factor, activin, platelet-derived growth factor, and prostaglandin E_2. Limited studies conducted with inhibitors to many of these growth-promoting factors have indicated partial mitigation of surgery-induced growth; however, it is likely that the response is multifactorial. Indeed, Hofer et al. [23] found that the combination of TGF-β and bFGF better replicated the impact of wound fluid on the growth of melanoma cells in vivo than either growth factor alone. While these studies have focused on surgery-stimulated cell proliferation, studies have not yet addressed potential mechanisms by which wound-associated factors may promote cell survival pathways to diminish the impact of chemotherapy.

In vivo imaging used in this study allowed us to monitor the change of tumor burden non-invasively. A potential concern regarding bioluminescent imaging in the abdominal cavity is that ascites formation at the time of imaging could underestimate the cell number due to dilution of luciferin substrate by excessive ascites [36]. However, none of the mice injected with ID8-L11 cells had obvious ascites during the three imaging sessions and a supra-saturating concentration of substrate was used.

While clinically relevant, there are limitations of our model that caution direct application to humans. As opposed to human high-grade serous ovarian cancer cells, ID8 cells do not bear a p53 mutation and have intact *BRCA1* and *BRCA2* expression [37]. It is possible that p53-mutated cells or cells with diminished functional BRCA1 respond differently. Indeed, HGSOC with diminished BRCA1 or BRCA2 expression typically have increased sensitivity to DNA damaging chemotherapeutics and restoration of BRCA1 in a BRCA1 deficient breast cancer cell line decreased cisplatin sensitivity in a xenograph model [38, 39]. Additionally, we administered only a single dose of cisplatin rather than a full course of treatments as would occur clinically. Also, the wound healing process in humans differs from that of mice. For example, wound healing of many animals, including the mouse, occurs via contraction rather than epithelization as in humans. However, similar to humans, incisional and excisional wounding in mice typically completes within 1–2 weeks post-injury [40], with many similarities in cellular and molecular responses to humans [41]. Lastly, our bioluminescence results showing residual tumor burden did not correlate with survival data. We relied chiefly on behavioral parameters and significant accumulation of ascites as surrogates of survival for humanitarian reasons. Thus, we feel that survival data are less informative in the context of the current study than our bioluminescence data.

One concern regarding early initiation of chemotherapy in clinical practice is wound complications or morbidity. We did not find wound complications or increased morbidity associated with early chemotherapy. These findings agree with a study investigating the effect of early post-operative chemotherapy on wound healing in patients with ovarian cancer [42]. In the study, early chemotherapy did not increase the risk of wound complications despite efforts to begin chemotherapy as soon as possible after cytoreductive surgery and neither the frequency of bowel resection nor type of fascial or skin closure adversely influenced the risk. In addition, early post-operative IP (EPIC) chemotherapy, which usually starts within 1 week after surgery, is not associated with increased morbidity in ovarian cancer [43]. Given the safety regarding early chemotherapy in animal and clinical studies, a clinical trial would be warranted to explore the feasibility and efficacy of perioperative vs. EPIC chemotherapy.

Conclusion

The results of this study indicate that surgical wounding enhanced peritoneal tumor burden in a syngeneic model of ovarian cancer. While administration of cisplatin at the time of surgical wounding mitigated the effect on tumor progression, the efficacy of this cisplatin appeared to be reduced. While direct relevance to humans is limited since the surgical wounding in this model did not include reducing tumor burden, these findings highlight the need for further studies investigating factors released at the time of surgery that impact tumor cell survival.

Abbreviations

bFGF: Basic fibroblast growth factor; HIPEC: Hyperthermic intraperitoneal chemotherapy; i.p: Intraperitoneally; PBS: Phosphate-buffered saline; POD: Post-operative day; TGF-β: Transforming growth factor beta; VEGF: Vascular endothelial growth factor

Acknowledgements

We thank Dr. Alexandre Hardy for technical assistance with in vivo imaging.

Funding

This project was funded by the Department of Obstetrics and Gynaecology, Mount Sinai Hospital/University Health Network Research Fund (2016–2017) and was supplemented by funds from the Princess Margaret Hospital Division of Gynecologic Oncology. AK was supported by CIHR grant MOP106679. The IVIS Spectrum In Vivo Imaging System used in this study was supported by The 3D (Diet, Digestive Tract, and Disease) Centre funded by the Canadian Foundation for Innovation and by the Ontario Research Fund, project numbers 19442 and 30961.

Authors' contributions

YL, a Gynecologic Oncology Surgical Fellow, performed the in vitro and in vivo studies and produced a first draft of the manuscript. AK transfected the ID8 cells with the luciferase expression construct, supervised all in vitro work, and generated the final version of the figs. YL, TM, and TJB conceived of and designed the study. TM secured the funding and TJB secured the animal care and use committee approval and oversaw all aspects of the work. AK, TM, and TJB made revisions to the manuscript. All authors read and approved the final manuscript.

Competing interests

The authors declare that they have no competing interests.

Author details

[1]Division of Gynecologic Oncology, Princess Margaret Hospital Cancer Centre, Toronto, ON, Canada. [2]Lunenfeld-Tanenbaum Research Institute at Sinai Health Systems, Mt. Sinai Hospital, 60 Murray Street, 6-10016-3, Toronto, ON M5T 3L9, Canada. [3]Department of Obstetrics and Gynecology, University of Toronto, Toronto, ON, Canada.

References

1. Baldwin LA, Huang B, Miller RW, Tucker T, Goodrich ST, Podzielinski I, DeSimone CP, Ueland FR, van Nagell JR, Seamon LG. Ten-year relative survival for epithelial ovarian cancer. Obstet Gynecol. 2012;120(3):612–8.
2. Coleman RL, Monk BJ, Sood AK, Herzog TJ. Latest research and treatment of advanced-stage epithelial ovarian cancer. Nat Rev Clin Oncol. 2013;10(4): 211–24.
3. Chi DS, Eisenhauer EL, Lang J, Huh J, Haddad L, Abu-Rustum NR, Sonoda Y, Levine DA, Hensley M, Barakat RR. What is the optimal goal of primary cytoreductive surgery for bulky stage IIIC epithelial ovarian carcinoma (EOC)? Gynecol Oncol. 2006;103(2):559–64.
4. Al Rawahi T, Lopes AD, Bristow RE, Bryant A, Elattar A, Chattopadhyay S, Galaal K. Surgical cytoreduction for recurrent epithelial ovarian cancer. Cochrane Database Syst Rev. 2013;2:CD008765.
5. Tewari KS, Java JJ, Eskander RN, Monk BJ, Burger RA. Early initiation of chemotherapy following complete resection of advanced ovarian cancer associated with improved survival: NRG oncology/gynecologic oncology group study. Ann Oncol. 2016;27(1):114–21.
6. Ceelen W, Pattyn P, Mareel M. Surgery, wound healing, and metastasis: recent insights and clinical implications. Crit Rev Oncol Hematol. 2014;89(1): 16–26.
7. Demicheli R, Retsky MW, Hrushesky WJ, Baum M, Gukas ID. The effects of surgery on tumor growth: a century of investigations. Ann Oncol. 2008; 19(11):1821–8.
8. Lange PH, Hekmat K, Bosl G, Kennedy BJ, Fraley EE. Acclerated growth of testicular cancer after cytoreductive surgery. Cancer. 1980;45(6):1498–506.
9. Retsky M, Demicheli R, Hrushesky W, Baum M, Gukas I. Surgery triggers outgrowth of latent distant disease in breast cancer: an inconvenient truth? Cancers (Basel). 2010;2(2):305–37.
10. Tyzzer EE. Factors in the production and growth of tumor metastases. J Med Res. 1913;28(2):309–32. 301
11. Simpson-Herren L, Sanford AH, Holmquist JP. Effects of surgery on the cell kinetics of residual tumor. Cancer Treat Rep. 1976;60(12):1749–60.
12. Gadducci A, Sartori E, Landoni F, Zola P, Maggino T, Maggioni A, Cosio S, Frassi E, LaPresa MT, Fuso L, et al. Relationship between time interval from primary surgery to the start of taxane- plus platinum-based chemotherapy and clinical outcome of patients with advanced epithelial ovarian cancer: results of a multicenter retrospective Italian study. J Clin Oncol. 2005;23(4): 751–8.
13. Biagi JJ, Raphael MJ, Mackillop WJ, Kong W, King WD, Booth CM. Association between time to initiation of adjuvant chemotherapy and survival in colorectal cancer: a systematic review and meta-analysis. JAMA. 2011;305(22):2335–42.
14. Fisher B, Gunduz N, Saffer EA. Influence of the interval between primary tumor removal and chemotherapy on kinetics and growth of metastases. Cancer Res. 1983;43(4):1488–92.
15. Roby KF, Taylor CC, Sweetwood JP, Cheng Y, Pace JL, Tawfik O, Persons DL, Smith PG, Terranova PF. Development of a syngeneic mouse model for events related to ovarian cancer. Carcinogenesis. 2000;21(4):585–91.
16. Greenaway J, Moorehead R, Shaw P, Petrik J. Epithelial-stromal interaction increases cell proliferation, survival and tumorigenicity in a mouse model of human epithelial ovarian cancer. Gynecol Oncol. 2008;108(2):385–94.
17. Yusa K, Zhou L, Li MA, Bradley A, Craig NL. A hyperactive piggyBac transposase for mammalian applications. Proc Natl Acad Sci U S A. 2011; 108(4):1531–6.
18. Mathe A, Komka K, Forczig M, Szabo D, Anderlik P, Rozgonyi F. The effect of different doses of cisplatin on the pharmacokinetic parameters of cefepime in mice. Lab Anim. 2006;40(3):296–300.
19. Hofstetter G, Concin N, Braicu I, Chekerov R, Sehouli J, Cadron I, Van Gorp T, Trillsch F, Mahner S, Ulmer H, et al. The time interval from surgery to start of chemotherapy significantly impacts prognosis in patients with advanced serous ovarian carcinoma - analysis of patient data in the prospective OVCAD study. Gynecol Oncol. 2013;131(1):15–20.
20. Bogden AE, Moreau JP, Eden PA. Proliferative response of human and animal tumours to surgical wounding of normal tissues: onset, duration and inhibition. Br J Cancer. 1997;75(7):1021–7.
21. Abramovitch R, Marikovsky M, Meir G, Neeman M. Stimulation of tumour growth by wound-derived growth factors. Br J Cancer. 1999; 79(9–10):1392–8.
22. Ramolu L, Christ D, Abecassis J, Rodier JF. Stimulation of breast cancer cell lines by post-surgical drainage fluids. Anticancer Res. 2014;34(7):3489–92.
23. Hofer SO, Shrayer D, Reichner JS, Hoekstra HJ, Wanebo HJ. Wound-induced tumor progression: a probable role in recurrence after tumor resection. Arch Surg. 1998;133(4):383–9.
24. Tagliabue E, Agresti R, Carcangiu ML, Ghirelli C, Morelli D, Campiglio M, Martel M, Giovanazzi R, Greco M, Balsari A, et al. Role of HER2 in wound-induced breast carcinoma proliferation. Lancet. 2003;362(9383):527–33.
25. Diegelmann RF, Evans MC. Wound healing: an overview of acute, fibrotic and delayed healing. Front Biosci. 2004;9:283–9.
26. Gunduz N, Fisher B, Saffer EA. Effect of surgical removal on the growth and kinetics of residual tumor. Cancer Res. 1979;39(10):3861–5.
27. Fisher B, Gunduz N, Coyle J, Rudock C, Saffer E. Presence of a growth-stimulating factor in serum following primary tumor removal in mice. Cancer Res. 1989;49(8):1996–2001.
28. Donaldson KL, Goolsby GL, Wahl AF. Cytotoxicity of the anticancer agents cisplatin and taxol during cell proliferation and the cell cycle. Int J Cancer. 1994;57(6):847–55.
29. Amin AT, Shiraishi N, Ninomiya S, Tajima M, Inomata M, Kitano S. Increased mRNA expression of epidermal growth factor receptor, human epidermal receptor, and survivin in human gastric cancer after the surgical stress of laparotomy versus carbon dioxide pneumoperitoneum in a murine model. Surg Endosc. 2010;24(6):1427–33.
30. Yan TD, Black D, Savady R, Sugarbaker PH. Systematic review on the efficacy of cytoreductive surgery combined with perioperative intraperitoneal chemotherapy for peritoneal carcinomatosis from colorectal carcinoma. J Clin Oncol. 2006;24(24):4011–9.
31. Lim MC, Chang S-J, Yoo HJ, Nam B-H, Bristow R, Park S-Y. Randomized trial of hyperthermic intraperitoneal chemotherapy (HIPEC) in women with primary advanced peritoneal, ovarian, and tubal cancer. J Clin Oncol. 2017; 35(15 suppl) Abstr 5520
32. van Driel WJ, Koole SN, Sikorska K, Schagen van Leeuwen JH, Schreuder HWR, Hermans RHM, de Hingh I, van der Velden J, Arts HJ, Massuger L et al. Hyperthermic intraperitoneal chemotherapy in ovarian Cancer. N Engl J Med 2018; 378(3):230–240.
33. Curigliano G, Petit JY, Bertolini F, Colleoni M, Peruzzotti G, de Braud F, Gandini S, Giraldo A, Martella S, Orlando L, et al. Systemic effects of surgery: quantitative analysis of circulating basic fibroblast growth factor (bFGF), vascular endothelial growth factor (VEGF) and transforming growth factor beta (TGF-beta) in patients with breast cancer who underwent limited or extended surgery. Breast Cancer Res Treat. 2005;93(1):35–40.
34. Ikeda M, Furukawa H, Imamura H, Shimizu J, Ishida H, Masutani S, Tatsuta M, Kawasaki T, Satomi T. Surgery for gastric cancer increases plasma levels of vascular endothelial growth factor and von Willebrand factor. Gastric Cancer. 2002;5(3):137–41.
35. Maniwa Y, Okada M, Ishii N, Kiyooka K. Vascular endothelial growth factor increased by pulmonary surgery accelerates the growth of micrometastases in metastatic lung cancer. Chest. 1998;114(6):1668–75.
36. Baert T, Verschuere T, Van Hoylandt A, Gijsbers R, Vergote I, Coosemans A. The dark side of ID8-Luc2: pitfalls for luciferase tagged murine models for ovarian cancer. J Immunother Cancer. 2015;3:57.
37. Walton J, Blagih J, Ennis D, Leung E, Dowson S, Farquharson M, Tookman LA, Orange C, Athineos D, Mason S, et al. CRISPR/Cas9-mediated Trp53 and Brca2 knockout to generate improved murine models of ovarian high-grade serous carcinoma. Cancer Res. 2016;76(20):6118–29.
38. Tagliaferri P, Ventura M, Baudi F, Cucinotto I, Arbitrio M, Di Martino MT, Tassone P. BRCA1/2 genetic background-based therapeutic tailoring of human ovarian cancer: hope or reality? J Ovarian Res. 2009;2:14.

39. Tassone P, Di Martino MT, Ventura M, Pietragalla A, Cucinotto I, Calimeri T, Bulotta A, Neri P, Caraglia M, Tagliaferri P. Loss of BRCA1 function increases the antitumor activity of cisplatin against human breast cancer xenografts in vivo. Cancer Biol Ther. 2009;8(7):648–53.

40. Ansell DM, Campbell L, Thomason HA, Brass A, Hardman MJ. A statistical analysis of murine incisional and excisional acute wound models. Wound Repair Regen. 2014;22(2):281–7.

41. Perez R, Davis SC. Relevance of animal models for wound healing. Wounds. 2008;20(1):3–8.

42. Kolb BA, Buller RE, Connor JP, DiSaia PJ, Berman ML. Effects of early postoperative chemotherapy on wound healing. Obstet Gynecol. 1992;79(6):988–92.

43. Goodman MD, McPartland S, Detelich D, Saif MW. Chemotherapy for intraperitoneal use: a review of hyperthermic intraperitoneal chemotherapy and early post-operative intraperitoneal chemotherapy. J Gastrointest Oncol. 2016;7(1):45–57.

10

Is adjuvant chemotherapy beneficial for patients with FIGO stage IC adult granulosa cell tumor of the ovary?

Dan Wang, Yang Xiang*, Ming Wu, Keng Shen, Jiaxin Yang, Huifang Huang and Tong Ren

Abstract

Background: To evaluate the association between adjuvant chemotherapy and clinical outcomes in patients with stage IC adult granulosa cell tumor (AGCT).

Methods: We performed a retrospective study of patients with stage IC AGCT diagnosed at our hospital from January 1985 to September 2015. We analyzed descriptive statistics, and performed univariate and multivariate and Kaplan–Meier survival analyses.

Results: Sixty stage IC AGCT patients were identified, including 28 in the no adjuvant chemotherapy group (NACG) and 32 in the adjuvant chemotherapy group (ACG). The median follow-up time was 88 months (range: 9–334 months). Sixteen patients developed recurrences, including nine in the NACG and seven in the ACG groups. Univariate analysis identified incomplete surgical staging and initial treatment place as associated with disease-free survival (DFS) ($P = 0.003$ and 0.038, respectively). Incomplete surgical staging remained a risk factor for recurrence in multivariate analysis (hazard ratio (HR) = 3.883, 95% confidence interval (CI): 1.123–13.430, $P = 0.032$). The 5-year DFS rates in the NACG and ACG groups were 76.3% and 87.5% respectively ($P = 0.197$). Adjuvant chemotherapy was thus not associated with improved DFS. Furthermore, the number of chemotherapy cycles was not associated with recurrence rate (≤3 cycles vs. > 3 cycles, HR = 0.613, 95% CI: 0.112–3.351, $P = 0.572$).

Conclusion: Administration of adjuvant chemotherapy does not improve DFS in patients with stage IC AGCT. Further studies with larger samples involving multi-institutional collaboration are needed to validate new treatment regimens for this disease.

Keywords: Adult granulosa cell tumor, Adjuvant chemotherapy, Stage IC

Background

Granulosa cell tumors (GCTs) are uncommon, accounting for only about 5% of all ovarian malignancies, but comprising 70% of ovarian sex cord-stromal tumors [1]. Most GCTs are adult GCTs (AGCTs), based on their clinical presentation and histological findings. AGCT comprises a clinically and molecularly unique subtype of ovarian malignancy with different behavior from other histological subtypes. The majority of AGCTs are diagnosed at an early stage and have a good prognosis, with 5- and 10-year overall survival rates of 98% and 84%, respectively [2]. However, AGCTs can occasionally be indolent, with a tendency to late relapse, associated with significant morbidity and difficult therapeutic choices.

Surgery is the cornerstone of treatment for AGCT, and patients with stage I AGCT have a favorable prognosis following surgical treatment alone, though the National Comprehensive Cancer Network guidelines (NCCN) recommend adjuvant chemotherapy for patients with advanced stage disease, or stage I disease with high risk factors. However, the definition of what constitutes a high risk factor remains unclear, and current evidence regarding the use of adjuvant chemotherapy in women with early stage AGCT is conflicting. Some studies have suggested that women might benefit from adjuvant chemotherapy [3, 4], while others failed

* Correspondence: xiangy@pumch.cn
Department of Obstetrics and Gynecology, Peking Union Medical College Hospital, Chinese Academy of Medical Science and Peking Union Medical College, No. 1 Shuaifuyuan Road, Dongcheng District, Beijing 100730, People's Republic of China

to show any effect of postoperative chemotherapy on survival or relapse rates [5, 6]. This lack of clear evidence regarding the benefit of adjuvant chemotherapy in early stage AGCT makes treatment decisions difficult.

According to the revised FIGO stage (2014), ovarian epithelial cancer stage IC can be subdivided into intraoperative rupture (IC1), capsule ruptured before surgery or tumor on ovarian surface (IC2), and malignant cells in ascites or peritoneal washings (IC3). This new FIGO staging provides a more precise definition of the risk in stage IC [7]. Indeed, patients with stage IC have a higher relapse rate and shorter median time to relapse compared with stage IA patients [8, 9]. Some authors suggest the use of adjuvant therapy in AGCT stage IC patients with preoperative rupture or malignant ascites [10], but there remains limited information regarding the role of adjuvant chemotherapy in stage IC [8, 11]. The aim of this study was thus to evaluate the association between adjuvant chemotherapy and disease-free survival (DFS) in patients with stage IC AGCT.

Methods

This study was approved by the ethics committee of our hospital. All patients diagnosed with AGCT at our hospital from January 1985 to September 2015 were reviewed. Sixty patients were diagnosed with FIGO stage IC AGCT.

Information was collected from all patients regarding age, menopausal status, tumor diameter, preoperative serum CA125, FIGO stage, type of surgery, adjuvant therapy, relapse characteristics, and relapse treatment and follow-up information. Follow-up information was obtained from outpatient files or by telephone interview with patients or their relatives. Tumor stage was based on the new staging system reports (FIGO staging system, FIGO Committee on Gynecologic Oncology, 2014) [7].

All patients underwent surgery. Fertility-sparing surgery was defined as preservation of the uterus and at least one ovary. Total abdominal hysterectomy and bilateral salpingo-oophorectomy was classified as radical surgery. Staging was considered complete when it included peritoneal washing, omentectomy (or omental biopsy), multiple peritoneal biopsies, and biopsy of any suspicious area. Pelvic and/or para-aortic lymphadenectomy were optional procedures, according to the surgeon's experience and the intraoperative findings.

The exact indications for adjuvant chemotherapy in the present study were unclear because of the retrospective nature of the study, and the decision to administer adjuvant chemotherapy was made by the attending physicians after discussion with the patients.

Statistical analysis

Statistical analysis was performed using SPSS version 15 (SPSS, Inc., Chicago, IL, USA). Patient demographics

and baseline characteristics were summarized using descriptive statistics. Patients were defined into no adjuvant chemotherapy group (NACG) and adjuvant chemotherapy group (ACG). Median values were compared using Mann–Whitney U-tests and frequency distributions were compared using χ^2 and Fisher's exact tests. The main objective of the study was to evaluate the association between adjuvant chemotherapy and disease-free survival (DFS), defined as the time from initial surgery to the first recurrence or date of censoring. DFS survival curves were obtained using the Kaplan–Meier method and compared using log-rank tests. A P value < 0.05 was considered statistically significant. Variables with $P < 0.05$ on univariate analysis were selected for multivariate analysis.

Results

Sixty patients with Stage IC AGCT were identified during the study period, including 28 in the NACG group and 32 in the ACG group. The median age at diagnosis was 41 years (range: 23–75 years). Their baseline characteristics are summarized in Table 1. The FIGO distributions were as follows: surgical spill in 34 patients (IC1), capsule ruptured before surgery or tumor on ovarian

Table 1 Clinical characteristics of AGCT in stage IC

	All patients N = 60	NACG N = 28 (%)	ACG N = 32 (%)	p
Age (median)	41.0	41.5	40.5	0.410
Tumor size (cm)	8	7	8.4	0.523
Serum Ca125(U / ml)	15.5	14.4	16.4	0.751
Menopause				0.744
Yes	14 (23.3)	6 (21.4)	8 (25.0)	
No	46 (76.7)	22 (78.6)	24 (75.0)	
FIGO stage (%)				0.944
IC1	34 (56.7)	16 (57.1)	18 (56.2)	
IC2-IC3	26 (43.3)	12 (42.9)	14 (43.8)	
Surgical procedure				0.605
Fertility surgery	30 (50.0)	15 (53.6)	15 (46.9)	
Radical surgery	30 (50.0)	13 (46.4)	17 (53.1)	
Staging operation				0.102
Yes	26 (43.3)	9 (32.1)	17 (53.1)	
No	34 (56.7)	19 (67.9)	15 (46.9)	
Lymphadenectomy				0.245
Yes	24 (40.0)	9 (32.1)	15 (46.9)	
No	36 (60.0)	19 (67.9)	17 (53.1)	
First operation at clinical				0.696
Our clinical	37 (61.7)	18 (64.3)	19 (59.4)	
Outer	23 (38.3)	10 (35.7)	13 (40.6)	

AGCT: adult granulosa cell tumor; ACG: adjuvant chemotherapy group; NACG: no adjuvant chemotherapy group surface in 23 patients (IC2), and malignant cells in ascites or peritoneal washings in three patients (IC3).

All patients underwent upfront surgery, including 26 (43.3%) who underwent complete surgical staging and 34 (56.7%) who did not. Twenty-four patients (40%) had pelvic and/or para-aortic lymphadenectomy during surgery and the removed lymph nodes were all negative for metastatic AGCT. Thirty-seven (61.7%) patients received surgical treatment in our center and 23 (38.3%) were operated on elsewhere and then referred for subsequent evaluation postoperatively.

Thirty-two (53.3%) patients received adjuvant chemotherapy, with a mean of 3.2 (range: 1–6) chemotherapy cycles. The chemotherapy regimens included bleomycin, etoposide, and cisplatin (BEP) in 11 patients; cisplatin, vincristine, bleomycin in seven; cisplatin and cyclophosphamide in four; paclitaxel and carboplatin (TC) in five; and other regimens in five patients. Among the 32 patients who received chemotherapy, eight (25%) received more than three cycles and 24 (75%) received three or fewer cycles.

Survival analysis

The median follow-up time was 88 months (range: 9–334 months). During the study period, sixteen patients (26.7%) experienced at least one recurrence, including nine in the NACG group and seven in the ACG group.

Among all patients with recurrences, the median time to recurrence was 66 months (range: 7–165 months).

The anatomic locations of the first recurrences included the pelvis alone in eight patients, the abdomen alone in two, and the pelvis plus abdomen in six. Thirteen patients underwent debulking surgery plus chemotherapy and three patients received surgical reduction alone. Eleven patients (69%) developed a second recurrence (4 pelvic plus abdominal relapse; 3 pelvic; 3 abdominal; 1 hepatic involvement) after a median time of 48 months from diagnosis of the first recurrence (range: 24–105 months). Five patients were treated with surgery, five with surgery plus chemotherapy, and one with palliative care.

The associations between clinical factors and DFS in the 60 patients with stage IC AGCT are shown in Table 2. According to univariate analysis, menopause, FIGO stage, adjuvant chemotherapy, and lymph node dissection were not associated with DFS, while surgical staging ($P = 0.003$) and initial treatment place ($P = 0.038$) were significantly associated with DFS (Fig. 1). Incomplete surgical staging (hazard ratio (HR) = 3.883, 95% confidence interval (CI): 1.123–13.430, $P = 0.032$) was still a significant predictive factor for recurrence in multivariate analysis. The 5-year DFS rates in the NACG and ACG groups were 76.3% and 87.5%, respectively ($P = 0.197$) (Fig. 2). Further analysis of the ACG subgroups revealed no association between the number of

Table 2 Univariate and multivariate analysis of patients in stage IC AGCT

Factors	5 year DFS rate (%)	Univariate		Multivariate	
		HR (95% CI)	P	HR (95% CI)	P
Menopause			0.065		
Yes	100	1			
No	75.4	0.183 (0.024–1.391)			
Surgery			0.003		0.032
Staging	93.8	1		1	
Unstaged	70.6	4.95 (1.557–15.792)		3.883 (1.123–13.430)	
Stage			0.971		
IC1	76.9	1			
IC2-IC3	80.8	1.019 (0.368–2.819)			
Adjuvant chemotherapy			0.197		
No	76.3	1			
Yes	87.5	0.517 (0.186–1.433)			
Initial treatment			0.038	0.345	0.345
Our clinical	91.9	1		1	
Outer	72.2	2.984 (1.012–8.799)		1.747 (0.549–5.562)	
Lymph node dissection			0.386		
Yes	87.8	1			
No	76.1	1.578 (0.557–4.472)			

AGCT: adult granulosa cell tumor; DFS: disease-free survival

Is adjuvant chemotherapy beneficial for patients with FIGO stage IC adult granulosa cell tumor..

89

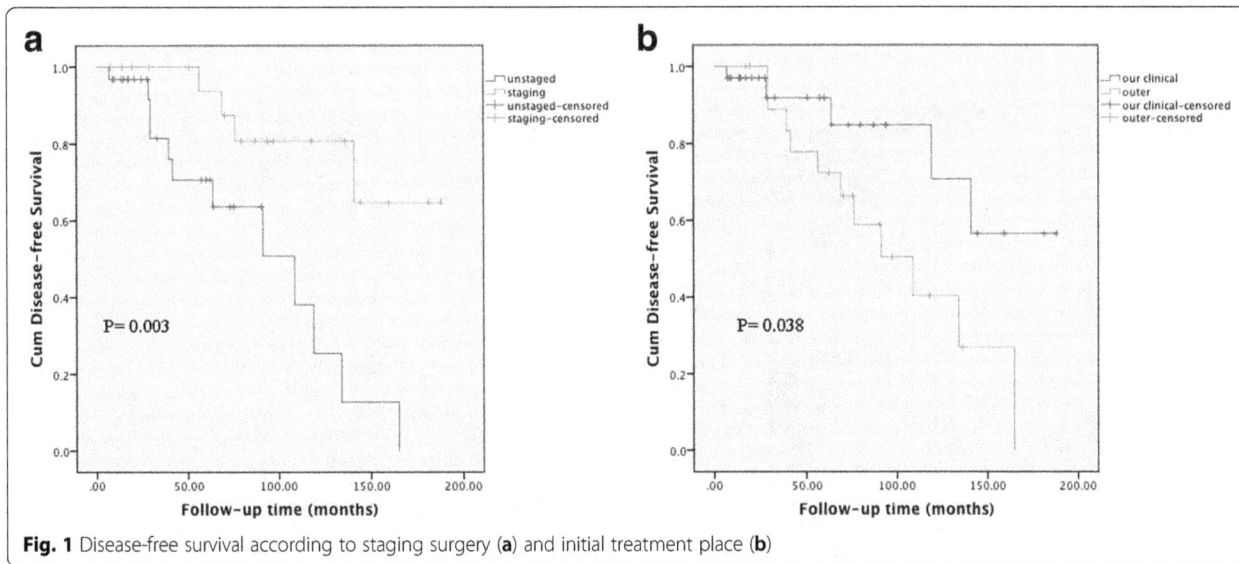

Fig. 1 Disease-free survival according to staging surgery (**a**) and initial treatment place (**b**)

chemotherapy cycles and the incidence of recurrence (≤3 cycles vs. >3 cycles, HR = 0.613, 95% CI: 0.112–3.351, $P = 0.572$) (Fig. 3).

Discussion

Adjuvant chemotherapy was not associated with improved DFS in the current cohort of 60 patients with stage IC AGCT. Furthermore, the number of cycles of chemotherapy was not associated with improved DFS among those patients who received postoperative chemotherapy.

AGCT is a late-relapse disease, and long-term follow-up is necessary to obtain reliable data [12]. The median follow-up time in our study was significantly longer than in other recent reports (88 months; range: 9–334 months) [3, 5], and the recurrence rate was 26.7%, which was consistent with previous reports [4, 13], suggesting that this was a realistic and representative reflection of the natural history of the disease.

NCCN guidelines suggest that adjuvant chemotherapy should be considered in patients with early-stage disease but with high risk factors (e.g., high mitotic index, tumor

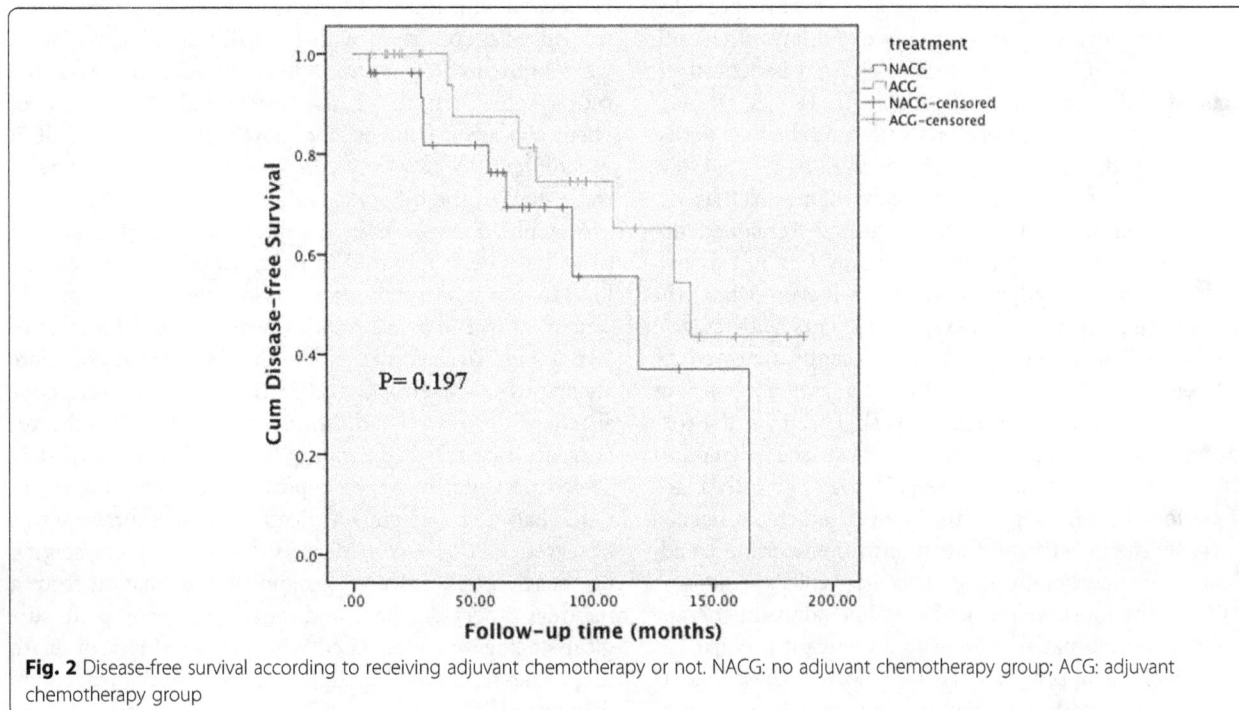

Fig. 2 Disease-free survival according to receiving adjuvant chemotherapy or not. NACG: no adjuvant chemotherapy group; ACG: adjuvant chemotherapy group

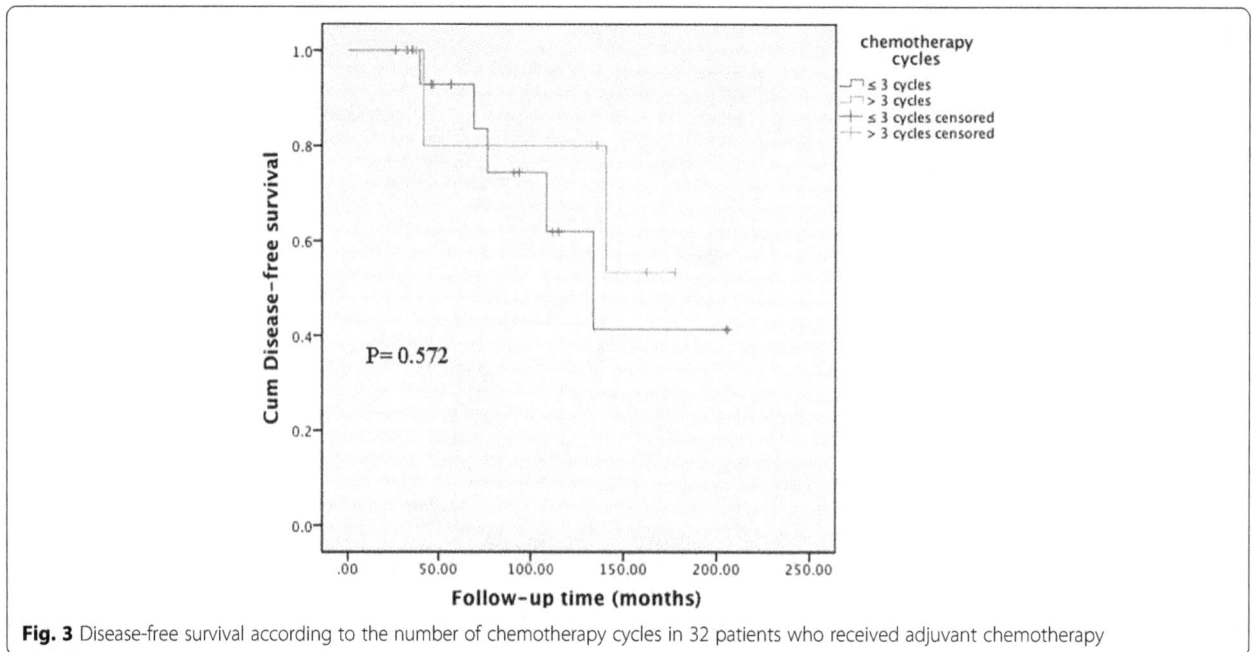

Fig. 3 Disease-free survival according to the number of chemotherapy cycles in 32 patients who received adjuvant chemotherapy

rupture, or incomplete surgical staging); however, our data do not appear to support this recommendation, and showed that adjuvant chemotherapy did not protect against recurrence in patients with AGCT. Adjuvant chemotherapy is not always administered in our practice, and almost half (46.7%) of all patients with stage IC disease did not receive adjuvant chemotherapy. However, the retrospective nature of the trial means that the reasons why these patients did not receive adjuvant chemotherapy were unknown. Previous studies have provided conflicting reports regarding the role of adjuvant chemotherapy in AGCT. Several studies showed beneficial effects of platinum-based treatments [3, 14, 15], though most of these included patients with advanced stage disease, which has a poorer prognosis than early stage disease, and unadjusted survival analyses meant that the role of chemotherapy in stage I disease remained obscure. However, adjuvant chemotherapy was not associated with a reduced recurrence rate, even when the survival analysis was restricted to patients with stage I AGCT [6, 12]. Mangili et al. also recently reported no difference in DFS between stage IC patients with or without adjuvant chemotherapy [11]. The potential toxicity of chemotherapy, including second acute leukemia [16] and cardiovascular disease [17], together with a lack of obvious benefit, suggest that more studies are needed to clarify the benefit and thus inform the decision to administer chemotherapy for early stage AGCT.

BEP is the most widely used first-line adjuvant therapy regimen among patients for whom adjuvant therapy has been deemed appropriate [18]. However, these agents are associated with potentially serious toxicities, such as myelosuppression and pulmonary disorders associated with bleomycin [19]. Prospective trials are therefore needed to assess the therapeutic ratio of regimens other than the widely used BEP. NCCN guidelines (category 2B) also recommend TC, and the Gynecologic Oncology Group is currently developing a randomized phase II trial to compare TC with BEP, with progression-free survival as the primary outcome (ClinicalTrials.gov Identifier NCT01042522). The expectation is that TC may be associated with reduced toxicity and similar progression-free survival compared with BEP. BEP and TC regimens were both used in some of our patients; however, the retrospective nature of the study and the variety of chemotherapy regimens and doses used means that it was difficult to draw any conclusions regarding the relative values of the different regimens in this study.

Age, FIGO stage, staging surgery, and initial treatment place have been reported as prognostic factors in AGCT [3, 12]. Surgical staging was associated with improved outcomes in the present series, with 5-year DFS rates of 93.8% and 70.6% in patients with and without complete staging, respectively ($P = 0.003$). These results were consistent with previous studies demonstrating that the recurrence rate was significantly increased in incompletely staged patients. In Park's report, completely staged patients had no recurrence or deaths, while recurrence was observed in 14.3% of patients without complete staging [3]. Seagle et al. analyzed prognostic information from a national cancer database and found that incomplete surgical staging was associated with increased risk of death [20]. These reports highlight the need for an accurate diagnosis at presentation.

Is adjuvant chemotherapy beneficial for patients with FIGO stage IC adult granulosa cell tumor..

91

Initial treatment outside was a risk factor for recurrence in univariate analysis (5-year DFS rate: 91.9% vs 72.2%), though this was not a significant factor in multivariate analysis. This may be explained by suboptimal surgical extent, delayed initiation of adjuvant treatment in high-risk patients, or an inaccurate pathological diagnosis.

This study raises questions over the importance of chemotherapy in patients with stage IC AGCT. The lack of any obvious benefit of adjuvant chemotherapy suggests that new effective treatment modalities are needed, based on a deeper understanding of the pathogenesis of AGCT. Shah et al. examined *FOXL2* gene mutations in ovarian granulosa cell tumors [21] and showed that *FOXL2* mutation was associated with increased CYP17 expression. Inhibition of this enzyme may thus reverse the effect of *FOXL2* mutation. Additional inhibition of CYP17 may be achieved by novel agents such as abiraterone and ketoconazole [22], and therapies targeting this mechanism may prove to be more useful and less toxic than traditional chemotherapy [5]. Other novel potential targets (vascular endothelial growth factor (VEGF), HER2) are being investigated. In an era of precision medicine, postoperative patient care and decisions about adjuvant chemotherapy can be individualized based on these immunohistochemical factors, such that patients whose GCTs show high expression levels of VEGF or HER2 can be treated with bevacizumab or trastuzumab/imatinib, respectively [23, 24].

The current study was limited by its retrospective nature, including heterogeneity in terms of staging and work-up, and variable chemotherapy regimens, as well as by the rarity of the disease. However, the present study included a relative large cohort of stage IC patients and the results thus contribute to the limited body of knowledge on this condition. Further studies in large series are needed to characterize patients with stage IC subtype who can be spared adjuvant chemotherapy, and to define the real risk factors in stage IC. However, prospective clinical trials are difficult and time-consuming given the rarity of the disease, its indolent nature, and its overall good prognosis in the early stage. International collaboration is therefore needed to generate large studies with the aim of validating new treatment regimens for patients with high-risk early stage AGCT.

Conclusions

Adjuvant chemotherapy does not improve DFS in patients with stage IC AGCT. Further clinical trials, including using novel agents, are needed to characterize patients with stage IC AGCT who can be spared adjuvant chemotherapy, and to define the real risk factors in this disease.

Abbreviations

ACG: Adjuvant chemotherapy group; AGCT: Adult granulosa cell tumor; BEP: Bleomycin, etoposide and cisplatin; DFS: Disease-free survival; FIGO: International Federation of Gynecology and Obstetrics; FOXL2: Forkhead Box L2.; HER2: Human epidermal growth factor receptor-2.; NACG: No adjuvant chemotherapy group.; NCCN: National ComprehensiveCancer Network.; PVB: Cisplatin, vincristine, bleomycin.; PC: Cisplatin, cyclophosphamide.; TC: Paclitaxel and carboplatin.; VEGF: Vascular endothelial growth factor.

Funding

No

Authors' contributions

DW have participated in the design of the study, analyzed the data, prepared the manuscript and revised it critically. MW, KS, JY, HH have participated for the acquisition and analysis of data. YX and TR have designed the study, responsed for the concept, analyzed the data and revised it critically for important intellectual content. All authors read and approved the final manuscript.

Competing interests

The authors declare that they have no competing interests.

References:

1. Schweppe KW, Beller FK. Clinical data of granulosa cell tumors. J Cancer Res Clin Oncol. 1982;104(1–2):161–9.
2. McConechy MK, Farkkila A, Horlings HM, Talhouk A, Unkila-Kallio L, van Meurs HS, et al. Molecularly defined adult granulosa cell tumor of the ovary: the clinical phenotype. J Natl Cancer Inst. 2016;108(11):djw134.
3. Park J-Y, Jin KL, Kim D-Y, Kim J-H, Kim Y-M, Kim K-R, et al. Surgical staging and adjuvant chemotherapy in the management of patients with adult granulosa cell tumors of the ovary. Gynecol Oncol. 2012;125(1):80–6.
4. Uygun K, Aydiner A, Saip P, et al. Clinical parameters and treatment results in recurrent granulosa cell tumor of the ovary. Gynecol Oncol. 2003;88(3): 400–3.
5. Meisel JL, Hyman DM, Jotwani A, Zhou Q, Abu-Rustumd NR, et al. The role of systemic chemotherapy in the management of granulosa cell tumors. Gynecol Oncol. 2015;136(3):505–11.
6. Karalok A, Turan T, Ureyen I, Tasci T, Basaran D, Koc S, et al. Prognostic factors in adult Granulosa cell tumor: a long follow-up at a single center. Int J Gynecol Cancer. 2016;26(4):619–25.
7. Ray-Coquard I, Brown J, Harter P, Provencher DM, Fong PC, Maenpaa J, et al. Gynecologic Cancer inter group (GCIG)consensus review for ovarian sex cord stromal tumors. Int J Gynecol Cancer 2014 ;24(9 Suppl 3):S42–S47.
8. Wilson MK, Fong P, Mesnage S, Chrystal K, Shelling A, Payne K, et al. Stage I granulosa cell tumours: a management conundrum? Results oflong-term follow up. Gynecol Oncol. 2015;138(2):285–91.
9. Bryk S, Färkkilä A, Bützow R, Leminen A, Tapper J, Heikinheimo M, et al. Characteristics and outcome of recurrence in molecularly defined adult-type ovarian granulosa cell tumors. Gynecol Oncol. 2016;143(3):571–7.
10. Schneider DT, Calaminus G, Wessalowski R, Pathmanathan R, Selle B, Sternschulte W, et al. Ovarian sex cordstromal tumors in children and adolescents. J Clin Oncol. 2003;21(12):2357–63.
11. Mangili G, Ottolina J, Cormio G, Loizzi V, De Iaco P, Pellegrini DA, et al. Adjuvant chemotherapy does not improve disease-free survival in FIGO stage IC ovarian granulosa cell tumors: The MITO-9 study. Gynecol Oncol. 2016;143(2):276–80.
12. Mangili G, Ottolina J, Gadducci A, Giorda G, Breda E, Savarese A, Candiani M, et al. Long-term follow-up is crucial after treatment for granulosa cell tumours of the ovary. Br J Cancer. 2013;109(1):29–34.
13. Thrall MM, Paley P, Pizer E, Garcia R, Goff BA. Patterns of spread and recurrence of sex cord-stromal tumors of the ovary. Gynecol Oncol. 2011; 122(2):242–5.

14. Pautier P, Gutierrez-Bonnaire M, Rey A, Sillet-Bach I, Chevreau C, Kerbrat P, et al. Combination of bleomycin, etoposide, and cisplatin for the treatment of advanced ovarian granulosa cell tumors. Int J Gynecol Cancer 200818(3): 446–452.

15. Savage P, Constenla D, Fisher C, Shepherd JH, Barton DP, Blake P, et al. Granulosa cell tumours of the ovary: demographics, survival and the management of advanced disease. Clin Oncol (R Coll Radiol). 1998;10(4): 242–5.

16. Howard R, Gilbert E, Lynch CF, Hall P, Storm H, Holowaty E, et al. Risk of leukemia among survivors of testicular cancer: a population-based study of 42,722 patients. Ann Epidemiol. 2008;18(5):416–21.

17. van den Belt-Dusebout AW, Nuver J, de Wit R, Gietema JA, ten Bokkel Huinink WW, Rodrigus PT, et al. Long-term risk of cardiovascular disease in 5-year survivors of testicular cancer. J Clin Oncol. 2006;24(3):467–75.

18. Schumer ST, Cannistra SA. Granulosa cell tumor of the ovary. J Clin Oncol. 2003;21(6):1180–9.

19. Homesley HD, Bundy BN, Hurteau JA, et al. Bleomycin, etoposide, and cisplatin combination therapy of ovarian granulosa cell tumors and other stromal malignancies: a gynecologic oncology group study. Gynecol Oncol. 1999;72(2):131–7.

20. Seagle B-LL, Ann P, Butler S, Shahabi S. Ovarian granulosa cell tumor: a National Cancer Database study. Gynecol Oncol. 2017;146(2):285–91.

21. Shah SP, Köbel M, Senz J, Morin RD, Clarke BA, Wiegand KC, et al. Mutation of FOXL2 in granulosa-cell tumors of the ovary. N Engl J Med. 2009;360(26): 2719–29.

22. Garcia-Donas J, Hurtado A, García-Casado Z, Albareda J, López-Guerrero JA, Alemany I, et al. Cytochrome P17 inhibition with ketoconazole as treatment for advanced granulosa cell ovarian tumor. J Clin Oncol. 2013;31(10):e165–6.

23. Tsoi M, Laguë MN, Boyer A, Paquet M, Nadeau MÈ, Boerboom D. Anti-VEGFA therapy reduces tumor growth and extends survival in a murine model of ovarian granulosa cell tumor. Transl Oncol. 2013;6(3):226–33.

24. Stern HM. Improving treatment of HER2-positive cancers: opportunities and challenges. Sci Transl Med2012;4 (127):127rv122.

11

Single and combined use of red cell distribution width, mean platelet volume, and cancer antigen 125 for differential diagnosis of ovarian cancer and benign ovarian tumors

Yuan-yuan Qin[†], Yang-yang Wu[†], Xiao-ying Xian, Jin-qiu Qin, Zhan-feng Lai, Lin Liao and Fa-quan Lin[*]

Abstract

Background: Cancer is widely believed to result from chronic inflammation, and red cell distribution width (RDW) and mean platelet volume (MPV) are considered as inflammatory markers for cancer. We investigated the values of RDW, MPV, and cancer antigen 125 (CA125), alone or in combination, for distinguishing between ovarian cancer and benign ovarian tumors.

Methods: The study included 326 patients with ovarian cancer, 290 patients with benign ovarian tumors, and 162 control subjects. Hematologic tests were performed at initial diagnosis.

Results: RDW was increased and MPV was decreased in the ovarian cancer group compared with the control and benign ovarian tumor groups. RDW was positively correlated and MPV was negatively correlated with cancer stage. Area under the curve (AUC) analysis for ovarian cancer versus benign ovarian tumors revealed that the specificity and sensitivity were increased for the combination of MPV and CA125 compared with either marker alone, and the specificity was increased for the combination of RDW and CA125, compared with either alone. The AUCs for RDW plus CA125 and MPV plus CA125 were significantly larger than for any of the markers alone.

Conclusions: In conclusion, combinations of the markers RDW, MPV, and CA125 may improve the differential diagnosis of ovarian cancer and benign ovarian tumors.

Keywords: Red cell distribution width, Mean platelet volume, Cancer antigen 125, Ovarian cancer

Background

Ovarian cancer is one of the most common malignant tumors of the gynecological system, with the highest mortality rate of all gynecological tumors [1]. The ovaries are located in the pelvic cavity and are thus relatively concealed, in addition to which early ovarian cancer lacks any obvious clinical manifestations and diagnostic methods, making it difficult to diagnose early and to distinguish from benign ovarian tumors. More than 70% of patients with ovarian cancer are therefore initially diagnosed at an

advanced stage, and the 5-year survival rate is only 30%. Ovarian cancer thus presents a serious threat to women's health [2]. Cancer antigen 125 (CA125) is a clinical ovarian tumor marker, but its sensitivity is relatively low and other markers are therefore needed to allow discrimination between early ovarian cancer and benign ovarian tumors.

The red cell volume distribution width (RDW) is a quantitative parameter indicating the size of the red blood cells. RDW reflects red cell volume heterogeneity and is usually measured as part of the whole blood cell count. Several studies have suggested that a high RDW may be closely related to endometrial, ovarian, and liver cancers [3–5]. Furthermore, activated platelets are involved in cancer

* Correspondence: fqlin1998@163.com
[†]Equal contributors
Department of Clinical Laboratory, The First Affiliated Hospital of Guangxi Medical University, Guangxi Zhuang Autonomous Region, Nanning, China

progression and metastases [6, 7]. Mean platelet volume (MPV) is a marker of activated platelets and has been associated with gastric, thyroid, and ovarian cancers [8–10]. Both RDW and MPV have recently been studied in various diseases. The aim of the current study was to investigate the roles of RDW, MPV, and CA125, either alone or in combination, for distinguishing between ovarian cancer and benign ovarian tumors.

Methods

Patients

We performed a retrospective study in patients diagnosed with ovarian cancer at the First Affiliated Hospital of Guangxi Medical University, China, from January 2015 to May 2017. Patients who had undergone complete surgical resection with a histologically confirmed diagnosis of ovarian cancer, and who were untreated before diagnosis were included in the study. Patients with diabetes mellitus, cardiovascular disease, kidney disease, blood disease, acute inflammation, anemia, recent iron therapy, venous thrombosis for > 6 months, and recent blood transfusions (within the last 3 months) were excluded. Patients with ovarian cancer were classified into groups according to cancer stage, in accordance with the standards established by the International Federation of Gynecology and Obstetrics in 2000 [11]. Patients diagnosed with benign ovarian tumors (mature ovarian teratoma, simple ovarian cyst, ovarian endometriosis) in our hospital during the same time period comprised the benign ovarian tumor group, and healthy subjects were selected as the control group. There were no marked differences in age among the three groups. This study was approved by the ethics committee of the First Affiliated Hospital of Guangxi Medical University, China.

Method

Venous blood (2 mL) was collected from each patient in the morning and placed in EDTA-K2 anticoagulation tubes and drying tubes. Whole blood cell parameters were determined using a Beckman Coulter LH 780 hematology analyzer (Beckman Coulter, Brea, CA, USA). The white blood cell count, absolute neutrophil count, absolute lymphocyte count, absolute monocyte count, hemoglobin concentration (Hb), blood platelet count (PLT), MPV, platelet distribution width (PDW), and RDW were obtained directly by the hematology analyzer. Serum CA125 levels were detected using a Roche E6000 analyzer (Roche Diagnostics, Basel, Switzerland).

Statistical analysis

All data were analyzed using SPSS 20.0 software (IBM Corp., Armonk, NY). Continuous variables are expressed as mean ± standard deviation or median (interquartile range), and categorical variables are expressed as numbers and percentages. Differences in baseline characteristics among the three groups were analyzed by one-way ANOVA. Differences in relevant indicators between two groups were compared using Tukey's test. Correlations between RDW and PDW and cancer stage in patients with ovarian cancer were analyzed by Spearman's correlation. Sensitivity and specificity were defined by receiver-operating characteristic curves, and differences in the area under the curve (AUC) were detected using MedCalc version 15.0. A P value of < 0.05 was considered statistically significant.

Results

A total of 326 patients with ovarian cancer (range 27–81 years) were included in this study. According to the grading standards, 118 patients (36.2%) had stage I cancer, 65 (19.9%) had stage II, 83 (25.5%) had stage III, and 60 (18.4%) had stage IV. A further 290 patients with benign ovarian tumors (range 20–71 years) and 162 healthy control subjects (range 22–62 years) were also included in the study. White blood cell count, absolute neutrophil count, absolute lymphocyte count, absolute monocyte count, Hb, PLT, MPV, PDW, RDW, and CA125 differed significantly among the three groups (Table 1).

RDW and MPV levels in patients with ovarian cancer or benign ovarian tumors and in healthy individuals are shown in Figs. 1 and 2. RDW was higher in the ovarian cancer group compared with both the control and benign ovarian tumor groups (cancer vs. benign ovarian tumors, $P < 0.001$; cancer vs. control, $P < 0.001$; benign ovarian tumors vs. control, $P < 0.001$; Tukey's test). However, MPV was lower in the ovarian cancer group compared with the control and benign ovarian tumor groups (cancer vs. benign ovarian tumor, $P < 0.001$; cancer vs. control, $P < 0.001$; benign ovarian tumor vs. control, $P < 0.001$; Tukey's test).

Correlations between cancer stage and RDW and MPV in patients with ovarian cancer are shown in Figs. 3 and 4. Correlation analysis demonstrated that RDW was positively correlated and MPV was negatively correlated with cancer stage.

Receiver-operating characteristic analysis was used to assess the AUCs for single and combined biomarkers (Table 2). RDW and MPV had high sensitivities for distinguishing between ovarian cancer and benign ovarian tumors (76.70% and 74.20%, respectively), while MPV and CA125 had high specificities (73.8% and 73.4%, respectively). The specificity and sensitivity increased when MPV and CA125 were combined, and the specificity increased when RDW and CA125 were combined. Moreover, the combination of RDW plus CA125 manifested a significantly larger AUC (0.844, 0.813–0.872) compared with RDW and CA125 alone ($P = 0.013$ and $P < 0.001$, respectively), and the combination of MPV and CA125

Table 1 Laboratory characteristics of the participants

Variables	ovarian cancer	benign ovarian tumors	controls	P-value
Number	326	290	162	
Age(years)	43.15 ± 11.59	43.18 ± 9.25	44.13 ± 6.90	0.544
W; (10⁹/L)	8.28 ± 4.01[a]	6.69 ± 2.25	6.33 ± 1.49[c]	<0.001
N; (10⁹/L)	6.11 ± 4.04[a]	4.12 ± 2.01	3.70 ± 1.12[c]	<0.001
L; (10⁹/L)	1.52 ± 0.68[a]	1.97 ± 0.67	2.07 ± 0.72[c]	<0.001
Mo; (10⁹/L)	0.49 ± 0.01[a]	0.45 ± 0.15	0.44 ± 0.15[c]	0.001
Hb; (g/L)	106.38 ± 19.53[a]	124.64 ± 13.13	128.14 ± 6.47[c]	<0.001
PLT; (10¹²/L)	216.50 ± 130.92[a]	239.68 ± 88.08	248.18 ± 64.8[c]	0.001
MPV; (fl)	8.19 ± 0.86[a]	9.31 ± 0.91[b]	9.64 ± 0.63[c]	<0.001
PDW;(%)	0.16 ± 0.01[a]	0.16 ± 0.02[b]	0.16 ± 0.01[c]	<0.001
RDW;(%)	0.16 ± 0.02[a]	0.14 ± 0.01[b]	0.13 ± 0.01[c]	<0.001
CA125; U/mL	68.85(32.20–385.05)[a]	23.15(14.43–37.76)	5.94(4.04–13.94)[c]	<0.001

Data are expressed as mean ± standard deviation or median (interquartile range)
W, white blood cell count; N, absolute neutrophil count; L, absolute lymphocyte count; Mo, absolute monocyte count; Hb, hemoglobin; PLT, blood platelet count;
MPV, mean platelet volume; PDW, platelet distribution width; RDW, red cell distribution width; CA125, cancer antigen 125
P values were calculated by one-way ANOVA tests
[a]Indicates a significant difference (P < 0.05) between ovarian cancer and benign ovarian tumors (Tukey's test)
[b]Indicates a significant difference (P < 0.05) between benign ovarian tumors and controls (Tukey's test)
[c]Indicates a significant difference (P < 0.05) between ovarian cancer and controls (Tukey's test)
10^9,10^9; 10^{12},10^12

manifested a significantly larger AUC (0.862, 0.833–0.889) compared with MPV and CA125 alone (both P < 0.001) (Fig. 5).

Discussion

Early diagnosis and treatment of ovarian cancer can improve the 5-year survival rate to > 90%, compared with < 50% in patients with a late diagnosis [12]. The main diagnostic methods for ovarian cancer are currently mainly gynecological examination, tumor marker detection, imaging, cytology, and histology, though all these tests have some limitations. The identification of early ovarian cancer markers is thus of great importance in terms of improving the diagnosis, treatment efficacy, and prognosis of patients. The results of the current study showed that RDW levels were significantly higher and MPV levels were significantly lower in patients with ovarian cancer compared with patients with benign ovarian tumors and healthy controls. Furthermore, various combinations of RDW, MPV, and CA125 were valuable for diagnosing ovarian cancer and distinguishing it from benign ovarian tumors.

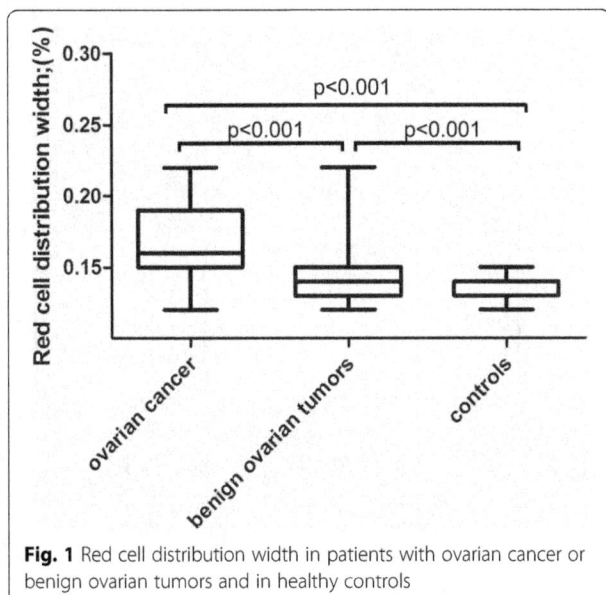

Fig. 1 Red cell distribution width in patients with ovarian cancer or benign ovarian tumors and in healthy controls

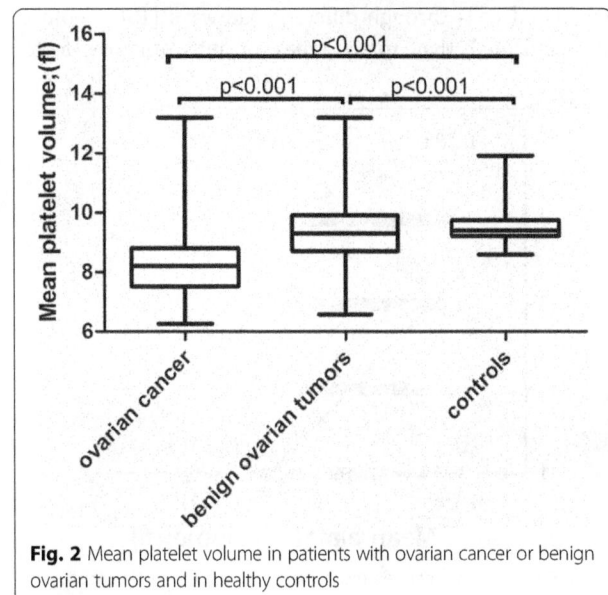

Fig. 2 Mean platelet volume in patients with ovarian cancer or benign ovarian tumors and in healthy controls

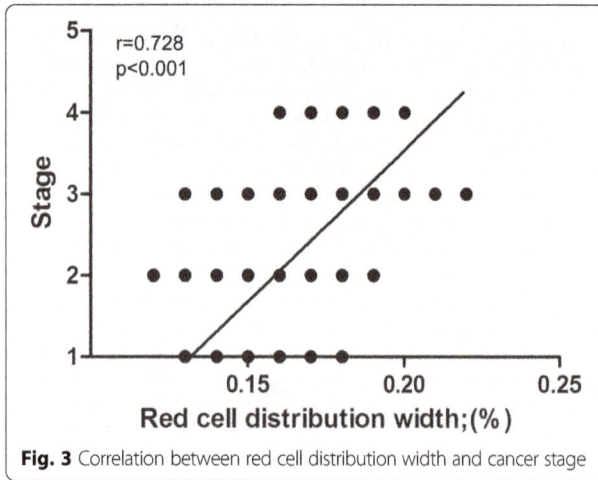

Fig. 3 Correlation between red cell distribution width and cancer stage

Table 2 Receiver operating characteristic curve analyses showing the utilities of single and combined markers for differentiating between ovarian cancer and benign ovarian tumors

Markers	Sensitivity	Specificity	+PV	-PV	AUC
RDW;(%)	76.70	70.30	74.40	72.90	0.823(0.791–0.852)
MPV;fl	74.20	73.80	76.10	71.80	0.823(0.790–0.852)
CA125;U/mL	71.80	73.40	75.20	69.80	0.772(0.737–0.804)
RDW + CA125	60.74	90.34	87.60	67.20	0.844(0.813–0.872)
MPV + CA125	74.85	82.07	82.40	74.40	0.862(0.833–0.889)

+PV, positive predictive value; -PV, negative predictive value; AUC, area under curve; RDW, red cell distribution width; MPV, mean platelet volume; CA125, cancer antigen 125

Cancer is widely believed to be the result of chronic inflammation [4]. Inflammatory cytokines have been shown to play a role in inhibiting the stimulatory effect of erythropoietin on bone marrow erythrocyte stem cells, anti-apoptosis, and cell maturation, thus causing more immature red blood cells to be released into the peripheral blood circulation, thereby increasing the heterogeneity of peripheral red blood cells and RDW [13]. Elevated RDW may also be associated with an increased rate of ineffective hematopoiesis caused by chronic inflammation. Hunziker et al. demonstrated that the inflammatory response and oxidative stress could affect erythropoiesis, and alter blood cell membrane deformability and erythrocyte half-life, thereby increasing RDW [14]. Ovarian cancer has certain characteristics of a chronic inflammatory disease, and levels of many cytokines, including tumor necrosis factor-a, interleukin (IL)-1, and IL-17, are unbalanced in patients with ovarian cancer,cytokines may affect the production, apoptosis, size, and fragility of red blood cells through different pathways [15]. Neote et al. confirmed that many types of inflammatory factor

receptors were expressed on the surface of red blood cells, and suggested that red blood cells were involved in the inflammatory process [16]. Patients with advanced ovarian cancer often have impaired gastrointestinal and immune functions, which may result in deficiencies of iron, folic acid, vitamin B12, and other red blood cell metabolites, various degrees of anemia; and an increased RDW.

MPV is a marker of platelet function and activation that can be determined easily during complete blood counts, with no additional cost. Various studies have identified MPV as a useful indicator in some inflammatory diseases, and it has been associated with disease activity and severity of inflammation [17]. Incebiyik et al. reported low MPV values in pelvic inflammatory disease, and emphasized its diagnostic value [18]. Reduced MPV levels have also been implicated in non-small cell lung cancer, multiple myeloma, and severe primary dysmenorrhea [19–21]. However,

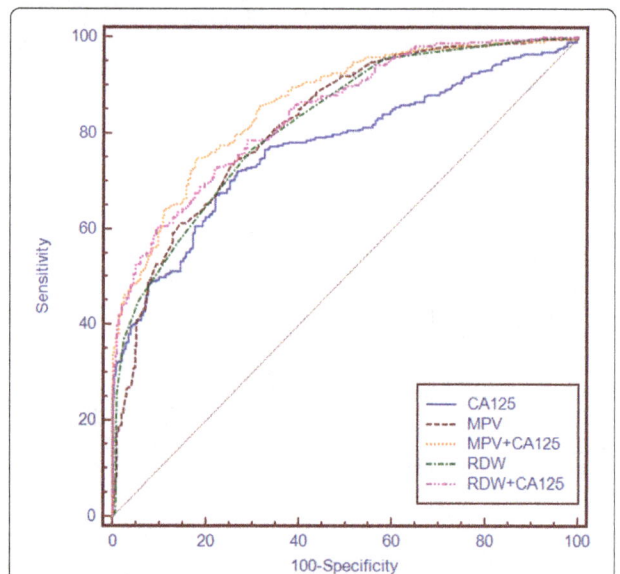

Fig. 4 Correlation between mean platelet volume and cancer stage

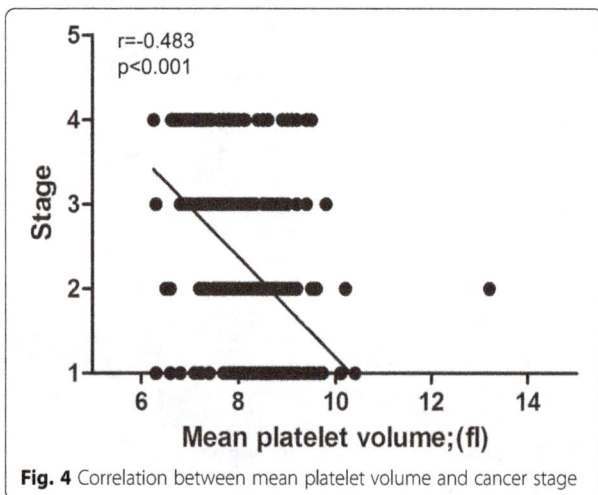

Fig. 5 Receiver-operator characteristics curves for RDW, MPV, and CA125 alone or combined showing sensitivity and 100-specificity for the differential diagnosis of ovarian cancer versus benign ovarian tumors. RDW, red cell distribution width; MPV, mean platelet volume; CA125, cancer antigen 125

the mechanism responsible for the low MPV in patients with ovarian cancer remains unclear. Inflammation and coagulation have been shown to mediate the immune response, which in turn plays an important role in tumor development, invasion, and metastasis [22]. Some factors, such as IL-1, IL-6, and granulocyte colony-stimulating factor can indirectly increase platelet production [23, 24], and considerable evidence suggests that IL-6 promotes tumorigenesis by regulating apoptosis, survival, angiogenesis, metastasis, and metabolism [25]. In addition, megakaryopoiesis and subsequent thrombopoiesis in cancer may be stimulated by granulocyte colony-stimulating factor and macrophage colony-stimulating factor, which can be secreted by tumor cells [26]. Both basic and clinical studies have found a link between malignancy and platelet abnormalities [27]. Platelets play a key role in regulating inflammation. Released inflammatory mediators increase platelet activation, leading to a subsequent change in MPV. The consumption of platelets at the inflammation site may be responsible for the decrease in MPV. Furthermore, the inflammatory environment can impair megakaryopoiesis, in turn causing the release of small platelets from the bone marrow [28].

CA125 is a commonly used biochemical marker for ovarian cancer diagnosis. However, CA125 levels may also be increased in patients with some benign gynecological lesions, such as endometriosis and pelvic inflammatory disease, making it prone to false positive results [29]. The current study showed that, compared with RDW, MPV, and CA125 alone, MPV combined with CA125 had higher sensitivity and specificity for distinguishing between ovarian cancer and benign ovarian tumors, and RDW combined with CA125 had higher specificity. The combinations of CA125 with RDW or MPV manifested significantly larger AUCs compared with RDW, MPV, and CA125 alone, suggesting that using these combined markers may improve the early detection of ovarian cancer and its differential diagnosis from benign ovarian tumors.

This study had some limitations. This was a relatively small retrospective study in patients with ovarian cancer, and the small sample size prevented us from drawing any firm conclusions about the correlations between RDW, MPV, and ovarian cancer. Further, large-scale prospective studies are therefore needed to confirm these results. Furthermore, this study only included Chinese participants, and the results therefore cannot be generalized to other ethnic groups. Nevertheless, to the best of our knowledge, this study provides the first evidence for the combined use of RDW, MPV, and CA125 for discriminating between ovarian cancer and benign ovarian tumors.

Conclusions

Early diagnosis of ovarian cancer and its distinction from benign ovarian tumors are essential for improving its prognosis. CA-125 alone is insufficient for this purpose, but combinations of RDW, MPV, and CA125 may facilitate the early detection and differential diagnosis of ovarian cancer compared with benign ovarian tumors.

Abbreviations

CA125: Cancer antigen 125; Hb: Hemoglobin; L: Absolute lymphocyte count; Mo: Absolute monocyte count; MPV: Mean platelet volume; N: Absolute neutrophil count; PDW: Platelet distribution width; PLT: Blood platelet count; RDW: Red cell distribution width; W: White blood cell count

Acknowledgments

We would like to thank Department of Clinical Laboratory,the First Affiliated Hospital of Guangxi Medical University,China.

Funding

This research did not receive any specific grant from funding agencies in the public, commercial, or not-for-profit sectors.

Authors' contributions

F-QL and Y-YQ conceived the idea and designed the study protocol. J-QQ contributed with provision of study material or patients. Z-FL, X-YX and LL collected, assembled data and interpreted the data; Y-YQ and Y-YW performed statistical analysis, wrote the manuscript. All authors read and approved the final manuscript.

Competing interests

The authors declare that they have no competing interests.

References

1. Siegel RL, Miller KD, Jemal A. Cancer statistics, 2015. CA Cancer J Clin. 2015;65(1):5–29.
2. Nam EJ, Yoon H, Kim SW, Kim H, Kim YT, Kim JH, et al. MicroRNA expression profiles in serous ovarian carcinoma. Clinical cancer research : an official journal of the American Association for Cancer Research. 2008;14(9):2690–5.
3. Kemal Y, Demirag G, Bas B, Onem S, Teker F, Yucel I. The value of red blood cell distribution width in endometrial cancer. Clin Chem Lab Med. 2015;53(5):823–7.
4. Qin Y, Wang P, Huang Z, Huang G, Tang J, Guo Y, et al. The value of red cell distribution width in patients with ovarian cancer. Medicine. 2017;96(17):e6752.
5. Koma Y, Onishi A, Matsuoka H, Oda N, Yokota N, Matsumoto Y, et al. Increased red blood cell distribution width associates with cancer stage and prognosis in patients with lung cancer. PLoS One. 2013;8(11):e80240.
6. Bambace NM, Holmes CE. The platelet contribution to cancer progression. Journal of thrombosis and haemostasis : JTH. 2011;9(2):237–49.
7. Goubran HA, Stakiw J, Radosevic M, Burnouf T. Platelet-cancer interactions. Semin Thromb Hemost. 2014;40(3):296–305.
8. Yun ZY, Li N, Zhang X, Zhang H, Bu Y, Sun Y, et al. Mean platelet volume, platelet distribution width and carcinoembryonic antigen to discriminate gastric cancer from gastric ulcer. Oncotarget. 2017;8(37):62600–5.
9. Yu YJ, Li N, Yun ZY, Niu Y, Xu JJ, Liu ZP, et al. Preoperative mean platelet volume and platelet distribution associated with thyroid cancer. Neoplasma. 2017;64:594–8.
10. Ma X, Wang Y, Sheng H, Tian W, Qi Z, Teng F, et al. prognostic significance of thrombocytosis, platelet parameters and aggregation rates in epithelial ovarian cancer. J Obstet Gynaecol Res. 2014;40(1):178–83.
11. Okines AF, Morris R, Hancock BW. An Evaluation of FIGO 2000: the first 5 years. The Journal of reproductive medicine. 2008;53(8):615–22.
12. Li J, Dowdy S, Tipton T, Podratz K, Lu WG, Xie X, et al. HE4 as a biomarker for ovarian and endometrial cancer management. Expert Rev Mol Diagn. 2009;9(6):555–66.

13. Forhecz Z, Gombos T, Borgulya G, Pozsonyi Z, Prohaszka Z, Janoskuti L. Red cell distribution width in heart failure: prediction of clinical events and relationship with markers of ineffective erythropoiesis, inflammation, renal function, and nutritional state. Am Heart J. 2009;158(4):659–66.

14. Hunziker S, Celi LA, Lee J, Howell MD. Red cell distribution width improves the simplified acute physiology score for risk prediction in unselected critically ill patients. Crit Care. 2012;16(3):R89.

15. Weiss G, Goodnough LT. Anemia Of chronic disease. N Engl J Med. 2005;352(10):1011–23.

16. Neote K, Darbonne W, Ogez J, Horuk R, Schall TJ. Identification Of a promiscuous inflammatory peptide receptor on the surface of red blood cells. J Biol Chem. 1993;268(17):12247–9.

17. Ozdemir R, Karadeniz C, Doksoz O, Celegen M, Yozgat Y, Guven B, et al. Are mean platelet volume and platelet distribution width useful parameters in children with acute rheumatic carditis? Pediatr Cardiol. 2014;35(1):53–6.

18. Incebiyik A, Seker A, Vural M, Gul Hilali N, Camuzcuoglu A, Camuzcuoglu H. May mean platelet volume levels be a predictor in the diagnosis of pelvic inflammatory disease? Wien Klin Wochenschr. 2014;126(13–14):422–6.

19. Gao L, Zhang H, Zhang B, Zhang L, Wang C. Prognostic Value of combination of preoperative platelet count and mean platelet volume in patients with resectable non-small cell lung cancer. Oncotarget. 2017;8(9):15632–41.

20. Zhuang Q, Xiang L, Xu H, fang F, Xing C, Liang B, et al. the independent association of mean platelet volume with overall survival in multiple myeloma. Oncotarget. 2016;7(38):62640–6.

21. Kabil Kucur S, Seven A, Yuksel KB, Sencan H, Gozukara I, Keskin N. Mean platelet volume, a novel biomarker in adolescents with severe primary dysmenorrhea. J Pediatr Adolesc Gynecol. 2016;29(4):390–2.

22. Babu SN, Chetal G, Kumar S. Macrophage Migration inhibitory factor: a potential marker for cancer diagnosis and therapy. Asian Pacific journal of cancer prevention : APJCP. 2012;13(5):1737–44.

23. Kemal Y, Yucel I, Ekiz K, Demirag G, Yilmaz B, Teker F, et al. elevated serum neutrophil to lymphocyte and platelet to lymphocyte ratios could be useful in lung cancer diagnosis. Asian Pacific journal of cancer prevention : APJCP. 2014;15(6):2651–4.

24. Mantovani A, Allavena P, Sica A, Balkwill F. Cancer-related inflammation. Nature. 2008;454(7203):436–44.

25. Kumari N, Dwarakanath BS, das a, Bhatt AN. Role of interleukin-6 in cancer progression and therapeutic resistance. Tumour biology : the journal of the International Society for Oncodevelopmental Biology and Medicine. 2016;37(9):11553–72.

26. Kowanetz M, Wu X, lee J, tan M, Hagenbeek T, Qu X, et al. granulocyte-colony stimulating factor promotes lung metastasis through mobilization of Ly6G+Ly6C+ granulocytes. Proc Natl Acad Sci U S A. 2010;107(50):21248–55.

27. Sierko E, Wojtukiewicz MZ. Platelets and angiogenesis in malignancy. Semin Thromb Hemost. 2004;30(1):95–108.

28. Gasparyan AY, Ayvazyan L, Mikhailidis DP, Kitas GD. Mean platelet volume: a link between thrombosis and inflammation? Curr Pharm Des. 2011;17(1):47–58.

29. Terry KL, Sluss PM, Skates SJ, Mok SC, Ye B, Vitonis AF, et al. Blood and urine markers for ovarian cancer: a comprehensive review. Dis Markers. 2004;20(2):53–70.

12

Discordant anti-müllerian hormone (AMH) and follicle stimulating hormone (FSH) among women undergoing in vitro fertilization (IVF): which one is the better predictor for live birth?

Shunping Wang[1,2], Yi Zhang[3], Virginia Mensah[1,2], Warren J. Huber III[1,2], Yen-Tsung Huang[3,4*] and Ruben Alvero[1,2*]

Abstract

Background: This study sought to clarify the roles of Anti-müllerian hormone (AMH) and follicle stimulating hormone (FSH) in predicting live birth, especially in patients with discordant AMH and FSH. A large IVF data set provided by eIVF®, consisting of 13,964 cycles with AMH, FSH, age, BMI, and birth outcomes were evaluated. Patients were categorized into four groups: Good prognosis group (AMH ≥1 ng/ml; FSH < 10 mIU/ml), Poor prognosis group (AMH < 1 ng/ml; FSH ≥10 mIU/ml), Reassuring AMH group (AMH ≥1 ng/ml; FSH ≥10 mIU/ml), and Reassuring FSH group (AMH < 1 ng/ml; FSH < 10 mIU/ml). The interaction between AMH, FSH, and their impact on live birth rate among these four groups was evaluated using Generalized Additive Mixed Modeling (GAMM).

Results: Analysis revealed a nonlinear relationship of AMH and FSH with live birth rate among all ages. Among the four groups, the good prognosis group had the highest live birth rate while the poor prognosis group had the lowest live birth rate (29.3% vs 13.1%, $p < 0.005$). In the discordant groups, the live birth rate of the reassuring AMH group was significantly higher than the reassuring FSH group (22.8% vs 15.6%, $p < 0.005$).

Conclusions: Although both FSH and AMH are widely use to assess the ovarian reserve in women undergoing evaluation for infertility, AMH appears to be superior to FSH among all age groups. This is particularly important for patients with discordant AMH and FSH where reassuring AMH is a better clinical predictor of cycle success.

Background

In women undergoing evaluation for infertility, ovarian reserve testing with anti-müllerian hormone (AMH) and follicle stimulating hormone (FSH) provides important prognostic information regarding reproductive outcomes. AMH is a peptide hormone produced by granulosa cells of early antral follicles and can be collected at any point during a woman's menstrual cycle [1–3]. Although no established cutoff for normal and abnormal AMH exists, it is generally accepted that AMH > 0.8–1.0 ng/ml are suggestive of normal ovarian reserve [4]. FSH is a hormone produced by the anterior pituitary and when elevated

above 10 mIU/ml, is suggestive of diminished ovarian reserve [5]. Both markers are affected by a woman's age: AMH decreases as age increases, while FSH increases as age increases. The American Society for Reproductive Medicine considers evaluation of both serum methods acceptable measures of ovarian reserve [6]. Although AMH and FSH are generally accepted as useful in predicting response to ovarian stimulation, existing evidence is controversial regarding the utility of both markers for the prediction of live birth [4, 5, 7–14].

In a retrospective review of 76 in vitro fertilization (IVF) cycles, Barad et al. found AMH to be a superior predictor of clinical pregnancy outcome compared to FSH [15]. Similarly, Nelson et al. evaluated 340 patients undergoing first IVF or Intracytoplasmic Sperm Injection (ICSI) cycles and found that AMH predicts live birth and anticipated

* Correspondence: ythuang@stat.sinica.edu.tw; ralvero@wihri.org
[3]Brown University School of Public Health, Providence, RI 02912, USA
[1]Brown University Warren Alpert Medical School, Providence, RI 02912, USA
Full list of author information is available at the end of the article

oocyte yield better than FSH and age [16]. Another retrospective analysis comparing multiple markers of ovarian reserve determined that AMH, antral follicle count, and quantity of oocytes retrieved were the most reliable predictors of live birth [17]. These studies, though compelling, are limited by small sample sizes and stringent inclusion criteria which limits their external validity. The question, therefore, of which ovarian reserve marker is a better predictor of live birth remains unanswered, leaving infertility specialists with limited evidence to guide their treatment decisions.

Clinicians additionally often encounter a discrepancy between the two markers—a situation which can affect the interpretation of a woman's likelihood of live birth. Leader et al. showed a frequency of AMH and FSH discordance of as many as 1 in 5 evaluations for female infertility [18]. In a small retrospective study, having an elevated FSH (> 10 mIU/ml) but reassuring AMH (> 0.6 ng/ml) was found to be significantly associated with higher oocyte yield, greater number of day 3 embryos, and lower cycle cancellation rates compared to women with random AMH levels < 0.6 ng/ml. Clinical pregnancy rate among this group was likewise higher, but the difference was not statistically significant [19]. Gleicher et al. similarly reported that among 115 female infertility patients with discordant AMH and FSH (normal age specific AMH with abnormal FSH), oocyte yield was diminished compared to their AMH/FSH concordant counterparts (normal age specific AMH and FSH) [20]. Still, when discordant results are encountered, there is a paucity of data regarding the prognostic relationship between AMH and FSH.

We sought to investigate this question of the clinical utility of AMH and FSH in a retrospective analysis of the eIVF® database, a multi-center dataset that encompasses over 140,000 cycles of assisted reproduction at over 60 fertility centers. The main objective of this study is to evaluate whether AMH or FSH is a better predictor of live birth among infertility patients of differing ages. Additionally, when AMH and FSH markers are discordant and confer potentially conflicting prognostic values, we determine which marker is a more reliable estimate of successful pregnancy outcome.

Methods
Patient selection
eIVF® is an electronic medical record software for clinical IVF settings designed by PracticeHwy.com (Dallas, Texas). The software package includes portals integrating clinical, administrative, and financial information. The dataset we obtained consisted of 144,044 fresh cycles from 60 centers in the United States from 2000 to 2016. Evaluation of this comprehensive de-identified dataset was determined to be exempt by the Women and Infants Institutional Review Board.

Figure 1 shows our CONSORT diagram for data processing. We excluded cycles which were incomplete, were non-autologous donor cycles, had unknown or missing cycle information, or contained outlier variables. Centers with less than 10 cycles were also excluded. Following application of these exclusion criteria, only 47,615 cycles remained in the dataset. Of note, since AMH has only been adopted in clinical use in the past few years, most cycles before 2010 were excluded because of missing AMH values. Thus our final dataset contained 13,790 autologous IVF cycles with known AMH, FSH, and confirmed determination of live birth.

The 13,790 cycles included for analysis were further subdivided into four groups using AMH = 1.0 ng/ml and FSH = 10.0 mIU/ml as cutoff values for normal/reassuring testing. Groups I and II represent a patient population with concordance between their AMH and FSH results. Group I included cycles from all good prognosis patients with AMH greater than or equal to 1.0 ng/ml and FSH less than 10 mIU/ml. Group II included cycles from patients considered poor responders based on AMH less than 1.0 ng/ml and FSH greater than or equal to 10 mIU/ml. Groups III and IV represent a patient population with discordance between their ovarian reserve markers. Group III included the cycles with AMH less than 1.0 ng/ml and with FSH less than 10 mIU/ml, while Group IV included cycles with AMH greater than or equal to 1.0 ng/ml and with FSH greater than or equal to 10 mIU/ml (Table 1). Our primary outcome of interest was live birth per cycle initiated.

Statistical analysis
Generalized additive mixed models (GAMM) were used to investigate the nonlinear fixed effects of AMH and FSH on live birth rate using penalized spline [21], while adjusting for the random effects of centers. AMH and FSH levels were transformed into log-scale before fitting the models because of their highly skewed distributions in our sample, and a small value, 0.7 was added to AMH and FSH levels before transformation to avoid taking logarithm of zero. GAMM were fit to delineate the marginal effects of AMH and FSH on live birth rate, adjusting for age. The joint effects of AMH and FSH were further characterized using two-dimensional spline under GAMM. The two-dimensional splines with AMH-by-FSH interaction and without were both explored to investigate the joint effects of AMH and FSH. All models were fitted through maximizing a penalized log-likelihood using R package mgcv. Based on the fitted models, we were able to predict the probability of live birth for a certain patient given one's AMH, FSH and age. To visualize the dose-response relationship

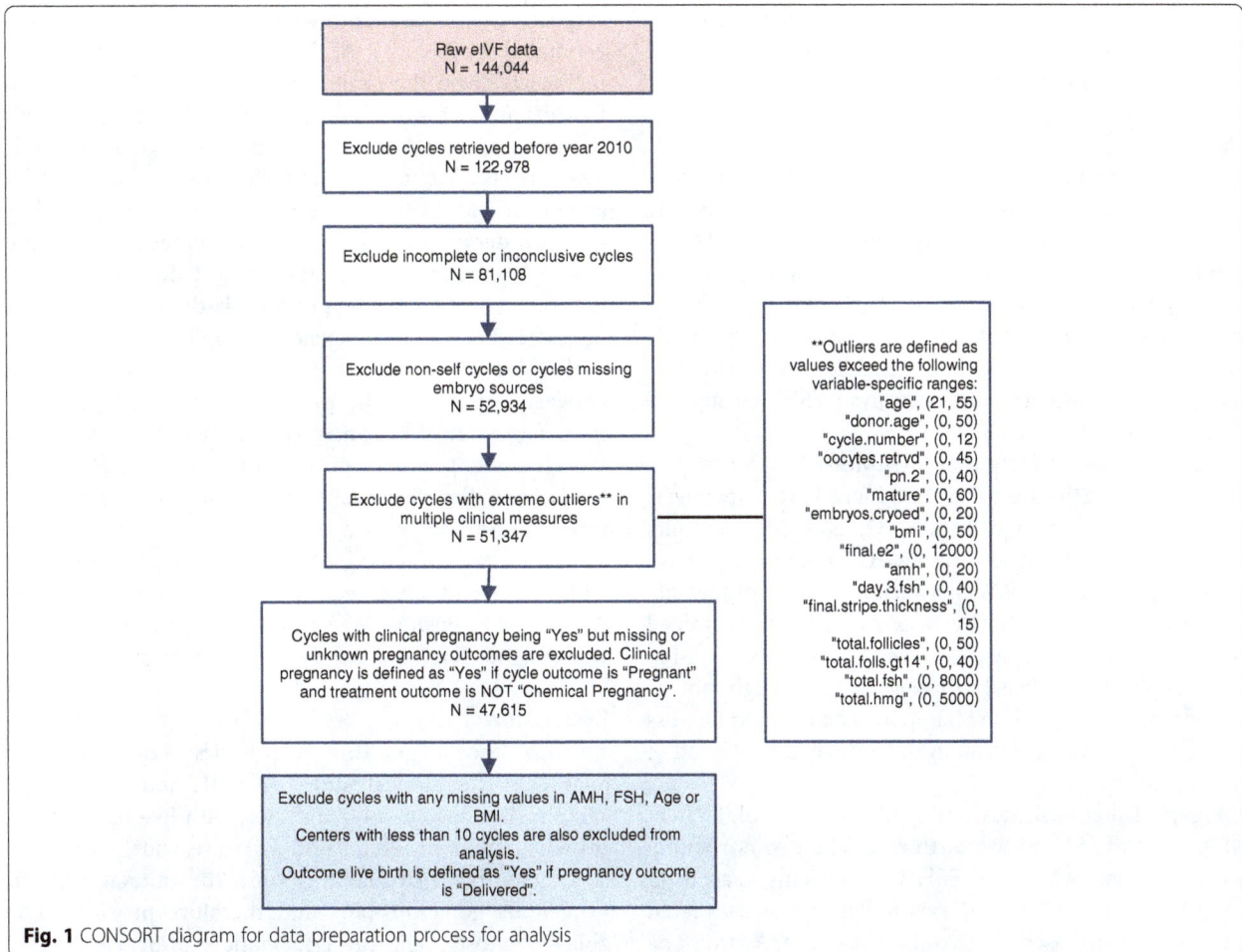

Fig. 1 CONSORT diagram for data preparation process for analysis

Table 1 Demographic characteristics and live birth rates of all four groups

All		Concordant		Discordant		
		Group I: Good Prognosis (AMH ≥ 1 & FSH < 10)	Group II: Poor Prognosis (AMH < 1 & FSH ≥ 10)	Group III: Reassuring FSH (AMH < 1 & FSH < 10)	Group IV: Reassuring AMH (AMH ≥ 1 & FSH ≥ 10)	
N	13,790	7997	1717	3271	805	
	Mean (SD)	Mean (SD)	Mean (SD)	Mean (SD)	Mean (SD)	P-values
Age	35.4 (4.7)	34.1 (4.5)	38.0 (4.1)	37.3 (4.3)	35.6 (4.4)	< 0.001
BMI	25.9 (6.0)	26.0 (6.0)	25.1 (5.2)	26.6 (6.3)	24.4 (4.9)	< 0.001
# of embryos transferred	1.7 (1.1)	1.8 (1.0)	1.5 (1.3)	1.8(1.2)	1.9 (1.2)	< 0.001
E2	2261 (1485)	2676 (1556)	1370 (973)	1690 (1151)	2240 (1243)	< 0.001
FSH (mIU/ml)	7.6 (3.8)	6.2 (2.0)	14.0 (4.4)	6.6 (2.2)	12.2 (3.1)	< 0.001
AMH (ng/ml)	2.4 (2.7)	3.6 (2.9)	0.4 (0.3)	0.5 (0.3)	2.3 (1.7)	< 0.001
Live Birth (%)	23.5%	29.1%[a,b,c]	12.8%[d, e]	15.4%[f]	22.7%	< 0.001

[a]Group I vs Group II. p-value < 0.001
[b]Group I vs Group III. p-value < 0.001
[c]Group I vs Group IV. p-value < 0.001
[d]Group II vs Group III. p-value 0.013
[e]Group II vs Group IV. p-value < 0.001
[f]Group III vs Group IV. p-value < 0.001

of AMH and/or FSH with respect to the probability of live birth, we plotted predicted probabilities given the corresponding AMH and FSH under each model.

Results

Table 1 presents the baseline characteristics of the four groups based on our previously defined cutoffs. The live birth rate for good prognosis patients (Group I) was significantly higher than patients with poor prognosis (Group II) (29.1% vs 12.8%; $p < 0.05$). Among the two discordant groups, patients with reassuring AMH (Group IV) had significantly higher live birth rate compared to patients with reassuring FSH (Group III) (22.7% vs 15.4%, $p < 0.05$).

Figure 2a and b show the GAMM established to predict the live birth rate using AMH and FSH respectively among patients of age 30, 35, 37, and 40 years old. Among all ages examined for AMH, there was a positive dose-response relationship between AMH and probability of live birth (Fig. 2a). Similarly, among all ages examined for FSH, there was a negative dose-response relationship between FSH and live birth (Fig. 2b), although not as significant as AMH. As AMH approached 6 ng/ml across all ages, there was a plateau in the estimated likelihood of live birth.

Figure 3 demonstrates our model for the joint effect of AMH and FSH on live birth rate. The two horizontal axes represent AMH and FSH values evenly spaced on log-scale, and the vertical axis indicates the estimated live birth rates based on two-dimensional GAMM. The predicted birth rates for patients with age 30, 35, 37, and 40 years old are shown in Fig. 3a, b, c, and d

respectively. Consistent with the prior trend, the estimated probability of live birth decreases as age increases, given the same AMH and FSH. Within each figure panel of specified age, the predicted live birth probability ascends rapidly with AMH when AMH is less than 8.2 ng/ml for fixed FSH. In comparison, for any given AMH value, the estimated live birth probability only decreases slightly as FSH increases from the lowest truncated value to the highest. In other words, the joint effect of AMH and FSH is dominated by that of AMH. The three-dimensional graphs provide a comprehensive visualization of dose-response relationship between any combination of AMH, FSH, and live birth rate. The joint effect analysis indicates that AMH is a more reliable predictor of live birth rate than FSH. Particularly in the discordant groups, a reassuring AMH (grey region) suggests a better likelihood of live birth compared to reassuring FSH (red region). Consistent with the trend observed in marginal models, higher AMH has a positive effect on live birth success rate while higher FSH and age demonstrate negative effects.

Discussion

To our knowledge, this is the first comprehensive analysis of the clinical utility of AMH and FSH with a sample size close to 14,000 cycles, with live birth as the primary outcome. AMH and FSH are widely accepted as predictors of ovarian response to stimulation with exogenous gonadotropins and therefore provide valuable prognostic clinical information prior to an IVF cycle start. Previous studies have reported on the utility of AMH and/or FSH as predictors of IVF cycle success

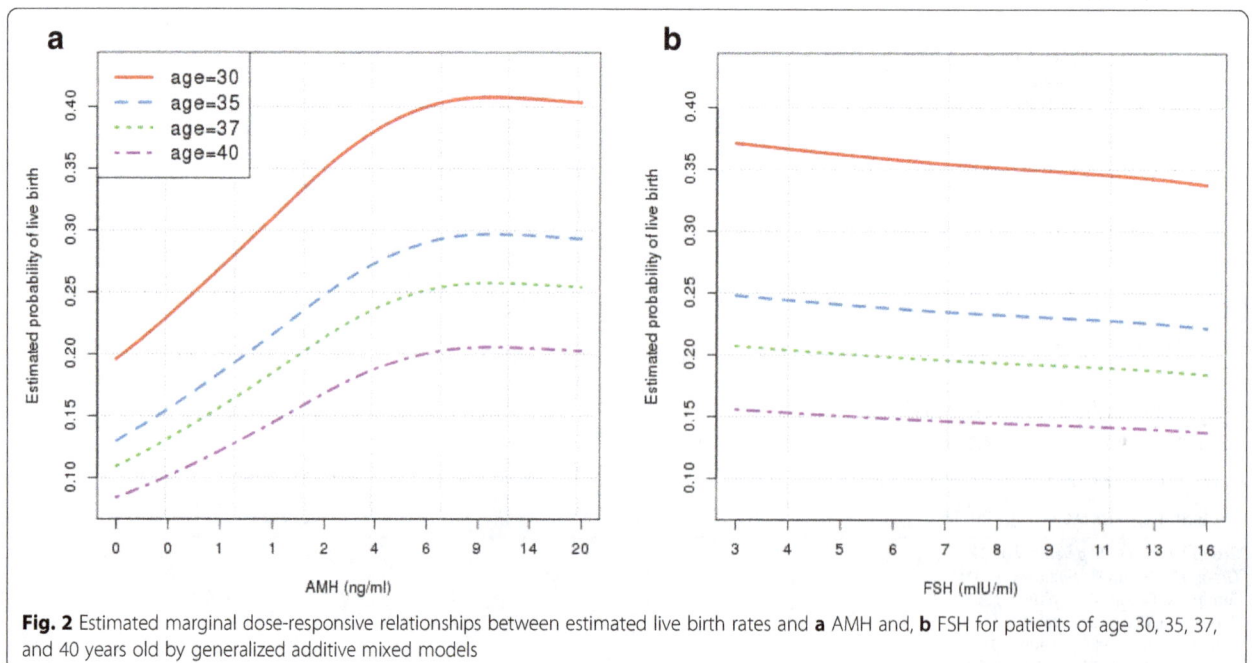

Fig. 2 Estimated marginal dose-responsive relationships between estimated live birth rates and **a** AMH and, **b** FSH for patients of age 30, 35, 37, and 40 years old by generalized additive mixed models

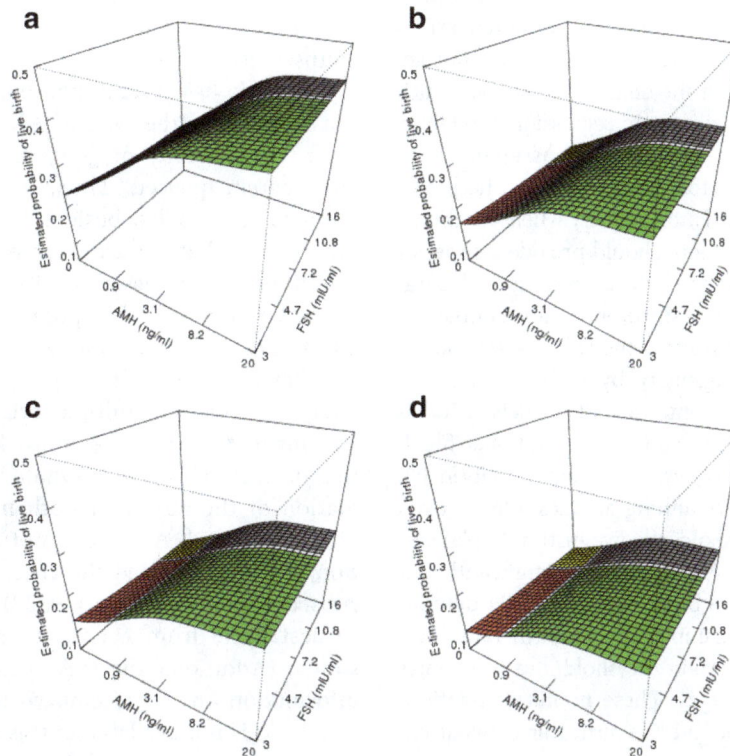

Fig. 3 Estimated joint effects of AMH and FSH on live birth rates by two-dimensional generalized additive mixed models for patients from different age groups. **a** 30 years old, **b** 35 years old, **c** 37 years old, and **d** 40 years old. Green: good prognosis (AMH ≥ 1 ng/ml & FSH < 10 mIU/ml); Yellow: poor prognosis (AMH < 1 ng/ml & FSH ≥ 10 mIU/ml); Red: FSH reassuring group (AMH < 1 ng/ml & FSH < 10 mIU/ml); Grey: AMH reassuring group (AMH ≥ 1 ng/ml & FSH > 10 mIU/ml)

defined by oocyte yield [22–24], number and quality of embryos [24], clinical pregnancy rate [22, 24], and live birth [17, 24, 25]. Our analysis advances these previous findings by suggesting that while both markers confer some prognostic value to the prediction of live birth, AMH is superior to FSH among all age groups. This is suggested by two principal findings in Fig. 3. First, the fact that irrespective of FSH value, a low AMH confers a lower likelihood of live birth among young patients. This live birth likelihood is even lower for older patients with low AMH. Additionally, in patients with high FSH, a high AMH rescues live birth probability (i.e. > 20%) across all age groups. Both findings suggest AMH is the more important determinant of pregnancy outcome than FSH.

Unsurprisingly, our study suggests live birth rates are highest in good prognosis cycles (Group I) and lowest in poor prognosis cycles (Group II). Prediction of cycle success is more difficult when AMH and FSH are discordant. In the 13,964 cycles we analyzed, AMH and FSH levels were discordant (Group IIII: AMH ≥1 ng/ml and FSH ≥10 mIU/ml and Group IV: AMH < 1 ng/ml and FSH < 10 mIU/ml) in 30% of cycles, compared to a 20% discordance between AMH and FSH in over 5300

women reported by Leader et al. Although this study clearly describes a high rate of discordance between AMH and FSH, it is limited by the absence of clinical outcomes. Gleicher et al. reported on the impact of AMH and FSH discordance on oocyte yield in a small prospective study of 350 IVF cycles [20]. In the discordant population, a normal AMH with abnormal FSH predicted a higher oocyte yield than a normal FSH with abnormal AMH. Although there were age dependent discrepancies, AMH was found to be a better clinical predictor of oocyte yield. In our study, a reassuring AMH predicted a higher live birth rate among discordant cycles, likewise suggesting that a normal AMH is a better clinical predictor of cycle success when AMH and FSH are discordant. We also examined the proportion PCOS, male factors, and the protocol types among the four groups (Additional file 1: Appendix 4, Table S1), but the role of these factors in the AMH/FSH-live birth rate association (e.g., as mediators, confounders, or effect modifiers) may require additional research.

Conventionally logistic regression models consisted of the first-order main effects of clinical measures are used to investigate the clinical utility of AMH and FSH in predicting IVF success rate. These parametric approaches make several assumptions about the data, such as underlying linear relationship and normally distributed errors between the predictors and outcomes, which may not accurately reflect the nature of the clinical measures. In this study we utilized a semiparametric regression modeling, penalized spline regression, to reduce the assumed linear relationship between predictors and outcome. The piecewise continuous polynomials, or splines, when combined with mathematical penalization, should provide a superior overall fit of the data compared to a conventional parametric approach. In addition, since our study sample are pooled from 26 IVF centers across the U.S., we also adjust for the center-level heterogeneity by including random intercept effects for each center in all models. Models without adjusting centers are shown in Additional file 1: Appendix 1. Our results suggest a nonlinear relationship of AMH and live birth rate among all ages. Once AMH levels reach a certain threshold, the live birth rate plateaus and further increases in AMH do not significantly increase the likelihood of live birth. Similarly, FSH demonstrates a nonlinear relationship with live birth rate: once FSH levels increase to a certain threshold, live birth rates decline for patients of all ages. These nonlinear relationships between AMH, FSH, and live birth mirror what clinicians often encounter in practice, but more importantly suggest that the ovarian reserve markers are associated with live birth in an age dependent manner. The statistical approach used in our study to evaluate AMH and FSH is flexible in characterizing non-linear dose-response relationship between predictors and outcomes, and thus provides an alternative analysis tool that could have been neglected in existing literature.

The marginal dose-response relationship of AMH or FSH with live birth rate (Fig. 2a and b), however, should be interpreted with certain caveats. For example, the marginal effect of AMH did not account for the effect contributed by FSH, and the high correlation of AMH and FSH may exert an undue influence, i.e., confounding on the AMH-live birth association. To address this issue, we further characterized the joint effect of AMH and FSH using GAMM with two dimensional splines where we were able to investigate the effect of one marker by adjusting for the other one. We also explored the possibility of expanding the above models to include potential confounder BMI, which resulted in very similar results (Additional file 1: Appendix 2). We applied the above prediction models to an internal dataset from patients at our center to test the model validity. The Receiver Operating Curve area under curve calculation equaled 0.67, suggesting age, AMH, and FSH alone are perhaps not sufficient to accurately predict the IVF success rate. Our group is therefore currently working on a more sophisticated model which incorporates demographic information and treatment outcomes, in order to better predict the likelihood of success with IVF and facilitate individualized patient counseling.

Our study has several inherent limitations. We could not control for the type of AMH or FSH assays used given the diversity of geographic areas encompassed and centers queried. Thus, there may be some variation to the results, besides the adjusted center-level differences, that we are unable to account for due to the differences in assay sensitivity and specificity. Another limitation is that poor prognosis patients may contribute a large proportion of cycles in this dataset: in other words, since poor prognosis patients are more likely to undergo multiple cycles before achieving a live birth, they may be more heavily represented in this dataset. This will inevitably lead to an underestimation of the ability of both markers to predict live birth likelihood. As an attempt to address this limitation, we re-performed the analysis presented but on a subset of population ($n = 9532$) consisted of only the earliest cycle from each patient and the results are similar (Additional file 1: Appendix 3). In addition, the information on day of embryo transfer (Day 2, Day 3, or Day 5) is not available in this database. It is possible that good prognosis and AMH reassuring groups may have higher percentage of Day 5 embryo transfer, although this should not affect our results. Lastly, although the eIVF database contains live birth rates for IVF cycles from 2000 to 2016, we only included cycles from 2010 to 2016 in our statistical analysis as AMH became a widespread test for ovarian reserve in 2010. Conversely, there are multiple strengths to this study including its large, heterogeneous patient population, geographic diversity, and comprehensive timeframe of IVF treatment cycles assessed. Furthermore, this study is unique in that it may be the largest study of its kind to evaluate live birth in a population of women in whom both AMH and FSH results were either concordant or discordant.

Conclusion

In conclusion, the ovarian reserve markers AMH and FSH are both associated with live birth probability, although AMH appears to be a stronger predictor especially in situations of discordant results. Although both demonstrate clear clinical utility for prognosis prediction in infertility patients, either marker evaluated alone or taken together are insufficient to predict a patient's likelihood of live birth. Prediction models which incorporate these markers in addition to other patient demographics and treatment response information are needed to provide accurate prognostic guidance for infertility specialists to facilitate patient counseling.

Additional file

Additional file 1: Figure S1. Estimated generalized additive mixed models (GAMMs) on different ages without adjusting for centers. A) AMH, and B) FSH. **Figure S2.** Joint model of AMH and FSH on predicting live birth rates without adjusting for centers. A) 30 year old, B) 35 year old, C) 37 year old, and D) 40 year old. **Figure S3.** Estimated generalized additive mixed models (GAMMs) on age and BMI. A) AMH, and B) FSH. **Figure S4.** Joint effect of AMH and FSH on predicting live birth rates for patients with four combination of age and BMI. **Figure S5.** Estimated generalized additive mixed models (GAMMs) using only first cycle of each patient. A) AMH, and B) FSH. **Figure S6.** Joint effect model of AMH and FSH on predicting live birth rate using only first cycle of each patient. A) 30 year old, B) 35 year old, C) 37 year old, and D) 40 year old. (DOCX 999 kb)

Abbreviations
AMH: anti-müllerian hormone; FSH: follicle stimulating hormone; GAMM: Generalized additive mixed models; IVF: in vitro fertilization

Acknowledgements
The authors thank PracticeHway.com Inc. for permission to use their data and are grateful for Jawid Rahimi and Victor Escott for their assistance in sorting and exporting data from eIVF. The authors also thank Richard Hackett for his comments that greatly improved the manuscript.

Funding
National Cancer Institute 5R03CA182937–02 (Y.-T.H.); Junior Research Awards in Genetics and Molecular Population Studies, Brown University (Y.-T.H. and Y.Z.).

Author's contributions
SW: contribution to the design of the study, acquisition of data, analysis and interpretation of data, and drafting the article. YZ: analysis and interpretation of data, revising the article critically for important intellectual content. VM and WJH: interpretation of data, revising the article critically for important intellectual content. Y-TH and RA: contribution to the concept of the study, interpretation of data, revising the article critically for important intellectual content. All authors approved the final version of the manuscript.

Competing interests
The authors declare that they have no competing interests.

Author details
[1]Brown University Warren Alpert Medical School, Providence, RI 02912, USA. [2]Women and Infants Fertility Center, Women and Infants Hospital of Rhode Island, 101 Dudley Street, Providence, RI 02905, USA. [3]Brown University School of Public Health, Providence, RI 02912, USA. [4]Institute of Statistical Science Academia Sinica, 128 Academia Road Sec. 2, Taipei 11529, Taiwan.

References
1. Broer SL, Broekmans FJM, Laven JSE, Fauser BCJM. Anti-Müllerian hormone: ovarian reserve testing and its potential clinical implications. Hum Reprod Update. 2014;20:688–701.
2. La Marca A, Stabile G, Artensio AC, Volpe A. Serum anti-Mullerian hormone throughout the human menstrual cycle. Hum Reprod Oxf Engl. 2006;21:3103–7.
3. Streuli I, Fraisse T, Chapron C, Bijaoui G, Bischof P, de Ziegler D. Clinical uses of anti-Müllerian hormone assays: pitfalls and promises. Fertil Steril. 2009;91:226–30.
4. Riggs RM, Duran EH, Baker MW, Kimble TD, Hobeika E, Yin L, et al. Assessment of ovarian reserve with anti-Müllerian hormone: a comparison of the predictive value of anti-Müllerian hormone, follicle-stimulating hormone, inhibin B, and age. Am J Obstet Gynecol. 2008; 199:202.e1–8.
5. Broekmans FJ, Kwee J, Hendriks DJ, Mol BW, Lambalk CB. A systematic review of tests predicting ovarian reserve and IVF outcome. Hum Reprod Update. 2006;12:685–718.
6. Practice Committee of the American Society for Reproductive Medicine. Testing and interpreting measures of ovarian reserve: a committee opinion. Fertil Steril. 2015;103:e9–17.
7. Blazar AS, Lambert-Messerlian G, Hackett R, Krotz S, Carson SA, Robins JC. Use of in-cycle antimullerian hormone levels to predict cycle outcome. Am J Obstet Gynecol. 2011;205:223.e1–5.
8. Elgindy EA, El-Haieg DO, El-Sebaey A. Anti-Müllerian hormone: correlation of early follicular, ovulatory and midluteal levels with ovarian response and cycle outcome in intracytoplasmic sperm injection patients. Fertil Steril. 2008;89:1670–6.
9. Seifer DB, MacLaughlin DT, Christian BP, Feng B, Shelden RM. Early follicular serum müllerian-inhibiting substance levels are associated with ovarian response during assisted reproductive technology cycles. Fertil Steril. 2002;77:468–71.
10. Verhagen TEM, Hendriks DJ, Bancsi LFJMM, Mol BWJ, Broekmans FJM. The accuracy of multivariate models predicting ovarian reserve and pregnancy after in vitro fertilization: a meta-analysis. Hum Reprod Update. 2008;14:95–100.
11. Broer SL, Mol B, Dólleman M, Fauser BC, Broekmans FJM. The role of anti-Müllerian hormone assessment in assisted reproductive technology outcome. Curr Opin Obstet Gynecol. 2010;22:193–201.
12. Tal R, Tal O, Seifer BJ, Seifer DB. Antimüllerian hormone as predictor of implantation and clinical pregnancy after assisted conception: a systematic review and meta-analysis. Fertil Steril. 2015; 103:119–130.e3.
13. Brodin T, Hadziosmanovic N, Berglund L, Olovsson M, Holte J. Comparing four ovarian reserve markers – associations with ovarian response and live births after assisted reproduction. Acta Obstet Gynecol Scand. 2015;94:1056–63.
14. Scott RT, Elkind-Hirsch KE, Styne-Gross A, Miller KA, Frattarelli JL. The predictive value for in vitro fertility delivery rates is greatly impacted by the method used to select the threshold between normal and elevated basal follicle-stimulating hormone. Fertil Steril. 2008;89:868–78.
15. Barad DH, Weghofer A, Gleicher N. Comparing anti-Müllerian hormone (AMH) and follicle-stimulating hormone (FSH) as predictors of ovarian function. Fertil Steril. 2009;91(4 Suppl):1553–5.
16. Nelson SM, Yates RW, Fleming R. Serum anti-Müllerian hormone and FSH: prediction of live birth and extremes of response in stimulated cycles–implications for individualization of therapy. Hum Reprod Oxf Engl. 2007;22:2414–21.
17. Lukaszuk K, Kunicki M, Liss J, Lukaszuk M, Jakiel G. Use of ovarian reserve parameters for predicting live births in women undergoing in vitro fertilization. Eur J Obstet Gynecol Reprod Biol. 2013;168:173–7.
18. Leader B, Hegde A, Baca Q, Stone K, Lannon B, Seifer DB, et al. High frequency of discordance between antimüllerian hormone and follicle-stimulating hormone levels in serum from estradiol-confirmed days 2 to 4 of the menstrual cycle from 5,354 women in U.S. fertility centers. Fertil Steril. 2012;98:1037–42.

13

Adipokine RBP4 drives ovarian cancer cell migration

Yanyan Wang[1,2], Yilin Wang[1] and Zhenyu Zhang[1*]

Abstract

Background: Obesity has been linked to several types of cancers including ovarian cancer. Retinol binding protein 4 (RBP4) is an adipokine that drives the development of hyperinsulinemia and type II diabetes in obesity patients and animals. Previously, we have identified RBP4 as a serum marker for ovarian cancer. Here we further explored the consequence of RBP4 upregulation in ovarian cancer cells and its molecular mechanism.

Results: Our results show that RBP4 is overexpressed in ovarian cancer cells to the same extent as in adipose tissues. The overexpression of RBP4 in ovarian cancer cells promotes cancer cell migration and proliferation. At molecular level, cancer progression factors MMP2 and MMP9 are induced in response to RBP4 overexpression. We further investigated which signaling pathways are utilized by RBP4 to activate ovarian cancer cell migration. We found RhoA/Rock1 pathway is turned on and CyclinD1 is upregulated in RBP4 overexpressed cells. Inhibition of RhoA/Rock1 pathway reduces the RBP4-induced MMP2 and MMP9 expression. The RBP4 action is depend on its associated ligand vitamin A/retinol acid (RA) and possibly involves similar pathways as for conferring insulin resistance. Moreover, we show that knockdown of RBP4 significantly reduce cancer cell migration and proliferation as well as expressions of oncogenic factors.

Conclusions: Our results indicated that RBP4 can drive ovarian cancer cell migration and proliferation via RhoA/Rock1 and ERK pathway. It suggests that RBP4 act as a oncogene in ovarian cancer cells. Thus, RBP4 could be a molecular bridge between obesity and cancers and a potential target for treating obese cancer patients.

Keywords: Ovarian cancer, Obesity, RBP4, Retinol acid, Migration

Background

Obesity is a well-established cancer risk factor and its occurrence is strongly associated with several types of cancers, including breast, colon, endometrial, ovarian, gastric, pancreatic and liver cancers [1, 2]. However, the molecular mechanisms that link obesity and cancers remain largely elusive. Identifying metabolites and secreted factors that connect increased fat mass to tumorigenesis is one of the central questions.

Retinol binding protein 4 (RBP4) is secreted by liver and adipose tissues [3, 4]. RBP4 acts as the major transporter for vitamin A/retinol acid (RA) in serum [3]. Under normal physical conditions, RA bound RBP4 circulates together with transthyretin (TTR) as a holo-

RBP-TTR complex [5]. Upon arrival, RA can either enter the targeted cell by passive diffusion or active transportation by Stimulated by RA 6 (STRA6) [6–10].

Besides its transportation function, RBP4 has recently been recognized as an adipokine [4]. Cumulative evidences showed that overexpression of RBP4 from adipose tissues promote hyperinsulinemia and type II diabetes [11–15]. Several pathways have been identified mediate RBP4 signaling [16]. RA and its oxidative products can activate retinoic acid receptors and retinoid X receptors and promote glucose production in liver [17]. RBP4 with RA can activate STRA6, which will then recruit and activate Janus kinase and the transcription factors STAT3 or STAT5 [18]. RBP4, independent of RA and STRA6, could promote pro-inflammatory responses possibly through pathways involving c-Jun N-terminal protein kinase (JNK)1, JNK2, or Toll-like receptor [19].

Ovarian cancer is the most lethal type of gynecological cancer in the world [20]. Ovarian cancers have a high

* Correspondence: zhenyuzhang2000@163.com
[1]Department of Gynaecology and Obstetrics, Beijing Chaoyang Hospital, Capital Medical University, No. 8 South Road, workers' Stadium, Chaoyang District, Beijing 100020, China
Full list of author information is available at the end of the article

occurrence rate in obesity peoples and obesity has been shown to promote ovarian cancer metastatic [21]. Recently, we found that RBP4 level is highly upregulated in ovarian cancer serum samples [22]. Overexpression of RBP4 had also been reported in liver, bone, and colon cancer cells [23–27]. However, the consequence of RBP4 overexpression on cancers and the mechanism of action of RBP4 in cancers are not clear.

We here investigated whether RBP4 is a tumorgenic factor that connects obesity and ovarian cancer. Our data showed that RBP4 was up-regulated in ovarian cancer cells and overexpression of RBP4 promoted cancer cell migration. The MMP-2 and MMP-9, key factors in cancer metastasis, were induced by RBP4 overexpression. We further identified RhoA/Rock1 pathway as mediators for RBP4 action. RhoA and Rock1 were overexpressed in response to RBP4 and inhibition of RhoA/Rock1 reduced MMP-2 and MMP-9 expression. The RBP4 action was dependent on its associated ligand RA. Moreover, knockdown of RBP4 greatly reduced cancer migration. Our data not only established RBP4 as a direct linkage between obesity and ovarian cancer, but also suggested RBP4 was a possible target for cancer treatment, especially in those associated with obesities.

Methods
Study samples
This study was approved by the Medical Ethical Committee of Beijing Chaoyang Hospital (Beijing, China). The written informed consents were obtained from all the participants enrolled in the study. Specimens were sampled from patients undergoing surgery for ovarian carcinoma or benign ovarian tissues at the Beijing Chaoyang Hospital.

All procedures were approved by the Animal Care and Use Committee of Beijing Chaoyang Hospital (Beijing, China). All experiment methods were performed in accordance with the relevant guidelines and regulations. In brief, healthy specific-pathogen-free (SPF) male SD rats were purchased from the Vital River. All rats were preserved under standard housing laboratory conditions. After one week of adaptation to the diet and the new environment, female SD rats were divided into two diet groups: the normal control (NC) group fed ad libitum a standard rodent chow, the high-fat (HF) group fed ad libitum a high-fat chow. After six weeks to induce obesity, the ovarian tissues were obtained after euthanasia.

Reagents
Antibodies against RBP4 (#ab109193), actin (#ab8226), RhoA (#ab187027), p-RhoA (#ab41435), ROCK1 (#ab45171), Erk (#ab54230), p-Erk (#ab51100), Cyclin D1 (#ab134175), MMP2 (#ab37150), MMP9 (#ab38898) were obtained from Abcam, USA. ROCK1 inhibitor Y27632

was purchased from Sigma, USA. All primers for qPCR were ordered from Invitrogen (Shanghai, China).

Human ovarian cancer cell line A2780 was obtained from Prof. Haiteng Deng laboratory [28, 29]. SKOV3 was preserved in our lab [30]. Cells were maintained in DMEM medium in incubator with 5% CO_2 at 37 °C.

Cell transfection
To upregulate the expression of RBP4, the human RBP4 full length cDNA was amplified and inserted into the pCMV-Flag vector, and a scramble sequence was inserted into the pCMV-flag vector as the control vector. To knock down the expression of RBP4, a RBP4 siRNA was designed and obtained from Jima Inc. (Shanghai, China). For transfection, the cells were seeded into 6-well plates. When cell confluency reached 50%, RBP4 siRNA or RBP4-pCMV-Flag was transfected into the cells using lipo2000 according to the manufacturer's instructions.

Western blotting
Cells were lysed in RIPA buffer with protease and phosphatase inhibitor cocktail. Equal amount of protein samples was loaded onto 12% SDS-PAGE and was then transferred to PVDF membranes. After blocking with 5% BSA for 1 h at room temperature, the membranes were incubated with primary antibodies at 4 °C overnight. Then, the membranes were incubated with horseradish peroxidase-conjugated secondary antibody (from Zhongshanjinqiao, China) for 1 h at room temperature. The protein bands were visualized by ChemiDoc XRS+ (BioRad, USA). Data analysis was done using Quantity one.

Quantitative reverse transcription- polymerase chain reaction (qRT-PCR)
Total RNA was isolated from the cells using trizol method. RNA was reverse transcribed using the Prime-Script RT Master Mix (B-Belife, China) according to the manufacturer's instructions. The PCR amplifications were performed using SYBR Premix Ex Taq II (B-Belife, China). The expression level of each sample was internally normalized against that of the glyceraldehyde 3-phosphate dehydrogenase (GAPDH). The relative quantitative value was calculated using $2^{-\Delta\Delta Ct}$ method. Each experiment was performed in triplicate. The primers used in real-time PCR were as follow: RBP4 F: AGGAGAACTTCGACAAGGCTC; RBP4 R: GAGAACTCCG CGACGATGTT; GAPDH F: GGAGCGAGATCCCTC-CAAAAT; GAPDH R: GGCTGTTGTCATACTTCT-CATGG; RHOA F: AGCCTGTGGAAAGACATGCTT; RHOA R: TCAAACACTGTGGGCACATAC; Rock1 F: AACATGCTGCTGGATAAATCTGG; Rock1 R: TGT ATCACATCGTACCATGCCT; cyclinD1(CCND1) F: GC TGCGAAGTGGAAACCATC; cyclinD1(CCND1) R:

CCTCCTTCTGCACACATTTGAA; ERK1 F: CTACA
CGCAGTTGCAGTACAT; ERK1 R: CAGCAGGATC
TGGATCTCCC; MMP2 F: TACAGGATCATTGGCTA-
CACACC; MMP2 R: GGTCACATCGCTCCAGACT;
MMP9 F: TGTACCGCTATGGTTACACTCG; MMP9
R: GGCAGGGACAGTTGCTTCT.

Immunohistochemistry
The expression of RBP4 was assessed using immunohis-
tological staining as described previously [20]. Briefly,
tissue samples were fixed and cut to 5 μm thick. RBP4
antibody was applied on the sections for 30 min and incubated overnight at 4 °C then shaking at room
temperature for 30 min. Antibody binding was amplified
using biotin and streptavidin HRP for 10 min each and
the complex was visualized using DAB. ALL sections
were assessed microscopically for positive DAB staining.
The immunostained sections were examined under microscopy and the expression level of RBP4 was scored
on the basis of the intensity of staining.

In vitro migration assay
A 24-well Transwell chamber (Corning, #3422, USA)
was used to examine the invasive ability of the ovarian cancer cells. Cells were suspended in DMEM
medium and were added into the upper Transwell
chamber. The lower Transwell chamber was filled
with DMEM medium supplemented with 10% FBS.
After incubation of 16 h at 37 °C, the non-migrated
cells were removed with a sterile cotton swab, and
the migrated cells were stained with 0.1% crystal violet for 20 min at room temperature. The numbers of
cells were calculated under a light microscope in five
random fields.

Proliferation assay
Cell proliferation was determined by MTT assay. Cells
were seeded at 1000 cells/well in a 96-well plate. After
incubation for indicated time, MTT was added into the
plate incubated for 4 h. The optical density (OD) was
measured 490 nm at designated time.

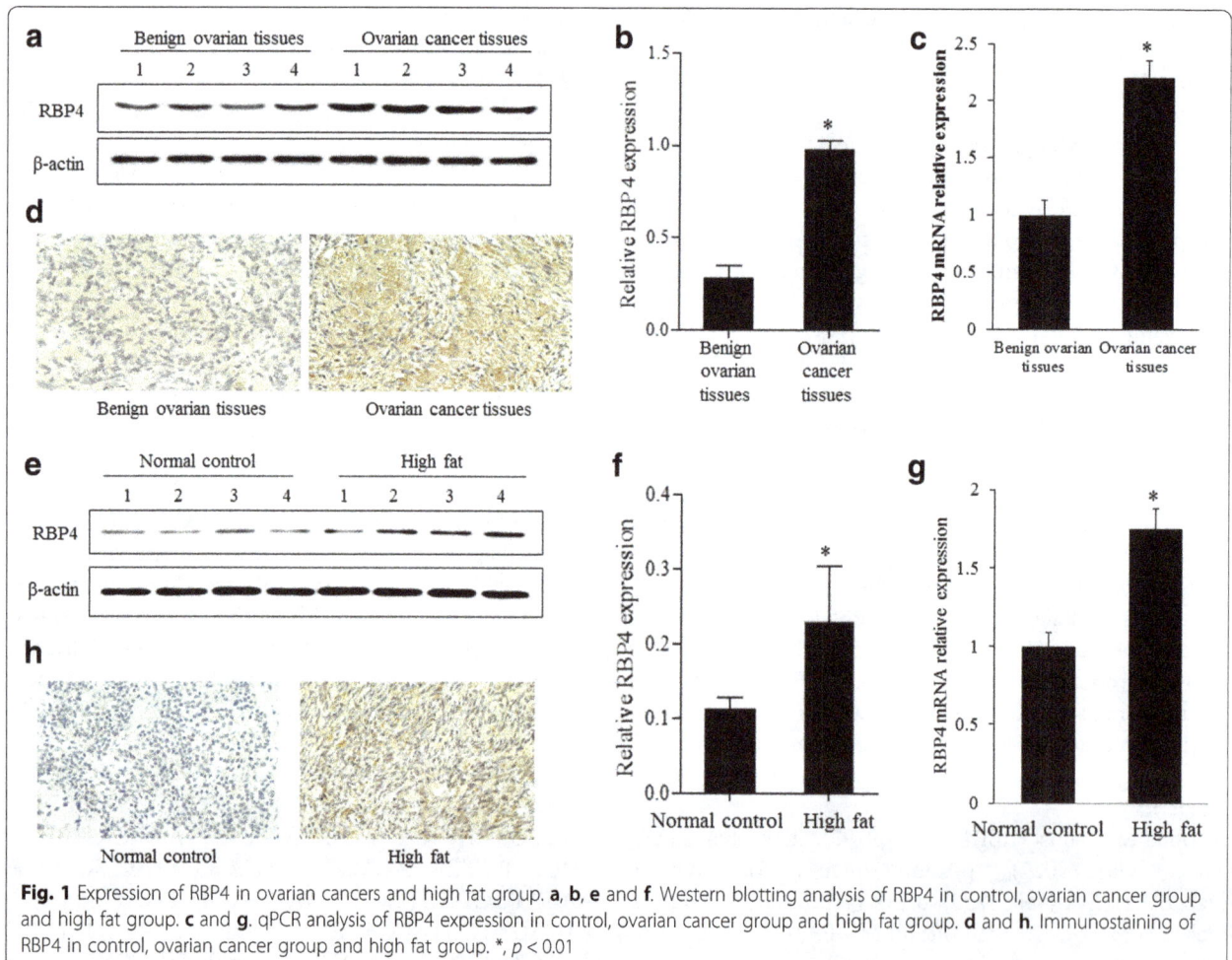

Fig. 1 Expression of RBP4 in ovarian cancers and high fat group. **a**, **b**, **e** and **f**. Western blotting analysis of RBP4 in control, ovarian cancer group and high fat group. **c** and **g**. qPCR analysis of RBP4 expression in control, ovarian cancer group and high fat group. **d** and **h**. Immunostaining of RBP4 in control, ovarian cancer group and high fat group. *, $p < 0.01$

Cell cycle analysis

Cell cycle distribution was analyzed by PI staining and flow cytometry. The 1×10^5 cells / well were seeded in 6-well plates. The cells were then harvested, fixed with 70% ice cold ethanol, and stored at 4 °C until analysis. After fixation, the cells were washed twice with cold phosphate-buffered saline (PBS) and centrifuged, following which the supernatants were removed. The pellet was resuspended and stained with PBS containing 50 µg/ml PI and 100 µg/ml RNaseA for 20 min in the dark. The cell cycle data were analyzed using Modifit software.

Statistical analysis

All the continuous variables were expressed as average ± standard deviation (SD). Student's t-test was used for the difference analysis. A P value of more than 0.01 was considered as statistical significance. Graphpad 5.0 software was used for all the statistical analyses.

Results

Expression of RBP4 in ovarian cancer tissues and obesity tissues

We first detected the RBP4 expression levels in ovarian cancer tissues. Western blot results showed that the RBP4

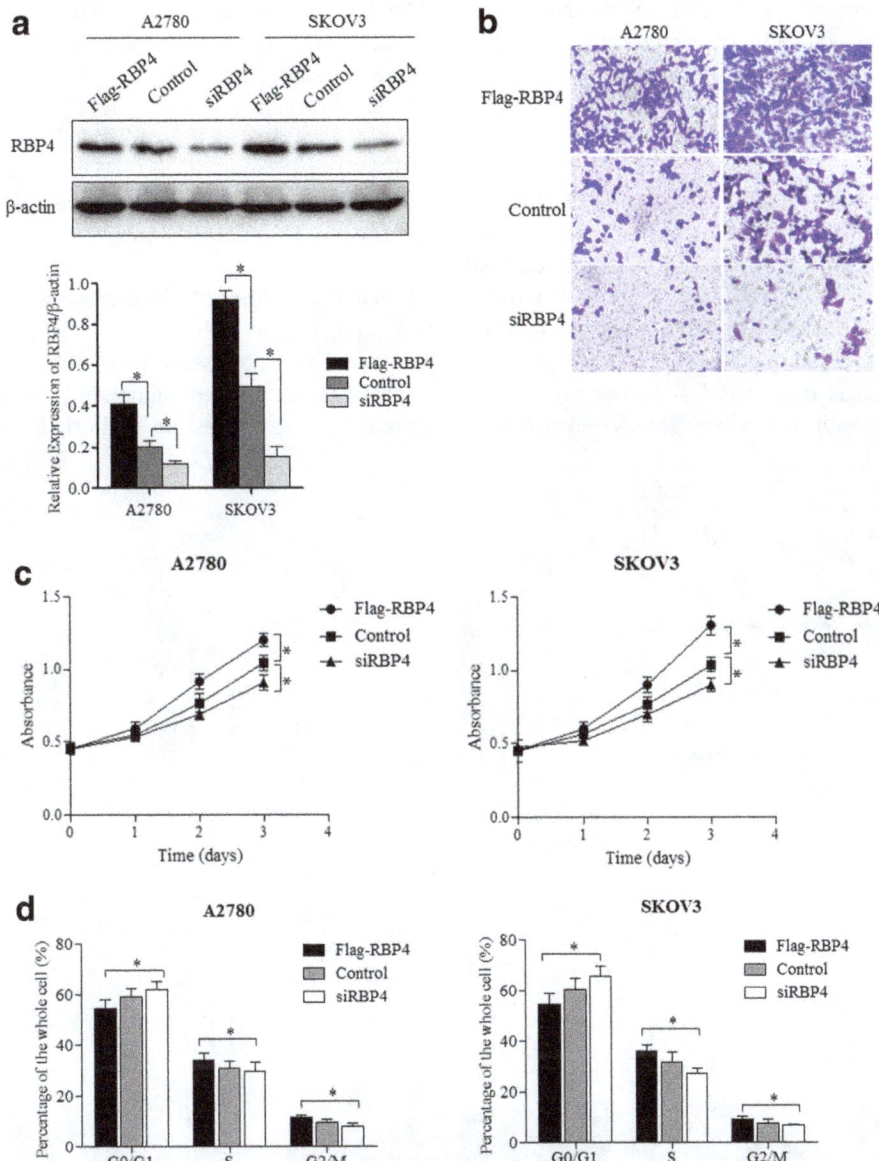

Fig. 2 RBP4 promotes ovarian cancer cell migration and proliferation. **a**. Western blot analysis of RBP4 levels in cells with Flag-RBP4 overexpression, RBP4 knockdown and control cells. **b**. Cell migration assays of RBP4 overexpression, control and RBP4 knockdown cells. **c**. Cell proliferation profile of cells with RBP4 overexpression, control and RBP4 knockdown cells. **d**. Cell cycle distribution of cells with Flag-RBP4 overexpression, control and RBP4 knockdown cells. *, $p < 0.01$

protein was upregulated by nearly 4-fold in ovarian cancer tissues comparing to the benign ovarian tissues (Fig. 1a-b). The higher expression of RBP4 was further verified by qRT-PCR experiment (Fig. 1c) and immunostaining (Fig. 1d). The mRNA level of RBP4, as revealed by qRT-PCR, was twofold higher in ovarian cancer tissues comparing to the benign ovarian tissues (Fig. 1c). The RBP4 level in cancer tissues, shown in brown, was significantly increased comparing to the benign ovarian tissues, which only exhibited weak staining (Fig. 1d). As a control, we created obese rat model by fed with a high-fat group rats and measured the expression level of RBP4 in ovarian tissues. Similarly as in previous report [4], the RBP4 level was elevated in ovarian tissues from the high fat (HF) group compared to the normal control (NC) group (Fig. 1e-h). The extent of RBP4 overexpression was comparable in ovarian cancer cells and in adipose tissues.

RBP4 promotes migration and proliferation of ovarian cancer cells

We used ovarian cancer cell line A2780 and SKOV3 to test the effects of RBP4 expression on ovarian cancer. Firstly, we confirmed the effect of RBP4 overexpression and knocked down in A2780 and SKOV3 cells (Fig. 2a). Then the transwell migration assays showed that RBP4 overexpression can greatly enhance cancer cell migration in both cell lines (Fig. 2b). In contrast, cancer cells were less mobile when RBP4 was knocked down with siRNA (Fig. 2b). We then carried

out proliferation assay to explore the effect of RBP4 expression on cell proliferation in A2780 and SKOV3 cells. The results showed that ovarian cancer cells with RBP4 overexpression grows faster than control cells, while the RBP4 knockdown inhibited cell proliferation (Fig. 2c). Finally, we analyzed the cell cycle distribution with respect to RBP4 expression. More cells were in S and G2/M phase when RBP4 overexpressed (Fig. 2d). Collectively, these results indicated that RBP4 promotes migration and proliferation of ovarian cancer cells.

RBP4 induces migration-related genes expression in ovarian cancer cells

We have shown that RBP4 overexpression can greatly stimulate ovarian cancer cell migration. Then, we tested the expression level of MMP2 and MMP9, which are essential for cancer metastasis [31]. Both protein and mRNA levels of MMP2 and MMP9 were elevated when RBP4 overexpressed in SKOV3 and A2780 cells (Fig. 3). The observation further confirmed the effect of RBP4 expression on cancer cell migration.

RBP4 activates RhoA/Rock1 pathways and cyclin D1

To explore how RBP4 exerts its effect on cancer cells, we tested the expression level of several key players in tumorigenesis related signaling. RBP4 overexpression stimulated the expression of both RhoA and Rock1. In

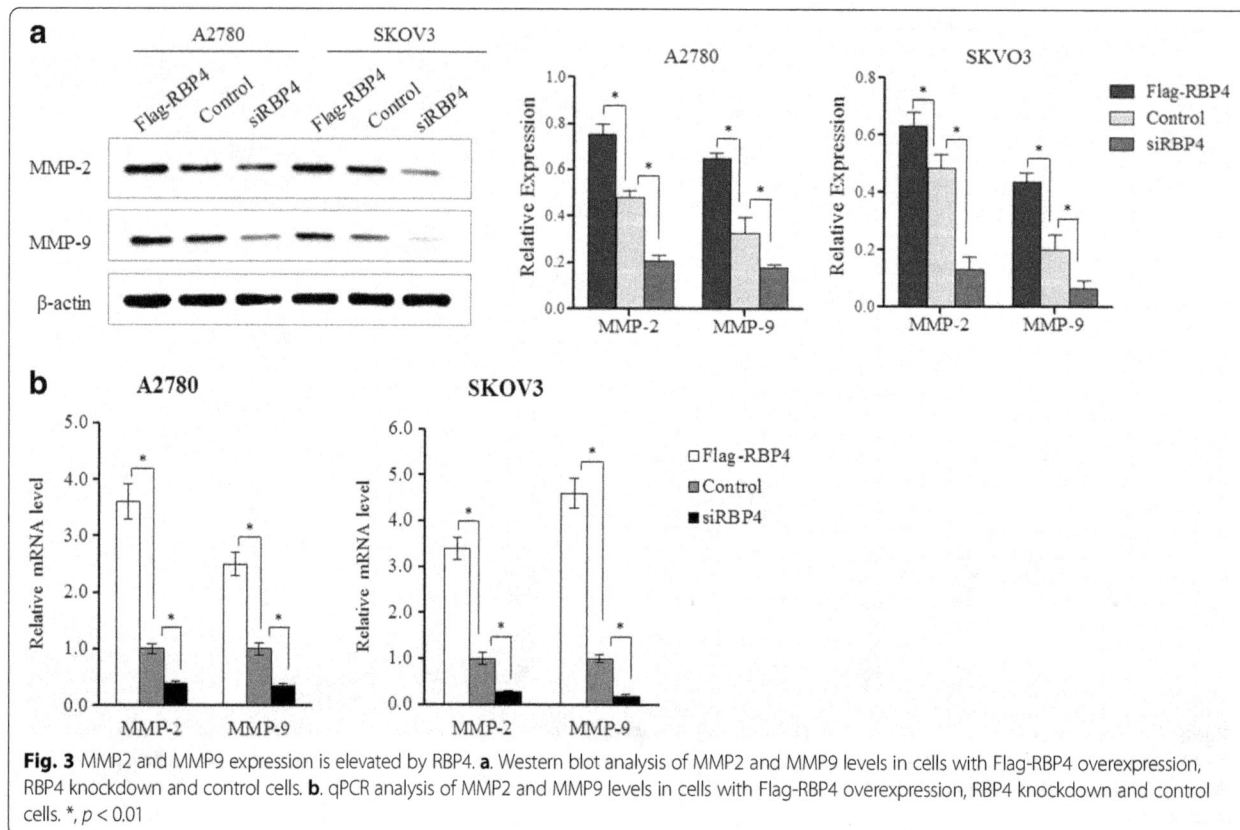

Fig. 3 MMP2 and MMP9 expression is elevated by RBP4. a. Western blot analysis of MMP2 and MMP9 levels in cells with Flag-RBP4 overexpression, RBP4 knockdown and control cells. b. qPCR analysis of MMP2 and MMP9 levels in cells with Flag-RBP4 overexpression, RBP4 knockdown and control cells. *, p < 0.01

RBP4 overexpression groups, the RhoA and Rock1 levels were elevated at both mRNA and protein level (Fig. 4a, b). Moreover, the p-RhoA level was also increased, revealed by western blotting. Similarly, the Cyclin D1 expression was promoted at both mRNA and protein level. Previously, overexpressed phospho-ERK triggerd ovarian cancer cell migration [32, 33]. Although the ERK expression level remained unchanged upon RBP4 overexpression, the phosphorylated ERK had been elevated by RBP4 overexpression (Fig. 4c, d). Interestingly, suppression of RBP4 expression significantly reduced the level of RhoA/Rock1 as well as Cyclin D1 comparing to control group (Fig. 4).

RBP4 action is partially dependent on RhoA1/rock pathway

Rock1 inhibitor Y-27632 had been shown to effectively inhibit Rock1 and its associated pathways [34]. To test if RBP4 induced cancer cell migration is RhoA/Rock1 dependent, we added Y-27632 to our RBP4 overexpression cells. Y-27632 can effectively reduce the MMP-2/MMP9 expression level even when RBP4 overexpressed. However, the level of MMP2/MMP9 with Y-27632 was still higher than control group. The results indicated that the RBP4 action was partially depending on Rock1 pathway (Fig. 5a and b).

RBP4 action is dependent on RA

RBP4 is a major RA transport protein [3]. We tested whether the RBP4 effect on ovarian cancer cells is RA dependent. In the absence of RA, the RBP4 overexpression had moderate stimulation on RhoA/Rock1 and Cyclin D1 expression (Fig. 6a, b). When RA was added, the RBP4 effect was stimulated. As a control, RA had little effect when RBP4 is suppressed. RA was partially transported through membrane transporter STRA6 and RBP4-RA complex had been shown to activate STRA6 and its associated signaling pathways [6–10]. We tested the expression level of STRA6 in ovarian cancer cells with qRT-PCR. The STRA6 mRNA level

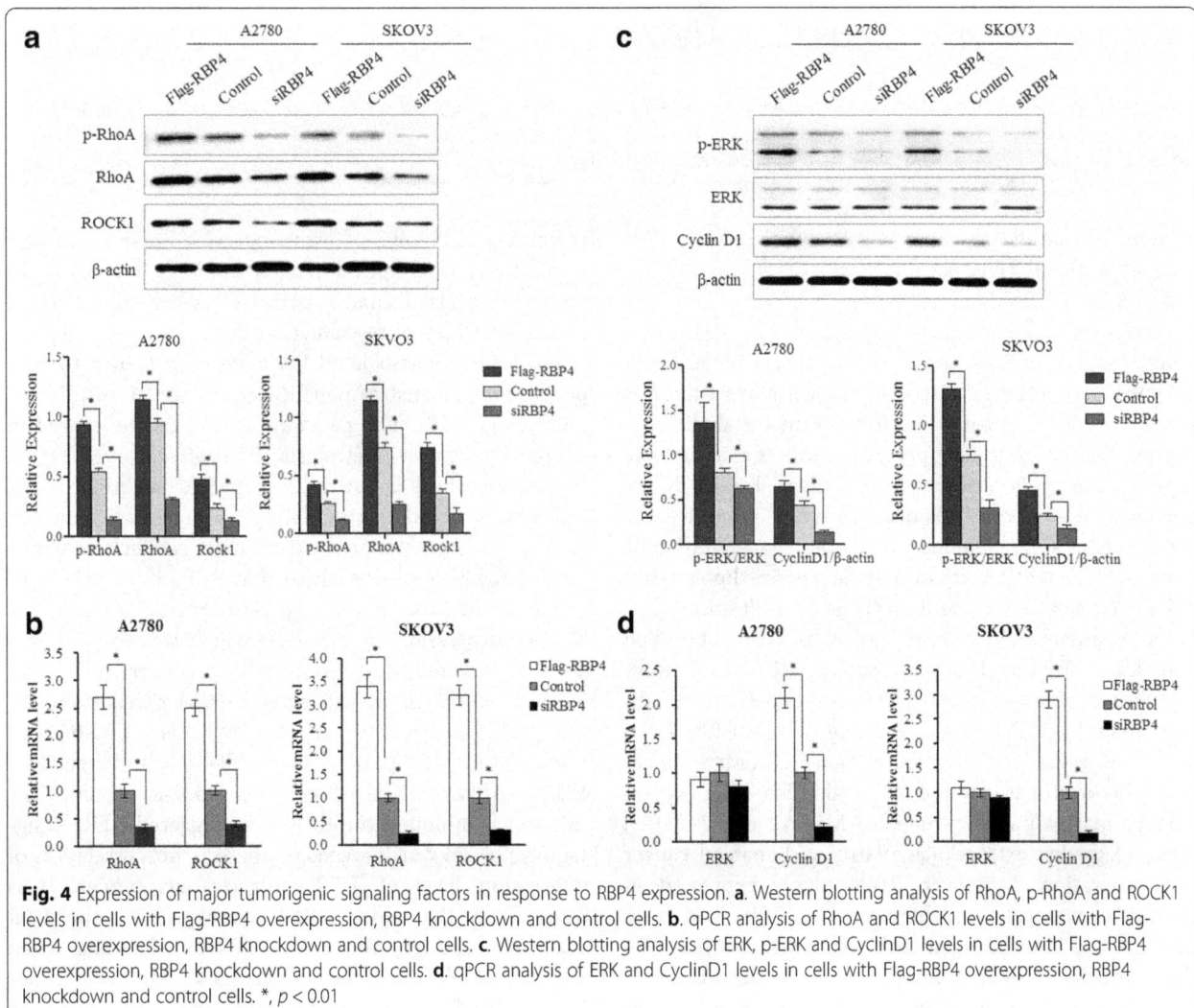

Fig. 4 Expression of major tumorigenic signaling factors in response to RBP4 expression. **a**. Western blotting analysis of RhoA, p-RhoA and ROCK1 levels in cells with Flag-RBP4 overexpression, RBP4 knockdown and control cells. **b**. qPCR analysis of RhoA and ROCK1 levels in cells with Flag-RBP4 overexpression, RBP4 knockdown and control cells. **c**. Western blotting analysis of ERK, p-ERK and CyclinD1 levels in cells with Flag-RBP4 overexpression, RBP4 knockdown and control cells. **d**. qPCR analysis of ERK and CyclinD1 levels in cells with Flag-RBP4 overexpression, RBP4 knockdown and control cells. *, $p < 0.01$

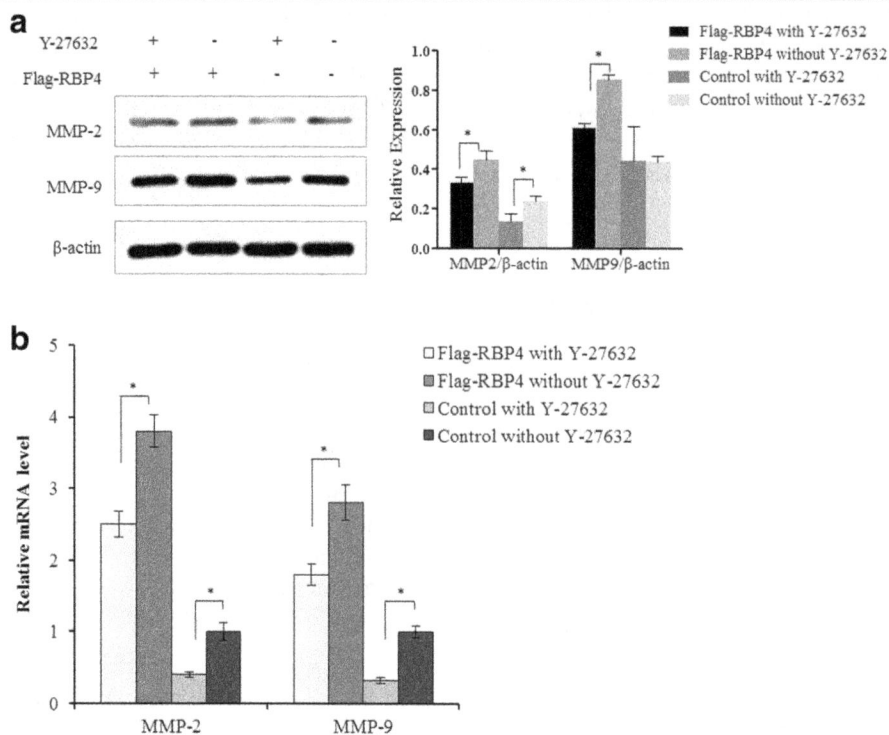

Fig. 5 RBP4 induced MMP-2 and MMP-9 overexpression is partially dependent on RhoA/Rock1 pathway. **a**. Effect of ROCK1 inhibitor Y-27632 on MMP2 and MMP9 expression examined by western blotting. **b**. Effect of ROCK1 inhibitor Y-27632 on MMP2 and MMP9 expression examined by qPCR. The cells were treated with Y-27632 (10 μm) for 24 h before harvesting. *, p < 0.01

stayed the same in either RBP4 overexpression or knockdown cells (Fig. 6c).

Discussion

Obese patients are associated with high cancer risk, poor prognosis and reduced response to anti-cancer therapies [1, 2]. Obesity is intrinsically linked with metabolic syndrome that can indirectly promote cancers as metabolic reprogramming is a hallmark of cancer. Especially for ovarian cancer, obesity has been shown to promote cancer metastasis [21]. Besides that obesity can indirectly affect cancer metastasis through increasing lipogenesis, enhancing vascularity, and decreasing infiltration [21]. Here, we established a direct molecular linkage between adipokine RBP4 and ovarian cancer. RBP4 is a well-established obesity factors that is overexpressed by adipose tissues [4]. We proved that high level of RBP4 can stimulate migration and proliferation of ovarian cancer cells. The overexpression of RBP4 stimulated the expression of matrix metalloproteinase MMP-2 and MMP-9, which degraded extracellular matrix and enabled cancer cells migration. Moreover, RBP4 highly expressed in ovarian cancer cells and high level of RBP4 had been documented in ovarian patient's serum samples [22]. We thus proposed that high level of RBP4, either from adipose tissues or cancer tissues, can promote cancer

metastasis and obesity signaling, vice versa. Although currently lack of clinical data, it would be interesting to survey if ovarian cancer patients have a high rate of obesity and insulin resistance.

RBP4 and its associated RA have been shown to trigger several downstream pathways to confer insulin resistance [16–19]. The pathways could also be shared in promoting cancer metastasis. The effect of RBP4 on tumor metastasis is RA dependent. RA has broad metabolic roles including stimulating lipogenesis [35], which has been shown to promote ovarian cancer metastasis [21]. It has been documented that RBP4 bound RA, but not apo RBP4 can induce signaling of STRA6 [18]. The STRA6 expression and its signaling has been proposed drive oncogenic transformation of cancer cells [34]. STRA6 expressed in the ovarian cancer cell lines, although its level was not affected by RBP4. STRA6 could mediate, at least part of the RBP4 effect. Circulating RBP4-RA was associated with their partner protein TTR [5], which inhibited the RBP4-RA triggered STRA6 signaling [7]. To our knowledge, there is no correlation of expression level of TTR with ovarian cancer. It is quite likely that when RBP4 overexpressed, the TTR was not enough to block STRA6 signaling even STRA6 level remained unchanged. On the other hand, RBP4 itself without RA can still promote

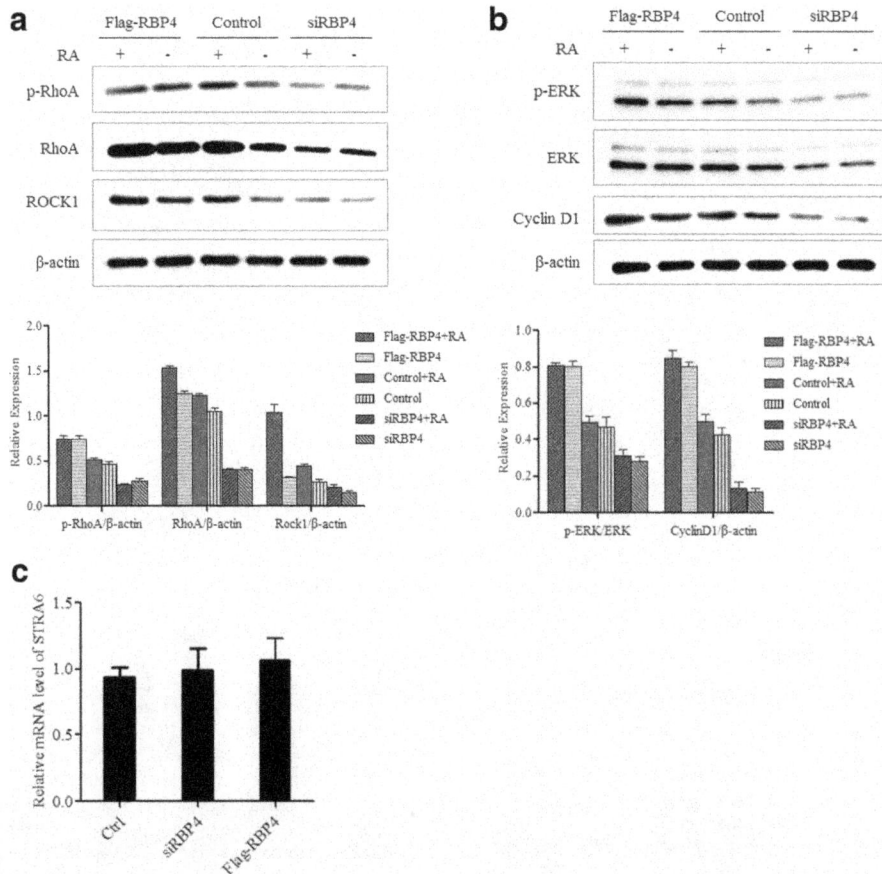

Fig. 6 RBP4 action is dependent on RA. **a**. Western blot analysis of RhoA, p-RhoA and ROCK1 levels in cells with or without RA. **b**. Western blot analysis of ERK, p-ERK and CyclinD1 levels in cells with or without RA. **c**. qPCR analysis of STRA6 levels in cells with Flag-RBP4 overexpression, RBP4 knockdown and control cells. *, $p < 0.01$

metastasis, although to a lesser degree. It has been shown RBP4, independent of RA and STRA6, can induce pro-inflammation reaction [19].

Adding to the existing knowledge, we showed that RhoA/Rock1 pathway was turned on in response to RBP4 overexpression. RhoA/Rock1 pathway played pivot roles in cell morphogenesis, adhesion, and motility and was often activated in malignant cancers [36]. Previous reports had shown that inhibition of RhoA/Rock1 suppressed MMP-2 and MMP-9 action [37–39]. Consistently, we observed that inhibiting RhoA/Rock1 pathway with Rock1 inhibitor Y-27632 can reduce RBP4 induced MMP-2 and MMP-9 overexpression, indicating that the migration effect of RBP4 was mediated by RhoA/Rock1 pathway. However, how RBP4 activated RhoA/Rock1 pathway was less clear. Considering RBP4 was mainly a secretive protein, novel membrane receptors was possibly involved in promoting RBP4 signaling. Further studies were in demand to fully elucidating the RBP4 signaling pathways that related to cancers.

We observed that knockdown of RBP4 can greatly suppress ovarian cancer cell migration and proliferation.

Considering RBP4 as a circulating protein, targeting RBP4 could be a relative easy option for ovarian cancer treatment, especially those associated with obesities.

Conclusion

In conclusion, this study described the function of RBP4 in driving ovarian cancer cell migration and proliferation. Moreover, the underlying molecular mechanism of RBP4 was activation of RhoA/Rock1 pathway and CyclinD1 expression. Therefore, RBP4 could be a molecular bridge between obesity and cancers and a potential target for treating obese cancer patients.

Abbreviations
RA: Vitamin A/retinol acid; RBP4: Retinol binding protein 4; STRA6: Stimulated by RA 6; TTR: Transthyretin

Acknowledgements
We thank Dr.Cui from Chinese Academy of Science for data analysis.

Funding
This work was supported by National Natural Science Foundation of China (81571455).

Authors' contributions

Yanyan Wang performed experiments, and wrote the manuscript; Yilin Wang contributed to data analysis. ZZ designed and supervised the project. All authors read and approved the final manuscript.

Competing interests

The authors declare that they have no competing interests.

Author details

[1]Department of Gynaecology and Obstetrics, Beijing Chaoyang Hospital, Capital Medical University, No. 8 South Road, workers' Stadium, Chaoyang District, Beijing 100020, China. [2]The First Affiliated Hospital of Jinzhou Medical University, No.2, people's street, Jinzhou 121001, China.

References

1. O'Flanagan CH, Bowers LW, Hursting SD. A weighty problem: metabolic perturbations and the obesity-cancer link. Horm Mol Biol Clin Invest. 2015; 23:47–57.
2. Iyengar NM, Hudis CA, Dannenberg AJ. Obesity and cancer: local and systemic mechanisms. Annu Rev Med. 2015;66:297–309.
3. Blaner WS. Retinol-binding protein: the serum transport protein for vitamin a. Endocr Rev. 1989;10:308–16.
4. Yang Q, Graham TE, Mody N, Preitner F, Peroni OD, Zabolotny JM, et al. Serum retinol binding protein 4 contributes to insulin resistance in obesity and type 2 diabetes. Nature. 2005;436:356–62.
5. Raghu P, Sivakumar B. Interactions amongst plasma retinol-binding protein, transthyretin and their ligands: implications in vitamin a homeostasis and transthyretin amyloidosis. Biochim Biophys Acta. 2004;1703:1–9.
6. Noy N. Retinoid-binding proteins: mediators of retinoid action. The Biochemical journal. 2000;348(Pt 3):481–95.
7. Berry DC, Croniger CM, Ghyselinck NB, Noy N. Transthyretin blocks retinol uptake and cell signaling by the holo-retinol-binding protein receptor STRA6. Mol Cell Biol. 2012;32:3851–9.
8. Terra R, Wang X, Hu Y, Charpentier T, Lamarre A, Zhong M, et al. To investigate the necessity of STRA6 upregulation in T cells during T cell immune responses. PLoS One. 2013;8:e82808.
9. Berry DC, Jacobs H, Marwarha G, Gely-Pernot A, O'Byrne SM, DeSantis D, et al. The STRA6 receptor is essential for retinol-binding protein-induced insulin resistance but not for maintaining vitamin a homeostasis in tissues other than the eye. J Biol Chem. 2013;288:24528–39.
10. Kawaguchi R, Yu J, Honda J, Hu J, Whitelegge J, Ping P, et al. A membrane receptor for retinol binding protein mediates cellular uptake of vitamin a. Science. 2007;315:820–5.
11. Graham TE, Yang Q, Bluher M, Hammarstedt A, Ciaraldi TP, Henry RR, et al. Retinol-binding protein 4 and insulin resistance in lean, obese, and diabetic subjects. N Engl J Med. 2006;354:2552–63.
12. Cho YM, Youn BS, Lee H, Lee N, Min SS, Kwak SH, et al. Plasma retinol-binding protein-4 concentrations are elevated in human subjects with impaired glucose tolerance and type 2 diabetes. Diabetes Care. 2006;29: 2457–61.
13. Lee DC, Lee JW, Im JA. Association of serum retinol binding protein 4 and insulin resistance in apparently healthy adolescents. Metab Clin Exp. 2007; 56:327–31.
14. Gavi S, Stuart LM, Kelly P, Melendez MM, Mynarcik DC, Gelato MC, et al. Retinol-binding protein 4 is associated with insulin resistance and body fat distribution in nonobese subjects without type 2 diabetes. J Clin Endocrinol Metab. 2007;92:1886–90.
15. Takebayashi K, Suetsugu M, Wakabayashi S, Aso Y, Inukai T. Retinol binding protein-4 levels and clinical features of type 2 diabetes patients. J Clin Endocrinol Metab. 2007;92:2712–9.
16. Fedders R, Muenzner M, Schupp M. Retinol binding protein 4 and its membrane receptors: a metabolic perspective. Horm Mol Biol Clin Invest. 2015;22:27–37.
17. Chambon P. A decade of molecular biology of retinoic acid receptors. FASEB journal: official publication of the Federation of American Societies for Experimental Biology. 1996;10:940–54.
18. Berry DC, Jin H, Majumdar A, Noy N. Signaling by vitamin a and retinol-binding protein regulates gene expression to inhibit insulin responses. Proc Natl Acad Sci U S A. 2011;108:4340–5.
19. Norseen J, Hosooka T, Hammarstedt A, Yore MM, Kant S, Aryal P, et al. Retinol-binding protein 4 inhibits insulin signaling in adipocytes by inducing proinflammatory cytokines in macrophages through a c-Jun N-terminal kinase- and toll-like receptor 4-dependent and retinol-independent mechanism. Mol Cell Biol. 2012;32:2010–9.
20. Selvaggi SM. Tumors of the ovary, maldeveloped gonads, fallopian tube, and broad ligament. Archives of pathology & laboratory medicine. 2000;124: 477.
21. Liu Y, Metzinger MN, Lewellen KA, Cripps SN, Carey KD, Harper EI, et al. Obesity contributes to ovarian Cancer metastatic success through increased lipogenesis, enhanced vascularity, and decreased infiltration of M1 macrophages. Cancer Res. 2015;75:5046–57.
22. Cheng Y, Liu C, Zhang N, Wang S, Zhang Z. Proteomics analysis for finding serum markers of ovarian cancer. Biomed Res Int. 2014;2014:179040.
23. Wang DD, Zhao YM, Wang L, Ren G, Wang F, Xia ZG, et al. Preoperative serum retinol-binding protein 4 is associated with the prognosis of patients with hepatocellular carcinoma after curative resection. J Cancer Res Clin Oncol. 2011;137:651–8.
24. Uehara H, Takahashi T, Izumi K. Induction of retinol-binding protein 4 and placenta-specific 8 expression in human prostate cancer cells remaining in bone following osteolytic tumor growth inhibition by osteoprotegerin. Int J Oncol. 2013;43:365–74.
25. Jiao C, Cui L, Ma A, Li N, Si H. Elevated serum levels of retinol-binding protein 4 are associated with breast Cancer risk: a case-control study. PLoS One. 2016;11:e0167498.
26. Abola MV, Thompson CL, Chen Z, Chak A, Berger NA, Kirwan JP, et al. Serum levels of retinol-binding protein 4 and risk of colon adenoma. Endocr Relat Cancer. 2015;22:L1–4.
27. Noy N, Li L, Abola MV, Berger NA. Is retinol binding protein 4 a link between adiposity and cancer? Horm Mol Biol Clin Invest. 2015;23:39–46.
28. Yu W, Qu H, Cao G, Liu C, Deng H, Zhang Z. MtHsp70-CLIC1-pulsed dendritic cells enhance the immune response against ovarian cancer. Biochem Biophys Res Commun. 2017;494:13–9.
29. Qu H, Chen Y, Cao G, Liu C, Xu J, Deng H, et al. Identification and validation of differentially expressed proteins in epithelial ovarian cancers using quantitative proteomics. Oncotarget. 2016;7:83187–99.
30. Bai H, Li H, Li W, Gui T, Yang J, Cao D, et al. The PI3K/AKT/mTOR pathway is a potential predictor of distinct invasive and migratory capacities in human ovarian cancer cell lines. Oncotarget. 2015;6:25520–32.
31. Gialeli C, Theocharis AD, Karamanos NK. Roles of matrix metalloproteinases in cancer progression and their pharmacological targeting. FEBS J. 2011;278: 16–27.
32. Tanaka Y, Terai Y, Tanabe A, Sasaki H, Sekijima T, Fujiwara S, et al. Prognostic effect of epidermal growth factor receptor gene mutations and the aberrant phosphorylation of Akt and ERK in ovarian cancer. Cancer Biol Ther. 2011;11:50–7.
33. Lok GT, Chan DW, Liu VW, Hui WW, Leung TH, Yao KM, et al. Aberrant activation of ERK/FOXM1 signaling cascade triggers the cell migration/ invasion in ovarian cancer cells. PLoS One. 2011;6:e23790.
34. Uehata M, Ishizaki T, Satoh H, Ono T, Kawahara T, Morishita T, et al. Calcium sensitization of smooth muscle mediated by a rho-associated protein kinase in hypertension. Nature. 1997;389:990–4.
35. Morikawa K, Hanada H, Hirota K, Nonaka M, Ikeda C. All-trans retinoic acid displays multiple effects on the growth, lipogenesis and adipokine gene expression of AML-I preadipocyte cell line. Cell Biol Int. 2013;37:36–46.
36. Narumiya S, Tanji M, Ishizaki T. Rho signaling, ROCK and mDia1, in transformation, metastasis and invasion. Cancer Metastasis Rev. 2009;28:65–76.
37. Chang HR, Huang HP, Kao YL, Chen SL, Wu SW, Hung TW, et al. The suppressive effect of rho kinase inhibitor, Y-27632, on oncogenic Ras/RhoA induced invasion/migration of human bladder cancer TSGH cells. Chem Biol Interact. 2010;183:172–80.
38. Chan CC, Wong AK, Liu J, Steeves JD, Tetzlaff W. ROCK inhibition with Y27632 activates astrocytes and increases their expression of neurite growth-inhibitory chondroitin sulfate proteoglycans. Glia. 2007;55:369–84.
39. Xue F, Takahara T, Yata Y, Xia Q, Nonome K, Shinno E, et al. Blockade of rho/ rho-associated coiled coil-forming kinase signaling can prevent progression of hepatocellular carcinoma in matrix metalloproteinase-dependent manner. Hepatology research: the official journal of the Japan society of. Hepatology. 2008;38:810–7.

14

Sialylation of EGFR by the ST6Gal-I sialyltransferase promotes EGFR activation and resistance to gefitinib-mediated cell death

Colleen M. Britain[1†], Andrew T. Holdbrooks[1†], Joshua C. Anderson[2], Christopher D. Willey[2] and Susan L. Bellis[1*]

Abstract

Background: The ST6Gal-I sialyltransferase is upregulated in numerous cancers, and high expression of this enzyme correlates with poor patient prognosis in various malignancies, including ovarian cancer. Through its sialylation of a select cohort of cell surface receptors, ST6Gal-I modulates cell signaling to promote tumor cell survival. The goal of the present study was to investigate the influence of ST6Gal-I on another important receptor that controls cancer cell behavior, EGFR. Additionally, the effect of ST6Gal-I on cancer cells treated with the common EGFR inhibitor, gefitinib, was evaluated.

Results: Using the OV4 ovarian cancer cell line, which lacks endogenous ST6Gal-I expression, a kinomics assay revealed that cells with forced overexpression of ST6Gal-I exhibited increased global tyrosine kinase activity, a finding confirmed by immunoblotting whole cell lysates with an anti-phosphotyrosine antibody. Interestingly, the kinomics assay suggested that one of the most highly activated tyrosine kinases in ST6Gal-I-overexpressing OV4 cells was EGFR. Based on these findings, additional analyses were performed to investigate the effect of ST6Gal-I on EGFR activation. To this end, we utilized, in addition to OV4 cells, the SKOV3 ovarian cancer cell line, engineered with both ST6Gal-I overexpression and knockdown, as well as the BxPC3 pancreatic cancer cell line with knockdown of ST6Gal-I. In all three cell lines, we determined that EGFR is a substrate of ST6Gal-I, and that the sialylation status of EGFR directly correlates with ST6Gal-I expression. Cells with differential ST6Gal-I expression were subsequently evaluated for EGFR tyrosine phosphorylation. Cells with high ST6Gal-I expression were found to have elevated levels of basal and EGF-induced EGFR activation. Conversely, knockdown of ST6Gal-I greatly attenuated EGFR activation, both basally and post EGF treatment. Finally, to illustrate the functional importance of ST6Gal-I in regulating EGFR-dependent survival, cells were treated with gefitinib, an EGFR inhibitor widely used for cancer therapy. These studies showed that ST6Gal-I promotes resistance to gefitinib-mediated apoptosis, as measured by caspase activity assays.

Conclusion: Results herein indicate that ST6Gal-I promotes EGFR activation and protects against gefitinib-mediated cell death. Establishing the tumor-associated ST6Gal-I sialyltransferase as a regulator of EGFR provides novel insight into the role of glycosylation in growth factor signaling and chemoresistance.

Keywords: β-galactoside α2-6 sialyltransferase 1 (ST6GAL1), Glycosylation, Epidermal growth factor receptor (EGFR) cell signaling, Gefitinib, Tumor cell biology, Kinomics, Tyrosine kinase

* Correspondence: bellis@uab.edu
†Equal contributors
[1]Department of Cell, Developmental, and Integrative Biology, University of Alabama at Birmingham, 350 McCallum Building, 1918 University Blvd, Birmingham, AL 35294, USA
Full list of author information is available at the end of the article

Background

It has long been known that tumor cells display an altered profile of cell surface glycans, however the functional role of glycosylation in regulating tumor cell behavior remains poorly-understood. The changes in tumor glycosylation are not random; instead, a select subset of glycans is consistently enriched in cancer cells. One of these elevated glycan structures is α2-6 linked sialic acid, which is added to N-glycosylated proteins by the ST6Gal-I sialyltransferase [1–3]. ST6Gal-I is upregulated in numerous cancers including ovarian, pancreatic, colon and breast [4–8], and high ST6Gal-I expression correlates with poor patient outcomes in several types of malignancies [5–8].

One of the central questions regarding ST6Gal-I's pro-tumorigenic activity is how changes in surface sialylation influence intracellular signaling cascades to modulate tumor cell behavior. We and others have reported that ST6Gal-I regulates the structure and function of a specific cohort of membrane receptors. As examples, ST6Gal-I-mediated sialylation of the β1 integrin drives tumor cell migration and invasion [9–12], whereas α2-6 sialylation of both the Fas and TNFR1 death receptors prevents apoptosis by blocking ligand-induced receptor internalization [13, 14]. ST6Gal-I-dependent sialylation also plays a prominent role in regulating the oligomerization of multiple receptors including CD45 [15] and PECAM [16]. Through its collective actions on diverse receptors, ST6Gal-I functions as a master regulator to control cell phenotype. In cancer cells, the upregulation of ST6Gal-I promotes hallmark cancer stem cell (CSC) behaviors including tumorspheroid growth, self-renewal, tumor-initiating potential and resistance to chemotherapy [4, 5, 17–19].

In the present study we identify another important receptor regulated by ST6Gal-I, the receptor tyrosine kinase, EGFR. OV4 ovarian cancer cells with enforced ST6Gal-I expression were subjected to an unbiased kinomics assay, which revealed that EGFR was one of the most differentially activated kinases in cells with upregulated ST6Gal-I. Specifically, EGFR tyrosine kinase activity was markedly enhanced in cells with high ST6Gal-I expression. Based on the kinomics results, we developed several cell model systems with either ST6Gal-I overexpression or knockdown to establish that EGFR is directly α2-6 sialylated by ST6Gal-I. Significantly, we find that ST6Gal-I-mediated sialylation of EGFR stimulates both the basal and EGF-induced activation of EGFR. Furthermore, α2-6 sialylation of EGFR regulates the viability of cells exposed to the EGFR inhibitor, geftinib. These results not only establish a new tumor-promoting function for ST6Gal-I, but also more broadly illuminate the importance of tumor glycans in fundamental tumor cell survival pathways.

Methods

Cell culture

For routine maintenance of cell lines, cells were grown in DME/F12 (OV4) or RPMI (SKOV3 and BxPC3) media supplemented with 10% fetal bovine serum (FBS – Atlanta Biologicals) and 1% antibiotic/antimycotics (Invitrogen). Cells were transduced with lentivirus encoding either the human ST6Gal-I gene (Genecopoeia) or shRNA against ST6Gal-I (Sigma, TRCN00000035432, sequence CCGGCGTGTGCTACTACTACCAGAACTC-GAGTTCTGGTAGTAGTAGCACACGTTTTTG).

Polyclonal populations of stably-transduced cells were isolated by puromycin selection. Overexpression or knockdown of ST6Gal-I was verified via immunoblot using anti-ST6Gal-I goat polyclonal antibody (R&D Systems, AF5924).

Kinomics assay

OV4 EV or OE cells were lysed by adding pre-chilled M-PER Mammalian Protein Extraction Reagent (Thermo-Scientific) containing protease and phosphatase inhibitors (Thermo Scientific). After a 30 min incubation on ice, the lysate was centrifuged at 14,000 rpm at 4 °C, and the supernatant immediately collected and stored at −80 °C. Global kinase activity (kinomic) profiling was performed in the UAB Kinome Core (www.kinomecore.com) using the PamStation®12 platform (PamGene, BV, The Netherlands) as previously described [20–25]. Briefly, lysates were loaded onto wells of 2% BSA blocked PamChips specific for the kinome analyzed – 15 μg lysate for the protein tyrosine kinase (PTK) chip and 2 μg lysate for the serine threonine kinase (STK) chip. Lysates were loaded along with standard kinase buffer (PamGene) containing ATP and FITC-labeled antibodies for detection of phosphorylated substrate probes. Both kinetic and end of reaction (end-level) peptide substrate phosphorylation image capture data was collected with Evolve software (PamGene) and analyzed using the BioNavigator (v. 6.2, PamGene). Upstream kinase prediction was performed using the UpKin upstream kinase prediction tool (PamGene) that calculates a normalized kinase statistic score and specificity score using data from the public phosphonet database (www.phosphonet.ca) to identify highly altered kinases that are displayed in bar graph and volcano plots [21, 22].

Immunoblotting

Cells were serum deprived for 2 h using media containing 1% FBS prior to treatment with 100 ng/mL rhEGF (R&D, 236-EG). Cells were treated for indicated times and lysed using radioimmune precipitation assay (RIPA) buffer supplemented with protease and phosphatase inhibitors. Total protein concentration was measured by BCA (Pierce). Samples were resolved by SDS-PAGE and

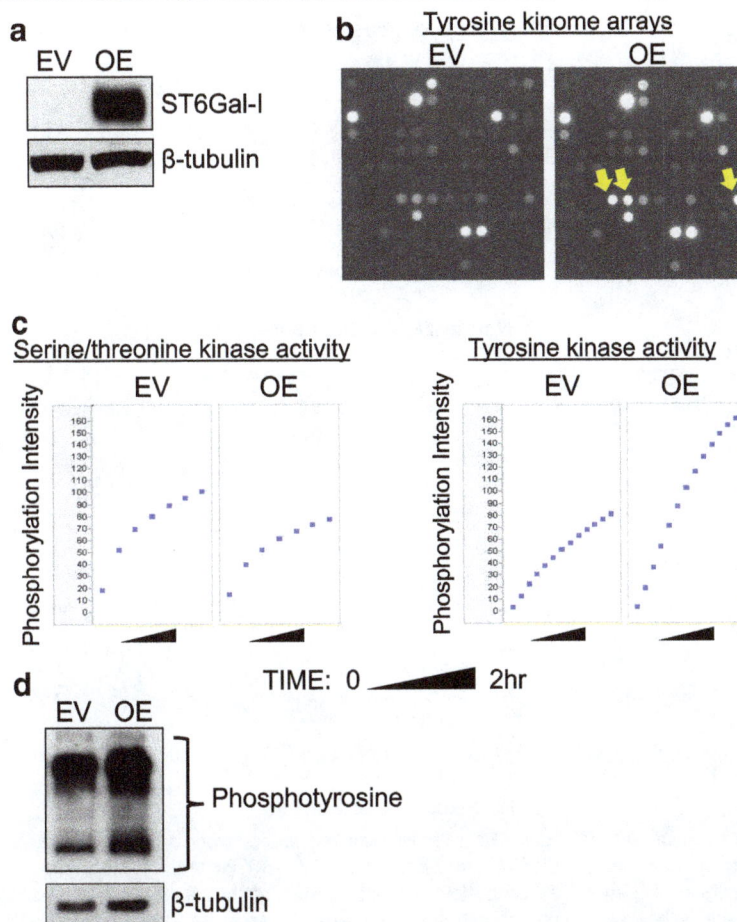

Fig. 1 ST6Gal-I promotes an increase in overall tyrosine kinase activity. **a.** OV4 cells were stably transduced with lentivirus encoding ST6Gal-I, and ST6Gal-I overexpression (OE) was confirmed by immunoblotting (EV = empty vector control). **b.** Whole array image capture at final prewash cycle number 92 of PTK array illustrating changes in tyrosine phosphorylation with qualitatively selected altered spots (yellow arrows) increased in ST6Gal-I OV4 OE cells as compared to EV cells. **c.** Whole chip comparative OE and EV array-mean phosphorylation intensity (y axis per cell) over time in the kinetic/prewash cycles (x axis per cell) for both the STK (left 2 panels) and PTK (right two panels) arrays. **d.** EV or OE cells were immunoblotted with an anti-phosphotyrosine antibody

transferred to polyvinylidene difluoride membranes. Membranes were incubated with 5% nonfat dry milk in TBS containing 0.1% Tween-20 (TBST). Immunoblots were probed with antibodies for p-EGFR (Y-1068, Cell Signaling Technology, cat #3777), or total EGFR (Cell Signaling Technology, cat #4267), followed by incubation with appropriate HRP-conjugated secondary antibodies (Cell Signaling Technologies). Protein loading was verified using anti-β-tubulin (Abcam, ab21058). Protein was detected by enhanced chemiluminescence using the ECL substrate from Pierce (cat# 32106). To visualize basal p-EGFR levels, which are lower than levels of EGF-induced p-EGFR, we optimized blotting conditions by increasing the total amount of protein loaded (> 40 µg) and prolonging film exposure times. We also used a more sensitive ECL reagent for the basal p-EGFR blots (SuperSignal West Dura from BioRad cat# 179-5060). In addition to immunoblotting for p-EGFR and total EGFR, OV4 cells were immunoblotted for total levels of tyrosine phosphorylation using an HRP-conjugated antibody

against phospho-tyrosine (BD Biosciences, cat #610011). Immunoblotting for p-EGFR was performed using three independently-prepared cell lysates, and densitometric quantification of bands from at least three independent blots was achieved using ImageJ software. All bands were normalized to their respective β-tubulin loading controls. Student's t test was employed to determine significance ($p < 0.05$).

SNA precipitation assay

250 µg of cell lysate was incubated with 150 µg of SNA-agarose (Vector Labs, cat# AL-1303). Samples were incubated at 4 °C overnight on a rotator. α2-6 sialylated proteins were then precipitated by centrifugation and washed 3 times with ice cold PBS. Precipitates were resolved by SDS-PAGE and immunoblotted for EGFR as described above.

Caspase 3/7 luminescence assay

Cells were seeded at equal densities into culture plates and allowed to adhere overnight. Prior to gefitinib

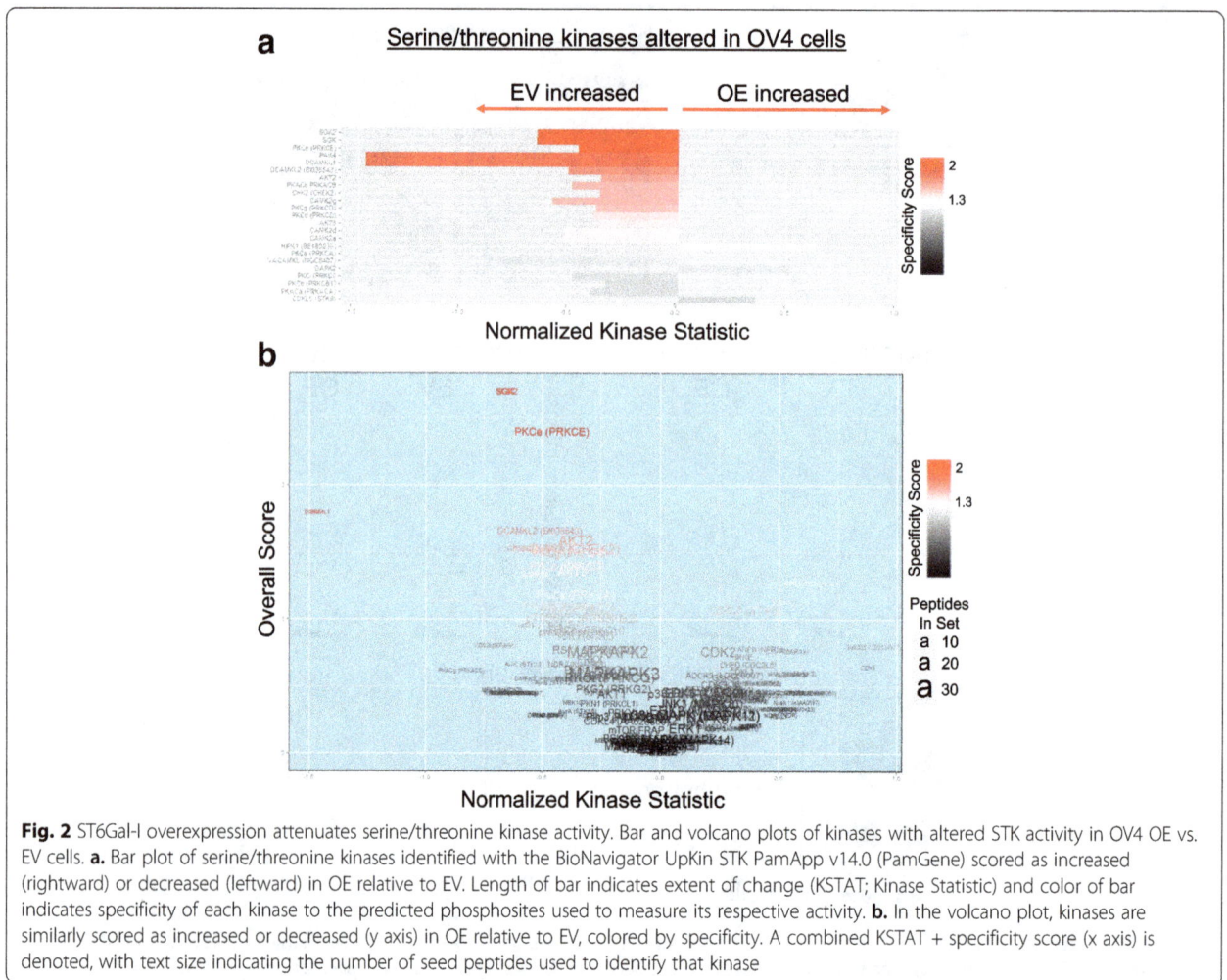

Fig. 2 ST6Gal-I overexpression attenuates serine/threonine kinase activity. Bar and volcano plots of kinases with altered STK activity in OV4 OE vs. EV cells. **a.** Bar plot of serine/threonine kinases identified with the BioNavigator UpKin STK PamApp v14.0 (PamGene) scored as increased (rightward) or decreased (leftward) in OE relative to EV. Length of bar indicates extent of change (KSTAT; Kinase Statistic) and color of bar indicates specificity of each kinase to the predicted phosphosites used to measure its respective activity. **b.** In the volcano plot, kinases are similarly scored as increased or decreased (y axis) in OE relative to EV, colored by specificity. A combined KSTAT + specificity score (x axis) is denoted, with text size indicating the number of seed peptides used to identify that kinase

treatment, cells were serum deprived in 1% FBS-containing media for 2 h and then treated with 1 µM gefitinib (Selleckchem, cat #S1025) for 24-72 h. Reconstituted Caspase-Glo 3/7 assay reagent (Promega, cat #G8093) was then added into each well, mixed via orbital shaker, and incubated at room temperature for 45 min. Luminescence was quantified with a BioTek Synergy H1 plate reader. The values represented were normalized to the caspase value for untreated cells. At least two independent experiments were conducted for each cell line.

Results

Kinomics assays reveal that ST6Gal-I overexpression switches signaling to favor tyrosine kinase activation

The OV4 ovarian cancer cell line is one of the few cancer lines that lacks detectable ST6Gal-I protein. To evaluate the role of ST6Gal-I in regulating kinase activity, ST6Gal-I was stably overexpressed (OE) in OV4 cells using a lentiviral vector (Fig 1a). An empty vector (EV) control cell line was also generated. As previously reported [26], OV4 OE cells have increased surface α2-6 sialylation relative to EV cells, as measured by SNA labelling and flow cytometry. SNA is a lectin that specifically recognizes α2-6 sialic acids.

To screen for potential changes in cell signaling consequent to forced ST6Gal-I expression, EV and OE cells were subjected to a kinomics assay. As shown in Fig. 1b, EV and OE cells displayed noticeable differences in the phosphorylation of select substrates (arrows), suggesting that ST6Gal-I modulates the activity of a distinct subset of kinases. Interestingly, OE cells exhibited a modest decrease in the net activity of serine/threonine kinases, compared with EV, cells (Fig. 1c, left panel), whereas OE cells had substantially increased tyrosine kinase activity (Fig. 1c, right panel). Enhanced tyrosine kinase activity in the OE line was confirmed by immunoblotting whole cell lysates with an anti-phosphotyrosine antibody that detects global changes in tyrosine kinase activity (Fig 1d).

We next evaluated the activity of specific serine/threonine kinases modulated by ST6Gal-I (Fig 2). In general, most of the serine/threonine kinases probed by the

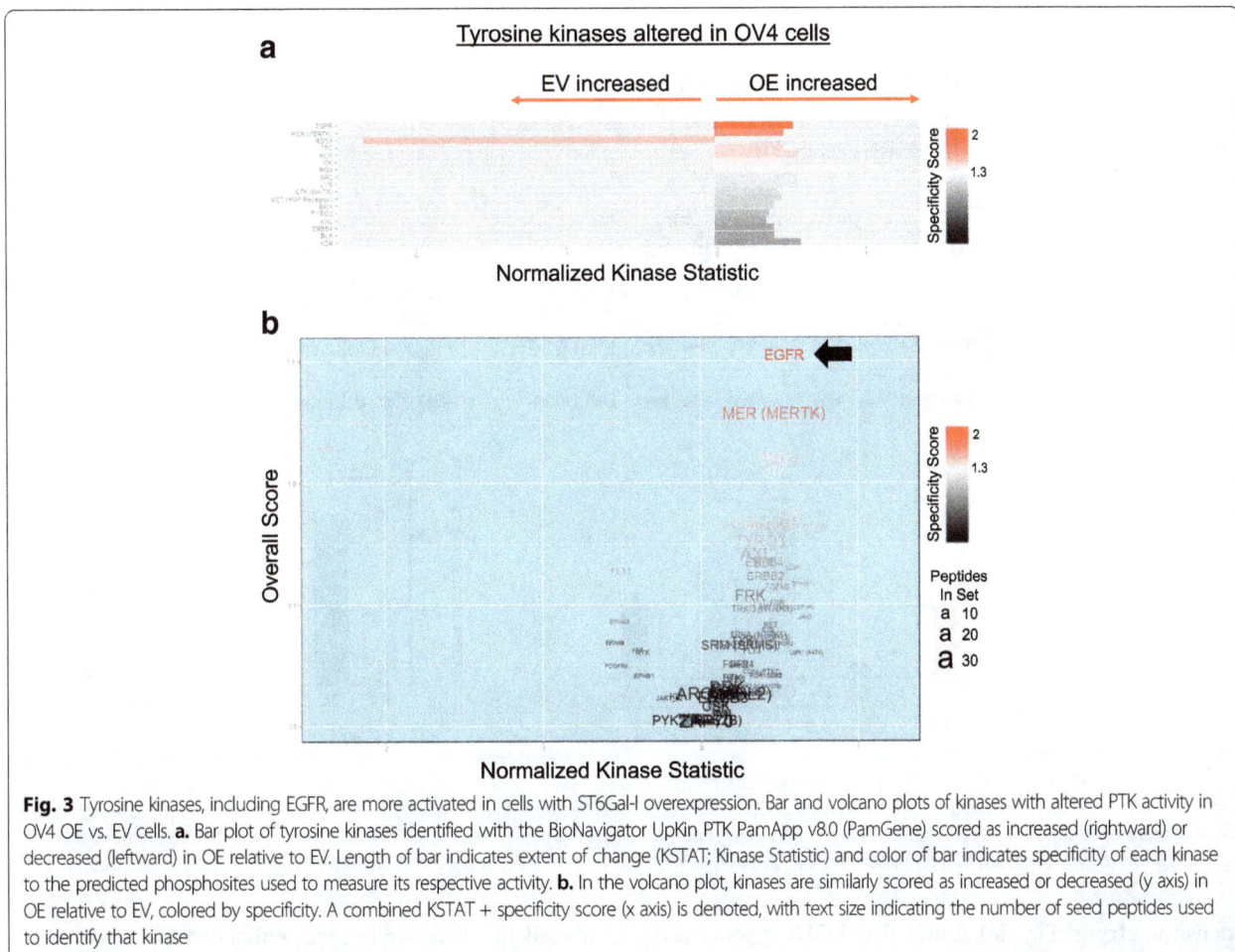

Fig. 3 Tyrosine kinases, including EGFR, are more activated in cells with ST6Gal-I overexpression. Bar and volcano plots of kinases with altered PTK activity in OV4 OE vs. EV cells. **a.** Bar plot of tyrosine kinases identified with the BioNavigator UpKin PTK PamApp v8.0 (PamGene) scored as increased (rightward) or decreased (leftward) in OE relative to EV. Length of bar indicates extent of change (KSTAT; Kinase Statistic) and color of bar indicates specificity of each kinase to the predicted phosphosites used to measure its respective activity. **b.** In the volcano plot, kinases are similarly scored as increased or decreased (y axis) in OE relative to EV, colored by specificity. A combined KSTAT + specificity score (x axis) is denoted, with text size indicating the number of seed peptides used to identify that kinase

kinomics assay exhibited increased activation in EV cells. The most prominent differentially activated kinases are shown in Fig. 2a. These include several members of the protein kinase C (PKC) and calcium-calmodulin-kinase-like (CAMKL) families. The specificity score measures the specificity of the kinase for its cognate peptides on the chip, with red indicating high specificity. The volcano plot in Fig. 2b relates the specificity score to the normalized kinase statistic score (i.e. relative kinase activity) to provide an overall score for kinase activation. Fig 3 depicts tyrosine kinase activity in EV and OV4 cells. Notably, nearly all of the tyrosine kinases screened were more active in OE cells (Fig. 3a). Many of these hyperactivated kinases are known to be associated with cell transformation, such as the non-receptor tyrosine kinases, src and lyn, and receptor tyrosine kinases, MET, ERBB4 and EGFR. As shown in the volcano plot (Fig. 3b), one of the most differentially-activated tyrosine kinases in OE vs. EV cells was EGFR (arrow).

ST6Gal-I overexpression in OV4 ovarian cancer cells increases basal and EGF-induced EGFR activation

Given that the kinomics assay pointed to enhanced EGFR activation in cells with forced ST6Gal-I

expression, we conducted additional analyses of this receptor. We first determined whether EGFR was a direct substrate for ST6Gal-I. To this end, cell lysates were incubated with agarose-conjugated SNA lectin to precipitate α2-6 sialylated proteins. These proteins were resolved by SDS-PAGE and immunoblotted for EGFR. As shown in Fig. 4a, α2-6 sialylated EGFR was clearly apparent in OE, but not EV, cells. The total amount of EGFR was equivalent in EV and OE cells, indicating that forced expression of ST6Gal-I did not alter EGFR expression. To assess the effects of EGFR sialylation on EGFR activation, cells were treated with EGF for up to 30 min, and then lysates were immunoblotted for p-EGFR (representative blot in Fig. 4b and corresponding densitometric analyses of blots from three independently-generated cell lysates in Fig 4c). At both 5 and 15 min following EGF stimulation, OE cells exhibited increased activation of EGFR relative to EV cells. In the blot depicted in Fig. 4b, p-EGFR levels in the untreated (UT) populations were below the limits of detection. We therefore optimized immunoblotting conditions to increase sensitivity (see Methods section), enabling visualization of basal p-EGFR. Fig. 4d

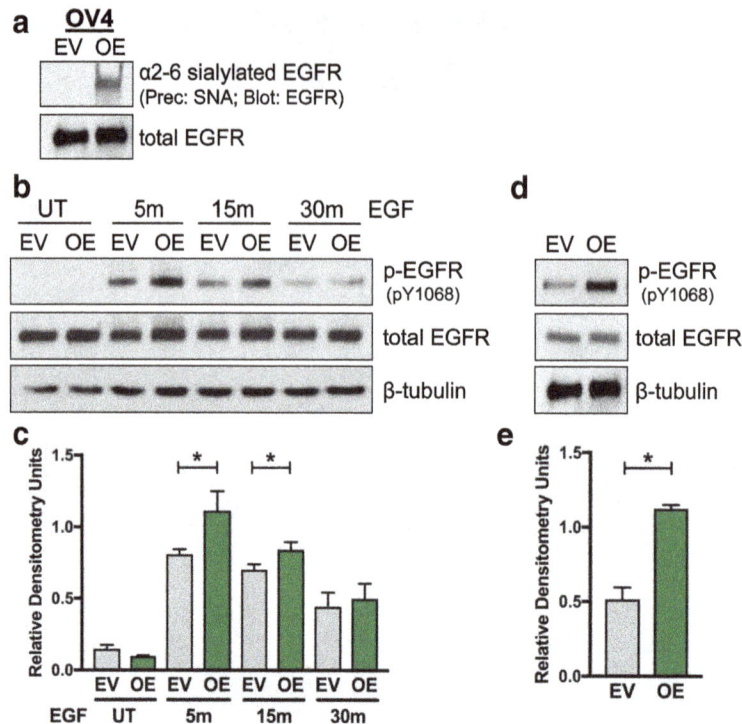

Fig. 4 EGFR phosphorylation is enhanced in OV4 ovarian cancer cells with ST6Gal-I overexpression. **a.** To measure levels of α2-6 sialylated EGFR, cell lysates were incubated with SNA-agarose. SNA is a lectin that specifically recognizes α2-6 sialic acids. Sialylated proteins were precipitated and then immunoblotted for EGFR. **b.** Representative p-EGFR immunoblot of EV or OE cells treated with EGF for 5, 15 and 30 min. **c.** Densitometric analysis of three independent blots of p-EGFR in EGF-treated OV4 cells, with values normalized to the β-tubulin loading control. **d.** Representative p-EGFR immunoblot of EV or OE cells to evaluate basal EGFR phosphorylation. **e.** Densitometric analysis of three independent blots of basal p-EGFR in OV4 cells. *, $p < 0.05$

(densitometry in Fig. 4e) shows that EGFR is more activated in the OE line even in the absence of exogenously-added EGF. These data are consistent with the kinomics assay, which was conducted on untreated cells.

ST6Gal-I activity regulates basal and EGF-induced EGFR activation in SKOV3 ovarian cancer cells

To determine whether sialylation-dependent regulation of EGFR was conserved across cancer cell lines, EGFR activity was examined in the SKOV3 ovarian cancer line. ST6Gal-I was either overexpressed (OE) in SKOV3 cells, or stably knocked-down (KD) using a shRNA-bearing lentiviral vector (Fig. 5a). SNA precipitation assays showed that, in comparison with EV control cells, EGFR had increased α2-6 sialylation in OE cells, and decreased α2-6 sialylation in KD cells. As with the OV4 line, manipulating ST6Gal-I expression in SKOV3 cells had no effect on total levels of EGFR. In correspondence with differential sialylation, basal p-EGFR was higher in SKOV3 OE vs. EV cells, whereas p-EGFR levels were greatly reduced in KD cells (densitometry for p-EGFR in Fig. 5b). Along with changes in basal activation, sialylation of EGFR regulated the response to EGF (representative blots in Fig. 5c and densitometry in Fig. 5d). EGF-

induced EGFR activation was enhanced in OE cells, but diminished in KD cells.

ST6Gal-I knockdown impairs basal and EGF-induced EGFR activation in BxPC3 pancreatic cancer cells

Recent studies suggest that ST6Gal-I has a similar function in multiple cancer types including ovarian, colon, and pancreatic adenocarcinoma. We therefore evaluated EGFR activation in a pancreatic cancer line, BxPC3. ST6Gal-I expression was knocked down (KD) in this line, which led to a loss in α2-6 sialylation of EGFR, as measured by SNA precipitation assay (Fig. 6a). Consistent with reduced EGFR sialylation, ST6Gal-I KD cells had dramatically decreased levels of basal activation of EGFR (densitometry for p-EGFR in Fig. 6b). As with basal activation, EGF-stimulated EGFR activation was suppressed by ST6Gal-I KD (representative blots in Fig. 6c and densitometry in Fig. 6d). Considering that elevated ST6Gal-I levels resulted in increased EGFR activation in all three cell lines, we next tested whether endogenous expression of ST6Gal-I correlates with p-EGFR in a side-by-side comparison of the lines. Fig. 6e shows that SKOV3 EV cells, which have the highest levels of ST6Gal-I of the three lines, exhibit the most pronounced basal activation of EGFR, whereas the

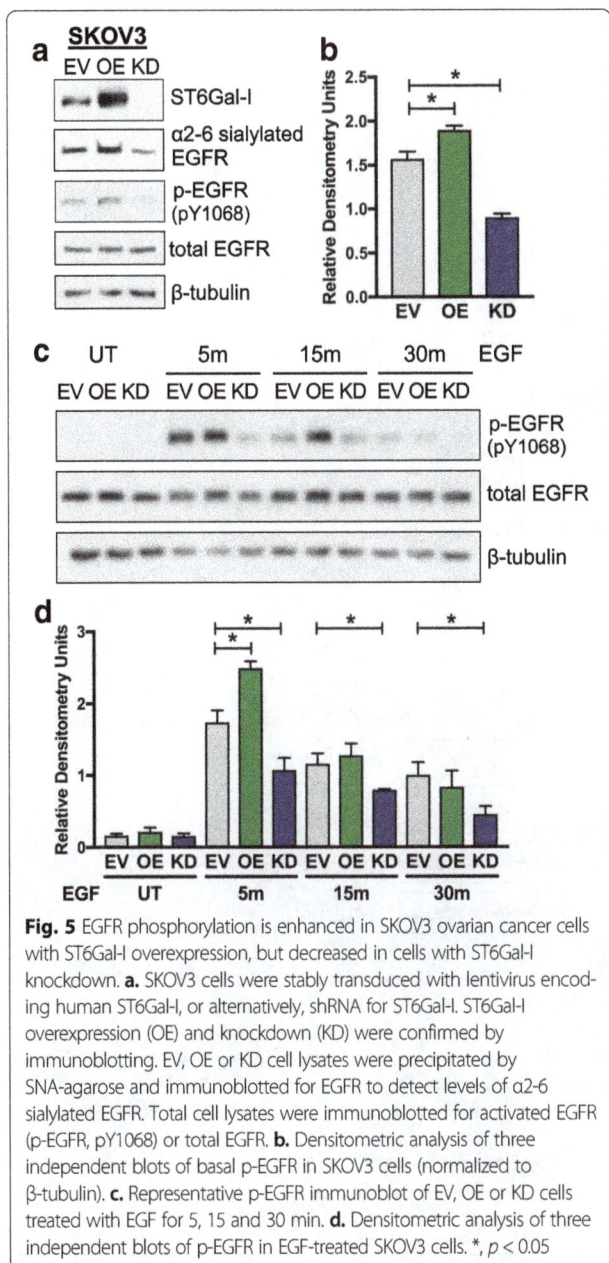

Fig. 5 EGFR phosphorylation is enhanced in SKOV3 ovarian cancer cells with ST6Gal-I overexpression, but decreased in cells with ST6Gal-I knockdown. **a.** SKOV3 cells were stably transduced with lentivirus encoding human ST6Gal-I, or alternatively, shRNA for ST6Gal-I. ST6Gal-I overexpression (OE) and knockdown (KD) were confirmed by immunoblotting. EV, OE or KD cell lysates were precipitated by SNA-agarose and immunoblotted for EGFR to detect levels of α2-6 sialylated EGFR. Total cell lysates were immunoblotted for activated EGFR (p-EGFR, pY1068) or total EGFR. **b.** Densitometric analysis of three independent blots of basal p-EGFR in SKOV3 cells (normalized to β-tubulin). **c.** Representative p-EGFR immunoblot of EV, OE or KD cells treated with EGF for 5, 15 and 30 min. **d.** Densitometric analysis of three independent blots of p-EGFR in EGF-treated SKOV3 cells. *, $p < 0.05$

lowest ST6Gal-I expressing cells, OV4 EV, display the least amount of basal p-EGFR. This finding suggests that, irrespective of the diverse genetic backgrounds of these three cell lines, there is correspondence between the level of ST6Gal-I activity and EGFR activation.

ST6Gal-I-mediated sialylation of EGFR regulates the viability of cells treated with gefitinib

The combined results in Figs 1, 2, 3, 4, 5 and 6 established that ST6Gal-I mediated sialylation of EGFR enhances its activation, as indicated by greater tyrosine kinase activity. To confirm the importance of ST6Gal-I in regulating EGFR-dependent cell survival, we examined

cell response to the EGFR inhibitor, gefitinib. In a prior study, it was shown that ST6Gal-I KD sensitizes cells to gefitinib-induced cell death [27]. Accordingly, OV4 EV and OE cells were treated with gefitinib, and then monitored for apoptosis using a caspase 3/7 activity assay. As shown in Fig. 7a, OV4 OE cells were resistant to gefitinib-mediated apoptosis. Contrarily, ST6Gal-I KD in BxPC3 cells enhanced gefitinib-induced cell death (Fig. 7b).

Discussion

Accumulating evidence suggests that ST6Gal-I is a potent survival factor, providing cancer cells with protection against a variety of microenvironmental assaults. Explicitly, α2-6 sialylation of select receptors inhibits galectin-mediated apoptosis [28–30], and ST6Gal-I also prevents cell death driven by TNFR1 [14, 31] and Fas [13]. In addition, ST6Gal-I protects tumor cells against cytotoxicity mediated by radiation [32] and chemotherapy drugs including cisplatin, gemcitabine and docetaxel [5, 17–19]. Furthermore, ST6Gal-I enables tumor cell survival under conditions of serum growth factor deprivation by enhancing Akt activation, and preventing tumor cell exit from the cell cycle [26].

In the current study, we describe a new survival function for ST6Gal-I in modulating the activity of EGFR. Utilizing an unbiased kinomics assay, we show that overall basal tyrosine kinase activity, a phenomenon well-known to contribute to malignant transformation [33–36], is profoundly elevated in cells with forced overexpression of ST6Gal-I. In particular, EGFR is one of the most highly activated of these tyrosine kinases. To substantiate this result, we manipulated ST6Gal-I expression in 3 different cancer cell lines, using both overexpression and knockdown approaches. In these models, EGFR was shown to be a direct substrate for ST6Gal-I-mediated sialylation, and in every case, α2-6-sialylation of EGFR increased both the basal and EGF-induced activation of EGFR. Thus, EGFR α2-6-sialylation is consistently correlated with increased tyrosine kinase activity despite the diverse genetic lesions present in the 3 distinct cancer lines. As well, ST6Gal-I-mediated EGFR sialylation protected tumor cells against gefitinib-induced cell death.

The role of sialylation in regulating EGFR has been previously investigated. Park et al. manipulated ST6Gal-I expression in colon carcinoma cells, and in concordance with our work, reported that EGFR sialylation prevented geftinib-induced cytotoxicity [27]. However, in contrast to our studies, α2-6 sialylation appeared to inhibit EGF-induced EGFR tyrosine phosphorylation [27]. The reason for this discrepancy is currently unclear. Other investigators have manipulated global sialylation to interrogate the functional effects on EGFR. Wong's group incubated cells with a sialidase enzyme that cleaves all sialic acid linkages (α2-3, α2-6 and α2-8) [37]. In this study, the removal of surface sialylation facilitated the formation of

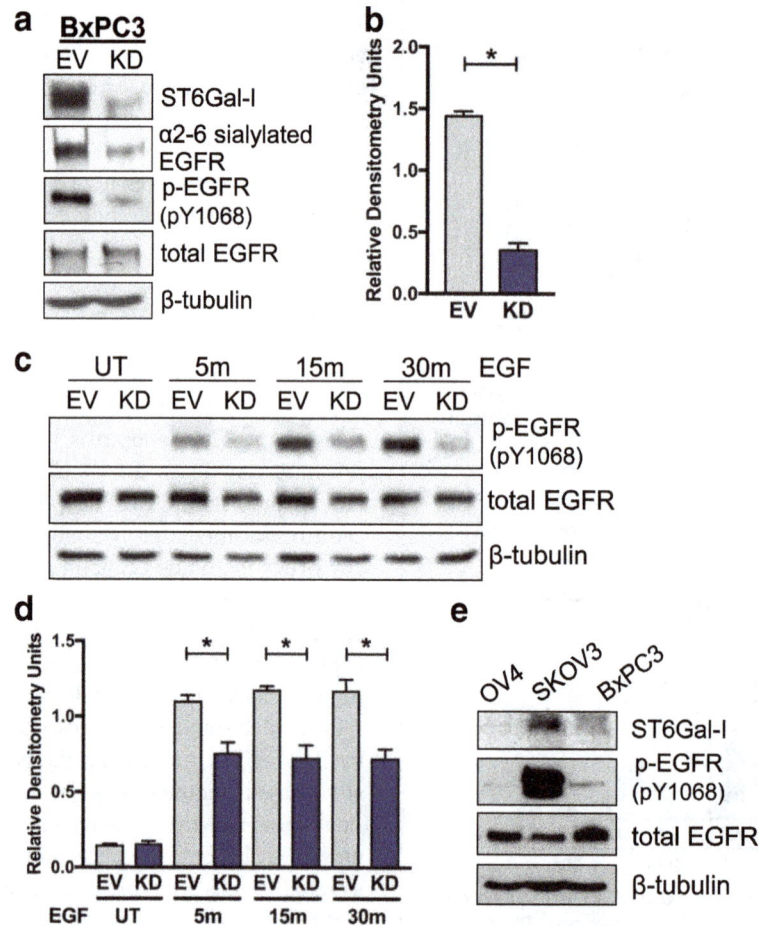

Fig. 6 Knockdown of ST6Gal-I diminishes EGFR phosphorylation in BxPC3 pancreatic cancer cells. **a.** Using lentivirus, BxPC3 cells were stably transduced with shRNA for ST6Gal-I, and ST6Gal-I knockdown (KD) was confirmed by immunoblotting. EV or KD cell lysates were precipitated by SNA agarose and immunoblotted for EGFR to detect α2-6 sialylated EGFR. Total cell lysates were immunoblotted for activated EGFR (p-EGFR, pY1068) or total EGFR. **b.** Densitometric analysis of three independent blots of basal p-EGFR in BxPC3 cells (normalized to β-tubulin). **c.** Representative p-EGFR immunoblot of EV or KD cells treated with EGF for 5, 15 and 30 min. **d.** Densitometric analysis of three independent blots of p-EGFR in EGF-treated BxPC3 cells. **e.** Total cell lysates from EV cells of the OV4, SKOV3 and BxPC3 lines were immunoblotted for ST6Gal-I, p-EGFR (Y1068) or total EGFR. *, $p < 0.05$

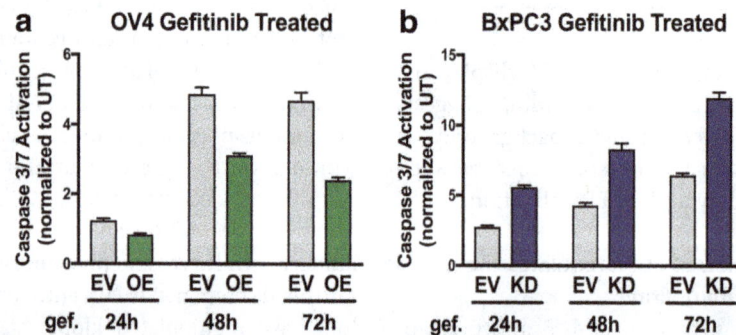

Fig. 7 ST6Gal-I activity protects cancer cells against gefitinib-mediated apoptosis. **a.** OV4 EV or OE cells and **b.** BxPC3 EV or KD cells were treated with gefitinib for 24, 48 and 72 h and analyzed for apoptosis via a luminescence assay that detects caspase 3 and 7 activity. Caspase activity in geftinib-treated cells was normalized to caspase activity in untreated cells. Data shown are from a representative experiment, with at least 2 independent experiments performed for each cell line. Graph depicts means ± S.D

EGF-induced EGFR dimers. This group further generated a recombinant, soluble EGFR protein and reported that sialidase-treated EGFR protein exhibited greater dimerization [38]. Yarema's group addressed the question of EGFR sialylation by incubating cells with a metabolic precursor of sialic acid that augments the intracellular pool of sialic acid, leading to enriched receptor sialylation [39]. The ensuing increase in EGFR sialylation was found to hinder EGFR's association with the extracellular galectin lattice, potentiating EGFR internalization. No changes in EGFR dimerization were observed in this latter study. Taken together, these studies highlight the importance of sialic acid in EGFR signaling, however there are some caveats associated with manipulating the global sialylation of tumor cells. First, complete removal of cell surface sialylation via sialidase treatment has profound effects on cell signaling, altering the activity of a myriad of receptors. Secondly, there is substantial evidence that the α2-3 and α2-6 sialic acid linkages are not always functionally equivalent. This is best exemplified by the activity of lectins such as galectins and siglecs that clearly discriminate between α2-3 and α2-6 sialylation. Finally, there is an extensive literature suggesting that α2-6 sialylation is particularly enriched in cancer cells [1–3] (and also stem cells [40, 41]). Our group has sought to model the tumor cell phenotype by examining the effect of selective ST6Gal-I upregulation, without grossly altering α2-3 sialylation. Through this approach, we find that high ST6Gal-I activity enhances EGFR activation, consistent with the vast literature suggesting that ST6Gal-I acts as a tumor-driver gene.

Further studies will be needed to better understand the effect of α2-6 sialylation on EGFR. EGFR has a complex mechanism of regulation involving receptor oligomerization, lipid raft localization, shedding, and dynamic partitioning between cellular compartments including the plasma membrane, endosome and nucleus [42–45]. Many of these processes are known to be influenced by EGFR glycan composition [39, 46–48]. Furthermore, glycosylation modulates the overall conformation of EGFR in the absence of ligand binding. For example, the N-glycans on two key Asn residues, Asn-420 and Asn 579, appear to maintain EGFR in a low affinity state. Ablation of Asn-420 glycosylation (via mutagenesis) leads to constitutive EGFR tyrosine phosphorylation and spontaneous oligomer formation [49]. Elimination of the Asn-579 site weakens auto-inhibitory tether interactions, and increases the number of preformed EGFR dimers in the absence of ligand [50]. It is tempting to speculate that the addition of the bulky, negatively-charged sialic acid at Asn-420 and/or Asn-570 could disrupt these critical auto-inhibitory interactions, potentiating basal EGFR activation.

Regardless of the mechanism by which α2-6 sialylation modulates EGFR structure (or potentially, localization), results herein are consistent with other studies indicating

that ST6Gal-I protects against gefitinib-induced cell death [27]. Gefitinib is widely-used in cancer therapy [51], and hence, the levels of ST6Gal-I expression in patient samples could be an important indicator of patient response to treatment. Intensive investigation is currently focused on how EGFR modifications affect the efficacy of EGFR inhibitors, however the role of EGFR glycosylation in drug response has received limited attention.

Conclusions

The collective data in this report indicate that up-regulation of ST6Gal-I, a common feature of cancer cells, promotes heightened activation of EGFR as well as resistance to gefitinib-induced cell death. Considering the immense contribution of EGFR to cancer [43, 52, 53], the establishment of α2-6 sialylation as a novel EGFR regulatory mechanism could advance a fundamental understanding of the relationship between growth factor signaling and cancer cell behavior.

Funding

These studies were supported by NIH grant R01 GM111093 (SLB). CMB was supported by a Predoctoral Fellowship funded by the T32 GM008111 Cell and Molecular Biology training grant. ATH was supported a Predoctoral Fellowship from the American Heart Association.

Authors' contributions

CMB and ATH were responsible for the acquisition and analysis of the data. JCA and CDW provided technical assistance with the kinomics assays and analysis of the data obtained from these experiments. CMB, ATH and SLB were responsible for the concept and design of this study, and together wrote the manuscript. All authors read and approved the final manuscript.

Competing interests

The authors declare that they have no competing interests.

Author details

[1]Department of Cell, Developmental, and Integrative Biology, University of Alabama at Birmingham, 350 McCallum Building, 1918 University Blvd, Birmingham, AL 35294, USA. [2]Department of Radiation Oncology, University of Alabama at Birmingham, 1700 6th Avenue South, Birmingham, AL 35233, USA.

References

1. Dall'Olio F, Chiricolo M. Sialyltransferases in cancer. Glycoconj J. 2001;18: 841–50.
2. Varki NM, Varki A. Diversity in cell surface sialic acid presentations: implications for biology and disease. Laboratory investigation; a journal of technical methods and pathology. Lab Investig. 2007;87(9):851–7.
3. Schultz MJ, Swindall AF, Bellis SL. Regulation of the metastatic cell phenotype by sialylated glycans. Cancer Metastasis Rev. 2012;31(3-4):501–18.
4. Swindall AF, Londono-Joshi AI, Schultz MJ, Fineberg N, Buchsbaum DJ, Bellis SL. ST6Gal-I protein expression is upregulated in human epithelial tumors and correlates with stem cell markers in normal tissues and colon cancer cell lines. Cancer Res. 2013;73(7):2368–78.
5. Schultz MJ, Holdbrooks AT, Chakraborty A, Grizzle WE, Landen CN, Buchsbaum DJ, et al. The tumor-associated glycosyltransferase ST6Gal-I regulates stem cell transcription factors and confers a cancer stem cell phenotype. Cancer Res. 2016;76(13):3978–88.

6. Hsieh CC, Shyr YM, Liao WY, Chen TH, Wang SE, Lu PC, et al. Elevation of beta-galactoside alpha2,6-sialyltransferase 1 in a fructoseresponsive manner promotes pancreatic cancer metastasis. Oncotarget. 2017;8(5):7691–709.

7. Lise M, Belluco C, Perera SP, Patel R, Thomas P, Ganguly A. Clinical correlations of alpha2,6-sialyltransferase expression in colorectal cancer patients. Hybridoma. 2000;19:281–6.

8. Recchi MA, Hebbar M, Hornez L, Harduin-Lepers A, Peyrat JP, Delannoy P. Multiplex reverse transcription polymerase chain reaction assessment of sialyltransferase expression in human breast cancer. Cancer Res. 1998;58:4066–70.

9. Christie DR, Shaikh FM, Lucas JA 4th, Lucas JA 3rd, Bellis SL. ST6Gal-I expression in ovarian cancer cells promotes an invasive phenotype by altering integrin glycosylation and function. J Ovarian Res. 2008;1(1):3.

10. Shaikh FM, Seales EC, Clem WC, Hennessy KM, Zhuo Y, Bellis SL. Tumor cell migration and invasion are regulated by expression of variant integrin glycoforms. Exp Cell Res. 2008;314(16):2941–50.

11. Lin S, Kemmner W, Grigull S, Schlag PM. Cell surface alpha 2,6 sialylation affects adhesion of breast carcinoma cells. Exp Cell Res. 2002;276(1):101–10.

12. Zhu Y, Srivatana U, Ullah A, Gagneja H, Berenson CS, Lance P. Suppression of a sialyltransferase by antisense DNA reduces invasiveness of human colon cancer cells in vitro. Biochim Biophys Acta. 2001;1536:148–60.

13. Swindall AF, Bellis SL. Sialylation of the Fas death receptor by ST6Gal-I provides protection against Fas-mediated apoptosis in colon carcinoma cells. J Biol Chem. 2011;286(26):22982–90.

14. Holdbrooks AT, Britain CM, Bellis SL. ST6Gal-I sialyltransferase promotes tumor necrosis factor (TNF)-mediated cancer cell survival via sialylation of the TNF receptor 1 (TNFR1) death receptor. J Biol Chem. 2017;Epub ahead of print.

15. Amano M, Galvan M, He J, Baum LG. The ST6Gal I sialyltransferase selectively modifies N-glycans on CD45 to negatively regulate galectin-1-induced CD45 clustering, phosphatase modulation, and T cell death. J Biol Chem. 2003;278(9):7469–75.

16. Kitazume S, Imamaki R, Ogawa K, Komi Y, Futakawa S, Kojima S, et al. Alpha2,6-sialic acid on platelet endothelial cell adhesion molecule (PECAM) regulates its homophilic interactions and downstream antiapoptotic signaling. J Biol Chem. 2010;285:6515–21.

17. Schultz MJ, Swindall AF, Wright JW, Sztul ES, Landen CN, Bellis SL. ST6Gal-I sialyltransferase confers cisplatin resistance in ovarian tumor cells. J Ovarian Res. 2013;6(1):25.

18. Chen X, Wang L, Zhao Y, Yuan S, Wu Q, Zhu X, et al. ST6Gal-I modulates docetaxel sensitivity in human hepatocarcinoma cells via the p38 MAPK/caspase pathway. Oncotarget. 2016;7(32):51955–64.

19. Chakraborty A, Dorsett KA, Trummell HQ, Yang ES, Oliver PG, Bonner JA, et al. ST6Gal-I sialyltransferase promotes chemoresistance in pancreatic ductal adenocarcinoma by abrogating gemcitabine-mediated DNA damage. J Biol Chem. 2018;293(3):984–94.

20. Duverger A, Wolschendorf F, Anderson JC, Wagner F, Bosque A, Shishido T, et al. Kinase control of latent HIV-1 infection: PIM-1 kinase as a major contributor to HIV-1 reactivation. J Virol. 2014;88(1):364–76.

21. Anderson JC, Taylor RB, Fiveash JB, de Wijn R, Gillespie GY, Willey CD. Kinomic alterations in atypical Meningioma. Med Res Arch 2015;3.

22. Gilbert AN, Shevin RS, Anderson JC, Langford CP, Eustace N, Gillespie GY, et al. Generation of microtumors using 3D human biogel culture system and patient-derived Glioblastoma cells for Kinomic profiling and drug response testing. J Vis Exp 2016;112.

23. Anderson JC, Willey CD, Mehta A, Welaya K, Chen D, Duarte CW, et al. High throughput Kinomic profiling of human clear cell renal cell carcinoma identifies Kinase activity dependent molecular subtypes. PLoS One. 2015;10(9):e0139267.

24. Ghosh AP, Willey CD, Anderson JC, Welaya K, Chen D, Mehta A, et al. Kinomic profiling identifies focal adhesion kinase 1 as a therapeutic target in advanced clear cell renal cell carcinoma. Oncotarget. 2017;8(17):29220–32.

25. Yang ES, Willey CD, Mehta A, Crowley MR, Crossman DK, Chen D, et al. Kinase analysis of penile squamous cell carcinoma on multiple platforms to identify potential therapeutic targets. Oncotarget. 2017;8(13):21710–8.

26. Britain CM, Dorsett KA, Bellis SL. The Glycosyltransferase ST6Gal-I protects tumor cells against serum growth factor withdrawal by enhancing survival signaling and proliferative potential. J Biol Chem. 2017;292(11):4663–73.

27. Park JJ, Yi JY, Jin YB, Lee YJ, Lee JS, Lee YS, et al. Sialylation of epidermal growth factor receptor regulates receptor activity and chemosensitivity to gefitinib in colon cancer cells. Biochem Pharmacol. 2012;83(7):849–57.

28. Fukumori T, Takenaka Y, Yoshii T, Kim HR, Hogan V, Inohara H, et al. CD29 and CD7 mediate galectin-3-induced type II T-cell apoptosis. Cancer Res. 2003;63(23):8302–11.

29. Toscano MA, Bianco GA, Ilarregui JM, Croci DO, Correale J, Hernandez JD, et al. Differential glycosylation of TH1, TH2 and TH-17 effector cells selectively regulates susceptibility to cell death. Nat Immunol. 2007;8(8):825–34.

30. Zhuo Y, Chammas R, Bellis SL. Sialylation of beta1 integrins blocks cell adhesion to galectin-3 and protects cells against galectin-3-induced apoptosis. J Biol Chem. 2008;283(32):22177–85.

31. Liu Z, Swindall AF, Kesterson RA, Schoeb TR, Bullard DC, Bellis SL. ST6Gal-I regulates macrophage apoptosis via alpha2-6 sialylation of the TNFR1 death receptor. J Biol Chem. 2011;286(45):39654–62.

32. Lee M, Park JJ, Lee YS. Adhesion of ST6Gal I-mediated human colon cancer cells to fibronectin contributes to cell survival by integrin beta1-mediated paxillin and AKT activation. Oncol Rep. 2010;23(3):757–61.

33. Blume-Jensen P, Hunter T. Oncogenic kinase signalling. Nature. 2001;411(6835):355–65.

34. Levitzki A, Gazit A. Tyrosine kinase inhibition: an approach to drug development. Science. 1995;267(5205):1782–8.

35. Regad T, Targeting RTK. Signaling pathways in cancer. Cancers (Basel). 2015;7(3):1758–84.

36. Vlahovic G, Crawford J. Activation of tyrosine kinases in cancer. Oncologist. 2003;8(6):531–8.

37. Yen HY, Liu YC, Chen NY, Tsai CF, Wang YT, Chen YJ, et al. Effect of sialylation on EGFR phosphorylation and resistance to tyrosine kinase inhibition. Proc Natl Acad Sci U S A. 2015;112(22):6955–60.

38. Liu YC, Yen HY, Chen CY, Chen CH, Cheng PF, Juan YH, et al. Sialylation and fucosylation of epidermal growth factor receptor suppress its dimerization and activation in lung cancer cells. Proc Natl Acad Sci U S A. 2011;108(28):11332–7.

39. Mathew MP, Tan E, Saeui CT, Bovonratwet P, Sklar S, Bhattacharya R, et al. Metabolic flux-driven sialylation alters internalization, recycling, and drug sensitivity of the epidermal growth factor receptor (EGFR) in SW1990 pancreatic cancer cells. Oncotarget. 2016;7(41):66491–511.

40. Hasehira K, Tateno H, Onuma Y, Ito Y, Asashima M, Hirabayashi J. Structural and quantitative evidence for dynamic glycome shift on production of induced pluripotent stem cells. Mol Cell Proteomics. 2012;11(12):1913–23.

41. Wang YC, Stein JW, Lynch CL, Tran HT, Lee CY, Coleman R, et al. Glycosyltransferase ST6GAL1 contributes to the regulation of pluripotency in human pluripotent stem cells. Sci Rep. 2015;5:13317.

42. Lambert S, Vind-Kezunovic D, Karvinen S, Gniadecki R. Ligand-independent activation of the EGFR by lipid raft disruption. J Invest Dermatol. 2006;126(5):954–62.

43. Normanno N, De Luca A, Bianco C, Strizzi L, Mancino M, Maiello MR, et al. Epidermal growth factor receptor (EGFR) signaling in cancer. Gene. 2006;366(1):2–16.

44. Perez-Torres M, Valle BL, Maihle NJ, Negron-Vega L, Nieves-Alicea R, Cora EM. Shedding of epidermal growth factor receptor is a regulated process that occurs with overexpression in malignant cells. Exp Cell Res. 2008;314(16):2907–18.

45. Tomas A, Futter CE, Eden ER. EGF receptor trafficking: consequences for signaling and cancer. Trends Cell Biol. 2014;24(1):26–34.

46. Azimzadeh Irani M, Kannan S, Verma C. Role of N-glycosylation in EGFR ectodomain ligand binding. Proteins. 2017;85(8):1529–49.

47. Fernandes H, Cohen S, Bishayee S. Glycosylation-induced conformational modification positively regulates receptor-receptor association: a study with an aberrant epidermal growth factor receptor (EGFRvIII/DeltaEGFR) expressed in cancer cells. J Biol Chem. 2001;276(7):5375–83.

48. Kaszuba K, Grzybek M, Orlowski A, Danne R, Rog T, Simons K, et al. N-Glycosylation as determinant of epidermal growth factor receptor conformation in membranes. Proc Natl Acad Sci U S A. 2015;112(14):4334–9.

49. Tsuda T, Ikeda Y, Taniguchi N. The Asn-420-linked sugar chain in human epidermal growth factor receptor suppresses ligand-independent spontaneous oligomerization. Possible role of a specific sugar chain in controllable receptor activation. J Biol Chem. 2000;275(29):21988–94.

50. Whitson KB, Whitson SR, Red-Brewer ML, McCoy AJ, Vitali AA, Walker F, et al. Functional effects of glycosylation at Asn-579 of the epidermal growth factor receptor. Biochemistry. 2005;44(45):14920–31.

51. Gui T, Shen K. The epidermal growth factor receptor as a therapeutic target in epithelial ovarian cancer. Cancer Epidemiol. 2012;36(5):490–6.

52. Raymond E, Faivre S, Armand JP. Epidermal growth factor receptor tyrosine kinase as a target for anticancer therapy. Drugs. 2000;60(Suppl 1):15–23. discussion 41-12

53. Slichenmyer WJ, Fry DW. Anticancer therapy targeting the erbB family of receptor tyrosine kinases. Semin Oncol. 2001;28(5 Suppl 16):67–79.

15

Preoperative assessment of ovarian tumors using a modified multivariate index assay

Hero A. Abdurrahman[1], Ariana Kh. Jawad[2*] ⓘ and Shahla K. Alalaf[3]

Abstract

Background: Preoperative differentiation between benign and malignant masses can be challenging. The aim of this research was to evaluate the performance of a modified multivariate index assay (MIA) in detecting ovarian cancer and to compare the effectiveness of gynecologist assessment, cancer antigen (CA) 125, and MIA for identifying ovarian masses with high suspicion of malignancy.

Results: This prospective observational study included 150 women with ovarian masses who underwent surgery in the Maternity Teaching Hospital from December 2014 to May 2016. Preoperative estimation of modified MIA, assessment by a gynecologist, and CA 125 level correlated with the surgical histopathology. A modified MIA was implemented because of lack of access to the software typically used. Among 150 enrolled women there were 30 cases of malignancy, including 8 cases (26%) of early-stage ovarian cancer and 22 cases (74%) of late-stage cancer. MIA showed high specificity (96.7%) in detecting cancer and a sensitivity of 70%, with a positive predictive value of 84% and a negative predictive value of 92.8%. No significant differences were detected between the MIA results and the histopathology results ($P = 0.267$). For early-stage ovarian cancer, the sensitivity of MIA was 100% compared with 75% for CA 125 alone.

Conclusion: MIA seems to be effective for evaluation of ovarian tumors with higher specificity and positive predictive value than CA 125 while maintaining high negative predictive value and with only a slightly lower overall sensitivity. For evaluation of early-stage ovarian cancer, MIA showed a much higher sensitivity that markedly outperformed CA 125 alone. This modified MIA strategy may be particularly useful in low resource setting.

Keywords: Multivariate index assay, CA 125, Ovarian, Tumor, Physician's assessment

Background

Ovarian cancer is the leading cause of mortality among all gynecologic cancers and the seventh most common cancer in females worldwide [1]. Approximately 10% of women will have some form of surgery for an ovarian mass during their lifetime, and although 20% of borderline ovarian tumors appear as simple cysts on ultrasound many of these tumors may proceed to malignancy later on [2]. Women with ovarian malignancies that are managed by specialized care provided by a gynecologic oncologist or in a specialized hospital have an improved mean survival time, making early diagnosis and rapid management of ovarian malignancy of paramount importance [3]. Radiologic and serum markers are relatively insensitive and as a result preoperative differentiation

between benign and malignant ovarian masses is problematic, especially in the differentiation of stage I epithelial ovarian cancer. No single ultrasound finding can differentiate between benign and malignant ovarian masses [2, 4].

Estimation of the risk of malignancy is essential when assessing ovarian masses, and the risk for malignancy has been assessed using 80 different models, including the Royal College of Obstetrician and Gynecologists guidelines. Simple models use discrete cutoff values, such as cancer antigen (CA) 125, pulsatility index, and resistive index [2, 5]. The American College of Obstetricians and Gynecologists and the Society of Obstetricians and Gynecologists of Canada have defined guidelines for the management of premenopausal women with a pelvic mass. These guidelines consider the following features suspicious for ovarian malignancy and warranting referral to a gynecological oncologist: serum CA 125 > 200 units/ml, ascites, evidence of abdominal

* Correspondence: aryianadr@yahoo.com
[2]Kurdistan Board for Medical Specialists, Kurdistan, Erbil, Iraq
Full list of author information is available at the end of the article

or distant metastasis, or a first-degree relative with ovarian or breast cancer [5, 6]. However, even in the presence of an ultrasonographically defined mass, serum CA 125 cannot reliably distinguish between a malignant or benign mass [7]. Furthermore, despite efforts to define factors that identify risk of malignancy a previous report showed that 30% of premenopausal women with ovarian cancer would not have been regarded as high risk using these guidelines [6].

As early-stage ovarian cancer carries a much more favorable prognosis than late-stage ovarian cancer there is an urgent need to identify subclinical disease. Serological markers are theoretically an ideal approach, but none of the available markers have 100% specificity and sensitivity [6]. The multivariate index assay (MIA) for ovarian cancer is composed of CA 125, beta 2-microglobulin, apolipoprotein A1 (ApoA1), transferrin, and prealbumin. These biomarkers are not used for screening but for evaluating women with a pelvic mass and can significantly improve the predictability of ovarian cancer so that patients can be referred to a subspecialist with expertise in managing ovarian cancer, thus improving clinical outcome [7]. A previous study showed that the MIA demonstrated higher sensitivity and lower specificity in detecting ovarian malignancies compared with physician assessment and CA 125 [8]. Another report showed that MIA demonstrated higher sensitivity and negative predictive value for ovarian malignancy compared with clinical impression and CA 125 in women with ovarian masses [7]. In our locality, gynecologists and general oncologists (there are no gynecologic oncologists in our locality) depend on clinical assessment, ultrasound, magnetic resonance imaging, and CA 125 level for evaluation of ovarian masses.

We aimed to introduce these biomarkers in our hospital but were unable to access the software needed for the MIA assay. Therefore, we conducted this study to evaluate the use of a modified MIA; specifically, we examined the application of a software-independent method using cut-off dependent risk classification to differentiate malignant from benign ovarian tumors and compared the effectiveness of this novel strategy with physician assessment and CA 125 for identification of ovarian masses with high suspicion of malignancy.

Methods

A prospective observational study was conducted on 150 women who were admitted for surgical management of ovarian masses in the Maternity Teaching Hospital, Erbil, Kurdistan, Iraq, from December 1 2014 to May 1 2016. The Maternity Teaching hospital is a tertiary referral hospital with 313 beds and the only public tertiary care hospital in Erbil Governorate (population of approximately 1,612,692). The hospital serves as a major

referral center for other public and private hospitals within Erbil Governorate and provides emergency obstetrics and gynecology service 24 h a day.

The criteria for inclusion in the study were as follows: female aged 18 years or older, a documented ovarian mass with planned surgical intervention within 3 months of imaging, not referred to an oncologist, and consent to undergo phlebotomy. The exclusion criteria were as follows: age less than 18 years, pregnancy, no planned surgical intervention, declined phlebotomy, or had a malignancy diagnosed in the previous 5 years. Menopause was defined as absence of menses for at least 12 months or age ≥ 50 years when the woman was unsure of her menses. All patients provided written informed consent. All patients were interviewed before the surgical intervention.

Preoperative venous blood (5–7 ml) was collected from each patient and placed in BD plastic vacutainer tubes with clot activators. Samples were transferred to the laboratory and centrifuged, and serum was separated as soon as possible to prevent hemolysis. Serum samples were stored at 2–8 °C for up to 2 days or frozen at –20 °C.

The MVI assay incorporates CA 125, beta 2 microglobulin, transferrin, transthyretin (prealbumin), and apolipoprotein A1. CA 125 was measured using the Elecsys CA 125 II tumor marker system (Fujirebio Diagnostics, Tokyo, Japan). The other four markers were measured on the Minineph system using Minineph kits (Binding Site Group, Birmingham, UK).

The OvaCalc software combines the value of each assay and uses the MVI assay algorithm to generate an ovarian risk malignancy index score that ranges from 0 to 10. A score of ≥5 in premenopausal women or a score of ≥4.4 in postmenopausal women indicates a high probability of malignancy. This software was not available to us due to policy decisions of the manufacturing company. The unavailability of the OvaCalc software forced us to use a modified MIA to assess the validity of these biomarkers in combination for screening ovarian tumors for malignancy. We decided to score the results of the assay as follows: positive cases (indicating a high risk of malignancy) were defined when three out of the five markers were positive, and negative cases (low risk of malignancy) were indicated when ≤2 markers were positive. In the individual assays, positive results were defined as CA 125 and beta 2 microglobulin values higher than normal ranges and apolipoprotein A1, transferrin, and prealbumin values lower than the normal ranges (Table 1).

For each patient, CA 125 was measured and analyzed as part of the MIA and alone. The CA 125 cutoff values were > 200 U/ml for premenopausal women and > 35 U/ml for postmenopausal women according to the published American College of Obstetrician and Gynecologists referral criteria [9].

Table 1 Laboratory ranges used for the multivariate index assay

Biomarkers	Ranges	Classifications
CA 125	Premenopausal, 200 IU/L Postmenopausal, 35 IU/L	Ranges above the upper limit regarded positive [11]
[a]β-2 microglobulin	1.22–2.46 g/L	Ranges above the upper limit regarded positive
[a]Transferrin	2.24–4.06 g/L	Level below the lower limit is regarded positive
[a]Apolipoprotein A1	1.24–2.02 g/L	Level below the lower limit is regarded positive
[a]Prealbumin	0.216–0.328 g/L	Level below the lower l imit is regarded positive

[a]Ranges obtained from The Binding Site Group kits

Normal ranges for the other four biomarkers were obtained from the leaflet provided with the kits (The Binding Site Group, Birmingham, UK) (Table 1).

This modified MVI assay could be used to screen for malignancy before the operation in our low resource setting.

Before surgery, the enrolling gynecologic surgeon performed preoperative assessment by asking the gynecologists whether they considered the ovarian tumor to be malignant based on available clinical information such as physical examination of the patient, family history of malignancy, results of imaging such as ultrasound, and laboratory tests including CA 125, but not the multivariate index assay. The answers were recorded as yes or no. Gynecologists were allowed to use any algorithm to determine their answer, but were not expected to explain how they reached their prediction. The gynecologists' opinions were recorded before surgery for all patients. During surgery, FIGO staging was used to surgically stage cases suspicious for cancer and the stage was recorded [10]. After surgery, results of histopathological examination were obtained for each patient from the histopathology department in the hospital laboratory.

Statistical analysis

Data were analyzed using the Statistical Package for Social Sciences (SPSS, version 22). Chi square test of association was used to compare between proportions. When the expected count of more than 20% of the cells in the table was less than 5 (which was attributed to small sample size in the cells of the table), Fisher's exact test was used [11]. The expected count of each cell of the table was calculated by multiplying the marginal totals and dividing this value by the grand total. McNemar test (2 × 2) was used when the results of the screening tests such as MIA or CA 125 were compared with a gold standard (the confirmatory test was the histopathological findings) of the same patient, as in Table 2.

Table 2 Assessing the accuracy of screening tests

		Histopathology results (gold standard)		P
		Positive	Negative	
Screening tests like MIA	Positive	TP	FP	TP + FP
	Negative	FN	TN	FN + TN
Total		TP + FN	FP + TN	Grand total

P value, determined by McNemar

TP true positive, TN true negative, FP false positive, FN false negative

$$\text{Sensitivity} = \text{TP}/(\text{TP} + \text{FN}) \times 100; \textbf{Specificity}$$
$$= \text{TN}/(\text{FP} + \text{TN}) \times 100; \textbf{Predictive value positive}$$
$$= (\text{PV}^+) : \text{TP}/(\text{TP} + \text{FP})$$
$$\times 100; \textbf{Predictive value negative } (\text{PV}^-)$$
$$: \text{TN}/(\text{FN} + \text{TN}) \times 100; \textbf{Total agreement}$$
$$= (\text{TP} + \text{TN})/\text{Grand total}$$

Microsoft Excel 2007 was used to plot the pie charts. A p value ≤0.05 was considered statistically significant.

Results

A total of 150 women with an ovarian mass were included in the study. The rate of malignancy was significantly higher among menopausal, grand multiparous, overweight, and obese women ($p < 0.001$) (Table 3).

Nearly one-third (30%) of the patients had serous cystadenoma, 18.7% had dermoid, and 12% had endometrioma (Table 4).

Approximately one-fourth of the cases (25.3%) were suspected to be malignant according to the opinion of the senior gynecologists prior to the operation, whereas 20% were proven to be malignant by histopathological examination (Table 5). Based on tumor markers, 30 and 16.7% of the masses were suspected to be malignant according to CA 125 and MIA test results, respectively.

The sensitivities of CA 125, MIA, and clinical assessment were 83.3, 70, and 70%, respectively (Table 6). When MIA and gynecologist assessment results were combined in parallel (if either or both of these tests was positive, the result of the test was considered positive), the sensitivity increased to 93.3% at the expense of specificity, which decreased to 82.5%. In general, MIA gave relatively high sensitivity (70%), specificity (96.7%), positive predictive value (84%), negative predictive value (92.8%), and total agreement (91.3%) compared with the other tests. There was no significant difference between MIA results and histopathology results ($p = 0.267$).

Out of the 150 cases sampled, 30 (19.9%) were malignant ovarian masses. Surgical staging of the 30 malignant ovarian masses determined that 13% were stage I, 13% were stage II, 37% were stage III, and 37% were stage IV

Table 3 Association of histopathological results with variables

Variables	Categories	Histopathological results						
		Malignant		Benign		Total		
		n	%	n	%	n	%	p
Menopausal status	Premenopausal	6	5.4	106	94.6	112	100.0	< 0.001
	Postmenopausal	24	63.2	14	36.8	38	100.0	
Parity	Nuliparous	8	16.7	40	83.3	48	100.0	0.001
	Multiparous [1–4]	4	7.4	50	92.6	54	100.0	
	Grandmultiparous (parity ≥5)	18	37.5	30	62.5	48	100.0	
Family history of CA (breast, ovary, colon)	Negative	29	20.4	113	79.6	142	100.0	1*
	Positive	1	12.5	7	87.5	8	100.0	
Combined OCP	Negative	27	19.1	114	80.9	141	100.0	0.384*
	Positive	3	33.3	6	66.7	9	100.0	
Fertility drugs	Negative	28	20.0	112	80.0	140	100.0	1*
	Positive	2	20.0	8	80.0	10	100.0	
Smoking	Negative	29	20.0	116	80.0	145	100.0	1*
	Positive	1	20.0	4	80.0	5	100.0	
Breast feeding	< 6 months	8	16.0	42	84.0	50	100.0	0.386
	≥ 6 months	22	22.0	78	78.0	100	100.0	
BMI (Kg/m²)	< 25	0	0.0	18	100.0	18	100.0	0.048
	25–29	14	26.9	38	73.1	52	100.0	
	≥ 30	16	20.0	64	80.0	80	100.0	

*By Fisher's exact test
OCP oral contraceptive pill, BMI body mass index, CA carcinoma

(Fig. 1). The sensitivities of CA 125 and MIA in detecting stage I and stage II cancers were 75 and 100%, respectively (Table 7). The specificities were 83.3 and 96.7%, respectively. No significant difference was detected between MIA and histopathology results (p = 0.0125).

The sensitivities of CA 125 and MIA in detecting stage III and stage IV tumors were 86.4 and 59.1%, respectively (Table 8). The specificities were 83.3 and 96.7%,

respectively. No significant difference was detected between MIA and histopathology results (p = 0.267).

Discussion

Early detection of ovarian cancer is very important to improve patient survival. The major challenge is how to identify masses with risk of malignancy, particularly in premenopausal women [2].

In the current study, the rate of ovarian malignancy was significantly higher among postmenopausal than premenopausal women, which is consistent with a previous report [12]. Although our study showed that the rate of ovarian cancer was higher among grand multiparous women (37.5%) than nulliparous women (16.7%), parity

Table 4 Distribution of patients by histopathological diagnosis

Histopathological diagnosis	Number	Percent
Serous cystadenoma	45	30.0
Dermoid	28	18.7
Endometrioma	18	12.0
Mucinous cystadenoma	16	10.7
Serous cystadenocarcinoma	14	9.3
Endometrioid adenocarcinoma	8	5.3
Hemorrhagic luteal cyst	7	4.7
Follicular cyst	6	4.0
Mucinous cystadenocarcinoma	3	2.0
Krukenberg's tumor	3	2.0
Granulosa cell cancer	2	1.3
Total	150	100.0

Table 5 Results of gynecologist assessment, CA 125, multivariate index assay, and histopathological findings in the cases (n = 150)

	Malignant		Benign	
	n	%	n	%
Gynecologist's assessment	38	25.3	112	74.7
CA 125	45	30.0	105	70.0
MIA	25	16.7	125	83.3
Histopathology results	30	20.0	120	80.0

CA cancer antigen, MIA multivariate index assay

Table 6 Validity of the tests and clinical assessment compared with histopathological results

	Sensitivity %	Specificity %	PPV %	NPV %	Agreement %	P*
CA 125	83.3	83.3	55.6	95.2	83.3	0.004
MIA	70	96.7	84	92.8	91.3	0.267
Gynecologist's assessment	70	85.8	55.3	92	82.7	0.169
MIA and/or Clinical	93.3	82.5	57.1	98	84.7	< 0.001

*By McNemar test
CA cancer antigen, MIA multivariate index assay

is generally considered a well-established protective factor for ovarian cancer [13]. Bodelon et al. found that among 623 women diagnosed with invasive epithelial ovarian cancer, 102 (16%) were nulliparous and 521 (84%) were parous [14]. Tsilidis et al. found that compared with nulliparous women; parous women had a 29% lower risk of ovarian cancer with an 8% reduction in risk for each additional pregnancy [15].

The rate of malignancy was significantly higher among overweight women (BMI 25–30; 26.9%) and obese women (BMI > 30; 20%) than among women with normal BMI (0%). Beehler et al. found that compared with underweight or normal (BMI ≤ 24.9) premenopausal women, obese (BMI > 30.0) premenopausal women had an approximately 2-fold increase in the risk for malignancy. Postmenopausal women, however, did not show the same tendency, with only a small, non-significant decrease in risk among the heaviest women [16].

Our research showed no significant association between the rate of malignancy and family history of cancer ($p = 1$), oral contraceptive pill (OCP) use for more than 1 year ($p = 0.384$), fertility drugs (ovulation induction > 12 cycles) ($p = 1$), smoking ($p = 1$), and breast feeding for more than 6 months ($p = 0.386$).

A meta-analysis by Havrilesky et al. showed an inverse association between OCP use and ovarian cancer [17]. Ovarian cancer risk was 25–28% lower in women with a

history of OCP use compared with never-users [18]. Risk was further reduced with longer duration of OCP use, and was decreased by more than 50% in women with more than 10 years of use [19, 20]. Ovarian cancer risk in OCP ever-users remained reduced for at least 30 years after the last use of OCPs, although the protection may diminish over time [21]. The insignificant result in our study may be related to the small number of women taking OCP.

Other studies revealed marked differences in the risk profiles of various histological types of ovarian cancer with regard to cigarette smoking [21, 22]. Current cigarette smoking increased the risk of invasive mucinous and borderline mucinous ovarian tumors, whereas former smoking increased the risk of borderline serous ovarian tumors [23]. No associations between smoking and risk of invasive serous and endometrioid ovarian cancer were observed [23].

Another study reported that breastfeeding was inversely associated with the risk of ovarian cancer; in particular, long-term breastfeeding (> 12 months) demonstrated a stronger protective effect [24].

Epithelial ovarian cancer has been described as a "silent killer", because advanced disease is found at initial diagnosis in more than 60% of cases. In Denmark, 74% of patients were diagnosed with FIGO stage III–IV disease, compared with 60–70% in Australia, Canada, Norway, and the UK [25]. Surgical staging of ovarian tumors operated on in a tertiary care hospital revealed that more than half (56%) of the patients had stage III–IV disease. On histology, papillary serous cystic adenocarcinoma was found to be the most common type (54%),

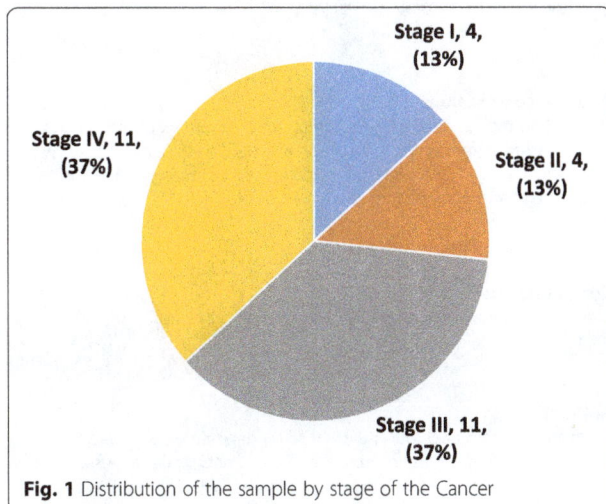

Fig. 1 Distribution of the sample by stage of the Cancer

Table 7 Sensitivity of CA 125 and MIA tests in detecting stage 1 and stage 2 ovarian cancers

		Stage I & II		Benign		Total		
		n	%	n	%	n	%	p
CA 125	Positive	6	75.0	20	16.7	26	20.3	< 0.001
	Negative	2	25.0	100	83.3	102	79.7	
MIA	Positive	8	100.0	4	3.3	12	9.4	0.0125
	Negative	0	0.0	116	96.7	116	90.6	
	Total	8	100.0	120	100.0	128	100.0	

CA 125 cancer antigen 125, MIA multivariate index assay

Table 8 Sensitivity of CA 125 and MIA tests in detecting stage 3 and stage 4 ovarian cancers

		Stage III & IV		Benign		Total		
		n	%	n	%	n	%	
CA 125	Positive	19	86.4	20	16.7	39	27.5	< 0.001
	Negative	3	13.6	100	83.3	103	72.5	
MIA	Positive	13	59.1	4	3.3	17	12.0	0.267
	Negative	9	40.9	116	96.7	125	88.0	
	Total	22	100.0	120	100.0	142	100.0	

CA 1

followed by mucinous 22%, endometrioid (10.6%), yolk sac (2.6%), dysgerminoma (4%), and adult granulosa cell tumor (5.3%) [26].

In one study, the individual accuracies of pelvic examination and serum CA 125 in discriminating between benign and malignant pelvic masses were approximately the same (76 and 77%, respectively) [27]. A systemic review by Kristen Pepin showed that the sensitivity of CA 125 in distinguishing between benign and malignant masses ranged from 61 to 90%, while the specificity ranged from 35 to 91%. The positive predictive value of CA 125 in women with an adnexal mass was 35 to 91%, and the negative predictive value was between 67 and 90% [28]. Miller et al. showed that replacing CA 125 with the MIA increased the sensitivity (77–94%) and negative predictive value (87–93%), while decreasing specificity (35–68%) and positive predictive value (40–52%) [29]. Similar trends were noted for premenopausal women and those with early-stage disease.

Our modified MIA demonstrated higher sensitivity and lower specificity compared with physician assessment and CA 125 in detecting ovarian malignancies. Such a noticeable improvement in sensitivity translates into a high negative predictive value, which is a clinically important measure to assure physicians and patients that the risk of malignancy will be low for patients who have a negative result by MIA. In fact, the 92.5% (149/161) sensitivity of MIA itself will produce a negative predictive value of 92.9% (156/168). The addition of MIA to clinical assessment brings significant improvement in sensitivity. This is, however, at the cost of reduced specificity [7]. Longoria et al. concluded that MIA combined with clinical assessment had significantly higher sensitivity (95.3%) compared with clinical assessment alone (68.6%) or CA 125-II (62.8%) [30]. In our research, MIA gave a higher specificity and negative predictive value compared with a study conducted by Bristoe et al., in which MIA demonstrated higher sensitivity and negative predictive value for ovarian malignancy compared with clinical impression and CA125-II [31].

MIA had a higher sensitivity than CA 125 in the detection of early-stage ovarian cancer (FIGO I & II),

which was consistent with the study by Ueland et al. [7]; however, this was not the case in the detection of late-stage ovarian cancers (FIGO III & IV), for which the specificity of MIA was higher than that of CA 125 [30].

This study had several limitations. One limitation was the lack of the OvaCalc software to calculate scores; however, this is counterbalanced by the major benefit that our modified method can be used in the absence of access to software, which is the case in certain clinical settings. Another limitation is the lack of gynecologic oncology specialists in our locality.

The main strength of our study is the adaptation of available resources for discriminating ovarian tumors in a clinical setting with limited resources. Another strength of the current study lies in the inclusion of all types of ovarian malignancies that are seen in general gynecology practice. Although MIA is not intended for screening or follow-up of cases of ovarian cancer, its efficacy was proven in detecting ovarian malignancy, especially in early stages, which may significantly improve early case referral to oncology surgeons and yield a better patient survival.

Conclusions

The modified MIA applied in this study resulted in sufficient diagnostic accuracy and appears to be highly effective for the detection of ovarian malignancy. This modified MIA strategy may be a useful method for application in developing countries.

Acknowledgements
We thank the Edanz Group (http://www.edanzediting.com/ac) for editing a draft of this manuscript.

Funding
This work was supported by the Kurdistan Board for Medical Specializations. Financial support was for academic purposes only.

Authors' contributions
AKJ advised project direction and participated in manuscript writing and revision. HAA performed data collection and data analysis, and helped with manuscript revision. SKA participated in manuscript writing and revision. All authors read and approved the final manuscript.

Competing interests
The authors declare that they have no competing interests.

Author details
[1]Maternity Teaching Hospital, Kurdistan, Erbil, Iraq. [2]Kurdistan Board for Medical Specialists, Kurdistan, Erbil, Iraq. [3]Department of Obstetrics and Gynecology, Hawler Medical University, College of Medicine, Kurdistan region, Erbil, Iraq.

References

1. Ferlay J, Soerjomataram I, Ervik M, Dikshit R, Eser S, Mathers C, et al. GLOBOCAN 2012 v1.1, Cancer Incidence and Mortality Worldwide: IARC Cancer Base No. 11. Lyon, France. 2014. http://globcan.iarc.fr. Accessed 16 Jan 2015.

2. Management of suspected ovarian masses in premenopausal women (green-top guideline No. 62). Royal College of Obstetrician and Gynecologists. 2011. http://www.rcog.org.uk/globlassets/guidelineslgtg_62-pdf. Accessed 24 Feb 2018.

3. Vernooij F, Heintz P, Witteveen E, van der Graaf Y. The outcomes of ovarian cancer treatment are better when provided by gynecologic oncologists and in specialized hospitals: a systematic review. Gynecol Oncol. 2007;105:801–12.

4. Sundar S, Reynolds K. Benign and malignant ovarian masses. In: Luesley DM, Baker PN, editors. Obstetrics and gynaecology: an evidence based text for MRCOG. 2nd ed. London: Hodder Arnold; 2010. p. 814–27.

5. Le T, Giede C, Salem S, Lefebvre G, Rosen B, Bentley J, et al. Initial evaluation and referral guidelines for management of pelvic/ovarian masses. J Obstet Gynaecol Can. 2009;31(7):668–80.

6. American College of Obstetricians and Gynecologists' Committee on Practice Bulletins. Practice bulletin No. 174: evaluation and Management of Adnexal Masses. Obstet Gynecol. 2016;128(5):e210–26.

7. Ueland F, DeSimone C, Seamon L, Miller R, Goodrich S, Podzielinski I, et al. Effectiveness of a multivariate index assay in the preoperative assessment of ovarian tumors. Obstet Gynecol. 2011;117:1289–97.

8. Kozak KR, Su F, Whitelegee JP, Faull K, Reddy S, Farias-Eisner R. Characterization of serum biomarkers for detection of early stage ovarian cancer. Proteomics. 2005;5:4589–96.

9. Graham L. ACOG releases guidelines on management of adnexal masses. Am Fam Physician. 2008;77:1320–3.

10. Mutch DG, Prat J. 2014 FIGO staging for ovarian, fallopian tube and peritoneal cancer. Gynecol Oncol. 2014;133(3):401–4.

11. Moorman PG, Calingaert B, Palmieri RT, Iversen ES, Bentley RC, Halabi S, et al. Hormonal risk factors for ovarian cancer in premenopausal and postmenopausal women. Am J Epidemiol. 2008;167:1059–69.

12. Adami HO, Lambe M, Persson I, Ekbom A, Adami HO, Hsieh CC, et al. Parity, age at first childbirth, and risk of ovarian cancer. Lancet. 1994;344:1250–4.

13. Bodelon C, Wentzensen N, Schonfeld SJ, Visvanathan K, Hartge P, Park Y, et al. Hormonal risk factors and invasive epithelial ovarian cancer risk by parity. Br J Cancer. 2013;109:769–76.

14. Tsilidis KK, Allen NE, Key TJ, Dossus L, Lukanova A, Bakken K, et al. Oral contraceptive use and reproductive factors and risk of ovarian cancer in the European prospective investigation into cancer and nutrition. Br J Cancer. 2011;105:1436–42.

15. Beehler GP, Sekhon M, Baker JA, Teter BE, McCann SE, Rodabaugh KJ, et al. Risk of ovarian cancer associated with BMI varies by menopausal status. J Nutr. 2006;136:2881–6.

16. Collaborative Group on Epidemiological Studies of Ovarian Cancer. Ovarian cancer and body size: individual participant meta-analysis including 25,157 women with ovarian cancer from 47 epidemiological studies. PLoS Med. 2012;9:e1001200.

17. Havrilesky LJ, Gierisch JM, Moorman PG, Coeytaux RR, Urrutia RP, Lowery WJ, et al. Oral contraceptive use for the primary prevention of ovarian cancer. Evid Rep Technol Assess. 2013;212:1–514.

18. Moorman PG, Havrilesky LJ, Gierisch JM, Coeytaux RR, Lowery WJ, Urrutia RP, et al. Oral contraceptives and risk of ovarian cancer and breast cancer among high-risk women: a systematic review and meta-analysis. J Clin Oncol. 2013;31:4188–98.

19. Parkin DM. Cancers attributable to exposure to hormones in the UK in 2010. Br J Cancer. 2011;105:S42–8.

20. Collaborative Group on Epidemiological Studies of Ovarian Cancer. Ovarian cancer and oral contraceptives: collaborative reanalysis of data from 45 epidemiological studies including 23,257 women with ovarian cancer and 87,303 controls. Lancet. 2008;371:303–14.

21. Collaborative Group on Epidemiological Studies of Ovarian Cancer. Ovarian cancer and smoking: individual participant meta-analysis including 28,114 women with ovarian cancer from 51 epidemiological studies. Lancet Oncol. 2012;13:936–45.

22. International Agency for Research on Cancer. 2017. List of classifications by cancer sites with sufficient or limited evidence in humans, volumes 1 to 120a. Available from http://monographs.iarc.fr/ENG/classification/Table4.pdf. Accessed 27 Feb 2018.

23. Faber MT, Kjaer SK, Dehlendorff C, Chang-Claude J, Andersen KK, Hogdall E, et al. Cigarette smoking and risk of ovarian cancer: a pooled analysis of 21 case-control studies. Cancer Causes Control. 2013;24:989–1004.

24. Li D, Du C, Zhang Z, Li G, Yu Z, Wang X, et al. Breastfeeding and ovarian cancer risk: a systematic review and meta-analysis of 40 epidemiological studies. Asian Pac J Cancer Prev. 2014;15:4829–37.

25. Maringe C, Walters S, Butler J, Coleman MP, Hacker N, Hanna L, et al. Stage at diagnosis and ovarian cancer survival: evidence from the international cancer benchmarking partnership. Gynecol Oncol. 2012;127:75–82.

26. Khan A, Sultana K. Presenting signs and symptoms of ovarian cancer at a tertiary care hospital. J Pak Med Assoc. 2010;60:260–2.

27. Schutter EM, Keneman P, Sohn C, Kristen P, Crombach G, Westermann R, et al. Diagnostic value of pelvic examination, ultrasound, and serum CA 125 in postmenopausal women with a pelvic mass. An international multicenter study. Cancer. 1994;74:1398–406.

28. Pepin K, Carmen M, Brown A, Dizon DS. CA 125 and epithelial ovarian cancer: role in screening, diagnosis, and surveillance. Am J Hematol Oncol. 2014;10:22–8.

29. Ware Miller R, Smith A, DeSimone CP, Seamon L, Goodrich S, Podzielinski I, et al. Performance of the American College of Obstetricians and Gynecologists' ovarian tumor referral guidelines with a multivariate index assay. Obstet Gynecol. 2011;117:1298–306.

30. Longoria TC, Ueland FR, Zhang Z, Chan DW, Smith A, Fung ET, et al. Clinical performance of a multivariate index assay for detecting early-stage ovarian cancer. Am J Obstet Gynecol. 2014;210:78.e1–9.

31. Bristow RE, Smith A, Zhang Z, Chan DW, Crutcher G, Fung ET, et al. Ovarian malignancy risk stratification of the adnexal mass using a multivariate index assay. Gynecol Oncol. 2013;128:252–9.

16

FOLR1 increases sensitivity to cisplatin treatment in ovarian cancer cells

Ming-ju Huang[1,2†], Wei Zhang[1†], Qi Wang[1], Zhi-jun Yang[1], Sheng-bin Liao[1] and Li Li[1*]

Abstract

Background: Whether there is a mechanistic link between FOLR1 and response to cisplatin has not been extensively examined. In this study, we determine the expression of FOLR1 in ovarian cancer and examine if FOLR1 levels influence response to cisplatin.

Results: (1) FOLR1 protein expression was lowest in normal ovarian tissue, higher in benign ovarian tumors, and highest in malignant tumors ($P < 0.01$). (2) FOLR1 expression was decreased in platinum drug-resistant ovarian tumors compared to sensitive tumors ($P < 0.01$). Consistent with this, FOLR1 expression in tumors progressing following cisplatin treatment was lower than levels in tumors in remission ($P < 0.01$). (3) FOLR1 was successfully overexpressed at both the mRNA and protein levels following transfection in SKOV3 cells. (4) SKOV3 cells with FOLR1 overexpression were the most sensitive to cisplatin treatment (IC50 = 3.60 μg/ml) and exhibited the highest inhibition rates in the presence of the drug ($P < 0.05$). (5) The rate of apoptosis of SKOV3 cells increased with cisplatin treatment in a dose- and time-dependent manner ($P < 0.05$). Cisplatin also induced S phase arrest in a concentration-dependent manner ($P < 0.05$). Apoptosis and S phase proportion were significantly altered by FOLR1 overexpression ($P < 0.05$).

Conclusion: FOLR1 may be a useful biomarker for ovarian cancer, and it may be useful as a therapeutic application to improve sensitivity to cisplatin treatment.

Keywords: Folate binding protein, Ovarian cancer, SKOV3 cells, Cisplatin, Apoptosis, Cell cycle, Multidrug resistance

Background

Ovarian cancer is a serious malignancy, with high mortality and a five-year survival rate of approximately 20% - 30% for the prevailing advanced presentations [1]. Survival in patients with ovarian cancer can be improved with early detection, thorough surgery, and improved sensitivity to cisplatin-based chemotherapy. Folate binding protein (FOLR1) is a member of the human folate binding protein family. The gene is located on chromosome 11q13.3-14.1. FOLR1 is a glycosyl phosphatidylinositol connected membrane glycoprotein, consisting of 257 amino acids. The protein is completely exposed to extracellular molecules and anchored at the cell membrane by GPI [2]. FOLR1 is involved in DNA replication and damage repair. Its expression levels are closely related with tumor progression and cell proliferation [3, 4]. FOLR1, also known as folate

receptor proteins, mediates cellular responses to folate, including cell division, proliferation, and tissue growth [5]. Few publications have reported on FOLR1 expression in ovarian tissue. Shen et al. found that FOLR1 expression was decreased in cisplatin-resistant tumors [6],but whether there is a mechanistic link between FOLR1 and response to cisplatin has not been extensively examined. In this study, we determine the expression of FOLR1 in ovarian cancer and examine if FOLR1 levels influence response to cisplatin. The data we provide here suggest that FOLR1 may be a useful predictive biomarker for cisplatin sensitivity in ovarian cancer.

Results

Expression of FOLR1 in normal ovary, benign ovarian tumors, and ovarian cancer

Expression of FOLR1 in normal, benign, and cancerous ovarian tissues was determined by Western blot. GAPDH was used as a loading control. Expression of FOLR1 was lowest in normal ovarian tissue. FOLR1 was

* Correspondence: LiLi@gxmu.edu.cn
†Equal contributors
[1]Department of Gynecology Oncology, Tumor Hospital of Guangxi Medical University, Nanning 530021, China
Full list of author information is available at the end of the article

more highly expressed in benign tumors and even higher in malignant disease ($P < 0.01$)(Fig. 1).

Expression of FOLR1 in cancerous ovarian tissue is correlated with clinicopathologic factors

FIOG (International Federation of Gynaecology and Obstetrics) system 2000 is used to determine the stages of malignant ovarian patients. The expression of FOLR1 in stage I-II is lower than that in stage III-IV and also lower in the well-differentiated than that in the low-differentiated ($P<0.05$). While there is no difference for expression of FOLR1 in the four different pathologic tissue, the significant difference does exist between the mucinous and the serous ($P<0.05$). The specific results are shown in Fig. 2.

Correlation of expression of FOLR1 with tumor metastasis and ascites

Expression of FOLR1 in cancerous ovarian tissue with metastasizing to distant lymph node and/or organ is higher than that without metastasis ($P<0.05$).However,there's no significance about correlation of expression of FORL1 with whether metastasizing to the greater omentum or having asites ($P > 0.05$). The specific results are shown in Fig. 3.

FOLR1 expression in ovarian cancer tissue is correlated with patient treatment efficacy and drug resistance

FOLR1 protein expression was highest in patients with complete remission (complete response, CR). FOLR1 expression decreased with decreased drug sensitivity (partial response, PR > stable disease, SD > progressive disease, PD). The difference in expression in CR, PR, and SD patients compared to PD patients was statistically significant ($P < 0.01$). The difference in expression in CR and PR patients compared to PD and SD patients was also significant ($P < 0.05$). However, there was no statistically

significant difference in expression in CR and PR patients compared to SD patients ($P > 0.05$). Expression of FOLR1 in platinum drug-resistant ovarian cancer was lower than in platinum drug-sensitive tumors ($P < 0.01$),and after further chemotherapy expression of FOLR1 in PD was still lower than that in remission ($p < 0.01$) (Fig. 4).

Correlation of expression of FOLR1 in ovarian cancer tissue with prognosis of patients

ROC curve that determines the relationship of FOLR-1 expression and nature of ovarian cancer demonstrates that maximum Youden index is 3.115. The specific result is shown in Fig. 5a.

Univariate analysis of Kaplan-Meier survival curve demonstrates that median overall survival time is 29.4 months for the positive group and 32.3 months for the negative group respectively, and the difference is not statistically significant ($P > 0.05$)(Fig. 5b).

COX multivariate analysis denies expression of FOLR-1 as an independent prognostic factor.

FOLR1 expression in transfected SKOV3 cells

RT-PCR and Western blot were performed to confirm overexpression of FOLR1 at both the mRNA and protein levels in SKOV3 cells following transfection. Neither FOLR1 mRNA nor protein was detected in the empty vector transfected group (pWPI-SKOV3) or in control cells (SKOV3) (Fig. 6).

Growth inhibition and apoptosis of SKOV3 cells treated with cisplatin

MTT assays were performed and IC_{50} values of each group were determined in the presence of cisplatin. The IC_{50} values of SKOV3, pWPI-SKOV3, pWPI-FOLR1-SKOV3 cells were 5.01, 4.96, and 3.60 µg/ml, respectively. The IC_{50} to cisplatin of the pWPI-FOLR1-SKOV3 group was significantly lower than the two control

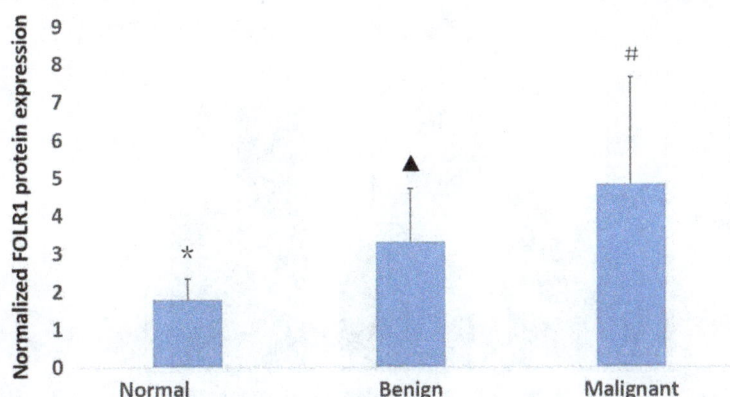

Fig. 1 Ovarian tissues expression of FOLR1 protein detected by western blot.*,$P = 0.000$,compared with benign;▲,$P = 0.002$,compared with malignant;#,$P = 0.000$,compared with normal

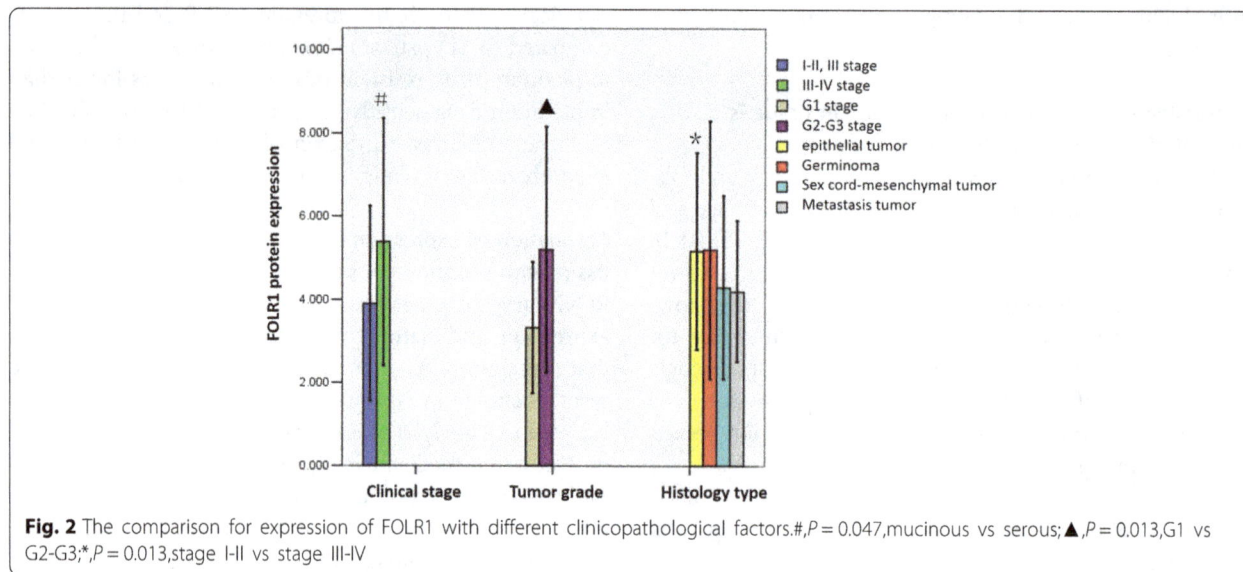

Fig. 2 The comparison for expression of FOLR1 with different clinicopathological factors.#,$P = 0.047$,mucinous vs serous;▲,$P = 0.013$,G1 vs G2-G3;*,$P = 0.013$,stage I-II vs stage III-IV

groups ($P < 0.05$). There was no significant difference in IC$_{50}$ between the two control groups ($P > 0.05$). For all groups, the growth inhibition rate in the presence of cisplatin increased in both a time- and dose-dependent manner. Apoptosis of cells in the three groups increased with cisplatin treatment in a similar manner. Under the same conditions, pWPI-FOLR1-SKOV3 cells displayed the highest growth inhibition rate compared to the other two groups ($P < 0.05$). Apoptosis also increased in each of the three groups in a dose- and time-dependent manner. Under the same conditions, pWPI-FOLR1-SKOV3 cells displayed the highest rates of apoptosis compared to the other groups ($P < 0.05$). There was no significant different between the two control groups ($P > 0.05$). The specific results are shown in Table 1.

Cell cycle analysis of cells treated with cisplatin

Flow cytometry showed that the proportion of pWPI-FOLR1-SKOV3 cells in S phase (no cisplatin treatment) was significantly higher than the proportion in the other two control groups ($P < 0.05$). For all three groups, treatment with cisplatin (1.8, 3.6, and 7.2 μg/ml), increased the percentage of cells in S phase in a dose-dependent manner ($P < 0.05$). Under the same conditions, the percentage of cells in S phase in the pWPI-FOLR1-SKOV3 group was highest compared to the other two groups ($P < 0.05$) (Fig. 7).

Concentration of residual cisplatin in cells detected by high performance liquid chromatography (HPLC)

The IC50 value in the pWPI-FOLR1-SKOV3 group was used as the reference concentration of cisplatin, and the

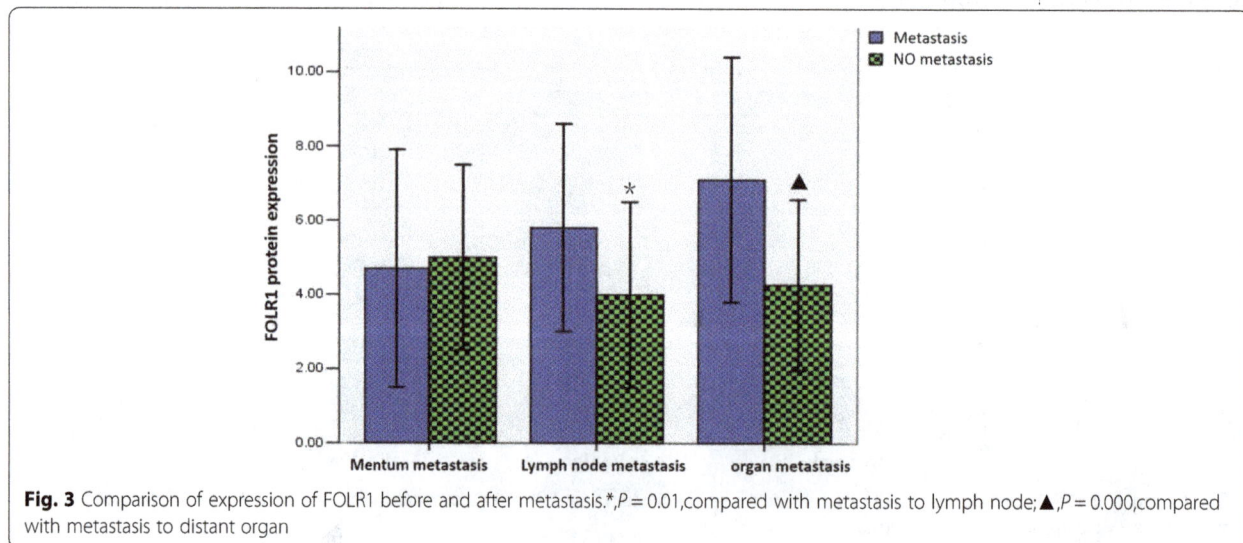

Fig. 3 Comparison of expression of FOLR1 before and after metastasis.*,$P = 0.01$,compared with metastasis to lymph node;▲,$P = 0.000$,compared with metastasis to distant organ

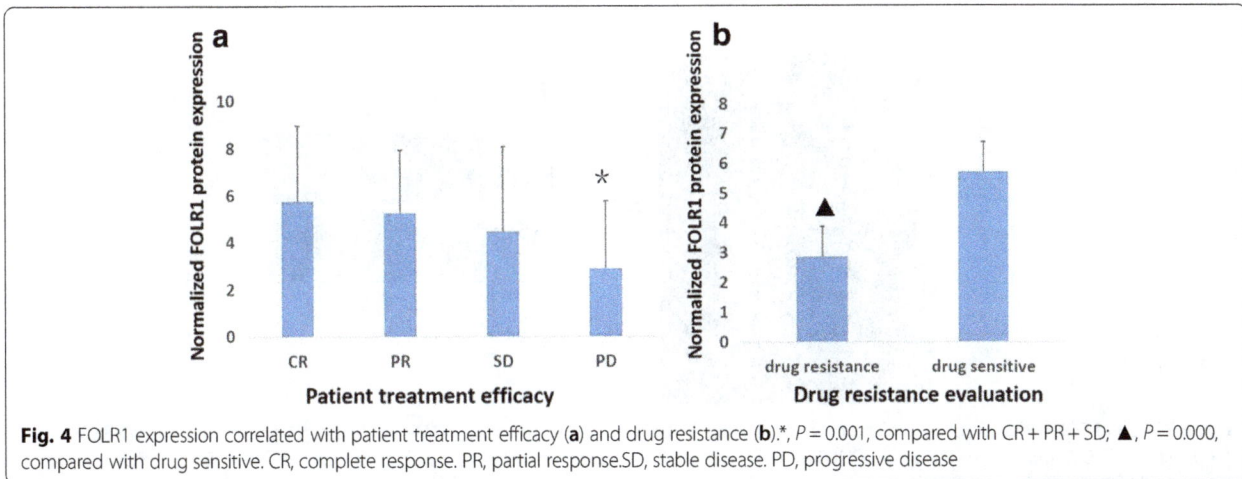

Fig. 4 FOLR1 expression correlated with patient treatment efficacy (**a**) and drug resistance (**b**).*, $P = 0.001$, compared with CR + PR + SD; ▲, $P = 0.000$, compared with drug sensitive. CR, complete response. PR, partial response.SD, stable disease. PD, progressive disease

same concentration of cisplatin was added to the three groups of cells, respectively. After 48 h of maturing they were used to detect the concentration of residual cispaltin in cells by HPLC (data not shown). Compared with standard curve, residual cisplatin concentration of the three groups were 1.543 ± 0.109 μg/10^6cells,1.487 ± 0.115 μg/10^6cells and 2.604 ± 0.205 μg/10^6cells,respectively. The pWPI-FOLR1-SKOV3 cells displayed the highest concentration compared to the other two groups ($P < 0.05$). There was no significant difference between the two control groups ($P > 0.05$). The specific results are shown in Fig. 8.

Discussion

In our previous study, we determined that FOLR1 was highly expressed in 160 ovarian tissue samples. This finding was consistent with another publications [7–9]. We find that FOLR1 is particularly high in cases of ovarian cancer, which suggests that FOLR1 may be useful as

a clinical diagnostic marker for the disease. Yuan et al. [10] showed that expression of FOLR1 in ovarian cancer was significantly higher than in either breast cancer or malignant mesothelioma. CA125 has been routinely used as a serum biomarker of ovarian cancer. However, it has proven to be a poor diagnostic indicator of sensitivity and specificity for early stage disease [11]. Thus, additional biomarkers are needed. Combined detection of CA125 and FOLR1 may be useful for the early diagnosis of ovarian cancer [12]. Such combination could also improve specificity and treatment response prediction [13].

Ovarian tumors are typically treated with cytoreductive surgery and platinum-based chemotherapy. However, long-term efficacy is limited. Yakirevich et al. [14] found that only 75% to 80% of epithelial ovarian cancers respond to chemotherapy, while the rest display primary resistance. Eventually, all patients develop chemotherapy

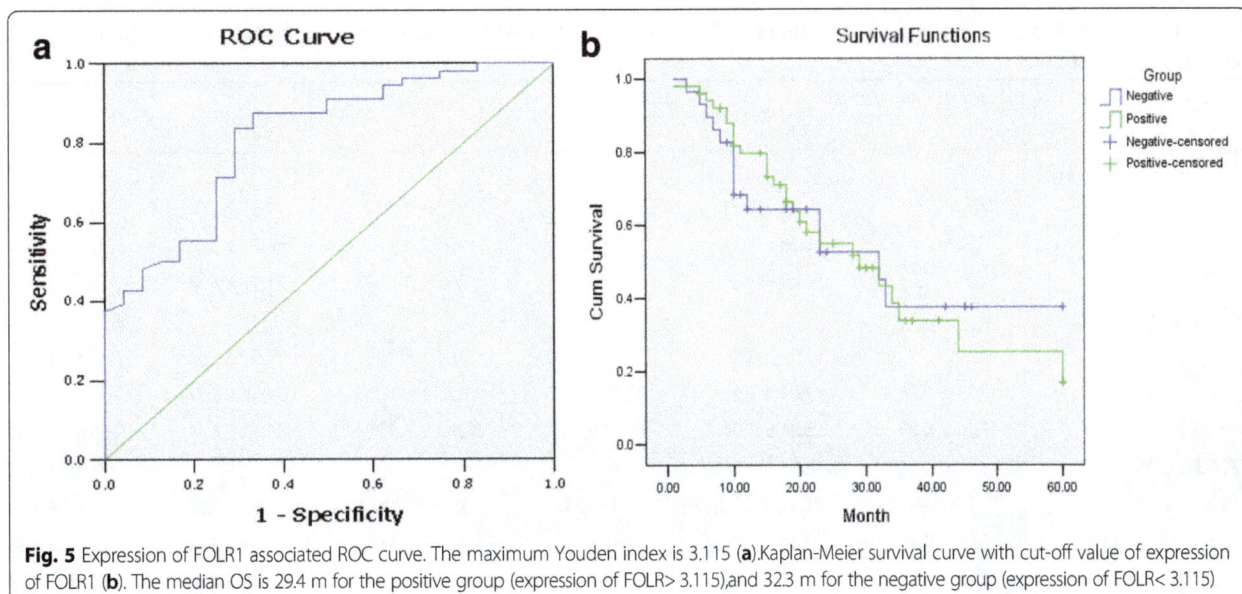

Fig. 5 Expression of FOLR1 associated ROC curve. The maximum Youden index is 3.115 (**a**).Kaplan-Meier survival curve with cut-off value of expression of FOLR1 (**b**). The median OS is 29.4 m for the positive group (expression of FOLR> 3.115),and 32.3 m for the negative group (expression of FOLR< 3.115)

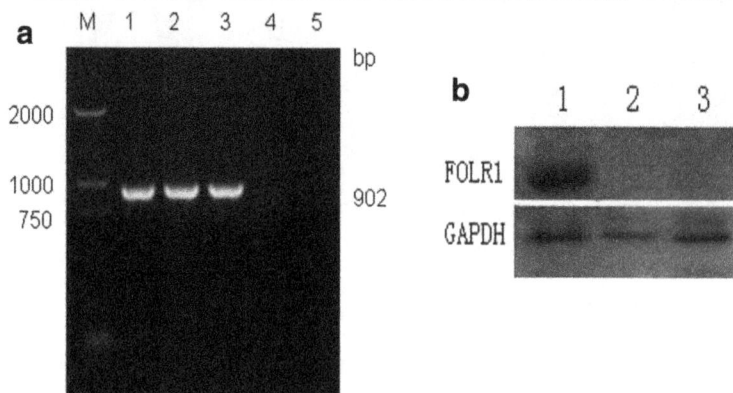

Fig. 6 RT-PCR of FOLR1 in each of the different groups (**a**) (lane M, DL2000 marker; lanes 1-3, rpWPI-FOLR1-SKOV3 group; lane 4, pWPI-SKOV3 group; lane 5, SKOV3 group). Expression of FOLR1 protein in different groups detected by Western blot (**b**) (lanes 1, rpWPI-FOLR1-SKOV3 group; lane 2, pWPI-SKOV3 group; lane 3, SKOV3 group)

drug resistance, which contributes to a low five-year survival rate and poor prognosis. We found that expression of FOLR1 is significantly reduced in drug-resistant ovarian tumors compared to drug-sensitive tumors. These findings are consistent with the finding that cisplatin-resistant cells display decreased levels of folate binding protein [6]. Decreased expression of FOLR1 in ovarian cancer cells is significantly associated with drug resistance. Thus, this may represent a mechanism of multi-drug resistance in the disease. Improvement of drug response has many potential benefits, including improving patient survival. We find that overexpression of FOLR1 in SKOV3 cells changes many of their biological properties, including cell cycle progression and apoptosis. SKOV3 cells overexpressing FOLR1 were the most sensitive to cisplatin treatment ($IC_{50} = 3.60$ μg/ml). These cells also displayed the most growth inhibition

following treatment. Our data show that high expression of FOLR1 in ovarian cancer cells increases sensitivity to cisplatin. We hypothesize that FOLR1 may promote ovarian cancer cell growth by transporting folic acid; it may also influence the response to cisplatin. However, more work is needed to determine the mechanism responsible for this effect. In the late 1990s, Gibb et al. [15] found that cisplatin induces apoptosis of ovarian cancer cells. Cisplatin is currently used as first-line chemotherapy for ovarian cancer treatment. Chemoresistance is associated with apoptosis and cell cycle changes. Resistance of ovarian cancer cells to chemotherapy-induced apoptosis is a primary reason for treatment failure [16, 17]. Cisplatin is induced by the endogenous mitochondrial pathway of apoptosis in ovarian cancer [18]. Here, we show that increased expression of FOLR1 increases sensitivity of ovarian cancer cells to

Table 1 Growth inhibition rate and apoptosis rate of each group of cells treated with different concentrations of cisplatin for different lengths of time

Group	Cases	Growth inhibition rate			Apoptosis rate		
		24 h	48 h	72 h	24 h	48 h	72 h
pWPI-FOLR1-SKOV 3 (μg/ml)							
1.8	12	8.86 ± 0.69	17.43 ± 0.91	30.29 ± 0.84	16.54 ± 2.58	24.84 ± 2.69	32.28 ± 2.97
3.6	12	18.52 ± 0.97	50.63 ± 1.31	64.28 ± 1.45	19.50 ± 2.71	50.08 ± 3.85	65.68 ± 4.03
7.2	12	32.24 ± 1.13	67.69 ± 1.24	79.38 ± 2.01	35.28 ± 3.59	71.44 ± 4.51	79.17 ± 4.58
pWPI-SKOV3 (μg/ml)							
1.8	12	6.54 ± 0.45	9.73 ± 0.67	15.79 ± 0.32	10.08 ± 2.19	14.89 ± 2.58	15.32 ± 2.61
3.6	12	12.89 ± 0.73	27.24 ± 0.85	38.21 ± 0.89	12.39 ± 2.06	27.61 ± 2.77	39.83 ± 3.19
7.2	12	19.26 ± 0.89	56.21 ± 1.04	69.77 ± 1.43	24.19 ± 2.78	58.80 ± 4.11	65.63 ± 3.91
SKOV3 (μg/ml)							
1.8	12	5.67 ± 0.48	8.35 ± 0.61	14.6 ± 0.45	9.27 ± 1.86	14.36 ± 2.56	17.72 ± 2.67
3.6	12	13.95 ± 0.56	24.59 ± 0.78	41.48 ± 0.75	11.27 ± 1.98	23.58 ± 2.49	40.64 ± 3.28
7.2	12	16.25 ± 0.67	57.73 ± 1.18	67.42 ± 1.51	23.62 ± 3.12	54.87 ± 4.10	68.64 ± 4.35

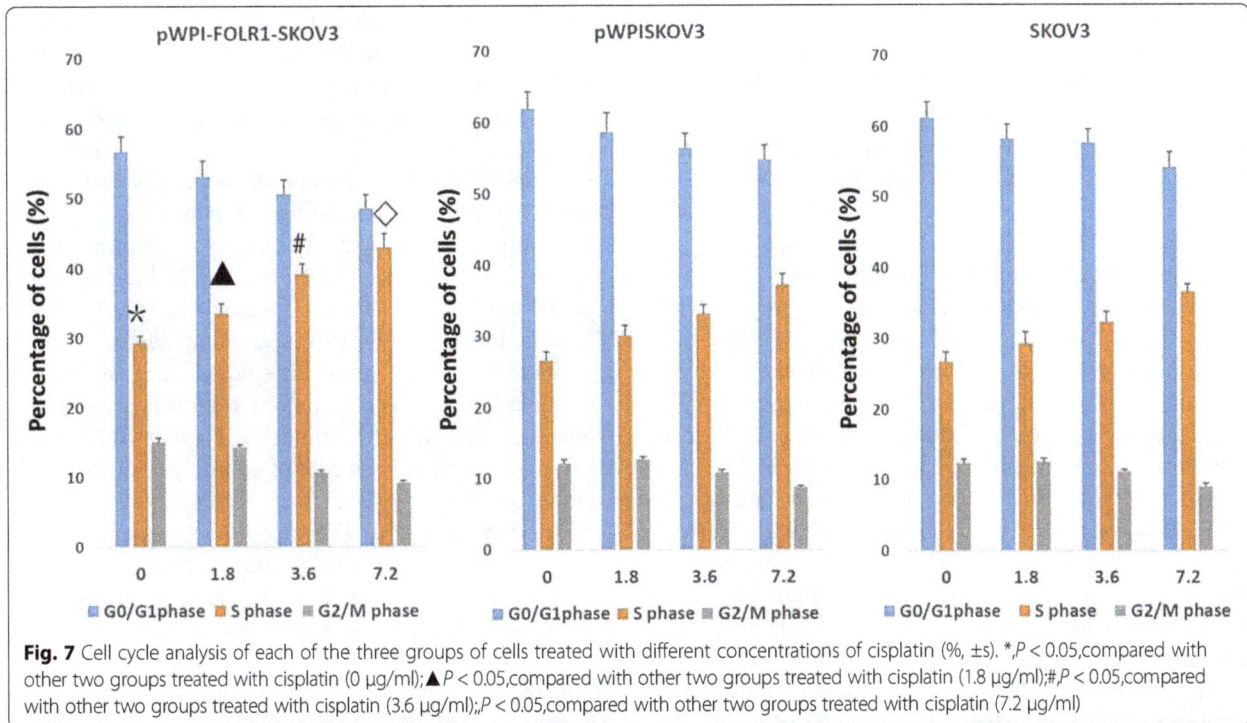

Fig. 7 Cell cycle analysis of each of the three groups of cells treated with different concentrations of cisplatin (%, ±s). *,$P < 0.05$,compared with other two groups treated with cisplatin (0 μg/ml);▲$P < 0.05$,compared with other two groups treated with cisplatin (1.8 μg/ml);#,$P < 0.05$,compared with other two groups treated with cisplatin (3.6 μg/ml);,$P < 0.05$,compared with other two groups treated with cisplatin (7.2 μg/ml)

cisplatin. We hypothesize that changes in FOLR1 expression and folate metabolism directly or indirectly contribute to cisplatin-induced apoptosis in ovarian cancer and influence cisplatin sensitivity. A main therapeutic goal is to limit multidrug resistance and improve the clinical efficacy of chemotherapy. This, in turn, would likely improve patient prognosis and survival.

Here, we find that, in the absence of cisplatin treatment, the proportion of cells overexpressing FOLR1 in S phase is significantly increased compared to the two control groups. One group reported that FOLR1 expression in ovarian cancer negatively correlated with the loss of the potential tumor suppressor gene caveolin [19].

Here, we find that treatment of SKOV3 cells with cisplatin resulted in S phase arrest. Those with FOLR1 overexpression showed the most dramatic increase in S-phase fraction following cisplatin treatment, consistent with the fact that this group was most sensitive to the chemotherapy. This is the first description of its kind, as there are no other publications describing a link between this pathway and folate metabolism.

In summary, we find that FOLR1 is highly expressed in ovarian cancer but is reduced following multidrug resistance. FOLR1 may be a useful biomarker for ovarian cancer, and it may be useful as a therapeutic application to improve sensitivity to cisplatin treatment [20].

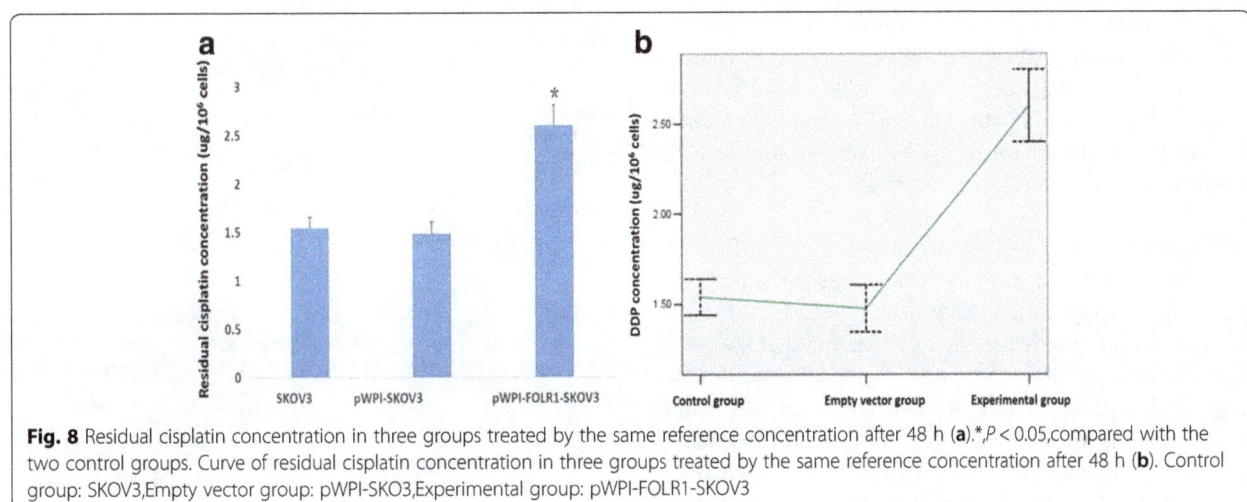

Fig. 8 Residual cisplatin concentration in three groups treated by the same reference concentration after 48 h (**a**).*,$P < 0.05$,compared with the two control groups. Curve of residual cisplatin concentration in three groups treated by the same reference concentration after 48 h (**b**). Control group: SKOV3,Empty vector group: pWPI-SKO3,Experimental group: pWPI-FOLR1-SKOV3

Conclusions

In summary, we find that FOLR1 is highly expressed in ovarian cancer but is reduced following multidrug resistance. FOLR1 may be a useful biomarker for ovarian cancer, and it may be useful as a therapeutic application to improve sensitivity to cisplatin treatment [20].

Methods

Detection of FOLR1 protein in ovarian tissue

All ovarian tissues were lysed, and protein samples were run by SDS-PAGE. Proteins were then transferred to PVDF membranes. Membranes were blocked for one hour at room temperature in PBS containing 5% milk/ 0.1% Tween. Membranes were then washed in PBS-Tween (0.1%) and incubated overnight with FOLR1 goat anti-human polyclonal antibody and goat anti-human GAPDH polyclonal antibody in PBS containing 5% milk at 4 °C. The next day, membranes were washed with PBS-Tween and incubated for two hours at room temperature with infrared fluorescent dye-labeled donkey anti-goat secondary antibody in PBS containing 5% milk. Blots were washed with PBS-Tween, and proteins were visualized using chemiluminescence reagents. The infrared fluorescence Odyssey imaging system was used to scan and analyze gray values and to calculate the relative expression of FOLR1.

Effect of cisplatin on SKOV3 cells

Full-length FOLR1 was PCR-amplified from pOTB7. Primer sequences contained EcoRI and XhoI sites. The amplified product was digested, purified, dephosphorylated, and then ligated into the pWPI vector to generate the recombinant plasmid pWPI-FOLR1. This recombinant plasmid was then transformed into *E. coli*, isolated, and sequenced. pWPI-FOLR1 was packaged with pCMV-dR8.74 and pMD2.G to produce lentivirus, which was used to infect SKOV3 cells. Flow cytometry using green fluorescence was performed to sort pWPI-FOLR1-SKOV3 positive cells. Control cells infected with lentivirus containing empty pWPI vector (pWPI-SKOV3) were generate in a similar manner. Untransfected SKOV3 cells were used as a blank control (SKOV3). Overexpression of FOLR1 was confirmed at the RNA and protein level by RT-PCR and Western blot, respectively.

MTT assay following cisplatin treatment

Cells were cultured for 24 h and then treated with increasing concentrations of cisplatin (0.5, 1, 2, 4, 8, 16, 32, and 64 μg/ml); treatment was maintained for 48 h. The growth inhibition rate of each sample was calculated. Half maximal inhibitory concentration (IC_{50}) software was used to obtain the IC_{50} of cisplatin in each of the three groups of cells. Concentration was normalized based on the IC_{50} of pWPI-FOLR1-SKOV3 cells treated with cisplatin. Concentrations of the three groups were $0.5 \times IC_{50}$, $1 \times IC_{50}$, and $2 \times IC_{50}$, and cells were cultured for 24 - 72 h. Values for each well were calculated, and the inhibition rate of cell growth was determined.

Flow cytometry to measure apoptosis and cell cycle progression following cisplatin treatment

Cells were cultured with increasing concentrations of cisplatin and incubated for 24, 48, and 72 h. PE-annexin V and 7-AAD (1 μl each) were mixed and added to cells. This was incubated for 15 min at room temperature in the dark. Next, 400 μl of ice-cold binding buffer was added and mixed gently before the cell preparations were examined by flow cytometry. Flow cytometry was then used to analyze the rate of apoptosis. For cell cycle analysis, cells were treated with cisplatin for 48 h. 1 μl RNA enzyme and 10 μl Triton X-100 were added to cells at room temperature for 30 min. Next, 1 μl PI was added and incubated at 4 °C for 30 min in the dark. Finally, flow cytometry was performed.

Statistical analysis

All experiments were performed at least three times, and statistical analysis was performed using SPSS13.0 software (SPSS Inc., Chicago, USA). The values were expressed as mean ± SD. ANOVA was used for comparisons made between more than two groups. Significance was set at $P < 0.05$. Dunnett's post hoc test was used to analyze multiple comparisons. P values of less than 0.05 ($P < 0.05$) were considered to be statistically significant.

Abbreviations

7-AAD: 7-amino-actinomycin; ANOVA: The analysis of variance; CA125: Cancer antigen 125; CR: Complete response; DDP: Cisplatin; DMEM: Dulbecco's modified eagle's medium; DMSO: Dimethyl sulfoxide; DNA: Deoxyribonucleic acid; EOC: Epithelial ovarian cancer; FIOG: International Federation of Gynaecology and Obstetrics; FOLR1: Folate binding protein; GAPDH: Glyceraldehyde 3-phosphate dehydrogenase; GPI: Glycosyl phosphatidylinositol; HPLC: High-performance liquid chromatography; IC_{50}: Half maximal inhibitory concentration; MDR: Multidrug resistance; mRNA: messenger RNA; MTT: 3-(4,5-dimethyl-2-thiazolyl)-2,5-diphenyl-2-H-tetrazolium bromide; PD: Progressive disease; PI: Propidium iodide; PR: Partial response; PVDF: Polyvinylidene fluoride; RNA: Ribonucleic acid; RT-PCR: Reverse transcription polymerase chain reaction; SD: Stable disease; SDS-PAGE: Sodium dodecyl sulphate-polyacrylamide gel electrophoresis

Acknowledgements

Not applicable.

Funding

The study was supported by the Guangxi Natural Science Foundation Nanning China. (Grant no. 2014jjAA40637). and the Ministry of Education Special Fund for Ph.D. Programs (Grant no. 20134503110009).

Authors' contributions

This study was conceived and designed by LL. HM-j and ZW finished the specific experiments. W-Q and YZ-j were in charge of specimens preparation.

LS finished this manuscript and submitting for publication. All authors read and approved the final manuscript.

Competing interests

The authors declare that they have no competing interests.

Author details

[1]Department of Gynecology Oncology, Tumor Hospital of Guangxi Medical University, Nanning 530021, China. [2]Department of Gynecology, Chongqing Three Gorges Central Hospital, Wanzhou District of Chongqing 404000, China.

References

1. Leitao MM Jr, Chi DS. Surgical management of recurrent ovarian cancer. Semin Oncol. 2009;36(2):106–11.
2. Ragoussis J, Senger G, Trowsdale J, Campbell IG. Genomic organization of the human folate receptor genes on chromosome 11q13. Genomics. 1992; 14(2):423–30.
3. Figini M, Ferri R, Mezzanzanica D, Bagnoli M, Luison E, Miotti S, Canevari S. Reversion of transformed phenotype in ovarian cancer cells by intracellular expression of anti folate receptor antibodies. Gene Ther. 2003;10(12):1018–25.
4. Ma DW, Finnell RH, Davidson LA, Callaway ES, Spiegelstein O, Piedrahita JA, Salbaum JM, Kappen C, Weeks BR, James J, et al. Folate transport gene inactivation in mice increases sensitivity to colon carcinogenesis. Cancer Res. 2005;65(3):887–97.
5. Sierra EE, Goldman ID. Recent advances in the understanding of the mechanism of membrane transport of folates and antifolates. Semin Oncol. 1999;26(2 Suppl 6):11–23.
6. Shen DW, Su A, Liang XJ, Pai-Panandiker A, Gottesman MM. Reduced expression of small GTPases and hypermethylation of the folate binding protein gene in cisplatin-resistant cells. Br J Cancer. 2004;91(2):270–6.
7. Dainty LA, Risinger JI, Morrison C, Chandramouli GV, Bidus MA, Zahn C, Rose GS, Fowler J, Berchuck A, Maxwell GL. Overexpression of folate binding protein and mesothelin are associated with uterine serous carcinoma. Gynecol Oncol. 2007;105(3):563–70.
8. Markert S, Lassmann S, Gabriel B, Klar M, Werner M, Gitsch G, Kratz F, Hasenburg A. Alpha-folate receptor expression in epithelial ovarian carcinoma and non-neoplastic ovarian tissue. Anticancer Res. 2008; 28(6A):3567–72.
9. Siu MK, Kong DS, Chan HY, Wong ES, Ip PP, Jiang L, Ngan HY, Le XF, Cheung AN. Paradoxical impact of two folate receptors, FRalpha and RFC, in ovarian cancer: effect on cell proliferation, invasion and clinical outcome. PLoS One. 2012;7(11):e47201.
10. Yuan Y, Nymoen DA, Dong HP, Bjorang O, Shih Ie M, Low PS, Trope CG, Davidson B. Expression of the folate receptor genes FOLR1 and FOLR3 differentiates ovarian carcinoma from breast carcinoma and malignant mesothelioma in serous effusions. Hum Pathol. 2009;40(10):1453–60.
11. Eltabbakh GH, Mount SL, Beatty B, Simmons-Arnold L, Cooper K, Morgan A. Factors associated with cytoreducibility among women with ovarian carcinoma. Gynecol Oncol. 2004;95(2):377–83.
12. Kurosaki A, Hasegawa K, Kato T, Abe K, Hanaoka T, Miyara A, O'Shannessy DJ, Somers EB, Yasuda M, Sekino T, et al. Serum folate receptor alpha as a biomarker for ovarian cancer: implications for diagnosis, prognosis and predicting its local tumor expression. Int J Cancer J Int Cancer. 2016;138(8): 1994–2002.
13. Chen YL, Chang MC, Huang CY, Chiang YC, Lin HW, Chen CA, Hsieh CY, Cheng WF. Serous ovarian carcinoma patients with high alpha-folate receptor had reducing survival and cytotoxic chemo-response. Mol Oncol. 2012;6(3):360–9.
14. Yakirevich E, Sabo E, Naroditsky I, Sova Y, Lavie O, Resnick MB. Multidrug resistance-related phenotype and apoptosis-related protein expression in ovarian serous carcinomas. Gynecol Oncol. 2006;100(1):152–9.
15. Gibb RK, Taylor DD, Wan T, O'Connor DM, Doering DL, Gercel-Taylor C. Apoptosis as a measure of chemosensitivity to cisplatin and taxol therapy in ovarian cancer cell lines. Gynecol Oncol. 1997;65(1):13–22.
16. Jeong JJ, Park N, Kwon YJ, Ye DJ, Moon A, Chun YJ. Role of annexin A5 in cisplatin-induced toxicity in renal cells: molecular mechanism of apoptosis. J Biol Chem. 2014;289(4):2469–81.
17. Feng X, Li L, Jiang H, Jiang K, Jin Y, Zheng J. Dihydroartemisinin potentiates the anticancer effect of cisplatin via mTOR inhibition in cisplatin-resistant ovarian cancer cells: involvement of apoptosis and autophagy. Biochem Biophys Res Commun. 2014;444(3):376–81.
18. Lin J, Spidel JL, Maddage CJ, Rybinski KA, Kennedy RP, Krauthauser CL, Park YC, Albone EF, Jacob S, Goserud MT, et al. The antitumor activity of the human FOLR1-specific monoclonal antibody, farletuzumab, in an ovarian cancer mouse model is mediated by antibody-dependent cellular cytotoxicity. Cancer Biol Ther. 2013;14(11):1032–8.
19. Bagnoli M, Canevari S, Figini M, Mezzanzanica D, Raspagliesi F, Tomassetti A, Miotti S. A step further in understanding the biology of the folate receptor in ovarian carcinoma. Gynecol Oncol. 2003;88(1 Pt 2):S140–4.
20. Xia W, Low PS. Folate-targeted therapies for cancer. J Med Chem. 2010; 53(19):6811–24.

17

Predicted luteal phase length has no influence on success of vitrified-warmed blastocyst transfer in natural cycle

M. Reljič[1*] and J. Knez[2]

Abstract

Background: This study evaluated the influence of menstrual cycle length, menstrual cycle variability and predicted luteal phase length on the success of vitrified-warmed blastocyst transfer in natural menstrual cycle using progesterone for luteal phase supplementation.

Methods: Consecutive women undergoing vitrified-warmed blastocyst transfer in natural menstrual cycle between January 2013 and December 2015 were included in this retrospective study. Patients' characteristics, clinical data and data about menstrual cycle length in the last year were collected from our database. Predicted luteal phase length (LPL) was defined as the period starting at ovulation (one day after positive urinary LH test) and ending on the last day before predicted menses, based on women's usual, minimal and maximal menstrual cycle length data. Logistic regression was used to identify the predictors significantly associated with live-birth.

Results: A total of 1195 FETs (frozen-thawed embryo transfers) resulted in 457 (38.24%) clinical pregnancies, 82 (17.94%), miscarriages and 371 live births (31.04%). There were no statistically significant differences in menstrual cycle length, menstrual cycle variability, day of LH surge, day of FET and predicted LPL between FET cycles resulting in live birth and those not resulting in live birth. In the multivariate logistic regression model, only women's age (OR 0.93, 95% CI: 0.90–0.96), transfer of morphologically optimal blastocysts (OR 2.17, 95% CI: 1.59–2.94) and endometrium thickness (OR 1.10, 95% CI: 1.03–1.17) were important independent prognostic factors for live birth.

Conclusion: Menstrual cycle length, menstrual cycle variability and predicted LPL do not seem to be an important factor influencing live birth after FET in natural cycles with progesterone supplementation. Results of our study suggest that FET should not be cancelled if LH surge is detected before or after the predicted period in natural cycle with progesterone supplementation.

Keywords: Predicted luteal phase length, Frozen embryo transfer, Blastocyst transfer, Natural cycle

Background

The transfer of frozen-thawed embryos (FET) has become an integral part of successful in vitro fertilization programs. With advances in cryopreservation techniques, this approach offers several important benefits to the patients, which include improved safety of the treatment and higher cumulative success rates. When transferring embryos, a receptive endometrium is a prerequisite for successful implantation and several protocols for endometrium

preparation can be used in patients undergoing FET. One of the commonly used approaches is natural cycle (NC) monitoring, where detection of ovulation is the reference for timing of embryo thawing and transfer [1]. The main advantages of NC over other protocols are avoidance of using multiple medications and low cost, although the timing of ovulation increases scheduling difficulties and cancelation rates [2]. Success rate of FET in NC depends on the appropriate patient selection. This is partly because cycle monitoring in women with irregular menstrual cycles is less feasible and more likely to result in canceling the embryo transfer. But even in women with regular and ovulatory cycles, the spontaneous conception rates are affected

* Correspondence: milan.reljic@guest.arnes.si
[1]Department for Reproductive Medicine and Gynaecological Endocrinology, Clinic for Gynecology and Perinatology, University Medical Centre Maribor, Ljubljanska 5, 2000 Maribor, Slovenia
Full list of author information is available at the end of the article

by menstrual cycle characteristics, such as menstrual cycle length, variability and luteal phase length [3–5]. It has been shown that even an isolated episode of short luteal phase may have an influence on reduced immediate fecundity in natural conception [3]. There is currently no data available showing a possible role of luteal phase length on the success of FET. The aim of our study was to determine whether predicted luteal phase length has an influence on the live birth rate in women undergoing FET in NC.

Methods

All women undergoing vitrified-warmed blastocyst transfer performed in natural cycle between 2013 and 2015 at the Department for Reproductive medicine and Gynecological Endocrinology, University Medical Centre Maribor were included in this retrospective study. According to our clinical practice all women undergoing FET are scheduled for a baseline pelvic ultrasound examination in the follicular phase of the menstrual cycle. Women with irregular menstrual cycles (< 24 or > 35 days), uterine pathology and hydrosalpinges visible on ultrasound were excluded from the analysis.

After observing the selection of the leading follicle and thickening of the endometrium on ultrasound, urinary LH tests were used twice daily to monitor the LH surge onset. FET was scheduled 5 or 6 days after positive morning and evening LH test. If the LH surge was not detected or if the results were inconclusive, the embryo transfer was canceled.

All expanded blastocysts were vitrified on day 5 or day 6 by using the combination of dimethyl sulfoxide (DMSO) and ethylene glycol cryoprotectants. Before vitrification blastocysts were graded according to our established grading system [6, 7]. In brief, the blastocyst was considered optimal if it was fully expanded and the blastocoel completely filled the embryo. Blastocysts were first exposed to equilibration media (7.5% DMSO/ethylene glycol) for 10 min and later to vitrification solution (15% DMSO/ethylene glycol) for 1 min (Irvine Scientific, Santa Ana, CA). Before vitrification, blastocysts were placed in closed straws (High security vitrification kit, Cryo Bio System, Paris, France). For thawing, the embryo carrier was expelled from the straw and quickly plunged into the thawing medium (1 M sucrose) for 1 min. Blastocysts were then transferred in dilution solution (0.5 M sucrose) 3 times for 3 min. They were cultured in recovery medium (Blast Assist System, Origio, Denmark) for at least 4 h before they were transferred into the uterus. Only blastocysts that had at least 50% intact blastomeres after thawing and started to re-expand were assessed suitable for transfer [7].

One or two vitrified-warmed blastocysts were transferred using clinical touch technique and Labotect catheters (Labotect GmbH, Labor-Technik-Göttingen, Germany).

The number of embryos transferred in each case depended on the quality of available embryos, the number of previous treatments, the number of embryos frozen in the same straw and according to the patient - doctor agreement.

Immediately prior to embryo transfer, pelvic ultrasound examination was performed to measure the endometrial thickness and evaluate the endometrial pattern. The endometrium thickness was measured in sagittal plane from one basal endometrial interface across the endometrial canal to the other basal surface. Secretory endometrial pattern was defined as an isoechoic and homogeneous hyperechoic endometrium with a non-prominent or absent central echogenic line.

According to our routine clinical practice, progesterone supplementation with 400 mg of micronized vaginal progesterone per day was started after FET. Serum β-hCG level measurement was scheduled 14 days after FET and ultrasound was performed 2 weeks later if the β-hCG levels were positive. Clinical pregnancy was defined as the presence of a gestational sac with a fetal heartbeat. Spontaneous miscarriage was defined as pregnancy loss after clinical confirmation of pregnancy. Live birth was recorded where one or more babies were born. The data on pregnancy outcome was collected by using a questionnaire.

Patients' characteristics clinical data and cycle outcome was collected from our database. The data about menstrual cycle length (usual, shortest, and longest) in the last year was collected as part of the routine infertility assessment. Predicted luteal phase length (LPL) was defined as the period starting at ovulation (one day after positive urinary LH test) and ending on the last day before predicted menses, based on women's usual, minimal and maximal menstrual cycle length data. A normal LPL was defined as 12–15 days, short as less than 12 days and long more than 15 days.

Patients' and cycles' characteristics were compared between the FET cycles resulting in live birth and FET cycles not resulting in live birth. Statistical analysis was performed with Statistica 8.0 data software system analysis (Stat Soft Inc., Tulsa, OK, USA). Mean and standard deviation for each continuous variable were calculated and Student's t test was used to compare these variables between both groups. Chi-square test was used in the evaluation of the categorical data. We have constructed univariate logistic regression models to test the predictive values of different patients' characteristics on the possibility of live birth. Variables proven statistically important by univariate logistic analysis were tested with multiple logistic regression model. Odds ratios and their 95% confidence intervals (CIs) were calculated. Live birth rates between cycles with predicted short, normal and long LPL were compared using Pearson chi-square test. P value < 0.05 was considered statistically significant.

The study was approved by our institutional review board.

Results

A total of 1195 FETs resulted in 457 (38.24%) clinical pregnancies, 82 (17.94%), miscarriages and 371 live births (31.04%). Women in cycles resulting in live birth were statistically significantly younger (33.20 ± 3.97 vs 34.46 ± 4.14 years, $p < 0.001$), had less previous unsuccessful IVF/ICSI attempts (1.68 ± 1.35 vs 1.87 ± 1.43, $p = 0.03$), thicker endometrium on the day of FET (10.38 ± 2.34 vs 9.95 ± 2.17 mm, $p = 0.004$), higher proportion of transferred blastocysts vitrified on day 5 (71.70% vs 64.56%, $p = 0.015$) and higher proportion of FET of optimal blastocysts (38.27% vs 20.14% $p < 0.001$) compared to women in cycles not resulting in live birth. There were no statistically significant differences between these two groups in the rate of secretory endometrial pattern, number of blastocysts transferred, cause of infertility, proportion of cycles with births after fresh embryo-transfer and in proportion of cycles with FET after freeze-all cycle (Table 1). There were also no statistically significant differences in usual, shortest and longest menstrual cycle length, menstrual cycle variability (maximum- minimum MC length), day of LH surge, day of FET and predicted LPL between FET cycles resulting in live birth and those not resulting in live birth (Table 2).

In the multivariate logistic regression model, only women's age (OR 0.93, 95% CI: 0.90–0.96), transfer of morphologically optimal blastocysts (OR 2.17, 95% CI: 1.59–2.94) and endometrium thickness (OR 1.10, 95% CI: 1.03–1.17) were important independent prognostic factors for live birth.

In 185 (15.48%) FET cycles, the predicted LPL was short (≤ 11 days), in 952 (79.67%) normal (12–15 days), and in 58 (4.85%) long (> 15 days) if the calculation was based on usual menstrual cycle length. If cycle variability

was taken into account then the proportion of predicted short, normal and long luteal phase length was different. However, there were no significant differences in live birth rate between these three groups, irrespective of whether the length of the luteal phase was predicted on the usual, minimum or maximum length (Table 3).

Discussion

Our data has shown that the predicted luteal phase length is not predictive of live birth after FET. The only important independent prognostic factors for live birth were women's age at the time of FET, transfer of morphologically optimal blastocysts and endometrial thickness, a finding that was also reported in previous studies [8, 9].

There are currently no other studies evaluating the influence of menstrual cycle characteristics on the outcome of FET in NC, but some observations that support this possibility come from studies on natural fertility. Based on these studies, menstrual cycle pattern, menstrual cycle length and variability are indicators of endocrine function and fertility potential of women. Usually menstrual cycle shortens with chronologic age and then there is an increase in variability at perimenopause [10]. Several authors have studied the association between menstrual cycle characteristics and spontaneous conception rate and discovered that shorter cycles are associated with reduced fecundability in women with regular cycles [4, 5, 10]. However, it was shown that adverse effect of short menstrual cycle length on fecundability was more pronounced in women with cycle length less than 25 days [10] and these women were not included in the present study.

Normal luteal phase length (LPL) is relatively fixed at 12–14 days [11]. Short LPL is often considered to be a clinical sign of luteal phase deficiency (LPD), which is an entity commonly associated with infertility [11]. LPD

Table 1 Clinical characteristics of FET cycles resulting in live birth and those not resulting in live birth

	FET resulting in live birth $N = 371$	FET NOT resulting in live birth $N = 824$	p-value
Age (mean ± SD)	33.20 ± 3.97	34.46 ± 4.14	< 0.001
Unexplained infertility (%, N)	17,52 (65)	15,29 (126)	NS
Tubal factor infertility (%, N)	22,37 (83)	26,46 (218)	NS
Male factor infertility (%, N)	42.31 (157)	42,84 (353)	NS
No. of previous IVF cycles (X ± SD)	1.68 ± 1.35	1.87 ± 1.43	0.03
Freeze all in previous cycle (%, N)	12.93 (48)	10.44 (86)	NS
Prior birth after fresh ET (%, N)	18.06 (67)	16.99 (140)	NS
No. of blastocysts transferred (X ± SD)	1.26 ± 0.44	1.23 ± 0.42	NS
ET of optimal blastocysts (%, N)	38.27 (142)	20.14 (166)	< 0.001
ET of blastocysts frozen on day 5 (%, N)	71.70 (266)	64.56 (532)	0.015
Endometrial thickness (mm, X ± SD)	10.38 ± 2.34	9.95 ± 2.17	0.004
Secretory endometrium pattern (%)	58.68	60.38	NS

ET embryotransfer

Table 2 Menstrual cycle characteristics in FET cycles resulting in live birth and those not resulting in live birth

	FET resulting in live birth N = 371	FET NOT resulting in live birth N = 824	p-value
Usual MC length (days)	28.17 ± 1.86	28.10 ± 1.67	NS
Min. MC length (days)	26.63 ± 2.42	26.74 ± 2.23	NS
Max. MC length (days)	30.20 ± 2.74	30.07 ± 2.70	NS
Max.- min. MC length (days)	3.68 ± 3.61	3.34 ± 2.68	NS
Day of cycle with LH surge	13.40 ± 2.16	13.32 ± 2.14	NS
Day of cycle with FET	19.26 ± 2.09	19.18 ± 2.09	NS
LPL predicted on usual MC length (days)	14.02 ± 1.92	13.91 ± 1.96	NS
LPL predicted on min. MC length (days)	12.41 ± 2.50	12.24 ± 2.71	NS
LPL predicted on max. MC length (days)	15.81 ± 2.53	15.73 ± 2.71	NS

MC menstrual cycle, LPL luteal phase length, *min* minimal, *max* maximal

can be caused by impaired corpus luteum function, resulting in the lack of adequate progesterone secretion or by inadequate response of endometrium to progesterone. Progesterone secretion in the luteal phase of menstrual cycle is crucial for secretory transformation of the endometrium leading to receptivity [12]. Therefore, women with short luteal phase may have impaired receptivity of the endometrium to implantation or lower capability to maintain a pregnancy [13]. Short luteal phase is not uncommon and was observed in 8.9–18.0% among normal cycling woman. In the present study, short luteal phase was predicted in 15.5% of cycles if calculation was based on woman's usual menstrual cycle length data. But if we take into account the menstrual cycle variability, the rate of cycles with predicted short luteal phase was between 2.6–32.0%. But regardless of the approach to calculation of the predicted LPL, there were no statistically significant differences between cycles with predicted short, normal and long luteal phases. One of the possible explanations could be that in the present study, luteal phase support was used. So even if LPD existed, it could be overcome by using micronized progesterone after embryo transfer. The benefit of luteal phase support in natural cycles has previously been demonstrated by Bjuresten et al. [14]. They concluded that women undergoing FET are often subfertile, and they may have suboptimal endometria during their natural cycles [14]. On the other hand, there is controversy in this field, since other authors did not confirm these findings and Groenewoud et al. in their meta-analysis concluded that currently there is too little evidence supporting a positive effect of luteal phase support in patients undergoing NC-FET [1, 15].

Limitations of the present study are its retrospective nature. The calculated predicted LPL is an entity that indirectly estimates the luteal phase length of the current cycle and this is a limitation of our study. Despite using multivariate regression models in the methodological approach to control for confounders, the presence of potential bias cannot be excluded. Self-reported data on menstrual cycle length and urinary LH tests could be unreliable. Luteal phase has been affected by progesterone supplementation after FET.

Conclusion

Menstrual cycle length, menstrual cycle variability and predicted LPL do not seem to play an important role for live birth rate after FET in natural cycles with progesterone supplementation. Results of our study also suggest that FET should not be cancelled if LH surge is detected before or after predicted period in natural cycle with progesterone supplementation. There is a need for further basic studies investigating the influence of luteal phase length on embryo implantation.

Table 3 Predicted luteal phase length in minimal, usual and maximal menstrual cycle length according to live birth rate

	Predicted short LPL (≤11 days)	Predicted normal LPL (12–15 days)	Predicted long LPL (> 15 days)	p- value
LPL predicted on min. MC length (%, N)	32.05 (383)	59.50 (711)	8.45 (101)	
Live birth rate	33.43 (128)	29.67 (211)	31.68 (32)	NS
LPL predicted on usual MC length (%, N)	15.48 (185)	70.79 (846)	13.72 (164)	
Live birth rate	34.59 (64)	30.39 (257)	30.49 (50)	NS
LPL predicted on max. MC length (%, N)	2.59 (31)	47.95 (573)	49.46 (591)	
Live birth rate	32.25 (10)	30.54 (175)	31.47 (186)	NS

MC menstrual cycle, LPL luteal phase length, *min* minimal, *max* maximal

Funding

The study was a part of research programme P3–0327 funded by the Slovenian Research Agency.

Authors' contributions

MR conceived and designed the study, performed the statistical analysis and drafted the manuscript. JK participated in data interpretation, in drafting the manuscript and edited the paper. Both authors read and approved the final manuscript.

Competing interests

The authors declare that they have no competing interests.

Author details

[1]Department for Reproductive Medicine and Gynaecological Endocrinology, Clinic for Gynecology and Perinatology, University Medical Centre Maribor, Ljubljanska 5, 2000 Maribor, Slovenia. [2]Department for Reproductive Medicine and Gynaecological Endocrinology, Clinic for Gynecology and Perinatology, University Medical Centre Maribor, Ljubljanska 5, 2000 Maribor, Slovenia.

References

1. Groenewoud ER, Cantineau AE, Kollen BJ, Macklon NS, Cohlen BJ. What is the optimal means of preparing the endometrium in frozen-thawed embryo transfer cycles? A systematic review and meta-analysis. Hum Reprod Update. 2013;19:458–70.
2. Greco E, Litwicka K, Arrivi C, Varricchio MT, Caragia A, Greco A, et al. The endometrial preparation for frozen-thawed euploid blastocyst transfer: a prospective randomized trial comparing clinical results from natural modified cycle and exogenous hormone stimulation with GnRH agonist. J Assist Reprod Genet. 2016;33(7):873–84.
3. Crawford NM, Pritchard DA, Herring AH, Steiner AZ. Prospective evaluation of luteal phase length and natural fertility. Fertil Steril. 2017;107:749–55.
4. Small CM, Manatunga AK, Klein M, Feigelson HS, Dominguez CE, McChesney R, et al. Menstrual cycle characteristics: associations with fertility and spontaneous abortion. Epidemiology. 2006;17:52–60.
5. Kolstad HA, Bonde JP, Hjøllund NH, Jensen TK, Henriksen TB, Ernst E, et al. Menstrual cycle pattern and fertility: a prospective follow-up study of pregnancy and early embryonal loss in 295 couples who were planning their first pregnancy. Fertil Steril. 1999;71:490–6.
6. Kovačič B, Vlaisavljević V, Reljič M, Čižek-Sajko M. Developmental capacity of different morphological types of day 5 human morulae and blastocysts. Reprod BioMed Online. 2004;8:687–94.
7. Kovačič B, Vlaisavljević V. Importance of blastocyst morphology in selection for transfer. In: Wu B, editor. Advances in embryo transfer. Rijeka: Intech; 2012. p. 161–77.
8. Veleva Z, Orava M, Nuojua-Huttunen S, Tapanainen JS, Martikainen H. Factors affecting the outcome of frozen-thawed embryo transfer. Hum Reprod. 2013;28(9):2425–31.
9. Salumets A, Suikkari AM, Mäkinen S, Karro H, Roos A, Tuuri T. Frozen embryo transfers: implications of clinical and embryological factors on the pregnancy outcome. Hum Reprod. 2006;21:2368–74.
10. Wise LA, Mikkelsen EM, Rothman KJ, Riis AH, Sorensen HT, Huybrechts KF, et al. A prospective cohort study of menstrual characteristics and time to pregnancy. Am J Epidemiol. 2011;174:701–9.
11. Practice Committee of the American Society for Reproductive Medicine. The clinical relevance of luteal phase deficiency: a committee opinion. Fertil Steril. 2012;98:1112–7.
12. Schliep KC, Mumford SL, Hammoud AO, Stanford JB, Kissell KA, Sjaarda LA, et al. Luteal phase deficiency in regularly menstruating women: prevalence and overlap in identification based on clinical and biochemical diagnostic criteria. J Clin Endocrinol Metab. 2014;99:1007–14.
13. Sonntag B, Ludwig M. An integrated view on the luteal phase: diagnosis and treatment in subfertility. Clin Endocrinol. 2012;77:500–7.
14. Bjuresten K, Landgren BM, Hovatta O, Stavreus-Evers A. Luteal phase progesterone increases live birth rate after frozen embryo transfer. Fertil Steril. 2011;95:534–7.
15. Lee VC, Li RH, Ng EH, Yeung WS, Ho PC. Luteal phase support does not improve the clinical pregnancy rate of natural cycle frozen–thawed embryo transfer: a retrospective analysis. Eur J Obstet Gynecol Reprod Biol. 2013;169:50–3.

18

Diagnostic value of the gynecology imaging reporting and data system (GI-RADS) with the ovarian malignancy marker CA-125 in preoperative adnexal tumor assessment

Michal Migda[1,3*] (ID), Migda Bartosz[2], Marian S. Migda[3], Marcin Kierszk[1], Gieryn Katarzyna[1] and Marek Maleńczyk[1]

Abstract

Objectives: The purpose of this study is to assess the preoperative evaluation of an adnexal mass using the GI-RADS classification and to verify whether CA-125 measurement can offer any additional benefits to the GI-RADS-based prediction of ovarian tumor malignancy.

Material and methods: In this study, we assessed a total of 215 women with an adnexal tumor using the GI-RADS classification combined with CA-125 measurement. All adnexal masses underwent histological verification.

Results: Of a total of 215 lesions, we classified 2 lesions as GI-RADS 2 (0.9%), 118 lesions as GI-RADS 3 (54.9%), 86 lesions as GI-RADS 4 (40.0%) and 9 lesions as GI-RADS 5 (4.2%). For GI-RADS 4–5 lesions, the sensitivity, specificity, PPV, NPV, ACC and OR were as follows: 94.3, 72.2, 52.6, 97.5, 77.7%, and 43.3 (CI 12.0–146), respectively. The corresponding parameters resulting from combining the GI-RADS classification with the CA-125 marker were as follows: 66.0, 93.8, 77.8, 89.4, 87.0%, and 29.6 (CI 12.6–69.6), respectively, with $p < 0.001$. For Ca-125 > 30 IU/mL alone, the results were as follows: 70.0, 80.3, 53.8, 89.1, 77.7%, and 9.5 (4.6–19.6), respectively, with $p < 0.0001$. Additionally, 47.8% of the patients had no symptoms, 36.5% had back pain, 5.2% had an increased abdominal size, 4.3% had menstrual irregularities and 2.6% had constipation. There were 152 benign and 18 malignant cases in the low risk group (GIRADS 1–3 and GIRADS 4 + CA-125 < 30 IU/mL) and 10 benign and 35 malignant tumors in the high-risk group (GIRADS 4 + CA125 > 30 IU/mL and GIRADS 5).

Conclusions: GI-RADS classification had good performance in discriminating ovarian tumors. The additional measurement of CA-125 improves the system specificity, PPV and ACC for preoperative adnexal tumor assessment.

Keywords: Gynecology imaging reporting and data system, Ca-125, Ultrasound, Ovarian tumor

Introduction

Ovarian cancer is the most lethal cancer among gynecological malignancies. It has been estimated that over 151,000 women died from this disease in 2012 worldwide [1]. In Poland, ovarian cancer is the second most frequently diagnosed malignancy of the female genital tract, with an incidence rate of 3600 new cases per year, and has the highest mortality among gynecological cancers, reaching 2600 deaths every year [2]. Sadly, nearly 70% of patients with ovarian cancer are diagnosed at an advanced stage, while the 5-year survival rate for patients with ovarian cancer may be as high as 90% when treated early [3]. It has been demonstrated that the survival of ovarian cancer patients is better when treatment is provided at specialized centers by gynecologists with expertise in gynecologic oncology [4]. To date, surgical treatment, chemotherapy, radiotherapy,

* Correspondence: mchmigda@gmail.com
[1]Clinical Unit of Obstetrics, Women's Disease and Gynecological Oncology, sw. Jozefa 53/59, United District Hospital, Collegium Medicum University of Nicolaus Copernicus in Toruń, Torun, Poland
[3]Civis Vita Medical Center, Torun, Poland
Full list of author information is available at the end of the article

biotargeted therapy and other technologies have improved. Screening tumor markers using gene chip technology by detecting the hypomethylation of certain genes may be potentially helpful in high-risk groups, such as BRCA1 and BRCA2 patients, but not in the general population [5]. Studies based on proteomics are based on appropriate protein analysis technology such as surface-enhanced laser desorption/ionization time-of-flight (TOF)-MS, which shows 100% sensitivity and 93.3% specificity, indicating that this approach is useful for diagnosing ovarian cancer [6]. A cytogenetic analysis study by Lagana showed that the progression of epithelial ovarian cancer is characterized by a series of combined epigenetic aberrations determined by loss of methylation of certain regions of DNA encoding genes such as the Ras-association domain-containing family 1 (RASSF1A) tumor suppressor, which is considered a new diagnostic development [7]. Additionally, technical improvement allows surgery on a patient with an early stage of ovarian carcinoma using laparoscopy or robot-assisted laparoscopy, making this an acceptable approach for this selected group [8]. The preoperative assessment of an adnexal mass is difficult, which leads to a disproportionate number of women with benign ovarian tumors being referred to specialized centers and, conversely, women with ovarian malignancy being inappropriately operated on in nonspecialized centers [4]. Ultrasonography is currently considered the primary imaging modality for identifying and characterizing adnexal masses [9]. Due to the subjective nature of the examination, there has been a need for standardized nomenclature and a definition of all tumor features evaluated by ultrasound. The International Ovarian Tumor Analysis provides consensus on ultrasonography nomenclature and definitions of all tumor features and has improved the discrimination of adnexal masses by including a quantitative assessment of some morphological features [10]. In 2009, based on the Breast Imaging Reporting and Data System (BI-RADS), Amor et al. proposed a Gynecology Imaging Reporting and Data System (GI-RADS) as a similar system to facilitate communication between sonographers and referring clinicians [11]. The contemporary diagnostic standard for ovarian cancer includes transvaginal ultrasound and the measurement of serum CA-125. A wide range of other diagnostic approaches is being investigated at present [1].

The purpose of this study was to assess the performance of the GI-RADS reporting system in the preoperative discrimination of adnexal masses in Polish women and to test whether the measurement of CA-125 can offer any additional benefits to the GI-RADS risk evaluation for the malignancy of ovarian tumors.

Materials and methods

This study was approved by the board of Clinical Unit of Obstetrics, Women's Disease and Gynecological Oncology, United District Hospital, Collegium Medicum University of Nicolaus Copernicus in Toruń, Poland. Over a 24-month period, we enrolled a total of 215 women with adnexal masses into the study. The inclusion criteria were primarily based on the clinical diagnosis of an adnexal mass followed by ultrasound confirmation at our tertiary center and the obtaining data indicating pathology. Patients with pregnancy, bilateral adnexal tumors or a malignancy diagnosis already established were excluded from the study.

Patients were assessed by an experienced examiner (500 scans a year) 2–3 days prior to surgery. Vaginal and transabdominal two-dimensional (2D) ultrasound examinations were performed using a Voluson E8 (GE Medical Systems, Zipf, Austria). Morphological features were examined according to GI-RADS and included unilateral involvement, the maximum diameter of the lesion, the wall thickness, septa, solid papillary projections, solid areas within the cyst, cystic content and ascites [6]. Color Doppler was used to assess peripheral or central vascularization.

Peripheral blood was collected for the measurement of serum CA-125 1 to 14 days prior to surgery. Blood was collected from all patients and stored in serum separator tubes. Automated analysis of CA-125 was performed by direct chemiluminescence using an Advia Centaur CA-125 II assay (Siemens Medical Solutions Diagnostics, Tarrytown, USA). Values were expressed in international units per milliliter (IU/mL).

A definitive histological diagnosis was obtained from surgical excision or a biopsy sample. Tumors were classified according to the WHO criteria [8]. Borderline tumors were considered malignant for the purposes of the present study. Statistical analysis was performed using the statistical software STATISTICA 10 (StatSoft Inc.). GI-RADS classification was combined with a CA-125 assay, and descriptive measures were calculated (for CA-125 > 30 IU/mL): sensitivity, specificity, positive predictive value (PPV), negative predictive value (NPV), accuracy (ACC), and odds ratio (OR) at a 95% confidence interval. In all cases of a categorical variable comparison, a Chi-squared test was used. In the case of GI-RADS, categories 2 and 3 were considered low-risk, while categories 4 and 5 were considered high-risk. Histological diagnosis was used as a gold standard. Continuous variables, such as age, were assessed using a Mann-Whitney U test. For all analyses, $p < 0.05$ was considered significant.

Results

The study was based on the analysis of 215 unilateral adnexal tumors. The average age of the patients was

47.2 years old (range = 13–89). The average age of the patients in the malignant tumor group was significantly higher than that in the benign tumor group: 60 years (range 36–89) vs 43.1 years (range 13–84), respectively, with a p-value of < 0.001 for both groups. We found a total of 53 masses to be malignant (24.7% of all adnexal tumors). In the 215 tumors, 2 lesions were classified as GI-RADS 2 (0.9%), 118 lesions were GI-RADS 3 (54.9%), 86 lesions were GI-RADS 4 (40.0%) and 9 lesions were GI-RADS 5 (4.2%). Table 1 shows all GI-RADS categories with the corresponding histological results. According to the GI-RADS classification, we had 2 cases of ovarian cancer that were classified in the low-risk category 3 (Table 1), of which one was in an asymptomatic 80-year-old woman and the other was in a 42-year-old woman with menstrual irregularities.

For GI-RADS classifications 4 and 5, the sensitivity, specificity, PPV, NPV, ACC and OR values were as follows: 94.3, 72.2, 52.6, 97.5, 77.7% and 43.3, respectively (CI 12.0–146). For the GI-RADS classification combined with the CA-125 marker, the sensitivity, specificity, PPV, NPV, ACC and OR values were as follows: 66.0, 93.8, 77.8, 89.4, 87.0% and 29.6, respectively (CI 12.6–69.6, $p < 0.001$). For Ca-125 > 30 IU/mL alone, the sensitivity, specificity, PPV, NPV, ACC and OR values were as follows: 70.0, 80.3, 53.8, 89.1, 77.7% and 9.5, respectively (CI 4.6–19.6, $p < 0.0001$) (Table 2).

GI-RADS classification had the highest sensitivity of all methods used. The application of Ca-125 measurement as

Table 1 GI-RADS classification according to specific histopathologic diagnoses

Histopathology	GI-RADS				N	%	% of malignant	% benign
	2	3	4	5				
adenocarcinoma ovary	0	2	36	6	44	20.5%	83.0%	
carcinoma papillare	0	0	0	1	1	0.5%	1.9%	
cystadenofibroma serosum proliferans	0	0	1	1	2	0.9%	3.8%	
cystadenoma mucinosum proliferans	0	0	1	0	1	0.5%	1.9%	
cystadenoma proliferans	0	1	3	1	5	2.3%	9.4%	
corpus luteum	1	1	0	0	2	0.9%		1.2%
corpus luteum hemorrhagicum	0	1	1	0	2	0.9%		1.2%
cystadenofibroma	1	1	5	0	7	3.3%		4.3%
cystadenofibroma mucinosum	0	1	2	0	3	1.4%		1.9%
cystadenofibroma serosum	0	4	2	0	6	2.8%		3.7%
cystadenoma mucinosum	0	4	1	0	5	2.3%		3.1%
cystadenoma serosum	0	2	0	0	2	0.9%		1.2%
cystis benigna	0	0	1	0	1	0.5%		0.6%
cystis follicularis	0	2	1	0	3	1.4%		1.9%
cystis lueinisans	0	2	0	0	2	0.9%		1.2%
cystis serosa	0	16	6	0	22	10.2%		13.6%
cystis serosa paraovarialis	0	11	0	0	11	5.1%		6.8%
cystis serosa paraoviducti	0	1	0	0	1	0.5%		0.6%
cystis serosum	0	1	0	0	1	05%		0.6%
cystis simplex	0	3	0	0	3	1.4%		1.9%
dermoidalna	0	2	0	0	2	0.9%		1.2%
endometrioma	0	35	7	0	42	19.5%		25.9%
fibrothecoma	0	1	6	0	7	3.3%		4.3%
folliculoma	0	0	2	0	2	0.9%		1.2%
hydrosalpinx	0	1	1	0	2	0.9%		1.2%
myoma pedunculated	0	1	0	0	1	0.5%		0.6%
ovarian abscess	0	0	1	0	1	0.5%		0.6%
teratoma	0	25	9	0	34	15.8%		21.0%
All	2	118	86	9	215	100.0%	100.0%	100.0%

N – number of cases

Table 2 Statistical analysis of GI-RADS classification and levels of the ovarian malignancy marker CA-125

Descriptive Statistics	Sensitivity	Specificity	PPV	NPV	ACC	OR	OR 95% CI	p-value
GI-RADS + CA 125 > 30 IU/mL	66.0%	93.8%	77.8%	89.4%	87.0%	29.6	12.6–69.6	< 0.00001
GI-RADS 4–5	94.3%	72.2%	52.6%	97.5%	77.7%	43.3	12.9–14.6	< 0.0000
CA-125 > 30 IU/mL	70.0%	80.3%	53.8%	89.1%	77.7%	9.5	4.6–19.6	< 0.0000

IU/ml international units per milliliter, *ACC* accuracy, *PPV* positive predictive value, *NPV* negative predictive value, *OR* odds ratio, *CI* confidence interval

an additional differentiation criterion improved the specificity of GI-RADS: 93.8% (with CA-125) vs 72.2% (without). Other descriptive statistics also seemed to have improved as well: a PPV of 77.8% vs 52.6% and an accuracy of 87% vs 77.7% with and without Ca-125, respectively. Unfortunately, the odds ratio decreased by approximately 30%, from 43.3 to 29.6. However, the odds ratio was still considerably higher for the combined measure than for Ca-125 alone: 29.6 vs 9.5.

The percentage of malignant tumors in our study was quite high (24.7%). The most frequent histological manifestation was adenocarcinoma (44 cases), which constituted approximately 83% of all the malignant cases. There were two malignant tumors classified as GI-RADS 3 ("probably benign"), which comprised 3.77% of all malignant cases. We classified a total of 42 lesions as "probably malignant" or "very probably malignant", which corresponded to 36 cases of GI-RADS 4 (85.7%) and 6 cases of GI-RADS 5 (13.6%), respectively. Among the malignant ovarian tumors, we diagnosed 9 cases (20.5% of the malignant cases, and 3.7% of the adnexal masses).

Regarding symptoms, 47.8% of patients were symptom-free and the rest had back pain (36.5%), increased abdominal size (5.2%), menstrual irregularities (4.3%) and constipation (2.6%) (Table 3). In the low-risk group (GIRADS 1–3 and GIRADS 4 with CA-125 < 30 IU/mL),

we report 152 benign and 18 malignant cases. In the high-risk group (GIRADS 4 with CA-125 > 30 IU/mL and GIRADS 5), we report 10 benign and 35 malignant tumors (Table 4).

Discussion

We found that using GI-RADS classification is not an effective method for predicting the malignancy of ovarian tumors when combined with CA-125 level measurement. When the GI-RADS system is combined with CA-125 levels of > 30 IU/ml, we report low sensitivity and high specificity for malignancy discrimination (66.0 and 93.8%, respectively). We also found that for GI-RADS 4 and 5, GI-RADS had higher sensitivity but lower specificity than for lower GI-RADS classifications: 94.3 and 72.2%, respectively. The results regarding GI-RADS performance are similar to those published by Zhang et al., despite the fact that the authors did not analyze the CA-125 levels as an additional marker for malignancy discrimination [12]. Following Amor et al., we support the statement that the GI-RADS classification system is useful for clinical decision-making and patient management [11, 13]. Due to the progress in the image quality and resolution of transvaginal ultrasound, image scores improve the objectivity and accuracy of ovarian tumor diagnosis [13]. Furthermore, ovarian tumor morphology assessment is subjective and requires the training and experience of sonographers to maintain a high quality of performance [14]. GI-RADS classification was developed in 2009 to simplify communication between sonographers and clinicians/gynecologists [11]. It is suggested that GI-RADS 4 and 5 cases be referred to a gynecological oncologist due to the 20% risk of malignancy [13]. Moszynski et al. highlight that the GI-RADS classification is a subjective measure, especially in the case of tumors classified as GI-RADS 4, which are considered to be difficult to assess [14]. Although there are other methods and scoring systems

Table 3 Clinical symptoms of women with adnexal masses

Clinical symptoms	GI-RADS				N	%
	2	3	4	5		
Lack of symptoms	1	64	44	1	110	47.8%
Back pain	1	50	32	1	84	36.5%
Increased abdomen size	1	0	6	5	12	5.2%
Menstrual irregularities[a]	0	3	5	2	10	4.3%
Constipation	0	2	3	1	6	2.6%
Weight loss	0	0	2	0	2	0.9%
Pain during intercourse[b]	0	2	0	0	2	0.9%
Nausea	0	1	0	0	1	0.4%
Leg swelling	0	0	1	0	1	0.4%
Frequent urination	0	0	1	0	1	0.4%
Urinary retention	0	0	1	0	1	0.4%
All	3	122	95	10	230	100.0%

[a]only for premenopausal women, [b]for sexually active women; *N* – number of cases

Table 4 Diagnostic performance of GI-RADS classification with CA-125

GI-RADS	Benign	Malignant
GI-RADS 1–3 and GI-RADS 4 + CA-125 < 30 IU/mL	152	18
GI-RADS 4 + CA-125 > 30 IU/mL and GI-RADS 5	10	35
All	162	53

to distinguish between malignant and benign ovarian tumors, these methods have complex scoring and regression of ultrasonographic findings and require combining the ultrasonographic results with laboratory indexes [10, 12, 15, 16]. More data is needed, however, for GI-RADS classification performance when used by nonexpert examiners.

The assessment of biomarkers may be a more objective method suitable for less-experienced ultrasonographers [14]. CA-125 is the most popular and widely used ovarian cancer marker, but its effectiveness in terms of ovarian cancer differential diagnosis is questionable [1, 4, 17–21]. While CA-125 is quite accurate among postmenopausal women, its many false-positive results in premenopausal patients are a main limitation [22]. Our cutoff value for CA-125 levels was 30 IU/ml, which can explain the low sensitivity (70%). Niemi et al. report a CA-125 sensitivity of 59.4% with a cutoff of 35 kU/ml, whereas Wang et al., using the same cutoff value, report a sensitivity and specificity of 85.9 and 85.2%, respectively [18]. The main reason for the late-stage increase in the CA-125 serum concentration could be the molecular weight of the protein, 200–1000 kDa, compared to that of human epididymis protein 4 (HE4), which is 25 kDa. The other clinical implication is the lack of specificity of CA-125 in patients with endometriosis. Thus, it is easy to misdiagnose ovarian endometriosis as ovarian cancer, which can lead to significant physical and physiological harm inflicted to patients [23]. Koneczny et al. report that the IOTA group LR1 and GI-RADS performed well when used by either experienced or less-experienced operators of ultrasound systems [24]. For prognostic models such as GI-RADS, very high sensitivity (94.6%) and good specificity (75.5%) for examiners at level III and level II (72.7 and 87.8%, respectively) was reported. Nevertheless, in our study, we report that combining GI-RADS with CA-125 measurements can yield improved values for diagnostic parameters such as sensitivity, specificity, PPV, NPV, ACC and OR, which were 66.0, 93.8, 77.8, 89.4, 87.0% and 29.6, respectively. A study by Lycke et al. reported that in postmenopausal women, RMI (> 200), ROMA (>/=29.9), CA-125 (> 35 U/ml), and HE4 (> 140 pmol/l) showed a sensitivity of 89, 91, 92, and 72% and a specificity of 80, 77, 80, and 92%, respectively. In premenopausal women, the sensitivity of RMI, ROMA (>/=11.6), CA125, and HE4 (> 70 pmol/l) was 87, 87, 96, and 83%, and the specificity was 90, 81, 60, and 91% [25], respectively. These results suggest that CA125 is superior to HE4 as a biomarker to identify women with ovarian cancer. HE4 is better at identifying benign lesions, which may help with differential diagnoses to guide the level of care and decrease overtreatment [25].

In evaluating the symptoms, we noticed that 47.8% of all cases were actually symptom-free. If present,

symptoms were nonspecific, such as back pain (36.5%), while an increased abdominal size was typical for GI-RADS 4 and 5 cases. Pitta et al. reported good discrimination of tumors based on the Ward agglomerative method for hierarchical clustering using the following symptoms: abdominal bloating and/or increased abdominal size, back pain, leg swelling, eating (unable to eat, feeling full quickly), feeling of abdominal mass, miscellaneous (fatigue and or difficulty breathing), digestion (indigestion and/or nausea/vomiting), bladder (urinary urge and/or frequent urination), and in combination with CA-125, this guidance should facilitate decision making for primary care physicians [4, 26]. In our opinion, this promising data presented by Pitta et al. enhanced further prospective research.

Our study has some limitations. First, this study was a retrospective study. Second, this study was based on data from only one health center, yielding a rather small cohort and possible examiner bias. Third, in our study, we had 2 ovarian cancers classified as low-risk (GI-RADS 3), of which one case was in a symptomless 80-year-old patient and the other case was in a 42-year-old patient with menstrual irregularities.

In conclusion, the GI-RADS classification showed good performance in discriminating ovarian tumors. GI-RADS is considered a useful tool for the management of patients with an adnexal mass who are referred to a tertiary center. When combined with the measurement of CA-125, the test specificity, PPV and ACC for the assessment of preoperative adnexal tumors is improved. Future studies should seek clinically sensitive imaging diagnostic methods for ovarian pathologies to establish an integrated, relatively specific system for early warning of tumors.

Abbreviations

CA-125: cancer antigen 125; GI-RADS: Gynecology imaging reporting and data system

Acknowledgments

We thank all of the patients for participating in the study.

Funding

None.

Authors' contributions

MM, Project development, data collection, and manuscript writing; MB, data analysis; MSM, data analysis and manuscript editing; MK, data collection; GK, manuscript editing; and MM, manuscript editing. All authors read and approved the final manuscript.

Competing interests

The authors declare that they have no competing interests.

Author details

[1]Clinical Unit of Obstetrics, Women's Disease and Gynecological Oncology, sw. Jozefa 53/59, United District Hospital, Collegium Medicum University of Nicolaus Copernicus in Toruń, Torun, Poland. [2]Department of Diagnostic Imaging, Second Faculty of Medicine with the English Division and the Physiotherapy Division, Medical University of Warsaw, Warsaw, Poland. [3]Civis Vita Medical Center, Torun, Poland.

References

1. Terlikowska KM, Dobrzycka B, Witkowska AM, Mackowiak-Matejczyk B, Sledziewski TK, Kinalski M, Terlikowski SJ. Preoperative HE4, CA125 and ROMA in the differential diagnosis of benign and malignant adnexal masses. J Ovarian Res. 2016;9(1):43.

2. Reports based on data of National Cancer Registry. The Maria Sklodowska-Curie Memorial Cancer Center. Department of Epidemiology and Cancer Prevention NCRAfh. In.; 2013. http://epid.coi.waw.pl/krn. Accessed 23 Mar 2016.

3. Aebi S, Castiglione M, Group EGW. Newly and relapsed epithelial ovarian carcinoma: ESMO clinical recommendations for diagnosis, treatment and follow-up. Ann Oncol. 2009;20(Suppl 4):21–3.

4. Pitta Dda R, Sarian Lo Fau - Barreta A, Barreta A Fau - Campos EA, Campos Ea Fau - Andrade LLdA, Andrade Ll Fau - Fachini AMD, Fachini Am Fau - Campbell LM, Campbell Lm Fau - Derchain S, Derchain S. Symptoms, CA125 and HE4 for the preoperative prediction of ovarian malignancy in Brazilian women with ovarian masses. BMC Cancer. 2013;18(13):423. https://doi.org/10.1186/1471-2407-13-423.

5. Dong X, Men X, Zhang W, Lei P. Advances in tumor markers of ovarian cancer for early diagnosis. Indian J Cancer. 2014;51(Suppl 3):e72–6.

6. Zhang WY, Zhu LR, Zheng YH, Zhou L, Zhang JZ, Wu JH, Liao QP. Study for drug-resistance of epithelial ovarian cancer by serum protein profiling. Zhonghua Yi Xue Za Zhi. 2009;89(19):1326–9.

7. Lagana AS, Colonese F, Colonese E, Sofo V, Salmeri FM, Granese R, Chiofalo B, Ciancimino L, Triolo O. Cytogenetic analysis of epithelial ovarian cancer's stem cells: an overview on new diagnostic and therapeutic perspectives. Eur J Gynaecol Oncol. 2015;36(5):495–505.

8. Bellia A, Vitale SG, Lagana AS, Cannone F, Houvenaeghel G, Rua S, Ladaique A, Jauffret C, Ettore G, Lambaudie E. Feasibility and surgical outcomes of conventional and robot-assisted laparoscopy for early-stage ovarian cancer: a retrospective, multicenter analysis. Arch Gynecol Obstet. 2016;294(3):615–22.

9. American College of O, Gynecologists. ACOG practice bulletin. Management of adnexal masses. Obstet Gynecol. 2007;110(1):201–14.

10. Alcazar JL, Pascual MA, Graupera B, Auba M, Errasti T, Olartecoechea B, Ruiz-Zambrana A, Hereter L, Ajossa S, Guerriero S. External validation of IOTA simple descriptors and simple rules for classifying adnexal masses. Ultrasound Obstet Gynecol. 2016;48(3):397–402.

11. Amor F, Vaccaro H, Alcazar JL, Leon M, Craig JM, Martinez J. Gynecologic imaging reporting and data system: a new proposal for classifying adnexal masses on the basis of sonographic findings. J Ultrasound Med. 2009;28(3):285–91.

12. Zhang T, Li F, Liu J, Zhang S. Diagnostic performance of the gynecology imaging reporting and data system for malignant adnexal masses. Int J Gynaecol Obstet. 2017;137(3):325–31.

13. Amor F, Alcazar JL, Vaccaro H, Leon M, Iturra A. GI-RADS reporting system for ultrasound evaluation of adnexal masses in clinical practice: a prospective multicenter study. Ultrasound Obstet Gynecol. 2011;38(4):450–5.

14. Moszynski R, Szubert S, Szpurek D, Michalak S, Sajdak S. Role of osteopontin in differential diagnosis of ovarian tumors. J Obstet Gynaecol Res. 2013; 39(11):1518–25.

15. Timmerman D, Testa AC, Bourne T, Ameye L, Jurkovic D, Van Holsbeke C, Paladini D, Van Calster B, Vergote I, Van Huffel S, et al. Simple ultrasound-based rules for the diagnosis of ovarian cancer. Ultrasound Obstet Gynecol. 2008;31(6):681–90.

16. Araujo KG, Jales RM, Pereira PN, Yoshida A, de Angelo Andrade L, Sarian LO, Derchain S. Performance of the IOTA ADNEX model in preoperative discrimination of adnexal masses in a gynecological oncology center. Ultrasound Obstet Gynecol. 2017;49(6):778–83.

17. Zhang F, Zhang ZL. The diagnostic value of transvaginal Sonograph (TVS), color Doppler, and serum tumor marker CA125, CEA, and AFP in ovarian Cancer. Cell Biochem Biophys. 2015;72(2):353–7.

18. Wang J, Gao J, Yao H, Wu Z, Wang M, Qi J. Diagnostic accuracy of serum HE4, CA125 and ROMA in patients with ovarian cancer: a meta-analysis. Tumour Biol. 2014;35(6):6127–38.

19. Hartman CA, Juliato CR, Sarian LO, Toledo MC, Jales RM, Morais SS, Pitta DD, Marussi EF, Derchain S. Ultrasound criteria and CA 125 as predictive variables of ovarian cancer in women with adnexal tumors. Ultrasound Obstet Gynecol. 2012;40(3):360–6.

20. Eagle K, Ledermann JA. Tumor markers in ovarian malignancies. Oncologist. 1997;2(5):324–9.

21. Andersen MR, Goff BA, Lowe KA, Scholler N, Bergan L, Dresher CW, Paley P, Urban N. Combining a symptoms index with CA 125 to improve detection of ovarian cancer. Cancer. 2008;113(3):484–9.

22. Niemi RJ, Saarelainen SK, Luukkaala TH, Maenpaa JU. Reliability of preoperative evaluation of postmenopausal ovarian tumors. J Ovarian Res. 2017;10(1):15.

23. Zheng LE, Qu JY, He F. The diagnosis and pathological value of combined detection of HE4 and CA125 for patients with ovarian cancer. Open Med. 2016;11(1):125–32.

24. Koneczny J, Czekierdowski A, Florczak M, Poziemski P, Stachowicz N, Borowski D. The use of sonographic subjective tumor assessment, IOTA logistic regression model 1, IOTA simple rules and GI-RADS system in the preoperative prediction of malignancy in women with adnexal masses. Ginekol Pol. 2017;88(12):647–53.

25. Lycke M, Kristjansdottir B, Sundfeldt K. A multicenter clinical trial validating the performance of HE4, CA125, risk of ovarian malignancy algorithm and risk of malignancy index. Gynecol Oncol. 2018.

26. Goff B. Symptoms associated with ovarian cancer. Clin Obstet Gynecol. 2012;55(1):36–42.

19

Low fertility may be a significant determinant of ovarian cancer worldwide

Wenpeng You[1]*(iD), Ian Symonds[1] and Maciej Henneberg[1,2]

Abstract

Background: Ageing, socioeconomic level, obesity, fertility, relaxed natural selection and urbanization have been postulated as the risk factors of ovarian cancer (OC56). We sought to identify which factor plays the most significant role in predicting OC56 incidence rate worldwide.

Methods: Bivariate correlation analysis was performed to assess the relationships between country-specific estimates of ageing (measured by life expectancy), GDP PPP (Purchasing power parity), obesity prevalence, fertility (indexed by the crude birth rate), opportunity for natural selection (I_{bs}) and urbanization. Partial correlation was used to compare contribution of different variables. Fisher A-to-Z was used to compare the correlation coefficients. Multiple linear regression (Enter and Stepwise) was conducted to identify significant determinants of OC56 incidence. ANOVA with post hoc Bonferroni analysis was performed to compare differences between the means of OC56 incidence rate and residuals of OC56 standardised on fertility and GDP respectively between the six WHO regions.

Results: Bivariate analyses revealed that OC56 was significantly and strongly correlated to ageing, GDP, obesity, low fertility, I_{bs} and urbanization. However, partial correlation analysis identified that fertility and ageing were the only variables that had a significant correlation to OC56 incidence when the other five variables were kept statistically constant. Fisher A-to-Z revealed that OC56 had a significantly stronger correlation to low fertility than to ageing. Stepwise linear regression analysis only identified fertility as the significant predictor of OC56. ANOVA showed that, between the six WHO regions, multiple mean differences of OC56 incidence were significant, but all disappeared when the contributing effect of fertility on OC56 incidence rate was removed.

Conclusions: Low fertility may be the most significant determining predictor of OC56 incidence worldwide.

Keywords: Ovarian cancer, Low fertility, Oxytocin, Significant predictor, Family well-being

Background

Ovarian Cancer (OC56, abbreviated as per the International Classification of Diseases published by the WHO) [1] ranks among the top ten most commonly diagnosed cancers and top five deadliest cancers in most countries [2, 3]. In 2015, OC56 was present in 1.2 million women and resulted in 161,100 deaths worldwide [4] . In the twenty-first century, a woman's overall lifetime risk of developing OC56 is around 1.6% [2, 5, 6], and her chance of dying of the disease is 1 in 100 [2, 6].

Although OC56 has been known to medical scientists for over 150 years [7], the aetiology of this lethal disease is not well understood. Most research on the aetiology of OC56 has focused on genetic and environmental carcinogenic factors, such as talc, pesticides, red meat and alcohol in diet, smoking, and herbicides. However, to date, none of these factors has been consistently shown to be a major risk factor for the development of OC56 [8]. Alternative hypotheses for the aetiology of the disease have also been suggested. Several studies have suggested that,

* Correspondence: wenpeng.you@adelaide.edu.au
[1]Adelaide Medical School, The University of Adelaide, Adelaide, SA, Australia
Full list of author information is available at the end of the article

obese women (those with a body mass index of at least 30 kg/m^2) may have a greater risk of developing OC56 because of their elevated levels of circulating estrogen [9–11]. An accumulation of somatic mutations has been suggested as the mechanism for the higher incidence of the disease in women over the age of 45 [9]. Urbanization may have improved public hygiene, sanitation and access to health care for women [12], but it has been associated with public health issues, including OC56 [13] due to the changes in occupational, dietary and exercise patterns [6, 12, 14, 15].

Natural selection, as one of the key mechanisms of evolution, differentiates phenotypes' survival and/or fertility that reflect genetic differences. The Biological State Index (I_{bs}) has been constructed to measure the opportunity for natural selection through differential mortality at the population level. The I_{bs} calculation combines life table function d_x (number of deaths at age x) with the age-specific completed relative fertility rate s_x (fraction of total fertility rate to a woman up to age x): $I_{bs} = 1 - \Sigma d_x s_x$ [16–21]. I_{bs} can be used as a way of measuring the opportunity for an individual born into a given population to pass on its genes to the next generation [17, 19, 22–24]. I_{bs} has been postulated to reflect changes in the mutation-selection balance as a result of the effect of improved healthcare on relaxing natural selection and thus measure the magnitude of accumulation of the deleterious genes [16], including those responsible for cancers such as OC56 [17], type 1 diabetes [18] and obesity [18, 19] in human populations.

The association between low fertility and OC56 risk has been well described and it has been postulated that this risk increases in women who have ovulated less over their lifetime either through infertility or administering the combined birth controls, such as contraceptive pills [6, 25–32].

To the best of our knowledge, despite that low fertility is a well-established risk factor for OC56, no research has compared the contributing effects of fertility to OC56 with other OC56 risk factors, such as ageing, I_{bs} (index of magnitude of OC56 genes accumulation in human populations), obesity and socioeconomic factors (GDP and urbanization).

There is significant variation in the incidence of OC56 between different geographic regions globally [2, 3, 33–35]. This phenomenon has also been observed in different populations [6, 13] within the same countries [36, 37]. A number of publications suggest that the disparity between regions and populations is related to socioeconomic level.

In this study, empirical macro-level data have been used to test the hypothesis that fertility (measured by the crude birth rate) is the principal determinant of developing OC56, and that it is fertility, instead of GDP, that is most important factor in shaping the regional variation of OC56 incidence rate.

Methods
Data sources
The following country specific data published by the agencies of the United Nations were analysed for this study.

1. The GLOBOCAN 2012 estimates of incidence rate of female OC56 [34].

GLOBOCAN provides contemporary population level estimates by cancer site and sex [2]. This project is conducted by the WHO research agency, the International Agency for Research on Cancer (IARC).

OC56 incidence rate is expressed as the number per 100,000 females who were diagnosed with OC56 in 2012. The age-standardized OC56 incidence rate was selected in the interest of the data comparability between countries.

2. The World Bank published data on crude birth rate, per capita GDP PPP and urbanization [38]

Crude birth rate (CBR) indicates the number of live births occurring during the year, per 1000 population estimated at midyear. CBR was used to index the fertility in this study over a 20 year period (1992) to reflect long exposure with delayed presentation of OC56. Terms "birth rate" and "fertility" are interchangeable in this paper.

Socio-economic level has been associated with OC56 risk [2, 34, 39, 40]. We chose per capita GDP purchasing power rate (GDP PPP in 2012 international $) because it takes into account the relative cost of local goods, services and inflation rates of the country.

Urbanization has been postulated as a major OC56 predictor [41, 42] because it represents the major demographic shift entailing lifestyle changes [12, 43, 44]. Urbanization is expressed with the country-specific percentage of total population living in urban areas in 2012.

3. The United Nations statistics division estimates of the life expectancy [45]

Country-specific life expectancy, which reflects ageing, has been well established to be correlated with OC56 incidence [46, 47]. Therefore, we selected life expectancy of older people (e_{65}, 2005–2010) [45] to index the ageing process at population level.

4. The magnitude of OC56 gene accumulation in a population indexed with the biological state index (I_{bs})

The country specific I_{bs} was downloaded from the previous publication [19]. It has been postulated that reduced natural selection (measured by I_{bs}) may have allowed accumulation of deleterious genes of non-communicable diseases [17–19], such as OC56 [17].

5. The WHO Global Health Observatory (GHO) data on obesity prevalence

Obese females may be at greater risk of developing OC56 than those who are not obese [48]. The country-specific percentage of the females aged 18+ with a BMI ≥ 30 kg/m^2 in 2010 was extracted from the GHO data repository [49].

Data selection
Country specific OC56 incidence rates, ageing, fertility, GDP, I$_{bs}$, obesity and urbanization were collated for all countries where data were available. We extracted OC56 incidence rates for 182 countries and then the other variables were matched individually with OC56.

Each country was treated as an individual study subject in the data analysis. Not all the countries (subjects) had information for all the variables.

The relevant United Nations agencies offer free online access to data required for the analyses in this study. No ethics approval was required as there were no individual patients involved in the study.

Data multicollinearity check
In order to avoid the inter-correlation between predictor variables, the multicollinearity statistics were calculated to test the correlations among the variables. Each variable was alternated as the dependent variable, and all the others were considered as the predictor variables in our analysis with the regression model. It was found that the collinearities between variables were not significant since only the tolerance of less than 0.20 and a VIF of more than 5 indicates a multicollinearity problem [50]. Values in our study were more than 0.20 and less than 5 respectively. Details are provided in Additional file 1.

Data analysis
To assess the population level determinants of OC56, the analysis proceeded in five steps.

1. Scatter plots were produced with the original data in Microsoft Excel® to explore and visualize the strength, shape and direction of correlations of OC56 to fertility and GDP respectively.
2. Data were logarithmed to improve their homoscedasticity for linear regression analyses. Bivariate (Pearson's r and nonparametric Spearman's rho) correlations were performed to evaluate the direction and strength of the correlations between all the variables of all the subjects and effects possible effects of non-normality of distributions on the strength of moment-product correlations.
3. Partial correlation analysis of Pearson's moment-product approach was performed. We alternated each of the six variables (ageing, fertility, GDP, I$_{bs}$, obesity and urbanization) as the independent predictor when all other five variables were included as the potential confounding factors. Fisher's r-to-z transformation was applied to assess the significance level of difference between pairs of correlation coefficients.
4. Standard multiple linear regression (enter) was performed to describe the correlations between the dependent variable (OC56) and the predicting variables. In order to explore if low fertility can partially explain why ageing, GDP, I$_{bs}$, obesity and urbanization are correlated with OC56, the enter multiple linear regression was performed to determine the correlations between OC56 incidence and the risk factors in two models: (1) when fertility was incorporated; and (2) excluded as a predicting variable Subsequently, standard multiple linear regression (Stepwise) was performed to select the predicting variable (s) which have the greatest influence on OC56 in two versions: (1) when fertility was incorporated and (2) excluded as a predicting variable.
5. The equations of the best fitting non-linear trendlines displayed in the scatter plots analysis of relationships between OC56 incidence and fertility ($y = 0.006 \times x^2 - 0.504x + 14.816$, $R^2 = 0.485$) and GDP PPP ($y = 0.7167x + 0.2225$, $R^2 = 0.2571$) were used to calculate and remove the contributing effects of GDP PPP on OC56 incidence rate respectively by using regressions of OC56 residuals around fertility and GDP PPP. This allowed us to create two new dependent variables, "Residual of OC56 standardised on fertility" and "Residual of OC56 standardised on GDP PPP"

Means of the OC56 incidence rate, the "Residuals of OC56 standardised on fertility" and "Residuals of OC56 standardised on GDP PPP" of all the countries were calculated for mean difference comparisons.

Analysis of variance (ANOVA) was conducted to detect the significant differences among the means of OC56 incidence rate, "Residual of OC56 standardised on fertility" and "Residual of OC56 standardised on GDP PPP" between the six WHO regions [51]. Further post-hoc (Bonferroni) tests were performed to identify the source (pairs) of significant differences.

Bivariate correlations, multiple linear regression analysis (Enter and Stepwise) and ANOVA were conducted with SPSS v. 24. The raw data were used for calculation of mean OC56 incidence rate and "Residual of OC56 standardised on fertility" and "Residual of OC56 standardised on GDP PPP". The significance was kept at the 0.05 level, but 0.01 and 0.001 levels were also reported. Standard multiple linear regression analysis criteria were set at probability of F to enter ≤0.05 and probability of F to remove ≥0.10.

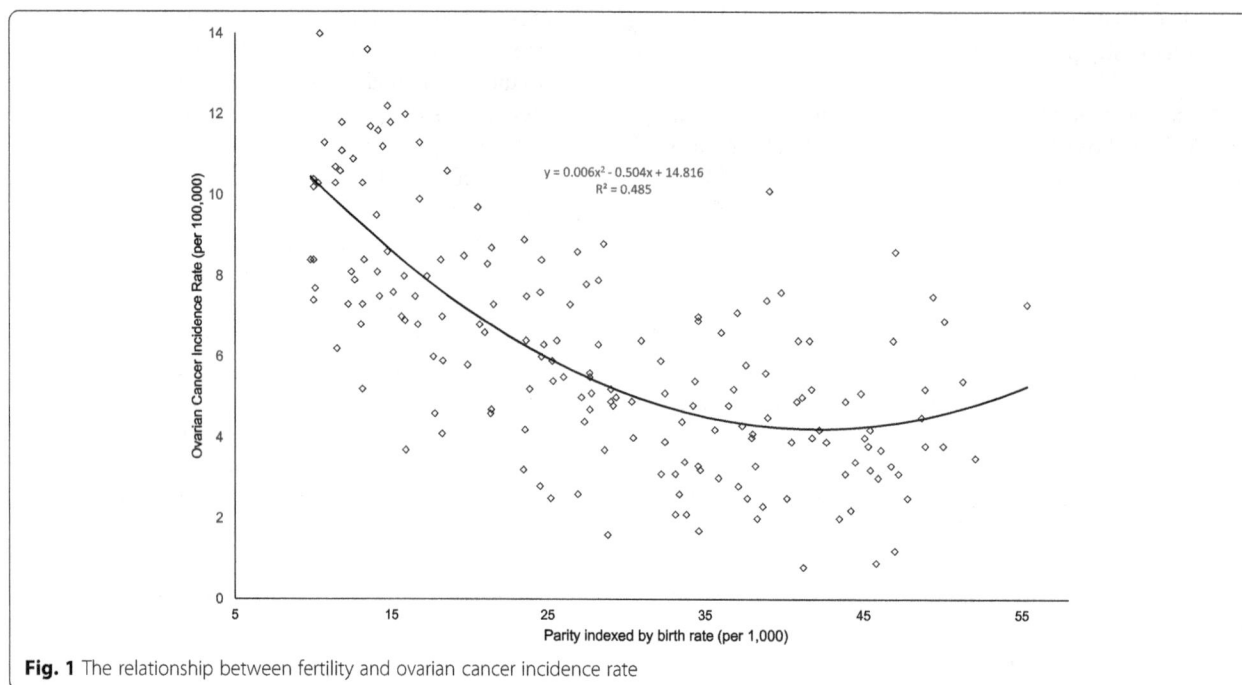

Fig. 1 The relationship between fertility and ovarian cancer incidence rate

Results

The relationship identified in the scatterplots between fertility and OC56 was noted to be polynomial with a strong, but inverse (negative) correlation ($R^2 = 0.485$, $p < 0.001$, $n = 179$, Fig. 1).

The strong relationship between fertility and OC56 identified in the scatterplots was confirmed by the subsequent nonparametric and Pearson r analyses based on the log-transformed data.

Globally, fertility was significantly and negatively correlated to OC56 incidence ($r = -0.632$ and rho = -0.655, $p < 0.001$ respectively in Pearson and non-parametric analyses) (Table 1).

It is also found that ageing, GDP, I_{bs}, obesity and urbanization had strong and significant correlations to OC56 incidence in both Pearson and non-parametric analyses respectively (Table 1).

The relationship between OC56 and each independent variable (ageing, fertility, GDP, I_{bs}, obesity and urbanization) was tested by keeping the other five variables statistically constant in partial correlation analysis. Fertility was the only predictor showing a substantial significant correlation ($r = -0.448$, $p < 0.001$) with OC56 independent of the other five variables (Table 2). Ageing showed significant, but weak correlation to OC56 ($r = -0.178$, $p < 0.05$). The Fisher r-to-z transformation revealed that OC56 was in significant stronger correlation with fertility than with ageing ($z = 2.68$, $p < 0.01$). GDP, I_{bs}, obesity and urbanization showed significant correlation to OC56 in the bivariate correlation analyses respectively. However, none of

Table 1 Pearson r (above the diagonal) and nonparametric "rho" (below the diagonal) correlation between all variables

	OC56	Ageing	Fertility	GDP	Ibs	Obesity	Urbanization
OC56	1	0.394***	−0.632***	0.507***	0.455***	0.189*	0.280***
Ageing	0.428***	1	−0.737***	0.748***	0.766***	0.322***	0.570***
Fertility	−0.655***	−0.769***	1	−0.772***	−0.712***	−0.338***	−0.557***
GDP PPP	0.531***	0.759***	−0.813***	1	0.742**	0.485***	0.713***
Ibs	0.602***	0.849***	−0.883***	0.858***	1	0.457***	0.551***
Obesity	0.169*	0.350***	−0.377***	0.453***	0.409***	1	0.484***
Urbanization	0.345***	0.657***	−0.628***	0.781***	0.711***	0.506***	1

The table shows the bivariate correlation between all the variables. *** $p < 0.001$; Country number: 167–182
Ovarian cancer (OC56) incidence rate is from the International Agency for Research on Cancer. Birth rate indexing fertility, GDP PPP and urbanization are from the World Bank. Ageing expressed as life expectancy (e_{65}) is from the United Nations. Obesity prevalence is from the World Health Organization
Biological State Index (I_{bs}) was downloaded from previous publications, which were calculated with the data of the world fertility form the UN Population Council and the WHO life tables

Table 2 Comparison of partial correlation coefficients between ovarian cancer incidence and each variable when the other five variables are controlled for

Variables	Fertility			Ageing			GDP			I_{bs}			Obesity			Urbanization		
	r	P	Df	R	p	df	r	p	df	r	p	df	r	p	df	r	p	df
Fertility	−0.448	< 0.001	160	–	–	–	–	–	–	–	–	–	–	–	–	–	–	–
Ageing	–	–	–	−0.178	0.023	160	–	–	–	–	–	–	–	–	–	–	–	–
GDP	–	–	–	–	–	–	0.148	0.060	160	–	–	–	–	–	–	–	–	–
I_{bs}	–	–	–	–	–	–	–	–	–	0.079	0.315	160	–	–	–	–	–	–
Obesity	–	–	–	–	–	–	–	–	–	–	–	–	−0.048	0.544	160	–	–	–
Urbanization	–	–	–	–	–	–	–	–	–	–	–	–	–	–	–	−0.131	0.095	160

The table shows partial correlations between Ovarian cancer (OC56) incidence between each variable while the other four variables are controlled for. - Controlled variable Ovarian cancer (OC56) incidence rate is from the International Agency for Research on Cancer. Fertility indexed by birth rate, GDP PPP and urbanization are from the World Bank. Ageing expressed as life expectancy (e_{65}) is from the United Nations. Obesity prevalence is from the World Health Organization Biological State Index (I_{bs}) was downloaded from previous publications, which were calculated with the data of the world fertility form the UN Population Council and the WHO life tables

these variables showed a significant correlation with OC56 independent of the other five predictors. This indicates that fertility is the only significant predictor of OC56 independent of the secondary association between OC56 incidence and I_{bs} (magnitude of OC56 accumulation) and environmental factors (ageing, fertility, GDP, obesity and urbanization).

Standard multiple linear regression (enter) analysis was applied to predict OC56 incidence when ageing, fertility, GDP, obesity and urbanization were included as the independent predicting variables.

When fertility was excluded as one of the independent variables, GDP PPP ($\beta = 0.471$, $p < 0.001$) and I_{bs} ($\beta = 0.250$, $p < 0.05$) were the two significant variables related to OC56 incidence. However, when fertility was included as an independent predictor, only the correlation between fertility and OC56 incidence was strong and significant. None of the other five predictors showed strong and significant correlation to OC56 (Table 3). Similarly, in a stepwise linear regression model, when fertility was not included as one of the

Table 3 Independent predictors of ovarian cancer incidence rate based on multiple linear regression modelling (Enter)

Variable	β	Std. Error	Sig.	β	Std. Error	Sig.
Fertility	–	–	–	−0.694	0.111	< 0.001
Ageing	−0.037	0.341	0.752	−0.207	0.309	0.052
GDP	0.471	0.055	< 0.001	0.163	0.052	0.174
I_{bs}	0.250	0.658	0.032	0.100	0.589	0.342
Overweight	−0.056	0.069	0.496	− 0.020	0.060	0.778
Urbanization	−0.122	0.105	0.211	−0.125	0.092	0.146

The table describes the multiple linear regression analysis (Enter) results including and excluding fertility as a predictor of breast cancer. df = 164; − excluded variable
Ovarian cancer (OC56) incidence rate is from the International Agency for Research on Cancer. Fertility indexed by birth rate, GDP PPP and urbanization are from the World Bank. Ageing expressed as life expectancy (e_{65}) is from the United Nations. Obesity prevalence is from the World Health Organization Biological State Index (I_{bs}) was downloaded from previous publications, which were calculated with the data of the world fertility form the UN Population Council and the WHO life tables

independent predictors, GDP and I_{bs} were selected as the variables having the greatest influence on the development of OC56. However, when fertility was included together with the other five independent variables, only fertility was selected as the most influential predictor of OC56 with the R^2 increase from 0.278 to 0.434. This suggested that GDP and I_{bs} did not appear to account for the major part of the impact on OC56 incidence. This finding supports our previous suggestion that fertility is the significant predictor of OC56 incidence in partial correlation analysis.

Table 4 showed that the mean OC56 incidence rate was lowest in Africa (4.19) and highest in Europe (8.70). The means of OC56 in the other four regions were 5.89 (Americas), 5.19 (Eastern Mediterranean), 5.90 (South East Asia) and 6.63 (Western Pacific). A post hoc Bonferroni analysis conducted on the multiple comparisons of means revealed that there were a number of significant differences in mean OC56 incidence rates between different WHO regions (Table 4). Mean of OC56 incidence in Europe was significantly greater than in Africa, Americas, East Mediterranean, South East Asia and West Pacific. Mean of OC56 in Americas was significantly greater than in Africa. The regions with greater means of fertility had lower means of OC56 incidence rates ($r = 0.985$, $p < 0.001$, $n = 6$).

A subsequent ANOVA with post hoc Bonferroni procedure performed on the means of "Residual of OC56 standardised on fertility" in different WHO regions showed there was no significant difference among and between regions (Table 4). Whilst the same procedure was performed on the means of "Residual of OC56 standardised on GDP PPP", the developed region, Europe still had the significantly higher "Residual of OC56 standardised on GDP PPP" than Africa, Americas and East Mediterranean (Table 4). The results from the post hoc Bonferroni tests conducted on comparisons between the WHO regions suggested that regional variations of OC56 incidence may only reach statistically significant levels if the contributing effect of their respective

Table 4 Comparison of mean differences of fertility, residuals of ovarian cancer (OC56) standardised on fertility and GDP PPP respectively between WHO regions

OC56 incidence rate			Residual of OC56 standardised on fertility			Residual of OC56 standardised on GDP		
I n Mean	J	Mean difference (I-J)	I n Mean	J	Mean difference (I-J)	I n Mean	J	Mean difference (I-J)
AF n = 46 Mean = 4.19	AM	−1.70*	AF n = 45 Mean = −0.29	AM	−0.16	AF n = 44 Mean = −0.15	AM	−0.03
	EM	−0.99		EM	−0.29		EM	1.03
	EU	−4.50***		EU	−0.30		EU	−2.15***
	SEA	−1.71		SEA	−0.67		SEA	−1.02
	WP	−2.44**		WP	−0.81		WP	−0.98
AM, n = 31 Mean = 5.89	AF	1.69*	AM n = 31 Mean = −0.13	AF	0.16	AM n = 29 Mean = −0.12	AF	0.03
	EM	0.70		EM	−0.13		EM	1.06
	EU	−2.81***		EU	−0.15		EU	−2.12**
	SEA	−0.01		SEA	−0.52		SEA	−0.99
	WP	−0.74		WP	−0.65		WP	−0.95
EM n = 22 Mean = 5.19	AF	0.99	EM n = 21 Mean = 0.001	AF	0.29	EM n = 18 Mean = −1.18	AF	−1.03
	AM	−0.70		AM	0.13		AM	−1.06
	EU	−3.51***		EU	−0.01		EU	−3.18***
	SEA	−0.71		SEA	−0.38		SEA	−2.05
	WP	−1.45		WP	−0.52		WP	−2.01
EU n = 50 Mean = 8.70	AF	4.50***	EU n = 49 Mean = 0.14	AF	0.30	EU n = 50 Mean = 2.00	AF	2.15***
	AM	2.81***		AM	0.15		AM	2.12**
	EM	3.51***		EM	0.01		EM	3.18***
	SEA	2.80*		SEA	−0.37		SEA	1.13
	WP	2.06*		WP	−0.50		WP	1.17
SEA n = 11 Mean = 5.90	AF	1.71	SEA n = 11 Mean = 0.38	AF	0.67	SEA n = 10 Mean = 0.87	AF	1.02
	AM	0.01		AM	0.52		AM	0.99
	EM	0.71		EM	0.38		EM	2.05
	EU	−2.80*		EU	0.37		EU	−1.13
	WP	−0.73		WP	−0.13		WP	0.04
WP n = 22 Mean = 6.63	AF	2.44**	WP n = 21 Mean = −0.01	AF	0.81	WP n = 19 Mean = 0.83	AF	0.98
	AM	0.74		AM	0.65		AM	0.95
	EM	1.45		EM	0.52		EM	2.01
	EU	−2.06*		EU	0.50		EU	−1.17
	SEA	0.73		SEA	0.13		SEA	−0.04

The mean difference comparison results conducted with One-way ANOVA Post hoc Bonferroni are reported. *$p < 0.05$, **$p < 0.01$, ***$p < 0.001$

Ovarian cancer (OC56) incidence rate is from the International Agency for Research on Cancer. Fertility indexed by birth rate, GDP PPP and urbanization are from the World Bank. Ageing expressed as life expectancy (e_{65}) is from the United Nations. Obesity prevalence is from the World Health Organization

Biological State Index (I_{bs}) was downloaded from previous publications, which were calculated with the data of the world fertility form the UN Population Council and the WHO life tables

fertility was included. In other words, except for fertility, the total contribution of the other OC56 risk factors to OC56 incidence may not be sufficient for the difference in mean rates to reach significance level. This result was supported by the findings identified in our previous partial correlation (Table 2) and multiple linear regression analyses (Table 3) that fertility is the critical risk factor for OC56.

Discussion

The worldwide secular trend of increased OC56 incidence may have multiple etiologies, which may act through multiple mechanisms at different magnitudes. By examining the correlations of OC56 with low fertility, ageing, GDP, I_{bs}, obesity and urbanization respectively, this study has shown that only fertility and aging were correlated with the OC56 incidence significantly, although the latter was not as strongly. Statistically, this may suggest that low fertility was the most significant risk factor for OC56 when compared to ageing, GDP, I_{bs}, obesity and urbanization. This finding is in agreement with three studies conducted by Hankinson et al. [32], Vachon et al. [31] and Cramer et al. [52] respectively which concluded that fertility is a significantly greater predictor of OC56 risk than other commonly used epidemiological variables.

The relationship between female reproductive performance and gynecological cancers has been known for over 300 years [30, 53]. Previous studies in multiple different populations have shown that nulliparous women have a 30–60% greater risk than parous women [52, 54]. Studies also reported that each additional full-term pregnancy lowers OC56 risk by approximately 15% [54, 55]. The mechanism of the influence of childbearing on reducing OC56 risk may be that full-term pregnancy, post-partum period and sometimes the subsequent lactation involve anovulation, suppress secretion of pituitary gonadotropins, lower levels of oestrogen [56–59], lessen exposure of the ovaries to chronic inflammation and mutation [60], and reduce proliferation of malignant transformations in the inclusion cysts and clefts which are invaginated and formed in the ovarian epithelium during ovulation [61].

Recent studies suggested that women with greater fertility may receive the protection against developing OC56 because:

1) They may produce more oxytocin [62–69] due to positive interactions between family members, especially those between spouses [64, 65, 70, 71]. Oxytocin may inhibit the progression of human ovarian carcinoma cells [28, 29].
2) They may have less stress due to more positive psychological well-being from greater family size, reduces stress levels. This may make their neuroendocrine and immune systems more efficient to reduce the risk of cancer (developing OC56) [72–75].
3) They are more likely to seek health service and maintain a healthy lifestyle [76–79], which may have their developing OC56 diagnosed earlier and removed in time.

This study revealed that low fertility determines the variation of OC56 incidence rate among the WHO regions. This finding contradicts the WHO and IARC's statement that socioeconomic level is the determinant of regional variation of OC56 incidence rate [2, 6, 34]. This may suggest that the correlation between fertility and socioeconomic status (SES) is spurious – caused by the correlation of both variables (SES and OC56 incidence) to the same one (fertility) [80–82].

The strength of this study is that it uses an ecological study approach, different from hitherto used approaches, to demonstrate that low fertility is a significant determinant of OC56 risk.

We need to note several limitations of this study:

1) Each country was considered as a whole subject for the ecological study. The country-specific data included in this study may be different from those collected from individual participants. Therefore, the correlations identified from the data analysis may not hold true for all the individuals to have the risk in OC56 development.
2) There may be some random errors that occurred when the United Nations and its agencies collected and aggregated data at country level. Data from developed countries may be more complete than those from developing countries.
3) There are different categories of OC56, but we could not differentiate them for the correlation analysis due to the unavailability of such data.

Conclusion

Low fertility appears to be a significant and strong determinant of OC56 risk independent of ageing, GDP, I_{bs}, obesity and urbanization. These findings may be helpful for governments, policy-makers, funders, clinicians and researchers when determining future screening and primary presentation strategies for the disease [32, 83, 84].

Abbreviations

FAO: The Food and Agriculture Organization of the United Nations; GDP PPP: Gross domestic product purchasing power parity; IARC: International Agency for Research on Cancer; I_{bs}: Biological State Index; OC56: Ovarian Cancer; UN: The United Nations; WHO: World Health Organization

Acknowledgments

The authors express appreciation to Jacques Ferlay from the International Agency for Research on Cancer of World Health Organization for his assistance in locating and defining the data.

Funding

The authors wish to thank the Mäxi Foundation, Switzerland for supporting this research.

Authors' contributions

WY conceived the hypothesis, and IS and MH consolidated the hypothesis. WY and MH conducted data analysis. All authors interpreted the data analysis results. IS and MH provided suggestions for WY to draft the manuscript. All authors reviewed, edited and approved the final manuscript.

Competing interests

The authors declare no competing of interest.

Author details

[1]Adelaide Medical School, The University of Adelaide, Adelaide, SA, Australia.
[2]Institute of Evolutionary Medicine, University of Zürich, 8057 Zurich, Switzerland.

References

1. IARC. Cancer. 2017 22 December 2017]; Available from: http://globocan.iarc.fr/Pages/cancer.aspx.

2. Ferlay J, et al. Cancer incidence and mortality worldwide: sources, methods and major patterns in GLOBOCAN 2012. Int J Cancer. 2015;136(5):E359–86.

3. Ferlay J, et al. Estimates of worldwide burden of cancer in 2008: GLOBOCAN 2008. Int J Cancer. 2010;127(12):2893–917.

4. Vos T, et al. Global, regional, and national incidence, prevalence, and years lived with disability for 310 diseases and injuries, 1990–2015: a systematic analysis for the global burden of disease study 2015. Lancet. 2016; 388(10053):1545–602.

5. Seiden MV. In: Longo DL KD, Jameson JL, Fauci AS, Hauser SL, Harrison LJ, editors. Gynecologic malignancies, in principles of internal medicine (18th ed.). New York: McGraw-Hill; 2012.

6. Reid BM, Permuth JB, Sellers TA. Epidemiology of ovarian cancer: a review. Cancer Biology & Medicine. 2017;14(1):9.

7. Vargas AN. Natural history of ovarian cancer. ecancermedicalscience. 2014;8:465.

8. The American Cancer Society. Do we know what causes ovarian Cancer? 2017; Available from: https://www.cancer.org/cancer/ovarian-cancer/causes-risks-prevention/what-causes.html.

9. Australian Government- Cancer Australia. What are the risk factors for ovarian cancer? 2017; Available from: https://ovarian-cancer.canceraustralia.gov.au/risk-factors.

10. Rodriguez C, et al. Body mass index, height, and the risk of ovarian cancer mortality in a prospective cohort of postmenopausal women. Cancer Epidemiology and Prevention Biomarkers. 2002;11(9):822–8.

11. Cauley JA, et al. The epidemiology of serum sex hormones in postmenopausal women. Am J Epidemiol. 1989;129(6):1120–31.

12. Allender S, et al. Quantification of urbanization in relation to chronic diseases in developing countries: a systematic review. J Urban Health. 2008;85(6):938–51.

13. Huang Z, et al. Incidence and mortality of gynaecological cancers: secular trends in urban shanghai, China over 40 years. Eur J Cancer. 2016;63:1–10.

14. Zhang X, Nicosia SV, Bai W. Vitamin D receptor is a novel drug target for ovarian cancer treatment. Curr Cancer Drug Targets. 2006;6(3):229–44.

15. Jordan SJ, et al. Does smoking increase risk of ovarian cancer? A systematic review. Gynecol Oncol. 2006;103(3):1122–9.

16. Stephan CN, Henneberg M. Medicine may be reducing the human capacity to survive. Med Hypotheses. 2001;57(5):633–7.

17. You W, H. M. Cancer incidence increasing globally: The role of relaxed natural selection. Evol Appl. 2017;00:1–13.

18. You W, Henneberg M. Relaxed natural selection contributes to global obesity increase more in males than in females due to more environmental modifications in female body mass. PloS one. 2018;13(7):e0199594.

19. Budnik A, Henneberg M. Worldwide increase of obesity is related to the reduced opportunity for natural selection. PLoS One. 2017;12(1):e0170098.

20. Henneberg M, Piontek J. Biological state index of human groups. Przeglad Anthropologiczny. 1975;XLI:191–201.

21. Henneberg M. Reproductive possibilities and estimations of the biological dynamics of earlier human populations. J Hum Evol. 1976;5:41–8.

22. You W, Henneberg M. Type 1 diabetes prevalence increasing globally and regionally: the role of natural selection and life expectancy at birth. BMJ Open Diabetes Research and Care. 2016;4(1):e000161.

23. You W, et al. Decreasing birth rate determining worldwide incidence and regional variation of female breast Cancer. Advances in Breast Cancer Research. 2018;07(01):1–14.

24. Staub K, et al. Increasing variability of body mass and health correlates in Swiss conscripts, a possible role of relaxed natural selection? Evol Med Public Health. 2018;2018(1):116–26. (accepted April 23, 2018)

25. Cancer Research UK. Ovarian cancer risks and causes. [Document] 2016 28/07/2016 13:29 20.08.2016]; Available from: http://www.cancerresearchuk.org.

26. McLemore MR, et al. Epidemiologic and genetic factors associated with ovarian cancer. Cancer Nurs. 2009;32(4):281.

27. Fraumeni JF, et al. Cancer mortality among nuns: role of marital status in etiology of neoplastic disease in women. J Natl Cancer Inst. 1969;42(3):455–68.

28. Imanieh MH, et al. Oxytocin has therapeutic effects on cancer, a hypothesis. Eur J Pharmacol. 2014;741:112–23.

29. Morita T, et al. Oxytocin inhibits the progression of human ovarian carcinoma cells in vitro and in vivo. Int J Cancer. 2004;109(4):525–32.

30. Britt K, Short R. The plight of nuns: hazards of nulliparity. Lancet. 2012; 379(9834):2322–3.

31. Vachon CM, et al. Association of parity and ovarian cancer risk by family history of breast or ovarian cancer in a population-based study of postmenopausal women. Epidemiology. 2002;13(1):66–71.

32. Hankinson SE, et al. A prospective study of reproductive factors and risk of epithelial ovarian cancer. Cancer. 1995;76(2):284–90.

33. Jayson GC, et al. Ovarian cancer. Lancet. 2014;384(9951):1376–88.

34. Ferlay, J., et al. GLOBOCAN 2012 v1.0, Cancer Incidence and Mortality Worldwide: IARC CancerBase No. 11 [Internet]. 2013 28.05.2016); Available from: http://globocan.iarc.fr.

35. Jemal A, et al. Global cancer statistics. CA Cancer J Clin. 2011;61(2):69–90.

36. Wei K, et al. Ovary cancer incidence and mortality in China, 2011. Chin J Cancer Res. 2015;27(1):38.

37. Horner M, et al. National Cancer Institute. Bethesda. MD. 1975-2006;2009

38. The World Bank Group. World Bank Open Data. 2016 12.07.2016]; Available from: http://data.worldbank.org/.

39. Ness RB, et al. Racial differences in ovarian cancer risk. J Natl Med Assoc. 2000;92(4):176.

40. Bertone-Johnson ER. Epidemiology of ovarian cancer: a status report. Lancet. 2005;365(9454):101–2.

41. Jin F, et al. Incidence trends for cancers of the breast, ovary, and corpus uteri in urban shanghai, 1972–89. Cancer Causes Control. 1993;4(4):355–60.

42. Lefkowitz ES, Garland CF. Sunlight, vitamin D, and ovarian cancer mortality rates in US women. Int J Epidemiol. 1994;23(6):1133–6.

43. Moore M, Gould P, Keary BS. Global urbanization and impact on health. Int J Hyg Environ Health. 2003;206(4):269–78.

44. WHO. Urbanization and health. WHO 2010 2010–12–07 15:20:05 2 November 2016]; Available from: http://www.who.int/bulletin/volumes/88/4/10-010410/en/.

45. United Nations, Department of Economic and Social Affairs, Population Division. World Population Prospects: The 2012 Revision, DVD Edition. 2013.

46. John EM, et al. Characteristics relating to ovarian cancer risk: collaborative analysis of seven US case-control studies. Epithelial ovarian cancer in black women. J Natl Cancer Inst. 1993;85(2):142–7.

47. Russo A, et al. Hereditary ovarian cancer. Crit Rev Oncol Hematol. 2009;69(1):28–44.

48. Engeland A, Tretli S, Bjørge T. Height, body mass index, and ovarian cancer: a follow-up of 1.1 million Norwegian women. J Natl Cancer Inst. 2003;95(16):1244–8.

49. WHO. Global Health Observatory, the data repository. WHO 2015 [11.26.2015]; Available from: http://www.who.int/gho/database/en/.

50. O'brien RM. A caution regarding rules of thumb for variance inflation factors. Quality & Quantity. 2007;41(5):673–90.

51. WHO. Global Health Risks Mortality and Burden of Disease Attributable to Selected Major Risks. Geneva: Geneva: World Health Organization; 2009.

52. Cramer DW, et al. Determinants of Ovarian Cancer Risk. I. Reproductive Experiences and Family History23. JNCI, Journal of the National Cancer Institute. 1983;71:711.

53. Ramazzini Ba. De morbis artificum Bernardini Ramazzini diatriba = Diseases of workers: the Latin text of 1713 revised, with translation and notes/by Wilmer Cave Wright. In: Wright WCet, B I, editors. Classics of Medicine Library Special edition/privately printed for the members of the Classics of Medicine Library. ed. Diseases of workers. Birmingham, Alabama: The Classics of Medicine Library; 1983.

54. Moorman PG, et al. Reproductive factors and ovarian cancer risk in African-American women. Ann Epidemiol. 2016;26(9):654–62.

55. Adami H-O, et al. Parity, age at first childbirth, and risk of ovarian cancer. Lancet. 1994;344(8932):1250–4.

56. Riman T, Nilsson S, Persson IR. Review of epidemiological evidence for reproductive and hormonal factors in relation to the risk of epithelial ovarian malignancies. Acta Obstet Gynecol Scand. 2004;83(9):783–95.

57. Casagrande J, et al. " Incessant ovulation" and ovarian cancer. Lancet. 1979;314(8135):170–3.

58. Fathalla M. Incessant ovulation and ovarian cancer–a hypothesis re-visited. Facts, views & vision in ObGyn. 2013;5(4):292.

59. WHO. Bulletin of the World Health Organization: The breast cancer conundrum, in Bull World Health Organ; 2013. p. 626–7.

60. Ness RB, et al. Factors related to inflammation of the ovarian epithelium and risk of ovarian cancer. Epidemiology. 2000;11(2):111–7.

61. Choi J-H, et al. Gonadotropins and ovarian cancer. Endocr Rev. 2007;28(4):440–61.

62. Kendrick KM. The neurobiology of social bonds. J Neuroendocrinol. 2004;16(12):1007–8.

63. Weisman O, Zagoory-Sharon O, Feldman R. Oxytocin administration to parent enhances infant physiological and behavioral readiness for social engagement. Biol Psychiatry. 2012;72(12):982–9.

64. Angeles L. Children and life satisfaction. J Happiness Stud. 2009;11(4):523–38.

65. Nan H, et al. Psychometric evaluation of the Chinese version of the subjective happiness scale: evidence from the Hong Kong FAMILY cohort. Int J Behav Med. 2014;21(4):646–52.

66. Carmichael MS, et al. Plasma oxytocin increases in the human sexual response. The Journal of Clinical Endocrinology & Metabolism. 1987;64(1):27–31.

67. Carmichael MS, et al. Relationships among cardiovascular, muscular, and oxytocin responses during human sexual activity. Arch Sex Behav. 1994;23(1):59–79.

68. Gordon G Jr, Burch RL, Platek SM. does semen have antidepressant properties? Arch Sex Behav. 2002;31(3):289–93.

69. Magon N, Kalra S. The orgasmic history of oxytocin: love, lust, and labor. Indian journal of endocrinology and metabolism. 2011;15(Suppl3):S156.

70. Insel TR, Hulihan TJ. A gender-specific mechanism for pair bonding: oxytocin and partner preference formation in monogamous voles. Behav Neurosci. 1995;109(4):782.

71. Young LJ, Murphy Young AZ, Hammock EA. Anatomy and neurochemistry of the pair bond. J Comp Neurol. 2005;493(1):51–7.

72. Antonova L, Mueller CR. Hydrocortisone down-regulates the tumor suppressor gene BRCA1 in mammary cells: a possible molecular link between stress and breast cancer. Genes Chromosomes Cancer. 2008;47(4):341–52.

73. Cohen S, Rodriguez MS. Pathways linking affective disturbances and physical disorders. Health Psychol. 1995;14(5):374–80.

74. Diener E, Chan MY. Happy people live longer: subjective well-being contributes to health and longevity. Applied Psychology: Health and Well-Being. 2011;3(1):1–43.

75. Williams RB, Schneiderman N. Resolved: psychosocial interventions can improve clinical outcomes in organic disease (pro). Psychosom Med. 2002;64:552–7.

76. Aizer AA, et al. Marital status and survival in patients with cancer. J Clin Oncol. 2013;31(31):3869–76.

77. Kim Y, et al. Psychological distress among healthy women with family histories of breast cancer: effects of recent life events. Psychooncology. 2005;14(7):555–63.

78. Peled R, et al. Breast cancer, psychological distress and life events among young women. BMC Cancer. 2008;8:245.

79. Bai A, et al. A survey of overall life satisfaction and its association with breast diseases in Chinese women. Cancer Med. 2016;5(1):111–9.

80. Myrskylä M, Kohler H-P, Billari FC. Advances in development reverse fertility declines. Nature. 2009;460(7256):741.

81. Galor O. The demographic transition: causes and consequences. Cliometrica. 2012;6(1):1–28.

82. Sinding SW. Population, poverty and economic development. Philosophical Transactions of the Royal Society B: Biological Sciences. 2009;364(1532):3023–30.

83. Whitaker L. The plight of nuns: hazards of nulliparity. Journal of Family Planning and Reproductive Health Care. 2012;38(2):116.

84. Kent A. Nuns and contraceptives. Reviews in Obstetrics and Gynecology. 2012;5(3–4):e166.

20

Live birth rate after human chorionic gonadotropin priming in vitro maturation in women with polycystic ovary syndrome

V. N. A. Ho[1], T. D. Pham[1], A. H. Le[1], T. M. Ho[1] and L. N. Vuong[1,2*]

Abstract

Background: In vitro maturation (IVM) has some advantages over conventional in vitro fertilization (IVF), particularly in polycystic ovary syndrome (PCOS) where the risk of ovarian hyperstimulation is high. We studied the live birth rate in a large series of PCOS women undergoing human chorionic gonadotropin (hCG)-priming IVM.

Methods: This retrospective study included women with PCOS aged 18–42 years undergoing IVM with hCG priming. We reported live birth rate after the first embryo transfer and cumulative live birth rate from embryos obtained in the IVM cycle. We also performed logistic regression to assess which factors predicted number of oocytes and live birth.

Results: We included 921 women (age 28.9±3.5 years, body mass index 21.8±3.1 kg/m^2, infertility duration 3.7±2.6 years, 81% primary infertility, 88% first IVF attempt, 94% ovulation induction failure). Live birth rate after the first embryo transfer was 31.7%, with a cumulative live birth rate from the cycle of 33.7%. High anti-Müllerian hormone levels predicted a high number of oocytes and a high oocyte maturation rate while the opposite was the case when luteinizing hormone levels were high.

Conclusions: In women with PCOS, hCG priming IVM was feasible and resulted in acceptable live birth rates.

Keywords: In vitro maturation, In vitro fertilization, Polycystic ovary syndrome, Cumulative live birth rate, Pregnancy outcomes

Background

Currently, in vitro fertilization (IVF) involves ovarian stimulation with supra-physiological doses of gonadotrophins in order to increase the oocyte yield, thus increasing the number of embryos. Gonadotrophins are expensive, and their use carries the risk of ovarian hyperstimulation syndrome (OHSS), particular in women with polycystic ovary syndrome (PCOS) women [1, 2].

In vitro maturation (IVM) involves collection of immature oocytes that are cultured in vitro until they reach the metaphase II (MII) stage prior to insemination and does not need controlled ovarian hyperstimulation (COH). Human IVM was first reported in 1991 in an unstimulated donor cycle [3], while the first live birth after IVM in a

woman with PCOS was reported in 1994 [4]. Although there were initially some concerns about IVM in terms of effectiveness and the risk of genetic abnormalities [5–8], recent studies have reported pregnancy rates after IVM comparable to IVF [9]. In addition, the risk of congenital abnormalities in IVM offspring does not appear to be increased [10–12].

The advantages of IVM over conventional IVF include lower cost (because it does not need ovarian hyperstimulation), the absence of OHSS and less inconvenience for women [13–17]. Absence of OHSS is particularly relevant for women with PCOS who are at high risk of OHSS during ovarian hyperstimulation during conventional IVF, but also have an increased risk of ovarian torsion and thromboembolism associated with high estradiol levels [1, 2, 18–20]. Therefore, IVM is a useful technique for women with PCOS [21]. Although other assisted reproductive medicine strategies, such as use

* Correspondence: drlan@yahoo.com.vn; lanvuong@ump.edu.vn
[1]IVFMD, My Duc Hospital, Ho Chi Minh City, Vietnam
[2]Department of Obstetrics and Gynecology, University of Medicine and Pharmacy at Ho Chi Minh City, Ho Chi Minh City, Vietnam

of gonadotropin-releasing hormone agonist (GnRHa) trigger and freeze-only cycles, have reduced the rate of OHSS in high-risk women [22–24], some cases of severe OHSS have still been reported when these strategies have been employed [25–27]. This is particularly relevant in women with PCOS undergoing IVF who are at high risk of OHSS.

Initial data suggested that outcomes after IVM in women with PCOS are at least as good as those in women without PCOS, but the total number of PCOS women treated with IVM is relatively small [28]. In addition, although there are some published data on clinical and ongoing pregnancy rates after IVM in PCOS women [21, 29–35], only three studies involving PCOS women have reported live birth rate [9, 30, 36]. Here, we report the live birth rate in PCOS women undergoing IVM, including predictors of live birth, number of oocytes retrieved and maturation rate after IVM.

Methods

Study design

This retrospective study was performed in My Duc hospital, a large private IVF center in Ho Chi Minh City, Vietnam. The study was carried out in accordance with the Declaration of Helsinki, and all patient information was handled confidentially. The confidential use of patient information for research purposes is exempt from ethical approval under Vietnamese law.

Subjects

To be eligible, women had to have PCOS diagnosed according to the Rotterdam criteria [37], be aged 18–42 years, and were undergoing IVM. Exclusion criteria included uterine abnormalities, and donor or preimplantation genetic screening/diagnosis cycles.

Stimulation, monitoring and oocyte pick-up

The same ovarian stimulation protocol was used in all patients. Oral contraceptive pills were given for two weeks to induce bleeding. Women received injections of follicle-stimulating hormone (FSH; Puregon, Merck Sharpe & Dohme) 100 IU/day on cycle days 3, 4 and 5. Ultrasound was performed on cycle day 5 to document follicular size and determine endometrial thickness. Women were given an injection of hCG 10,000 IU on cycle day 6 (independent of follicle size), and oocyte pick-up (OPU) was scheduled 36 h thereafter.

In vitro maturation protocol

After OPU, all oocytes were placed in pre-maturation medium for 2 h. They were then transferred to maturation medium (Origio, Denmark) and cultured for 20 h, after which mature oocytes underwent intra-cytoplasmic sperm injection (ICSI). In the remaining oocytes, maturation was

re-checked after another 4 h, with ICSI performed in any additional mature oocytes.

Embryo transfer

Fresh embryo transfer (ET) was performed 3 days (day 2, 4-cell embryos) or 4 days (day 3, 8-cell embryos) after OPU based on patient preference. Any additional embryos were frozen on the day of scheduled embryo transfer. When successful pregnancy did not occur, a frozen ET was planned. In frozen ET cycles, the endometrium was prepared using oral estradiol valerate 8 mg/day starting from the second or third day of the menstrual cycle. Endometrial thickness was monitored from day 6 onwards, and vaginal progesterone 800 mg/day was started when endometrial thickness reached ≥8 mm. A maximum of three embryos were thawed on the day of ET, two or three days after the start of progesterone depending on the stage of embryo freezing. Two hours after thawing, surviving embryos were transferred into the uterus. The number of embryos transferred was dependent on the number available and patient preference. In fresh and frozen cycles, a serum beta hCG test was performed 2 weeks after ET. Luteal support with estradiol 4 mg/day and vaginal progesterone 800 mg/day was continued up to at least 7 weeks of gestation.

Outcomes

We studied the live birth (birth of at least one newborn after 24 weeks' gestation that exhibits any sign of life) rate after the first ET. We also report the number of oocytes retrieved, maturation rate, fertilization rate, OHSS rate, implantation rate, positive pregnancy test (serum hCG level > 5 mIU/mL), clinical pregnancy (at least one gestational sac on ultrasound at 7 weeks), ongoing pregnancy (pregnancy continuing past 20 weeks' gestation), ectopic pregnancy (presence of a gestational sac outside the uterine cavity shown on sonography or laparoscopy) and miscarriage (pregnancy loss at < 12 weeks and from 12 to 24 weeks). In case of ongoing pregnancy, we reported preterm delivery, birth weight (grams), and any congenital anomaly. We also report median time to achieve live birth, and the cumulative live birth rate at 12 months after the IVM cycle.

Statistical analysis

Outcomes after the first ET are reported using descriptive statistics. We constructed Kaplan-Meier curves to estimate cumulative live birth rates. Univariate and multivariate logistic regression analyses were performed to identify predictive variables of live birth after the first ET. Univariate and multivariate linear regression analyses were also performed to identify predictive variables for the number of oocytes retrieved and for the maturation rate. All variables with p values of < 0.25 in the univariate analysis were included in the multivariate analyses to identify independent predictors of live birth after IVM. All analyses were performed using the R statistical package (R version 3.3.3).

Results

Participants

A total of 921 PCOS women underwent IVM between April 2014 and October 2016 (mean age 28.9 ± 3.5 years, body mass index [BMI] 21.8±3.1 kg/m^2, infertility duration 3.7±2.6 years) (Fig. 1, Table 1), The majority of women had primary infertility, were undergoing their first IVF attempt, and had ovulation induction failure as the indication for IVM (Table 1).

Controlled ovarian stimulation

The mean number of oocytes retrieved per woman was almost 15, nearly all embryos were Day 2, and maturation and fertilization rates were both approaching 70% (Table 2). The proportion of oocytes that were mature at the time of collection was about 7% (Table 2). No cases of OHSS were recorded.

Treatment outcomes

The live birth rate after the first IVM cycle ET was 31.7% (32.0% after fresh ET and 28.0% after frozen ET). The clinical pregnancy rate was higher (43.5%) but 10.3% of all pregnancies ended with miscarriage (Table 3). Additional embryo transfers were performed in 94 women. In the 12 months after the IVM cycle, 974 ETs were performed

(fresh and/or frozen) in 873 women. The cumulative live birth rate was 33.7% (Fig. 2, Table 3). The median time to achieve live birth was 8.7 months. No babies were born with congenital abnormalities.

Predictors of live birth

While a number of factors were significant predictors of live birth in the univariate analysis (including age, BMI, duration of infertility, and number of IVF attempts), only the number of embryos available for transfer and the number of embryos transferred were significant independent predictors of live birth after IVM on multivariate logistic regression analysis (Table 4). After transfer of a single embryo, the live birth rate was 80% lower than when two embryos were transferred ($p = 0.032$) but transferring three embryos did not significantly improve the live birth rate compared with transferring two embryos.

Predictors of number of oocytes and maturation rate

Factors significantly correlated with the number of oocytes on multivariate analysis were BMI, anti-Müllerian hormone (AMH) level, luteinizing hormone (LH) level, number of previous IVF attempts, and ovulation induction failure as the indication for IVM (Table 6). When BMI, AMH and the number of previous IVF attempts were higher, the number of oocytes retrieved was higher ($p < 0.001$, $p < 0.001$ and $p = 0.006$, respectively) (Table 5). Conversely, as LH increased the number of oocytes decreased ($p = 0.03$) (Table 5). PCOS women with ovulation

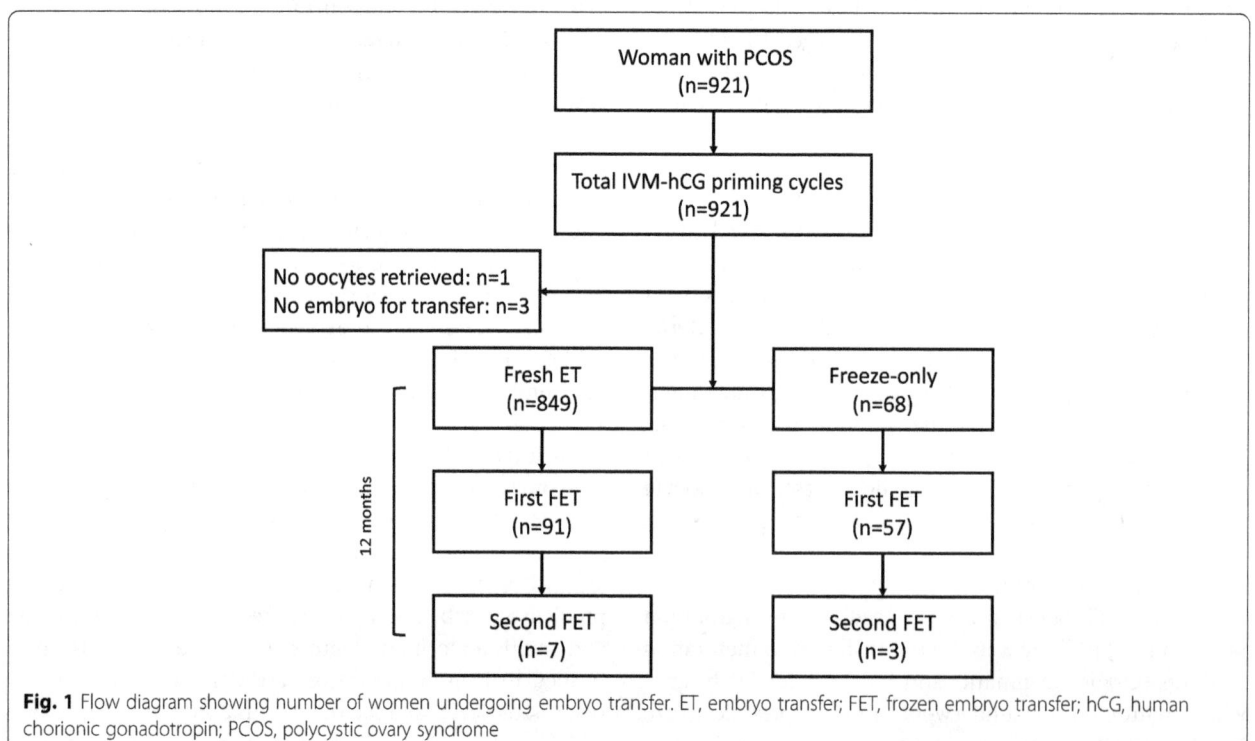

Fig. 1 Flow diagram showing number of women undergoing embryo transfer. ET, embryo transfer; FET, frozen embryo transfer; hCG, human chorionic gonadotropin; PCOS, polycystic ovary syndrome

Table 1 Demographic and clinical characteristics of participants at baseline

Characteristics	Participants ($n = 921$)
Age, years	28.9 ± 3.5
Body mass index, kg/m^2	21.8 ± 3.1
Anti-Müllerian hormone, ng/mL	12.3 ± 3.6
Antral follicle count, n	34.3 ± 18.3
Follicle-stimulating hormone[a], IU/mL	8.5 ± 1.9
Progesterone[a], ng/mL	0.7 ± 1.8
Luteinizing hormone[a], IU/L	14.3 ± 6.9
Free testosterone index[a]	5.2 ± 4.7
Menstrual cycles, n (%)	
Amenorrhea	52 (5.6)
Oligomenorrhea	850 (92.3)
Regular	19 (2.0)
Polycystic ovaries on ultrasound, n (%)	
Both ovaries	777 (84.4)
One ovary	144 (15.6)
Duration of infertility, years	3.7 ± 2.6
Type of infertility, n (%)	
Primary	747 (81.1)
Secondary	174 (18.9)
Number of IVF attempts, n, (%)	
1	814 (88.4)
2	80 (8.7)
3	27 (2.9)
Indications for IVM, n (%)	
Tubal factors	18 (2.0)
Male factors	13 (1.4)
Ovulation induction failure	862 (93.6)
Previous OHSS with COH	18 (2.0)
Other	10 (1.1)

Values are mean ± standard deviation, or number of women (%)
COH, controlled ovarian hyperstimulation, *IVF* in vitro fertilization, *IVM* in vitro maturation, *OHSS* ovarian hyperstimulation syndrome
[a]Hormone levels were assessed at the first physician visit, on the second day of progestogen-induced bleeding

Table 2 Laboratory outcomes

	Participants ($n = 921$)
Number of oocytes retrieved[a]	14.9 ± 8.9
Number of oocytes matured at collection	1.1 ± 2.3
Proportion of mature oocytes at collection, %	7.2 ± 14.5
Maturation rate, %	71.2 ± 14.5
Fertilization rate, %	68.2 ± 22.1
Number of embryos[b]	6.0 ± 3.6
Stage of embryos, n (%)	
Day 2	908 (98.6)
Day 3	9 (1.0)
Number of frozen embryos	1.5 ± 2.2

Values are mean ± standard deviation, or number (%)
[a]One woman without oocytes; [b]Three women without embryos

induction failure had a significantly higher number of oocytes than those with tubal factor indications for IVM ($p = 0.004$) (Table 5). BMI ($p < 0.001$), AMH ($p = 0.01$) and number of previous IVF attempts ($p = 0.008$) were also significant predictors of the maturation rate on multivariate analysis, with similar relationships to those for oocyte number (Table 5).

Discussion

The results of this retrospective analysis show that acceptable live birth rates can be achieved in women with PCOS after IVM with hCG priming. The live birth rate after IVM was close to that with conventional IVF. There are a number of possible reasons for this. Firstly, we have been doing IVM for nearly 12 years so have a good level of experience and competency with this technique. Secondly, the IVF rate at our center is slightly lower than that at other centers because we transfer day 3 embryos rather than blastocysts.

A limited number of previous studies have reported the live birth rate after IVM in women with polycystic ovary morphology or PCOS. In one of these, the cumulative live birth rate per oocyte collected (80 cycles of IVM in 56 women) was 41.3% [9]. In another study, the live birth rate per oocyte collected was also slightly higher, at 42.4% [30]. In our study, the live birth rate after the first embryo transfer, and cumulative live birth rate for one IVM cycle were lower (31.7% and 33.7%, respectively). However, direct comparison between ours and previous studies is difficult because both the previous studies did not use hCG priming (which facilitates fresh embryo transfer), and transferred a single blastocyst using fresh [30] or used fresh and frozen ET [9]. Fresh transfer of day 2 or day 3 embryos rather than blastocysts could be one potential explanation for the difference in live birth rate between the current study and existing data.

The live birth rate in our study was comparable to the 34.6% reported with fresh transfer of one or two day 3 embryos after IVM and ICSI in PCOS women from Canada and Turkey [36], and nearly twice that reported after frozen transfer of one or two day 3 embryos in women with PCOS in a European retrospective study (16.2%) [38]. Given that these studies and ours transferred day 3 embryos after IVM, the reasons underlying the lower live birth rate in the European study are not clear. Importantly, the live birth rate achieved after IVM based on the results of this analysis was comparable to that achieved with conventional IVF in similar women from Vietnam [39, 40].

Table 3 Pregnancy outcomes

	Overall[a] ($n = 873$)	Type of first embryo transfer	
		Fresh ($n = 823$)	Frozen ($n = 50$)
Number of embryos transferred	2.5 ± 0.6	2.5 ± 0.6	2.5 ± 0.6
After first embryo transfer			
Live birth, n (%)	277 (31.7)	263 (32.0)	14 (28.0)
Singleton	175/277 (63.2)	165/263 (62.7)	10/14 (71.4)
Twins	102/277 (36.8)	98/263 (37.3)	4/14 (28.6)
Positive beta hCG, n (%)	438 (50.2)	417 (50.7)	21 (42.0)
Clinical pregnancy, n (%)	380 (43.5)	361 (43.9)	19 (38.0)
Ongoing pregnancy, n (%)	286 (32.8)	272 (33.0)	14 (28.0)
Implantation, %	25.1	25.3	20.7
Ectopic pregnancy, n (%)	12 (1.4)	11 (1.3)	1 (2.0)
Miscarriage (before 12 weeks), n (%)	81 (9.3)	76 (9.2)	5 (10.0)
Miscarriage (between 12 and 24 weeks), n (%)	9 (1.0)	9 (1.1)	0 (0.0)
Birth weight, g			
Singleton	2980.7 ± 733.4	2951.3 ± 737.2	3433.3 ± 625.0
Twins	2325.8 ± 545.5	2302.1 ± 538.1	2412.5 ± 513.2
At 12 months			
Total number of embryo transfers, n (%)[b]			
1	779 (89.2)		
2	87 (10.0)		
3	7 (0.8)		
Live birth, n (%)	294 (33.7)		
Singleton	192/294 (65.3)		
Twins	102/294 (34.7)		
Positive beta hCG, n (%)	508 (58.2)		
Clinical pregnancy, n (%)	440 (50.4)		
Ongoing pregnancy, n (%)	326 (37.3)		
Implantation, %	25.6		
Ectopic pregnancy, n (%)	14 (1.6)		
Miscarriage (before 12 weeks), n (%)	102 (11.6)		
Miscarriage (between 12 and 24 weeks), n (%)	9 (1.0)		
Birth weight, g			
Singleton	2969.9 ± 737.3		
Twins	2307.2 ± 536.0		

Values are mean ± standard deviation, or number (%)

[a]Thirty-three women were lost to follow-up after the first transfer, 11 did not undergo embryo transfer, one woman had no oocytes retrieved, and three women had no embryos to transfer

hCG human chorionic gonadotropin

[b]A total of 1007 transfers were performed, but no follow-up data were available for 33, meaning that data from 974 transfers are reported

We identified the number of embryos available for transfer and the number of embryos transferred as significant independent predictors of live birth after IVM on multivariate logistic regression analysis, consistent with existing data [36, 41]. In our study, up to three embryos were transferred. The transfer of three embryos in some cases was based on earlier data suggesting that IVM embryos are not usually as good as IVF embryos. However, data from this analysis suggested that the transfer of more than two embryos did not result in significantly higher live birth rate. Data from a small study suggest that acceptable live birth rates can be achieved after IVM with single blastocyst transfer [9]. Although we found that additional variables were statistically

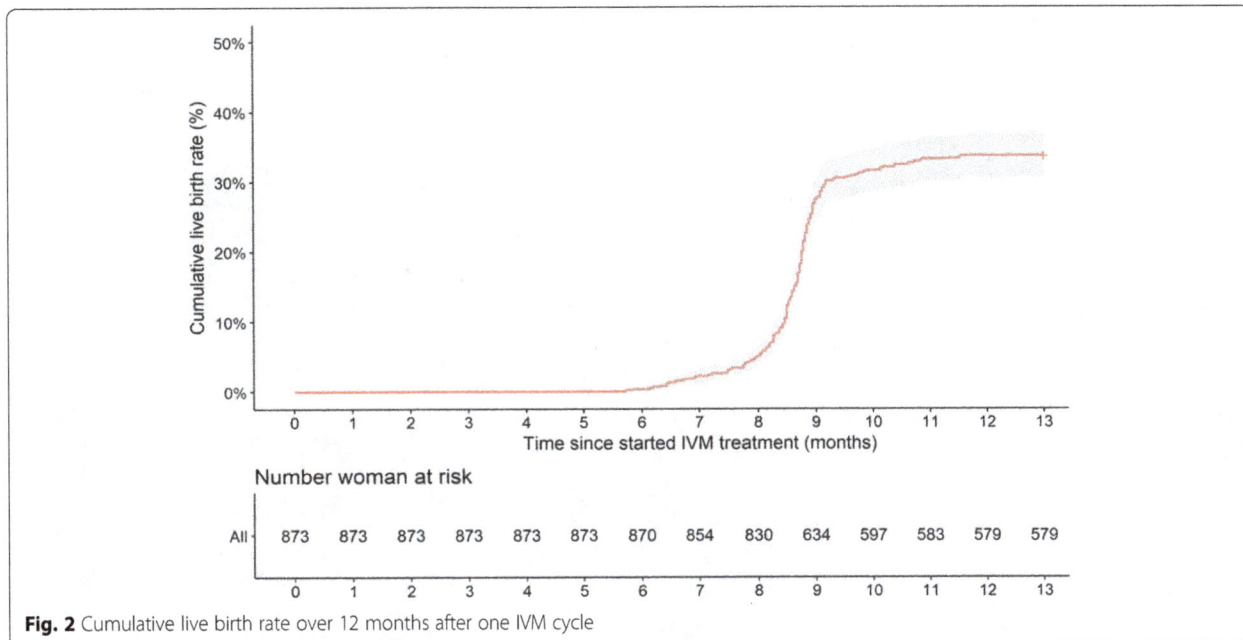

Fig. 2 Cumulative live birth rate over 12 months after one IVM cycle

significant predictors of live birth in univariate analyses, these did not persist in the multivariable model, possibly because the number of embryos and the number of embryos transferred are such strong and direct predictors of pregnancy and live birth.

Collection of a good number of oocytes is the first step in the IVM procedure and their maturation is essential so that there are a good number of embryos to transfer. To facilitate selection of suitable candidates prior to starting IVM, pretreatment factors associated with relevant procedural metrics are needed. This was the rationale for our analysis of predictive factors for number of oocytes and maturation rate.

Associations between serum AMH and/or AFC and live birth have been reported previously [29, 42], but these variables were not significant independent predictors of live birth in our analysis. However, we did identify significant associations between AMH and both the number of oocytes and the oocyte maturation rate. Conversely, these parameters decreased significantly when levels of LH were high. The reason for this is unclear given that a positive association between LH and AMH serum levels, independent of serum androgen levels, has been reported previously [43]. Baseline LH in our study (14.3 IU/L) was higher than that in patients from a previous similar study (9.1 IU/L) [29], but the importance of this remains to be determined. In a previous model to identify PCOS women suitable for IVM, the presence of at least eight cumulus oocyte complexes was identified as being associated with a higher number of good quality embryos and a better ongoing pregnancy rate [29]. Duration of infertility has previously been reported

as a significant predictor of live birth after IVM [36]. Although infertility duration was a significant predictor of live birth on univariate analysis, this association did not persist in the multivariate model. However, we did identify significant independent associations between the number of previous IVF attempts and both oocyte number and maturation rate.

BMI was not a significant predictor of live birth after IVM but was significantly associated with the number of oocytes retrieved during the procedure. This is in contrast to data from a retrospective cohort study that failed to find any association between BMI and the number and quality of oocytes in PCOS women undergoing IVM [44]. The influence of BMI on IVM is an important area for future study, particularly with respect to potential ethnic differences, because Asian women with PCOS are usually lean and have a lower BMI than Western PCOS populations [45].

In 2013, an American Society of Reproductive Medicine (ASRM) committee described IVM as "an experimental procedure" that should only be performed "in specialized centers for carefully selected patients", and that candidates for this approach to infertility treatment include those at risk for OHSS and women with PCOS [46]. Our study was conducted at a specialist center and in the target groups described and showed the potential for live birth rates after IVM to approach those achieved with traditional IVF. There is also much debate about how IVM is defined, and there is not yet any consensus about a standard protocol for IVM. The ASRM committee recently defined IVM as "maturation in culture of immature oocytes after their recovery from follicles

Table 4 Factors influencing the live birth rate after first embryo transfer after in vitro maturation

Predictive factors	Live births (n = 277)	No live births (n = 596)	Univariate analysis Odds ratio (95% CI)	p-value	Multivariate analysis Odds ratio (95% CI)	p-value
Pretreatment factors (n = 873)[b]						
Age, years[a]	28.1 ± 3.5	29.1 ± 3.5	0.94 (0.90, 0.98)	0.004	0.97 (0.93, 1.02)	0.254
Body mass index, kg/m^2[a]	21.5 ± 2.8	22.0 ± 3.2	0.94 (0.90, 0.99)	0.019	0.95 (0.90, 1.00)	0.06
Anti-Müllerian hormone, ng/mL[a]	12.5 ± 3.6	12.2 ± 3.6	1.02 (0.98, 1.06)	0.304	–	–
Antral follicle count – n	34.3±17.9	34.4±18.5	1.00 (0.99, 1.01)	0.96	–	–
Follicle-stimulating hormone, IU/mL	8.6 ± 1.9	8.5 ± 1.8	1.03 (0.95, 1.11)	0.524	–	–
Progesterone, ng/mL	0.8 ± 1.9	0.7 ± 1.8	1.01 (0.93, 1.09)	0.761	–	–
Luteinizing hormone, IU/L	14.3 ± 6.9	13.5 ± 6.7	1.02 (1.00, 1.04)	0.105		
Free testosterone index	4.5 ± 5.6	4.6 ± 5.2	1.00 (0.97, 1.02)	0.786	–	–
Menstrual cycles, n (%)						
Amenorrhea	15 (5.4)	33 (5.5)	Ref		–	–
Oligomenorrhea	256 (92.4)	551 (92.4)	1.02 (0.56, 1.97)	0.946	–	–
Regular	6 (2.2)	12 (2.0)	1.10 (0.33, 3.43)	0.871	–	–
Polycystic ovaries on ultrasound, n (%)						
Both ovaries	228 (82.3)	488 (81.9)	Ref		–	–
One ovary	49 (17.7)	108 (18.1)	0.97 (0.67, 1.41)	0.88	–	–
Duration of infertility, years[a]	3.3 ± 2.3	3.8 ± 2.7	0.92 (0.86, 0.98)	0.011	0.95 (0.89, 1.02)	0.161
Type of infertility, n (%)						
Primary	229 (82.7)	479 (80.4)	Ref		–	–
Secondary	48 (17.3)	117 (19.6)	0.86 (0.59, 1.24)	0.419	–	–
Number of IVF attempts, n (%)						
1	259 (93.5)	514 (86.2)	Ref		–	–
2	11 (4.0)	64 (10.7)	0.34 (0.17, 0.63)	0.001	0.60 (0.32, 1.09)	0.105[c]
3	7 (2.5)	18 (3.0)	0.77 (0.30, 1.80)	0.566	–	–
Indications for IVM, n (%)						
Tubal factors	3 (1.1)	14 (2.3)	Ref		–	–
Male factors	2 (0.7)	11 (1.8)	0.85 (0.10, 6.01)	0.869	–	–
Ovulation induction failure	267 (96.4)	550 (92.3)	2.27 (0.73, 9.89)	0.202	1.92 (0.92, 4.38)	0.097
Previous OHSS with COH	3 (1.1)	14 (2.3)	1.00 (0.16, 6.24)	0.99	–	–
Others	2 (0.7)	7 (1.2)	1.33 (0.15, 9.99)	0.779	–	–
Treatment factors (n = 873)[b]						
Number of oocytes retrieved[a]	15.6 ± 8.4	14.7 ± 9.1	1.01 (0.99, 1.03)	0.182	0.98 (0.95, 1.01)	0.286
Number of mature oocytes after IVM[a]	9.1 ± 5.0	8.5 ± 5.3	1.02 (0.99, 1.05)	0.109	0.97 (0.92, 1.02)	0.212
Number of embryos available for transfer[a]	6.8 ± 3.6	5.7 ± 3.6	1.09 (1.05, 1.13)	< 0.001	1.14 (1.07, 1.22)	< 0.001
Mean number of embryos transferred[a]	2.6 ± 0.5	2.5 ± 0.6	1.55 (1.20, 2.01);	0.001		
Number of embryos transferred, n (%)						
1 embryo transferred	2 (0.7)	34 (5.7)	0.14 (0.02, 0.47)	0.008	0.20 (0.03, 0.69)	0.032
2 embryos transferred	104 (37.5)	247 (41.4)	Ref	–	Ref	–
3 embryos transferred	171 (61.7)	315 (52.9)	1.29 (0.96, 1.73)	0.092	1.25 (0.92, 1.69)	0.152
Embryo transfer method, n (%)						
Fresh	263 (94.9)	560 (94.0)	Ref		–	–
Freeze-only	14 (5.1)	36 (6.0)	0.83 (0.43, 1.53)	0.56	–	–

CI confidence interval, *COH* controlled ovarian hyperstimulation, *IVF* in vitro fertilization, *IVM* in vitro maturation, *OHSS* ovarian hyperstimulation syndrome
[a]Parameters analyzed as continuous variables; odds ratio values are per unit increase
[b]Thirty-three women were lost to follow-up after the first transfer, and 11 did not undergo embryo transfer, one woman had no oocytes retrieved, and three women had no embryos to transfer

Table 5 Factors influencing oocyte maturation ($n = 920$) and the number of oocytes retrieved ($n = 921$) after in vitro maturation

	Oocyte maturation				Oocytes retrieved			
	Univariate analysis		Multivariate analysis		Univariate analysis		Multivariate analysis	
	β	p-value	β	p-value	β	p-value	β	p-value
Age, years	0.001	0.99	–	–	0.11	0.19	−0.08	0.31
Body mass index, kg/m^2	−0.1	0.70	–	–	0.845	< 0.001	0.85	< 0.001
Anti-Müllerian hormone, ng/mL	0.31	0.15	0.32	< 0.001	0.28	0.001	0.36	< 0.001
Antral follicle count, n	0.07	0.27			0.002	0.88		
Follicle stimulating hormone, IU/mL	0.26	0.53	–	–	0.14	0.39	–	–
Progesterone, ng/mL	0.35	0.41	–	–	−0.17	0.31	–	–
Luteinizing hormone, IU/L	0.48	< 0.001	−0.11	0.01	−0.09	0.04	−0.09	0.03
Free testosterone index	0.44	0.002	−0.05	0.37	−0.03	0.62	–	–
Menstrual cycles, n (%)								
Amenorrhea	Ref	Ref	–	–	Ref	Ref	–	–
Oligomenorrhea	−6.68	0.05	−0.82	0.53	−0.82	0.54	–	–
Regular	−5.74	0.36	–	–	−3.96	0.11	−3.97	0.08
Polycystic ovaries on ultrasound, n (%)								
Both ovaries	Ref	Ref	–	–	Ref	Ref	–	–
One ovary	0.92	0.65	–	–	−1.06	0.26	–	–
Duration of infertility, years	0.21	0.48	–	–	−0.02	0.86	–	–
Type of infertility, n (%)								
Primary	Ref	Ref	Ref	Ref	Ref	Ref	Ref	Ref
Secondary	−5.79	0.003	1.15	0.13	1.38	0.07	1.17	0.11
Number of IVF attempts, n (%)								
1	Ref	Ref	Ref	Ref	Ref	Ref	Ref	Ref
2	−7.65	0.005	1.33	0.21	1.63	0.13	1.74	0.11
3	−5.77	0.21	4.71	0.008	4.51	0.01	4.84	0.006
Indications for IVM, n (%)								
Tubal factors	Ref	Ref	–	–	Ref	Ref	–	–
Male factors	−0.60	0.94	–	–	−2.24	0.49	–	–
Ovulation induction failure	−1.19	0.83	–	–	3.92	0.07	4.05	0.004
Previous OHSS with COH	−6.72	0.38	–	–	5.12	0.09	2.22	0.38
Others	−0.90	0.80	–	–	− 0.90	0.80	–	–

COH controlled ovarian hyperstimulation, IVF in vitro fertilization, IVM in vitro maturation, OHSS ovarian hyperstimulation syndrome

which may or may not have been exposed to FSH but were not exposed to either LH or hCG prior to retrieval to induce meiotic resumption." Use of hCG priming does not fulfil these criteria. However, this approach has been used by some centers because it was reported to improve oocyte maturation, development potential and outcomes [47–50]. However, data from a randomized controlled trial show that this was not associated with any difference between hCG-primed and non-primed IVM cycles in terms of subsequent embryo developmental competence [51]. Furthermore, despite an overall low quality of available evidence, a Cochrane review concluded that hCG-priming had no effect on pregnancy, miscarriage or live birth rates

with IVM using day 2–3 embryos, although well-designed randomized clinical trials in this area are required [52].

The hCG priming approach was the most common protocol at our institution over the period from which study data were analyzed. One of the advantages of using hCG priming is that fresh embryo transfer is possible due to the direct effects of hCG on the endometrium [53]. A disadvantage of hCG priming is that oocytes are at different levels of maturity at OPU, meaning that there is a need to do multiple checks for maturation and then perform several rounds of ICSI whenever mature oocytes are detected [54], both of which increase the laboratory workload and procedural costs. There is a need for more randomized controlled trials comparing hCG-priming and non-hCG-priming IVM to provide reliable data on the comparative effectiveness, complications, time to pregnancy, neonatal health, safety, costs and cost effectiveness of the two approaches. Additional research is required to define the optimal protocol for IVM. Whichever protocol is used, IVM is increasingly being associated with acceptable pregnancy outcomes and provides a promising alternative ART approach for specific groups of women that is efficient, convenient, safe and more financially accessible for many couples.

The retrospective design of this study was the most important limitation; however a large number of patients were included. In addition, pregnancy-related complications (e.g. pre-eclampsia, diabetes mellitus) were not documented. The age range of included patients was wide, but there were few patients at either end of the range, with the majority of patients being aged between 23 and 35 years. Our findings are only applicable to the specific approach taken to IVM in this study. The transfer of day 2 embryos is not commonly practiced in many IVF centers, however, there is actually no standard protocol for IVM and we are currently working to find out the optimal protocol for doing IVM. Since the period over which data were collected, the IVM protocol used at our center has changed, and now uses a non-hCG approach with transfer of two day 3 embryos, which is closer to modern ART practice. Although differences in IVM protocols are common, making comparison between studies and consensus difficult, IVM should continue to be studied because it is a promising ART technique. A key strength of this study is the large sample size, although the number of women in some subgroups used to analyze predictors of live birth was small. To the best of our knowledge, this is the largest study of IVM in PCOS to date and one of only a few to report live birth rate and cumulative live birth rate. Better understanding of IVM will improve its application in clinical practice and help with selecting women more likely to have a positive outcome. Improvements in IVM techniques are also contributing to better outcomes with this important ART technique [55]. In addition, because it can be performed rapidly without hormonal stimulation, IVM is a promising technique for preserving fertility in women with cancer who require gonadotoxic antineoplastic therapy [56].

Conclusions

The live birth rate after IVM in women with PCOS was acceptable and similar to that after IVF. IVM is a convenient option in these women and may be a feasible and effective alternative to IVF. Women with a high AMH and low LH at baseline appear to be most suitable for IVM, and transfer of two embryos gives a good result in terms of live birth rate.

Authors' contributions

VNAH and LNV were involved in study design, data collection, manuscript drafting, critical discussion and final approval of the manuscript. TDP was involved in data collection, analysis, critical discussion and final approval of the manuscript. AHL and TMH were involved in data collection, critical discussion and final approval of the manuscript.

Competing interests

The authors declare that they have no competing interests.

References

1. Brinsden PR, Wada I, Tan SL, Balen A, Jacobs HS. Diagnosis, prevention and management of ovarian hyperstimulation syndrome. Br J Obstet Gynaecol. 1995;102(10):767–72.
2. MacDougall MJ, Tan SL, Jacobs HS. In-vitro fertilization and the ovarian hyperstimulation syndrome. Hum Reprod. 1992;7(5):597–600.
3. Cha KY, Koo JJ, Ko JJ, Choi DH, Han SY, Yoon TK. Pregnancy after in vitro fertilization of human follicular oocytes collected from nonstimulated cycles, their culture in vitro and their transfer in a donor oocyte program. Fertil Steril. 1991;55(1):109–13.
4. Trounson A, Wood C, Kausche A. In vitro maturation and the fertilization and developmental competence of oocytes recovered from untreated polycystic ovarian patients. Fertil Steril. 1994;62(2):353–62.
5. Kerjean A, Couvert P, Heams T, Chalas C, Poirier K, Chelly J, Jouannet P, Paldi A, Poirot C. In vitro follicular growth affects oocyte imprinting establishment in mice. Eur J Hum Genet. 2003;11(7):493–6.
6. Nogueira D, Staessen C, Van de Velde H, Van Steirteghem A. Nuclear status and cytogenetics of embryos derived from in vitro-matured oocytes. Fertil Steril. 2000;74(2):295–8.
7. Young LE, Fernandes K, McEvoy TG, Butterwith SC, Gutierrez CG, Carolan C, Broadbent PJ, Robinson JJ, Wilmut I, Sinclair KD. Epigenetic change in IGF2R is associated with fetal overgrowth after sheep embryo culture. Nat Genet. 2001;27(2):153–4.
8. Zhang XY, Ata B, Son WY, Buckett WM, Tan SL, Ao A. Chromosome abnormality rates in human embryos obtained from in-vitro maturation and IVF treatment cycles. Reprod BioMed Online. 2010;21(4):552–9.
9. Walls ML, Hunter T, Ryan JP, Keelan JA, Nathan E, Hart RJ. In vitro maturation as an alternative to standard in vitro fertilization for patients diagnosed with polycystic ovaries: a comparative analysis of fresh, frozen and cumulative cycle outcomes. Hum Reprod. 2015;30(1):88–96.
10. Buckett WM, Chian RC, Holzer H, Dean N, Usher R, Tan SL. Obstetric outcomes and congenital abnormalities after in vitro maturation, in vitro fertilization, and intracytoplasmic sperm injection. Obstet Gynecol. 2007;110(4):885–91.
11. Chian RC, Xu CL, Huang JY, Ata B. Obstetric outcomes and congenital abnormalities in infants conceived with oocytes matured in vitro. Facts Views Vis Obgyn. 2014;6(1):15–8.
12. Fadini R, Mignini Renzini M, Guarnieri T, Dal Canto M, De Ponti E, Sutcliffe A, Shevlin M, Comi R, Coticchio G. Comparison of the obstetric and perinatal outcomes of children conceived from in vitro or in vivo matured oocytes in in vitro maturation treatments with births from conventional ICSI cycles. Hum Reprod. 2012;27(12):3601–8.
13. Choi MH, Lee SH, Kim HO, Cha SH, Kim JY, Yang KM, Song IO, Koong MK, Kang IS, Park CW. Comparison of assisted reproductive technology outcomes in infertile women with polycystic ovary syndrome: in vitro maturation, GnRH agonist, and GnRH antagonist cycles. Clin Exp Reprod Med. 2012;39(4):166–71.
14. Das M, Son WY, Buckett W, Tulandi T, Holzer H. In-vitro maturation versus IVF with GnRH antagonist for women with polycystic ovary syndrome: treatment outcome and rates of ovarian hyperstimulation syndrome. Reprod BioMed Online. 2014;29(5):545–51.
15. Ellenbogen A, Shavit T, Shalom-Paz E. IVM results are comparable and may have advantages over standard IVF. Facts Views Vis Obgyn. 2014;6(2):77–80.
16. Gremeau AS, Andreadis N, Fatum M, Craig J, Turner K, McVeigh E, Child T. In vitro maturation or in vitro fertilization for women with polycystic ovaries? A case-control study of 194 treatment cycles. Fertil Steril. 2012;98(2):355–60.
17. Huang JY, Chian RC, Tan SL. Ovarian hyperstimulation syndrome prevention strategies: in vitro maturation. Semin Reprod Med. 2010;28(6):519–31.
18. Koita-Kazi I, Serhal P. Thrombosis and hemostatic aspects of assisted conception. In: Cohen H, O'Brien P, editors. Disorders of Thrombosis and Hemostatis in Pregnancy. London: Springer; 2012.

19. Krishnan S, Kaur H, Bali J, Rao K. Ovarian torsion in infertility management - missing the diagnosis means losing the ovary: a high price to pay. J Hum Reprod Sci. 2011;4(1):39–42.

20. Ou YC, Kao YL, Lai SL, Kung FT, Huang FJ, Chang SY, ChangChien CC. Thromboembolism after ovarian stimulation: successful management of a woman with superior sagittal sinus thrombosis after IVF and embryo transfer: case report. Hum Reprod. 2003;18(11):2375–81.

21. Child TJ, Phillips SJ, Abdul-Jalil AK, Gulekli B, Tan SL. A comparison of in vitro maturation and in vitro fertilization for women with polycystic ovaries. Obstet Gynecol. 2002;100(4):665–70.

22. Al-Inany HG, Youssef MA, Aboulghar M, Broekmans F, Sterrenburg M, Smit J, Abou-Setta AM. GnRH antagonists are safer than agonists: an update of a Cochrane review. Hum Reprod Update. 2011;17(4):435.

23. Lainas TG, Sfontouris IA, Zorzovilis IZ, Petsas GK, Lainas GT, Alexopoulou E, Kolibianakis EM. Flexible GnRH antagonist protocol versus GnRH agonist long protocol in patients with polycystic ovary syndrome treated for IVF: a prospective randomised controlled trial (RCT). Hum Reprod. 2010;25(3):683–9.

24. Tiitinen A, Husa LM, Tulppala M, Simberg N, Seppala M. The effect of cryopreservation in prevention of ovarian hyperstimulation syndrome. Br J Obstet Gynaecol. 1995;102(4):326–9.

25. Fatemi HM, Popovic-Todorovic B, Humaidan P, Kol S, Banker M, Devroey P, Garcia-Velasco JA. Severe ovarian hyperstimulation syndrome after gonadotropin-releasing hormone (GnRH) agonist trigger and "freeze-all" approach in GnRH antagonist protocol. Fertil Steril. 2014;101(4):1008–11.

26. Ling LP, Phoon JW, Lau MS, Chan JK, Viardot-Foucault V, Tan TY, Nadarajah S, Tan HH. GnRH agonist trigger and ovarian hyperstimulation syndrome: relook at 'freeze-all strategy. Reprod BioMed Online. 2014;29(3):392–4.

27. Gurbuz AS, Gode F, Ozcimen N, Isik AZ. Gonadotrophin-releasing hormone agonist trigger and freeze-all strategy does not prevent severe ovarian hyperstimulation syndrome: a report of three cases. Reprod BioMed Online. 2014;29(5):541–4.

28. Siristatidis C, Sergentanis TN, Vogiatzi P, Kanavidis P, Chrelias C, Papantoniou N, Psaltopoulou T. In vitro maturation in women with vs. without polycystic ovarian syndrome: a systematic review and meta-analysis. PLoS One. 2015; 10(8):e0134696.

29. Guzman L, Ortega-Hrepich C, Polyzos NP, Anckaert E, Verheyen G, Coucke W, Devroey P, Tournaye H, Smitz J, De Vos M. A prediction model to select PCOS patients suitable for IVM treatment based on anti-Mullerian hormone and antral follicle count. Hum Reprod. 2013;28(5):1261–6.

30. Junk SM, Yeap D. Improved implantation and ongoing pregnancy rates after single-embryo transfer with an optimized protocol for in vitro oocyte maturation in women with polycystic ovaries and polycystic ovary syndrome. Fertil Steril. 2012;98(4):888–92.

31. Child TJ, Abdul-Jalil AK, Gulekli B, Tan SL. In vitro maturation and fertilization of oocytes from unstimulated normal ovaries, polycystic ovaries, and women with polycystic ovary syndrome. Fertil Steril. 2001; 76(5):936–42.

32. Ellenbogen A, Atamny R, Fainaru O, Meidan E, Rotfarb N, Michaeli M. In vitro maturation of oocytes: a novel method of treatment of patients with polycystic ovarian syndrome undergoing in vitro fertilization. Harefuah. 2011;150(11):833–6. 876

33. Shalom-Paz E, Almog B, Wiser A, Levin I, Reinblatt S, Das M, Son WY, Hananel H. Priming in vitro maturation cycles with gonadotropins: salvage treatment for nonresponding patients. Fertil Steril. 2011;96(2):340–3.

34. Shalom-Paz E, Holzer H, Son W, Levin I, Tan SL, Almog B. PCOS patients can benefit from in vitro maturation (IVM) of oocytes. Eur J Obstet Gynecol Reprod Biol. 2012;165(1):53–6.

35. Soderstrom-Anttila V, Makinen S, Tuuri T, Suikkari AM. Favourable pregnancy results with insemination of in vitro matured oocytes from unstimulated patients. Hum Reprod. 2005;20(6):1534–40.

36. Tannus S, Hatirnaz S, Tan J, Ata B, Tan SL, Hatirnaz E, Kenat-Pektas M, Dahan MH. Predictive factors for live birth after in vitro maturation of oocytes in women with polycystic ovary syndrome. Arch Gynecol Obstet. 2018;297(1): 199–204.

37. Rotterdam ESHRE/ASRM-sponsored PCOS consensus workshop group. Revised 2003 consensus on diagnostic criteria and long-term health risks related to polycystic ovary syndrome (PCOS). Hum Reprod. 2004;19(1):41–7.

38. Ortega-Hrepich C, Stoop D, Guzman L, Van Landuyt L, Tournaye H, Smitz J, De Vos M. A "freeze-all" embryo strategy after in vitro maturation: a novel approach in women with polycystic ovary syndrome? Fertil Steril. 2013; 100(4):1002 7.

39. Vuong LN, Dang VQ, Ho TM, Huynh BG, Ha DT, Pham TD, Nguyen LK, Norman RJ, Mol BW. IVF transfer of fresh or frozen embryos in women without polycystic ovaries. N Engl J Med. 2018;378(2):137–47.

40. Vuong NL, Pham DT, Phung HT, Giang HN, Huynh GB, Nguyen TTL, Ho MT. Corifollitropin alfa vs recombinant FSH for controlled ovarian stimulation in women aged 38-42 years with a body weight >=50kg: a randomized controlled trial. Hum Reprod Open. 2017:2017(3):1–11.

41. Dahan M, Hatirnaz E, Tan S, Ata B, Ozer A, Kanat-Pektas M, Hatirnaz S. Predicotrs of pregnancy outcomes in women with polycystic ovary syndrome who performed in-vitro maturation (IVM) of oocytes [abstract P-386]. Fertil Steril. 2016; 106(3, Suppl):e251.

42. Seok HH, Song H, Lyu SW, Kim YS, Lee DR, Lee WS, Yoon TK. Application of serum anti-Mullerian hormone levels in selecting patients with polycystic ovary syndrome for in vitro maturation treatment. Clin Exp Reprod Med. 2016;43(2):126–32.

43. Catteau-Jonard S, Pigny P, Reyss AC, Decanter C, Poncelet E, Dewailly D. Changes in serum anti-mullerian hormone level during low-dose recombinant follicular-stimulating hormone therapy for anovulation in polycystic ovary syndrome. J Clin Endocrinol Metab. 2007;92(11):4138–43.

44. Shalom-Paz E, Marzal A, Wiser A, Almog B, Reinblatt S, Tulandi T, Holzer H. Effects of different body mass indices on in vitro maturation in women with polycystic ovaries. Fertil Steril. 2011;96(2):336–9.

45. Zhao Y, Qiao J. Ethnic differences in the phenotypic expression of polycystic ovary syndrome. Steroids. 2013;78(8):755–60.

46. Practice Committees of the American Society for Reproductive Medicine and the Society for Assisted Reproductive Technology. In vitro maturation: a committee opinion. Fertil Steril. 2013;99(3):663–6.

47. Kim MK, Park EA, Kim HJ, Choi WY, Cho JH, Lee WS, Cha KY, Kim YS, Lee DR, Yoon TK. Does supplementation of in-vitro culture medium with melatonin improve IVF outcome in PCOS? Reprod BioMed Online. 2013;26(1):22–9.

48. Siristatidis CS, Vrachnis N, Creatsa M, Maheshwari A, Bhattacharya S: In vitro maturation in subfertile women with polycystic ovarian syndrome undergoing assisted reproduction. Cochrane Database Syst Rev 2013;(10): CD006606.

49. Son WY, Yoon SH, Lim JH. Effect of gonadotrophin priming on in-vitro maturation of oocytes collected from women at risk of OHSS. Reprod BioMed Online. 2006;13(3):340–8.

50. Farsi MM, Kamali N, Pourghasem M. Embryological aspects of oocyte in vitro maturation. Int J Mol Cell Med. 2013;2(3):99–109.

51. Zheng X, Wang L, Zhen X, Lian Y, Liu P, Qiao J. Effect of hCG priming on embryonic development of immature oocytes collected from unstimulated women with polycystic ovarian syndrome. Reprod Biol Endocrinol. 2012;10:40.

52. Reavey J, Vincent K, Child T, Granne IE. Human chorionic gonadotrophin priming for fertility treatment with in vitro maturation. Cochrane Database Syst Rev. 2016;11:Cd008720.

53. Fanchin R, Peltier E, Frydman R, de Ziegler D. Human chorionic gonadotropin: does it affect human endometrial morphology in vivo? Semin Reprod Med. 2001;19(1):31–5.

54. Son WY, Tan SL. Laboratory and embryological aspects of hCG-primed in vitro maturation cycles for patients with polycystic ovaries. Hum Reprod Update. 2010;16(6):675–89.

55. Sanchez F, Lolicato F, Romero S, De Vos M, Van Ranst H, Verheyen G, Anckaert E, Smitz JEJ. An improved IVM method for cumulus-oocyte complexes from small follicles in polycystic ovary syndrome patients enhances oocyte competence and embryo yield. Hum Reprod. 2017; 32(10):2056–68.

56. Chang EM, Song HS, Lee DR, Lee WS, Yoon TK. In vitro maturation of human oocytes: its role in infertility treatment and new possibilities. Clin Exp Reprod Med. 2014;41(2):41–6.

21

Mass spectrometry-based proteomics techniques and their application in ovarian cancer research

Agata Swiatly, Szymon Plewa, Jan Matysiak and Zenon J. Kokot[*]

Abstract

Ovarian cancer has emerged as one of the leading cause of gynecological malignancies. So far, the measurement of CA125 and HE4 concentrations in blood and transvaginal ultrasound examination are essential ovarian cancer diagnostic methods. However, their sensitivity and specificity are still not sufficient to detect disease at the early stage. Moreover, applied treatment may appear to be ineffective due to drug-resistance. Because of a high mortality rate of ovarian cancer, there is a pressing need to develop innovative strategies leading to a full understanding of complicated molecular pathways related to cancerogenesis. Recent studies have shown the great potential of clinical proteomics in the characterization of many diseases, including ovarian cancer. Therefore, in this review, we summarized achievements of proteomics in ovarian cancer management. Since the development of mass spectrometry has caused a breakthrough in systems biology, we decided to focus on studies based on this technique. According to PubMed engine, in the years 2008–2010 the number of studies concerning OC proteomics was increasing, and since 2010 it has reached a plateau. Proteomics as a rapidly evolving branch of science may be essential in novel biomarkers discovery, therapy decisions, progression predication, monitoring of drug response or resistance. Despite the fact that proteomics has many to offer, we also discussed some limitations occur in ovarian cancer studies. Main difficulties concern both complexity and heterogeneity of ovarian cancer and drawbacks of the mass spectrometry strategies. This review summarizes challenges, capabilities, and promises of the mass spectrometry-based proteomics techniques in ovarian cancer management.

Keywords: Ovarian cancer, Proteomics, Biomarkers, Drug-resistance, Diagnostics

Background
Ovarian cancer

Ovarian cancer (OC) causes about 125,000 deaths each year, which corresponds to over 4% of women cancer deaths worldwide [1, 2]. Only 5–10% of the OC cases are hereditary [3, 4]. OC tumors generally originate from other gynecological tissues than ovaries. Interestingly, tumors involves the ovary tissue secondarily [5]. However, despite several hypotheses of the OC origin, understanding its pathogenesis is still insufficient. Therefore, it has become a widely researched topic in the field of molecular sciences, which may influence modern medicine. Unfortunately, even though progress is made in prevention, development of novel tools for

early diagnosis and improvement of pharmacological therapies, the survival rate for OC remains poor. Patients often experience some symptoms but these are ignored or overlap with other ailments. Premalignant phase is difficult to recognize. A lack of sufficient screening options results in late detection. Despite successful surgery and appropriate treatment based on intravenous or intraperitoneal platinum- and taxane-based chemotherapy, diagnosis at advanced stages lowers 5-year survival rate to 27% [6]. This is caused by at least two factors: disease extension and biological differences in widely disseminated tumors [7]. Currently, less than 40% of all diagnosed OC cases are cured. However, if the diagnosis was made at the first stage of the disease, treatment could be limited to a surgical intervention alone [8].

* Correspondence: zkokot@ump.edu.pl
Department of Inorganic and Analytical Chemistry, Poznan University of Medical Sciences, Grunwaldzka 6 Street, 60-780 Poznań, Poland

Proteomics in cancer biomarker discovery

The improvement in –omics sciences, genomics, proteomics, metabolomics, has opened a new research chapter, which is expected to develop novel tools for early diagnosis, treatment monitoring or population screening [9, 10]. Fundamentally, cancerogenesis is associated with a genetic defect and epigenetic changes [11]. Many studies suggest that germline mutations in Breast Cancer Gene 1 (BRCA1) (17q21, chromosome 17: base pairs 43,044,294 to 43,125,482) and Breast Cancer Gene 2 (BRCA2) (13q12.3, chromosome 13: base pairs 32,315,479 to 32,399,671) are associated with a risk of breast and ovarian cancer [12]. Moreover, in epithelial OC some sporadic BRCA1 and BRCA2 mutations may occur, including BRCA1 hypermethylation [13]. Currently, it is thought that BRCA could be a useful prognostic marker only in combination with other biomarkers [14]. Since proteins are expressed by genes, and they are functional factors in phenotype characterization, the study of proteome profiles may yield information crucial for cancer research. Predictive markers could increase our understanding of molecular processes and pathological mechanisms, which is a dire need in modern medicine [15]. Sporadic molecular mutations that occur during abnormal cellular proliferation result in changes in protein secretion, modification or degradation. Therefore, in-depth proteomics analysis of various biosamples (e.g., serum, plasma, urine, tissues) obtained from cancer patients may facilitate the study of tumorigenesis, therapy monitoring, and development of novel targeted treatments. However, biomarker discovery might be challenging, bearing in mind that biomarker should improve currently used diagnostic methods, increase their sensitivity and specificity, provide optimal treatment, correspond to disease stage, and also be easily available in biofluids [16].

So far, proteomics methods have revealed thousands of potential cancer biomarkers. Most of the proteins suggested in the literature as clinically useful molecules are still awaiting proper validation. Hypothesis-testing is one of the most critical aspects of the cancer research. Another challenge in biomarker discovery is standardization and optimization of protocols. Some approaches are characterized by low precision and reproducibility, which is associated with poor study design [17]. Moreover, there are also biological challenges like sample variability or cancer heterogeneity. Nevertheless, a few biomarkers have been successfully implemented into clinical practice. To date, American Food and Drug Administration approved Cancer Antigen 125 (CA125) and human epididymis protein 4 (HE4) as circulating OC biomarkers for therapy monitoring and recurrence identification [18]. However, these tests have some inherent limitations, and their sensitivity and specificity should be increased, especially for patients with early stage of the tumor.It has been proved that

combination of existing biomarkers with additional markers in one discriminatory model may improve their performance [19]. Therefore, it may be suggested that proteomics is a chance to develop novel tools that will significantly reduce the OC mortality rate.

Mass spectrometry techniques in clinical proteomics

The use of contemporary mass spectrometry (MS) represented a significant breakthrough in proteomics analysis. Since fast-evolving MS-techniques have a great impact on biomedical science, this innovative technology was introduced into clinical research [20]. Recently, matrix-assisted laser desorption/ionization (MALDI), and surface-enhanced laser desorption/ionization (SELDI) connected with time-to-flight (TOF) detector as well as electrospray ionization (ESI) have been extensively used in clinical proteomics [21–23]. Linking MS techniques with liquid chromatography (LC) or capillary electrophoresis allows for obtaining high resolution spectral proteomic patterns from numerous sample types [24–27]. These methods have already been reported as accurate tools for discovering multi-component classifiers, which significantly discriminate cancer samples from control biofluids or tissues. A crucial step in every analytical experiment is the choice of an optimal approach. Bearing in mind complexity of biological samples, the proper methodology should be chosen with respect to both sample pretreatment and MS-based strategy [28]. Initially, MS was used in clinical proteomics only to identify proteins and peptides. Today, the introduction of technical advances allows also for quantitative investigations.

This review presents proteomics strategies based on MS techniques used in OC research. We summarize successes of the proteomics in OC management and discuss challenges associated with biomarker discovery and proteome analysis. Moreover, we discuss improvements in MS strategies and prospects for effective diagnosis and treatment of OC. The use of proteomics and mass spectrometry in the ovarian cancer studies in the years 2008–2017 is presented in the Fig. 1. It was prepared based on PubMed engine (http://www.ncbi.nlm.nih.gov/pubmed/) using the following keywords: "ovarian cancer and proteomics and mass spectrometry" and "ovarian cancer and proteomics". In the years 2008–2010 the number of studies concerning OC proteomics was increasing, and since 2010 it has been approximately at the same level. While, the contribution of the MS techniques in these studies is significant over the years.

Characterization of proteins in the OC development

The study of differentially expressed proteins in biosamples derived from OC patients or cell lines may improve early detection, treatment, and prognosis. MS-based

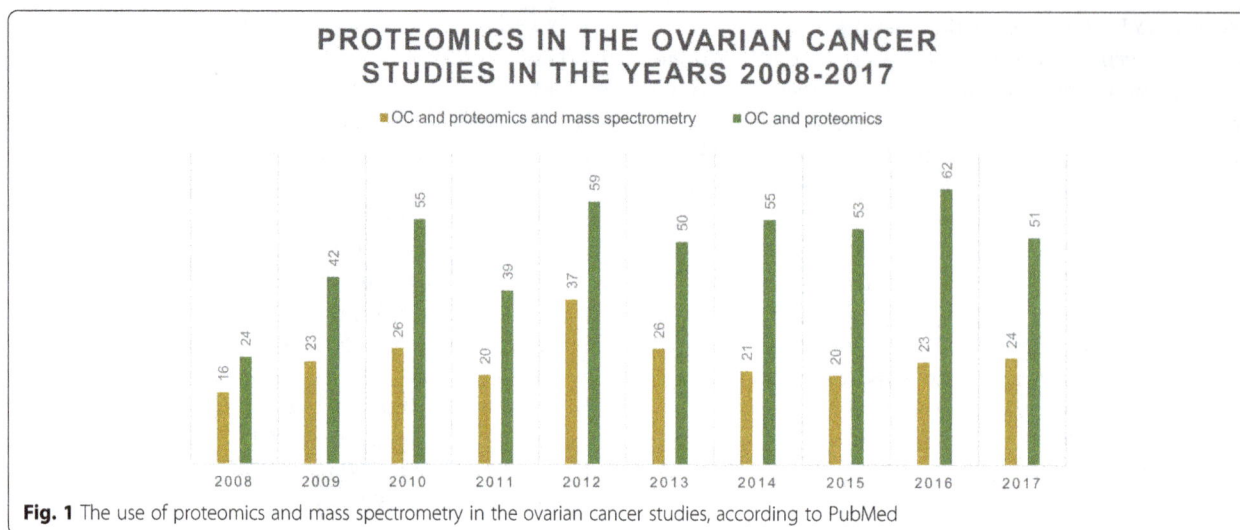

Fig. 1 The use of proteomics and mass spectrometry in the ovarian cancer studies, according to PubMed

proteomics techniques are widely employed to search sensitive and specific biomarkers, which, especially in combination with current diagnostic methods, may contribute to the detection of early stage OC. Moreover, identifying a relationship between overexpressed protein and dysfunctions in the cell cycle such as angiogenesis, apoptosis or proliferation, may be important for the development of novel therapies. Inhibition of the expression of significant proteins is a common method used to stop oncogenesis. Additionally, specific profiles of the proteins may indicate prognosis for the patients and help with proper treatment recommendations. Therefore, in this chapter, we discuss different MS-based strategies used in the clinical proteomics and their achievements in the field of the OC.

Protein-peptide profiling

Petricoin et al. were the first who introduced low-molecular-weight protein profiling into cancer proteomics [29]. Discovery and identification of proteomic patterns that reflect specific health conditions have become promising tools in clinical investigations. Both MALDI-TOF and SELDI-TOF MS are soft ionization techniques that cause minimal fragmentation of the obtained ions. Therefore, they are mainly used for protein profiling in low mass range. The resulting profiles may contain even thousands of data points – registered ions (mass/charge ratio - m/z), which are subjected to sophisticated data analysis. Bioinformatic tools select the most discriminative m/z features, based on varying peaks intensities/areas, and define proteomic pattern characteristic for the study groups of samples. Subsequently, the differentiating peaks may be identified as proteins using tandem MS or protein databases. However, the identification process is omitted in some papers and the results are presented only as the m/z values [16]. Protein-peptide

profiling offers various advantages, like a discovery of multi-marker panels, which usually demonstrate a higher level of discriminatory information comparing with single markers, or quick analysis of large groups of samples [30].

Protein-peptide profiling studies involve inexpensive and minimally invasive procedure of collecting blood and its components like serum or plasma. Moreover, other blood tests, which determine important factors and provide information about general patient condition, can be routinely performed in clinical laboratories. Biofluids represent the overall pathophysiological status of a studied individual [31]. Therefore, serum and plasma protein-peptide profiling has become a popular strategy in the field of ovarian cancer. In 2002, Petricoin et al. used SELDI-TOF MS to analyze serum samples from ovarian cancer patients and control group that contained healthy individuals and women with benign tumors [29]. A combination of a genetic algorithm and cluster analysis resulted in the selection of five m/z features: 534, 989, 2111, 2251, and 2465. The obtained discriminative panel significantly differentiated the study groups (sensitivity of 100%, specificity of 95%, and positive predictive value of 94%).

Further proteomic studies suggested that the use of a proper sample preparation method is required in order to detect aberrations in low abundance proteome. It is expected that potential biomarkers are mostly present at low concentrations, which disturbs their detection. For example, albumin, immunoglobulins, complement system proteins and transferrin are high-abundant blood proteins that represent about 99% of all serum proteins. Remaining 1% may be a rich source of yet unknown biomarkers [32]. To overcome the problem of high-abundance proteins, different strategies have been applied in OC biomarker discovery: immobilized metal affinity capture (IMAC) technology [33], immunodepletion [34], magnetic beads

[35], solid-phase extraction [19], biomarker enrichment kits [30], and anion exchange chromatography [36]. Table 1 presents m/z ratios and proteins identified as potential OC serum biomarkers. Despite application of purification techniques, most of the identified proteins are still highly abundant ones, such as apolipoprotein A1 or complement component 3. Moreover, these proteins seem to be unspecific, as they are also differently expressed in various types of cancer [37, 38]. However, the features of these proteins might be used to create multivariate predictive models, especially in combination with two common OC biomarkers – CA125 and HE4. Recently, a new OC diagnostic test was proposed – OVA 1, which is based on determination of serum levels of five different factors: CA125, apolipoprotein A1, beta-2-macroglobulin, transferrin, and transthyretin [39]. Therefore, protein-peptide profiling studies may be not a proper strategy to discover single useful biomarkers but they could contribute to developing multifactor tests.

Quantitative proteomics

Recently, new quantitative strategies of protein analysis have enjoyed huge attention. Since a discovery that proteomic changes under specific physiological conditions may help elucidate disease mechanisms and identify crucial

Table 1 M/z features (peptides) proposed as potential OC biomarkers in protein-peptide profiling studies

m/z	Identified protein	Ref.
1082.24; 1087.80; 1066.08; 1277.19; 1293.36; 1897.52; 4466.86; 4467.05; 4469.14; 4962.52; 8601.58; 8601.64; 11,693.29; 11,735.91; 17,105.23	no identification	[34]
5486; 6440; 13,720		[35]
28,043	apolipoprotein A1	[36]
12,828	transthyretin	[36]
2898.54		[30]
2210.80		[19]
3272	inter-α-trypsin inhibitor heavy chain H4	[36]
2582.35; 3027.57		[30]
2082.73; 3158.75		[19]
1041.68	keratin 2a	[30]
1224.68	glycosyltransferase-like 1B	[30]
1690.94; 1777.97; 1865.01; 2021.11	complement component 3 precursor	[30]
1505.24; 2023.17		[19]
1739.93	complement component 4A preproprotein	[30]
1966.91	casein kinase II alpha 1 subunit isoform a	[30]
2115.05	D-amino-acidoxidase	[30]
2345.19	transgelin 2	[30]
3239.55	fibrinogen alpha chain isoform alpha preproprotein	[30]
1945.38	kininogen – 1	[19]

biomarkers, a sensitive and accurate method for this purpose has been sought for. MS-based proteomics strategies may be divided into: "top-down" and "bottom-up" proteomics. In this review, we focus on the "bottom-up" strategy that is most common in clinical proteomics. The classical "bottom-up" strategy is based on staining proteins and two-dimensional electrophoresis. Stained spots of different abundance are digested, excised and identified mainly using MS techniques. Unfortunately, this strategy has many restrictions, as not all types of proteins are suitable for in-gel separation. Moreover, gel-to-gel variability made this method not significantly reproducible [40]. Due to these limitations, the classical approach seems to be often unreliable and quantitative analysis might be difficult to achieve. Therefore, the introduction of LC coupled with MS facilitated utilization of a novel "bottom-up" approach. A typical analysis starts with enzymatic (usually tryptic) digestion of the study proteins. Then the resulting short peptides are separated by LC, and eluates are further analyzed with tandem MS.

Recently two gel-free "bottom-up" strategies have been developed: isotopic labeling (like chemical isotopic labeling, isobaric tagging, metabolic isotopic labeling) and label-free analysis [41, 42]. In the label-based approach, peptides are linked with various tags in which ion signals correspond to relative peptide abundance in the analyzed sample. The most common labeling strategies include: SILAC (stable isotope labeling by amino acids in cell culture), ICAT (Isotope-coded affinity tag), iTRAQ (isobaric Tags for Relative and Absolute Quantification) and TMT (Tandem Mass Tags). Contrary to that, label-free analysis is based on precursor or spectral count. This approach has become popular due to a simpler sample preparation method and higher dynamic range as compared with labeling techniques [24]. The improvement of label-free approach consists in the advance of high-resolution mass spectrometer such as Orbitrap as well as TOF instruments [42].

Apart from the division into label-based and label-free methods presented in Fig. 2, two groups of "bottom-up" proteomics can be distinguished: discovery proteomics and targeted proteomics. The discovery proteomics is also called "shotgun" strategy, and it represents data-dependent acquisition. A considerable advantage of this method is a possibility to analyze thousands of proteins in one run. However, "shotgun" methods are usually characterized by low repeatability of peptide identification, which may be overcome by applying the targeted approach. Targeted proteomics techniques are mainly based on multiple-, selected- or parallel reaction monitoring, which results in sensitive and reproducible quantification of predefined proteins [42]. In the last few years, a third kind of acquisition has been developed: data-independent acquisition (DIA). During DIA analysis

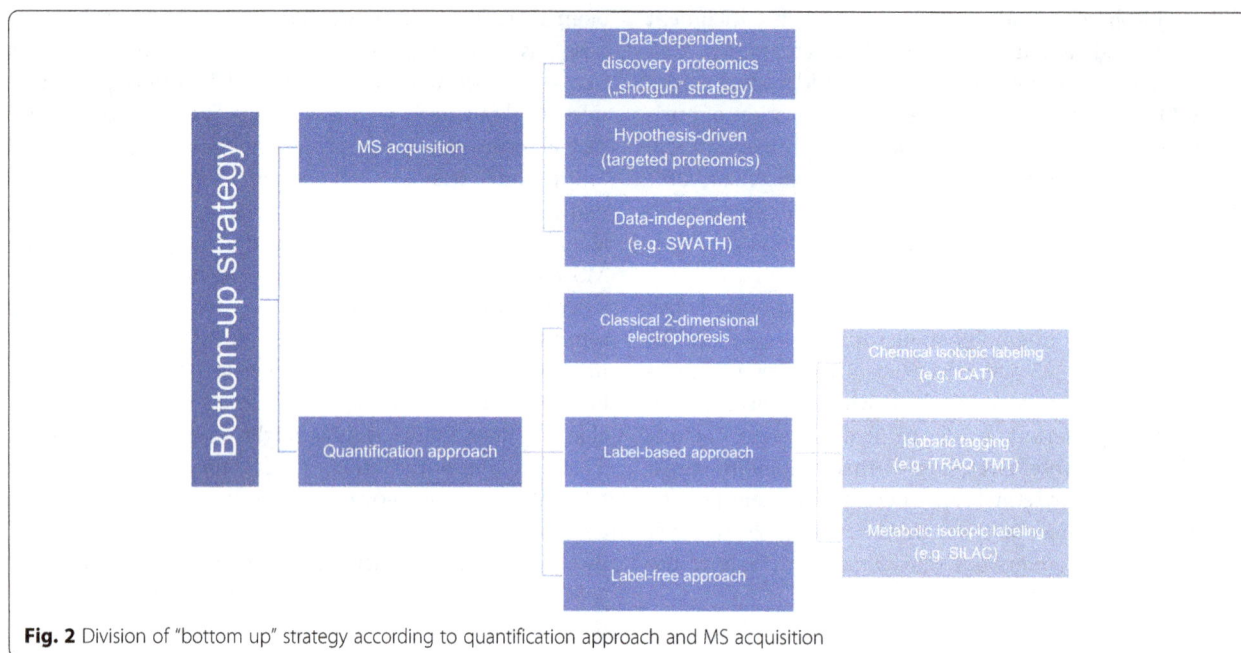

Fig. 2 Division of "bottom up" strategy according to quantification approach and MS acquisition

precursor ions from determined m/z isolation window are deterministically fragmented. Recently, sequential window acquisition of all theoretical mass spectra (SWATH) (exemplified by DIA) has become a popular approach for biomarker discovery based on spectral libraries and targeted data analysis [43].

Many different quantitative strategies have been applied in the ovarian cancer proteomics. The most commonly performed analysis of ovarian cell lines are based on SILAC strategy. Isotope label is bound directly to the proteins during their synthesis. One of the first studies in this field compared the usefulness of classical two-dimensional electrophoresis coupled with SILAC strategy for describing urokinase plasminogen activator influence on OC cells. It proved that labeling technique is characterized by low quantitative variation. Moreover, this research demonstrated that urokinase plasminogen activator is capable of changing the expression of some proteins like thioredoxin, annexin IV, and fatty acid binding protein 3 in the OC cells [44]. Another study suggested that calcium-activated chloride channel regulator 1 and chloride channels may be potential OC therapeutic targets [45]. SILAC strategy was also used to investigate oxidative stress in the OC cells, which is an important issue in developing novel photodynamic therapy agents [46]. It was also revealed that epithelial-mesenchymal transition activated by epidermal growth factor modifies metabolic processes and cell cycle control. Therefore, it is associated with OC development and progression [47].

Another approach widely used in OC characterization is isobaric tagging: TMT and iTRAQ [48]. These techniques allow for simultaneous identification as well as relative quantification of proteins in multiple samples. Isobaric tagging patterns are mainly focused on an analysis of proteolytic digestion of proteins and peptides. ITRAQ labeling combined with tandem MS techniques enabled a selection of a few potential OC biomarkers: serum amyloid A-4 [49], astacin-like metalloendopeptidase [49], protein S100-A11, Keratin type II cytoskeletal 8, inorganic pyrophosphatase, isocitrate dehydrogenase [50], legumain [51], and protein Z [52]. Moreover, iTRAQ analysis was proved to be a useful method to track changes in proteins during a transition from benign to malignant tumor-like PI3K/Akt signaling pathway [53]. Another study aimed at comparing protein expression of ovarian cancer and endometrial high-grade serous carcinomas in both tissue samples and cell lines. Both tumors exhibited similar protein profiles [54]. TMT is much less popular in the field of OC proteome. Sinclair J. et al. combined this technique with two-dimensional electrophoresis, two-dimensional LC, and MS techniques: MALDI-TOF, electrospray quadrupole time-of-flight (Q-TOF) and Orbitrap to analyze proteome of two OC cell line models. A set of potential OC biomarkers was proposed for further examination. Additionally, the utility of the selected biomarker – human active and pro-matrix metalloprotease-10, was examined using immunoassays to determine the level of this protein in human serum [55].

Although label-based strategies still remain the gold standard of quantitative proteomics, label-free methods have recently become more widespread. Therefore, LC combined with tandem MS was used to analyze plasma, ovary, and oviduct tissue samples from healthy and OC in chickens. The results were further compared to PCR and western blot analysis of human cell culture. Ovostatin 2 level was elevated in all the chicken samples as well as in human OC mRNA and cell lines [56]. The label-free analysis was also used in order to discover changes in protein expression and molecular/biological pathways in serum and tissues derived from malignant OC compared with benign tumors. Apolipoprotein AI and serotransferrin levels were reduced in both serum and tissue from patients with malignant OC tumor. Moreover, analysis of the interactome, which comprise the whole set of molecular interactions in a cell, and the pathways suggested a potential role of Poly(rC)-binding protein 1 in OC pathogenesis [57].

Although quantitative proteomics studies have significantly contributed to the discovery of OC protein patterns and cellular signaling networks, the approach has some limitations. SILAC method is mainly dedicated for cell line studies, which prevents human samples analysis [41]. The use of isobaric tagging patterns may be restricted by isotopic contaminations or background interference. Moreover, a common problem is co-isolation and fragmentation of some contamination ions together with the targeted precursor ion. Other drawbacks of the label-based approaches include high cost of the reagents and laborious sample preparation [16]. The major disadvantage of label-free methods is their low reproducibility. Additionally, they require extensive data processing and advanced statistical analysis [58].

Post-translational modifications

One of the challenges of the proteomic analysis is the proteome complexity, which results not only from high dynamic range of the biological samples but also from a wide variety of post-translational modifications e.g. glycosylation, ubiquitination, or phosphorylation. Many studies have proved that various types of cancers are associated with aberrations in protein modifications. Therefore, recent studies have focused on this field of proteomics to provide novel information on the disease development. In order to detect post-translational modifications and define their structures, sensitive MS methods are required like MALDI-TOF or LC-ESI (ESI - electrospray ionization) combined with dissociation techniques [59].

Protein glycosylation is undeniably a common and complex modification, responsible for several biological processes, like cell communication, signaling, adhesion, protein folding or solubility [6, 60]. There are two main categories of glycosylation depending on glycan attachments: N- and O- glycans. Analysis and characterization of glycans may be challenging due to glycan variety and structure complexity [61]. To overcome this limitation, it is necessary to use targeted isolation and enrichment methods as well as sensitive detection techniques. Several methods have been proposed as glycoprotein affinity enrichment techniques: lectin chromatography, hydrazide chemistry, hydrophilic interaction liquid chromatography, or capture via immobilized titanium dioxide and boronic acid. Glycomics based on MS analysis has been successfully used to characterize the proteome of OC patients [60, 62]. A comparison of glycosyltransferases involved in N-linked pathway in OC and normal ovarian tissues allowed for identification of OC-specific glycoproteins and glycosylation aberrations. Selected glycoproteins in patient sera were verified using immunoprecipitation and microarray. Results pointed out periostin and thrombospondin as potential OC markers with cancer-specific glycosylation [63]. Furthermore, N-linked sialylated glycoproteins were examined in OC and healthy controls sera. It was suggested that haptoglobin, PON1, and zinc-alpha-2-glycoprotein might have specific sialylation aberrations of the glycopeptides in the OC samples [64]. Glycomic strategies were also used to analyze proximal fluids derived from OC patients: ascites and malignant ovarian cyst fluids. Sialome (sialic acid that contains glycoproteins) of OC was identified, including a set of 13 sialoglycopeptides proposed as novel biomarkers [65]. The importance of the post-translational research was demonstrated in a study focused on CA125 N-glycan forms. Differentiations between CA125 glycoforms from OC patients and controls may improve sensitivity and specificity of this widely used biomarker [66]. Recently, a novel methodology, coupling HILIC-UPLC and microarray for affinity-based study of cancer-associated glycans in OC cell lysates, was proposed. A structure of monoclonal A4 antibody was revealed. Understanding the antibody cancer-specific binding to glycans may simplify its use as a diagnostic indicator [67].

The intracellular signaling networks are mainly based on reversible protein phosphorylation. It is a highly dynamic post-translational modification responsible for e.g. metabolism, apoptosis, homeostasis or proliferation [68]. Phosphoproteins, like glycoproteins, are usually present in biological samples at low concentrations. Consequently, a number of enrichment strategies have been proposed: immunoprecipitation, immobilized metal affinity chromatography, metal-oxide affinity chromatography, chemical modification, magnetic beads or hydroxyapatite chromatography [68, 69]. Recent studies have revealed the potential of phosphorylation profiling in oncogenesis characterization. Proteomic strategies have resulted in the discovery of targets of kinase inhibitors [70]. However, this approach is still out of favor according to OC studies. Research published by Francavilla et al. described phosphoproteomics as a promising strategy for understanding molecular determinants of OC. An analysis of epithelial cells collected from OC and healthy patients showed that cyclin-dependent kinase 7 (CDK7) controls cell proliferation. Therefore, inhibition of CDK7 may contribute to the development of efficient therapeutic strategies [71].

Although post-translational modification analysis seems to be an accurate and effective strategy for biomarker discovery and understanding cell signaling networking, there are some limitations that should be considered. Firstly, the modifications have to be subjected to chemical or enzymatic release. For example, ionization of native glycans is very poor [60]. Generally, phospho- and glyco-proteins are present in biosamples at low concentrations, so sufficient enrichment methods are required [72]. Moreover, reliable study results usually require derivatization. Sample preparation might be an issue mainly due to post-translational modification heterogeneity [73]. Finally, MS techniques have a limited dynamic range and minor modifications cannot be detected. Even though, when proper detection is achieved, accurate spectra interpretation and protein structure construction are challenging [72].

Protein and peptide tissue imaging

Human biofluids are usually characterized by high dynamic range, which complicates biomarker discovery process. As tissue samples are poor in proteins but rich in specific molecules related to disease, direct analysis of cancer tumors seems to be a promising approach. Standard tissue analysis is mainly based on immune-histochemistry (IHC) and histology. Nevertheless, deep proteomic tumor analysis may facilitate resolving the issues associated with OC diagnosis. The lack of significant biomarkers is not the only problem. Histological analysis usually confirms the disease and allows for tumor stage classification as per FIGO system. Further patient treatment depends on proper stage determination. However, staging is not sufficient as a prognostic parameter, and proper grade classification is an additional useful factor. Grading is assigned using light microscopy, which is rather subjective and not significantly reproducible. Therefore, new analytical methods are required to improve grading system and discover effective biomarkers. There are two rapidly evolving strategies to analyze proteins and peptides in tumor tissue: classical strategy and tissue imaging [74]. Classical proteomics such as LC-MS may be used to generate a molecular fingerprint of disease [75, 76]. These methods allow for identification of hundreds to thousands of proteins and peptides. However, the spatial distribution of specific molecules is lost in this kind of analysis as samples need to be homogenized. Recently, a direct MS analysis of tissue sections has become possible due to development of MALDI imaging mass spectrometry (MALDI-IMS) [77]. When coupled with histological analysis, MALDI-IMS may provide information not only about tissue proteome but also about the distribution of lipids, metabolites or xenobiotics. The use of MALDI technology requires a selection of matrix solution that coats tissue samples either with spray

coating or with automatic matrix spotter. Firstly, MALDI-IMS was used to analyze fresh frozen tissue sections but this kind of material is usually not available during standard diagnostic setting. Thus, strategies focused on formalin fixed and paraffin embedded (FFPE) materials have been successfully adapted.

A number of MALDI-IMS analyses have been conducted in the field of OC. A comparison of MALDI profiling, MALDI-IMS, and IHC analysis enabled identification of Reg-Alpha Fragment of the 11S proteasome activator complex as a potential OC biomarker. The protein was present in OC tumor and absent in benign tissues [78]. Moreover, hierarchical cluster analysis was applied to prove that MALDI-IMS is effective in differentiation of tissue regions [79]. MALDI-IMS was also proved to be a useful strategy in the OC interface zone analysis. Plastin 2 and peroxiredoxin 1 were identified as upregulated proteins in tumor region as compared with a normal tissue [80]. Recently, a novel methodology focused on N-glycan analysis in FFPE OC tissue has been proposed. Imaging technology combined with ESI MS was used to generate images of N-glycan structure distribution in tissue sections [81]. Another interesting approach is a combination of MALDI-IMS with top-down microproteomics. An analysis of benign, tumor and necrotic-fibrotic regions derived from OC biopsy specimens allowed for detection of promising novel biomarkers. The proposed methodology may contribute to identification of proteins that are usually lost during conventional proteomics analysis [82].

MALDI-IMS is potentially a revolutionary technique in pathology. Recently, tremendous improvement has been made in the field of sample preparation and instrumentation. However, the technique still poses a few challenges. First, there are no studies confirming its utility in clinical settings. Second, sample preparation and measurement methodology should be proved to be reproducible and robust in different laboratories. For better understanding of MALDI-IMS results, the integration with other –omics studies like transcriptomics still needs improvement [77, 79].

Proteomics in treatment response

Cytoreductive surgery coupled with chemotherapy based on paclitaxel, carboplatin, cisplatin, often in combination with taxanes, is the most common OC treatment option. A decision on postoperative chemotherapy depends on the risk of the tumor recurrence, stage, and grade. OC subtypes respond differently to treatment and chemo-resistance may occur as a serious side effect [6, 83]. According to statistics, even 25% of patients experience platinum resistance, and in 50–60% of cases cancer resistance develops during the treatment [84]. Investigation of chemotherapy mechanisms and discovery of factors responsible for chemotherapy response and resistance provide a selection of alternative therapies or chemo-sensitizing agents [85]. Unfortunately, individual agents offer rather low response rate: 5–20%. As a result, patients often have to choose between continuation of chemotherapy or supportive care only [84]. Drug resistance may occur due to pharmacokinetic, tumor-specific aberrations and microenvironment of the tumor [86]. Discovery of chemo-resistant biomarkers may improve personalized medicine and therapy planning. Therefore, a number of previously discussed techniques: MALDI-TOF MS, LC-MS/MS, SILAC, iTRAQ, label-free quantitation, ICAT, were proposed to identify new biomarkers and investigate proteome changes during OC treatment [85]. Previously identified chemo-resistance biomarkers are presented in Table 2.

MALDI-TOF MS strategy was first used to identify chemo-resistant biomarkers in a comparative analysis of platinum-sensitive and platinum-resistant cell lines. Five differentially expressed proteins were identified and further validated [87]. Another study focused on the same cell culture analysis discovered five new mitochondrial proteins potentially involved in chemo-resistance mechanisms. It was suggested that mitochondrial defects may be associated with drug resistance [88]. MALDI-TOF MS combined with LC-MS/MS analysis demonstrated that proteins responsible for metabolism, stress response, and apoptosis, are differentially expressed in paclitaxel sensitive and resistant OC cell lines. Moreover, one of disulfide isomerases was found to play an essential role in chemo-resistance [89]. Lee et al. also used a combination of two techniques: MALDI-TOF MS and LC-MS/MS and identified two potential chemo-resistant biomarkers in OC cells [90]. As glycosylation is often connected with cancer development, analysis of glycoproteins was used to discover useful biomarkers. Abnormalities in the expression of four glycoproteins were found to be characteristic of chemo-resistance cases [91].

A study utilizing label-free LC-MS/MS strategy confirmed that mitochondrial proteomic changes are important in both platinum [88] and cisplatin resistance [92]. Therefore, abnormalities in the concentration of three proteins were found to be characteristic of cisplatin-resistant OC cell line [92]. Moreover, the label-free approach confirmed that elevated levels of TXNDC17 in both OC cell and tissues are associated with paclitaxel resistance. The study additionally demonstrated the relationship between TXNDC17, poor prognostic factors, and short survival rate [93].

Recently, isotopic labeling has also been widely used in the investigation of drug resistance. SILAC analysis proved that, as in the case of platinum [88] and cisplatin resistance [92], doxorubicin resistance is partially caused by changes in mitochondria [94]. ICAT technique was applied in the study of cisplatin resistance. Changes in protein expression in chemo-resistant cells were

compared with mRNA expression levels [95]. Furthermore, another study based on ICAT-MS/MS analysis integrated with RNA analysis pointed out 16 protein changes in the chemo-resistant OC tissues. These results triggered a conclusion that chemotherapy response and resistance are determined by a set of proteins from following classes: extracellular-matrix, junction or cell adhesion proteins [96]. ITRAQ strategy turned out to be a useful approach in multidrug-resistance investigations [97]. Moreover, iTRAQ technique revealed that major histocompatibility complex class I peptide repertoire of OC cells is associated with the pathological condition of the cell and may become a new treatment target also in chemo-resistant cancers [98]. Advanced bioinformatics approach contributed to establishing prediction models based on iTRAQ analysis results. It was proved that proteomic profiles of OC may provide information on platinum drug responses [99].

The studies on the chemoresistance mechanism are very promising and may improve the treatment and prognosis of patients with OC. However, there is still a lot of work ahead [86]. Firstly, many analyses are conducted only on cell lines. An appropriate clinical material is limited and difficult to obtain [85]. Therefore, all encouraging results should be verified using OC tissue. Despite high-throughput technologies, there is still no significant biomarker to predict a treatment response [85]. Moreover, many cancers may develop resistance to different drugs and therapies [6].

Challenges for biomarker research in clinical proteomics

Although clinical proteomics did contribute to understanding of complicated molecular pathways of several diseases including OC, only few information and findings are significant enough to be translated into clinical settings. A great effort was made to introduce new, sensitive biomarkers to clinical practice. However, most of them did not meet the validation requirements. Currently, there seem to be a great number of studies focused on searching for marker candidates. Over the past decades, clinical proteomics has encountered some obstacles and challenges, which should be overcome in the future. In this chapter, we discussed the general challenges associated with the MS-based analysis of biomarkers. Drawbacks characteristic for the specific methods are presented in the particular chapters.

The first issue to deal with at the beginning of the research is experimental design. The sample size is often inadequate to draw any meaningful conclusions and to obtain significant statistical power. Selection and building of suitable statistical methods and models is an essential part of the experiment. Moreover, in order to ensure the necessary impact of the analysis, the study groups should be properly selected. Factors such as age,

Table 2 Drug-resistance markers in OC identified by MS-based proteomic techniques

Chemoresistance markers	MS technique	Ref.
Annexin 3; Destrin; Cofilin1; Gluthathione-S transferase omega 1; Cytosolic NADP+ dependent isocitrate dehydrogenase	MALDI-TOF	[87]
ATP synthase subunit alpha; Peroxiredoxin 3; Prohibitin; Electron transfer flavoprotein subunit alpha; Aldehyde dehydrogenase X	MALDI-TOF	[88]
ERp57	MALDI-TOF ESI-Q-TOF	[89]
Tumor rejection antigen (gp96) 1; Triose phosphate isomerase; Palmitoyl-protein thioesterase1 precursor; ER-associated DNAJ	MALDI-TOF ESI-Q-TOF	[91]
Aldehyde dehydrogenase 1 family, member A1; Annexin A1; Heterogeneous Nuclear Ribonucleoproteins A2; Rho GDP dissociation inhibitor	MALDI-TOF LC-MS/MS	[90]
Activated leukocyte cell adhesion molecule; A kinase anchoring protein 12; Nestin	Orbitrap	[92]
Thioredoxin domain containing 17	Orbitrap	[93]
Mitochondrial topoisomerase I	Orbitrap	[94]
Cell recognition molecule CASPR3; S100 protein family members; Junction adhesion molecule Claudin 4; CDC42-binding protein kinase beta	ESI-MS/MS	[95]
P53 binding protein 1; Catenin delta 1 and plakoglobin; EGF-containing fibulin-like extracellular matrix protein 1; Voltage-dependent anion-selective channel protein 1	HPLC-ESI-MS/MS	[96]
Pyruvate kinase isozymes M1/M2; Heat Shock Protein Family D	ESI-Q-TOF	[97]

diet, medication, etc. may have a crucial influence on the experiment [100]. Discovery of a sensitive and specific OC biomarker requires analysis and comparisons of several groups of samples including healthy controls, inflammatory controls, benign adnexal masses, early OC stage, and preferably other malignancies than OC. Proteins selected as relevant OC markers should be further compared with CA125 and HE4, and their utility as OC markers should be confirmed in longitudinal monitoring. Finally, for proper assessment of sensitivity and specificity, the selected markers need to be applied to blinded large study sets. Most of the experiments include only pilot analysis and omits another important step – expanding the study groups and sample size.

Another crucial factor in every proteomic experiment is the quality of clinical samples quality. The best way to collect samples is to create a biobank with all epidemiologic and genetic data. Samples should be collected in the conditions compatible with MS method and immediately frozen (e.g., in liquid nitrogen), preferably with the addition of protease inhibitors. One of the main pitfalls is the influence of inappropriate storage temperature and freeze-thaw cycles on the protein degradation. Endogenous contaminations with salts or lipids, and even inappropriate type of sample tube may affect the result of the experiment [101]. Therefore, in order to obtain the highest sample quality, a good communication between proteome scientists and clinical staff is necessary and all aspects of samples collection should be discussed.

Over the past years, unsuccessful efforts have been undertaken to discover OC screening method, including a unique proteomic signature. One of the main reasons for ineffective investigations is the limitations of MS methods. Despite significant progress in MS techniques, high dynamic proteome range still occurs as a major challenge. The most relevant proteins are usually present in biological samples in low concentrations, and their detection remains very difficult when high abundant proteins coexist. The most frequently used types of sample are serum and plasma. Since ten high abundant serum/plasma proteins account for about 90% of the total proteins, examination of all low concentrated proteins – the promising source of biomarkers is a huge challenge. To reduce the overall sample complexity, several methods have been proposed, including pre-fractionation, depletion or enrichment. However, proteomic techniques are still not sufficient to detect low abundant molecules. Although they are able to simplify the protein mixture, major blood components remain highly concentrated. Moreover, some depletion methods and other preanalytical steps lead to the removal of relevant proteins due to non-specific-bounds [16]. Therefore, the issue of low-abundance proteins analysis should be studied in the near future.

Even though MS-based techniques have been used in proteome science for a long time, there are still no uniform workflows and procedures. Therefore, inter-laboratory variability and low reproducibility often occur [16]. Another analytical challenge is statistical analysis and interpretation of the results containing hundreds, sometimes even thousands, of peptides and proteins. A typical result of the proteomic experiment is a list of interferences containing peptide-spectrum matches. Each interference is characterized by a score, which shows the confidence of correct identification. However, to avoid false-positive results, significant bioinformatics strategy may be a crucial step. P-value is not suitable for multiple testing of a database search, and need to be improved, usually by false discovery rate calculations [102].

Moreover, multiple comparisons require the use of proper corrections (e.g., Bonferroni correction, determination of the q-value) [72].

Past decade of MS-based research revealed many obstacles associated with biomarker discovery. Thus, more restrictions are required for each further analysis. Every experiment data should be validated with other complementary method like ELISA or western blot. Further analysis need to be also conducted using an external set of samples to ensure the reliability of the obtained results. Moreover, presented studies should be no longer limited to the list of differentially expressed proteins and peptides. Identified molecules need to be connected into one network and they need to explain complicated disease mechanisms. These steps are necessary for the future implementation of biomarker assessment to clinical practice.

Despite many challenges in biomarker studies, there are already two multimarker tests: OVA 1 and ROMA (risk of ovarian malignancy algorithm) approved by the Food and Drug Administration for OC diagnosis. Therefore, it should be expected that the current studies constitute a solid basis for creating new reliable diagnostic tools in the future. The addition of sophisticated MS techniques, like MALDI-IMS, to methods commonly used in the clinics, may be a step forward to significantly improve diagnosis and treatment.

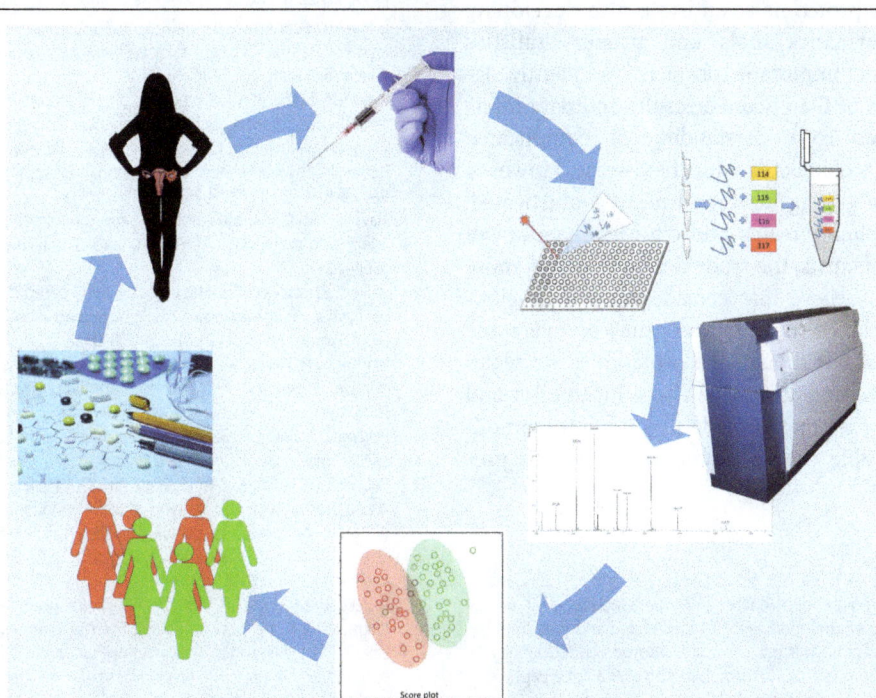

Fig. 3 Development of novel, innovative diagnostics methods, therapies or drug response monitoring based on proteomics techniques

Conclusions

Since OC is responsible for thousands of deaths each year, there is a dire need to improve diagnostics as well as treatments strategies. Elucidating the mechanisms and molecular pathways during carcinogenesis may contribute to developing novel targeted therapies and personalized medicine. Proteomics, as a rapidly evolving branch of science, may be essential in novel biomarkers discovery, therapy decisions, progression prediction, and monitoring of drug response or resistance. This review presents main proteomics techniques based on MS that provide information on molecular mechanisms of the OC. Many limitations of particular approaches have also been discussed. The first challenge is the heterogeneity and diverse origins of the OC. It should be taken into account during basic and clinical studies design. Another difficulty is a limited access to biological samples, especially OC tissues. Studies based on the OC cell lines should be verified using tumor tissues. The next issue that should be considered is low inter-laboratory reproducibility of the results. There are many studies proposing different OC biomarkers but usually none further research is conducted to confirm the proposals. Moreover, there are still some improvements necessary in MS techniques. Analytical protocols need to be standardized to introduce a reproducible and high-throughput analysis. Lack of uniform workflow leads to false-positive results associated for example with sample collection errors. Moreover, high dynamic range of compounds in biological samples is an issue that is still not solved. A great challenge for proteome scientists is also developing significant bioinformatics tools and proper statistics strategies. Another important obstacle, frequently ignored, is validation of the obtained results and data interpretation that lead to understanding of complicated molecular pathways connected with the disease. However, current studies are getting more and more sophisticated. Due to multidisciplinary teams and close cooperation of clinical staff and scientists, the study design becomes more advanced. Authors believe that considering fast development of MS techniques, all drawbacks may be overcome in the next few years. Although the proteomics strategies still require optimization, they have also a lot to offer and in the near future they may provide insights into complicated and inaccessible cancer proteomics, which is presented in the Fig. 3.

Abbreviations

BRCA 1: Breast Cancer Gene 1; BRCA 2: Breast Cancer Gene 2; CA125: Cancer Antigen 125; CDK7: cyclin-dependent kinase 7; DIA: data-independent acquisition; ESI: electrospray ionization; FFPE: formalin fixed and paraffin embedded; HE4: human epididymis protein 4; ICAT: Isotope-coded affinity tag; IHC: immune-histochemistry; IMAC: immobilized metal affinity capture; IMS: MALDI imaging mass spectrometry; iTRAQ: isobaric Tags for Relative and Absolute Quantification; LC: liquid chromatography; m/z: mass/charge ratio; MALDI: matrix assisted laser desorption/ionization; MS: mass spectrometry;

OC: ovarian cancer; Q-TOF: quadrupole time-of-flight; ROMA: risk of ovarian malignancy algorithm; SELDI: surface-enhanced laser desorption/ionization; SILAC: stable isotope labeling by amino acids in cell culture; SWATH: sequential window acquisition of all theoretical mass spectra; TMT: Tandem Mass Tags; TOF: time-to-flight

Funding

The project was supported by the Polish National Science Centre (2014/15/B/NZ7/00964).

Authors' contributions

A.S. and S.P. executed and drafted the manuscript. J.M. and Z.J.K made critical discussion about the study and designed structure of the manuscript. All authors have read and approved the manuscript submitted.

Competing interests

The authors declare that they have no competing interests.

References

1. Zhang B, Barekati Z, Kohler C, Radpour R, Asadollahi R, Holzgreve W, et al. Proteomics and biomarkers for ovarian cancer diagnosis. Ann Clin Lab Sci. 2010;40:218–25.
2. Poersch A, Grassi ML, Carvalho VP, Lanfredi GP, Palma Cde S, Greene LJ, et al. A proteomic signature of ovarian cancer tumor fluid identified by highthroughput and verified by targeted proteomics. J Proteomics. 2016;145:226–36.
3. Bast Jr RC, Hennessy B, Mills GB. The biology of ovarian cancer: new opportunities for translation.
4. Longuespée R, Boyon C, Desmons A, Vinatier D, Leblanc E, Farré I, et al. Ovarian cancer molecular pathology. Cancer Metastasis Rev. 2012;31:713–32.
5. Reid BM, Permuth JB, Sellers TA. Epidemiology of ovarian cancer: a review. Cancer Biol Med. 2017;14:9–32.
6. Elzek MA, Rodland KD. Proteomics of ovarian cancer: functional insights and clinical applications. Cancer Metastasis Rev. 2015;34:83–96.
7. Vaughan S, Coward JI, Bast RC, Berchuck A, Berek JS, Brenton JD, et al. Rethinking ovarian cancer: recommendations for improving outcomes. Nat Rev Cancer. 2011;11:719–25.
8. Hays JL, Kim G, Giuroiu I, Kohn EC. Proteomics and ovarian cancer: integrating proteomics information into clinical care. J Proteome. 2010;73: 1864–72.
9. Parker CE, Borchers CH. Mass spectrometry based biomarker discovery, verification, and validation – quality assurance and control of protein biomarker assays. Mol Oncol. 2014;8:840–58.
10. Matthews H, Hanison J, Nirmalan N. "Omics"-informed drug and biomarker discovery: opportunities. Challenges and Future Perspectives Proteomes. 2016;4:28.
11. Herceg Z, Hainaut P. Genetic and epigenetic alterations as biomarkers for cancer detection, diagnosis and prognosis. Mol Oncol. 2007;1:26–41.
12. Rebbeck TR, Mitra N, Wan F, Sinilnikova OM, Healey S, McGuffog L, et al. Association of type and location of BRCA1 and BRCA2 mutations with risk of breast and ovarian cancer. JAMA. 2015;313:1347–61.
13. Gee ME, Faraahi Z, McCormick A, Edmondson RJ. DNA damage repair in ovarian cancer: unlocking the heterogeneity. J Ovarian Res. 2018;11:50.
14. Ardekani AM, Liotta LA, Petricoin EF. Clinical potential of proteomics in the diagnosis of ovarian cancer. Expert Rev Mol Diagn. 2002;2:312–20.
15. Sajic T, Liu Y, Aebersold R. Using data-independent, high resolution mass spectrometry in protein biomarker research: perspectives and clinical applications. Proteomics Clin Appl. 2014.
16. Hajduk J, Matysiak J, Kokot ZJ. Challenges in biomarker discovery with MALDI-TOF MS. Clin Chim Acta. 2016.

17. Meehan KL, Rainczuk A, Salamonsen LA, Stephens AN. Proteomics and the search for biomarkers of female reproductive diseases. Reproduction. 2010; 140:505–19.

18. Romagnolo C, Leon AE, Fabricio ASC, Taborelli M, Polesel J, Del Pup L, et al. HE4, CA125 and risk of ovarian malignancy algorithm (ROMA) as diagnostic tools for ovarian cancer in patients with a pelvic mass: an Italian multicenter study. Gynecol Oncol. 2016;141:303–11.

19. Swiatly A, Horala A, Hajduk J, Matysiak J, Nowak-Markwitz E, Kokot ZJ. MALDI-TOF-MS analysis in discovery and identification of serum proteomic patterns of ovarian cancer. BMC Cancer. 2017;17.

20. Imperlini E, Santorelli L, Orrù S, Scolamiero E, Ruoppolo M, Caterino M. Mass spectrometry-based Metabolomic and proteomic strategies in organic Acidemias. Biomed Res Int. 2016;2016:9210408.

21. Merlos Rodrigo MA, Zitka O, Krizkova S, Moulick A, Adam V, Kizek R. MALDI-TOF MS as evolving cancer diagnostic tool: a review. J Pharm Biomed Anal. 2014;95:245–55.

22. Tabb DL. Quality assessment for clinical proteomics. Clin Biochem. 2013; 46:411–20.

23. Albalat A, Husi H, Stalmach A, Schanstra JP, Mischak H. Classical MALDI-MS versus CE-based ESI-MS proteomic profiling in urine for clinical applications. Bioanalysis. 2014;6:247–66.

24. Sandin M, Chawade A, Levander F. Is label-free LC-MS/MS ready for biomarker discovery? PROTEOMICS - Clin Appl. 2015;9:289–94.

25. Collins MA, An J, Hood BL, Conrads TP, Bowser RP. Label-free LC-MS/MS proteomic analysis of cerebrospinal fluid identifies protein/pathway alterations and candidate biomarkers for amyotrophic lateral sclerosis. J Proteome Res. 2015;14:4486–501.

26. Tsai T-H, Song E, Zhu R, Di Poto C, Wang M, Luo Y, et al. LC-MS/MS-based serum proteomics for identification of candidate biomarkers for hepatocellular carcinoma. Proteomics. 2015;15:2369–81.

27. Stalmach A, Husi H, Mosbahi K, Albalat A, Mullen W, Mischak H. Methods in Capillary Electrophoresis Coupled to Mass Spectrometry for the Identification of Clinical Proteomic/Peptidomic Biomarkers in Biofluids. 2015. p. 187–205.

28. Dittrich J, Becker S, Hecht M, Ceglarek U. Sample preparation strategies for targeted proteomics via proteotypic peptides in human blood using liquid chromatography tandem mass spectrometry. PROTEOMICS - Clin Appl. 2015;9:5–16.

29. Petricoin EF, Ardekani AM, Hitt BA, Levine PJ, Fusaro VA, Steinberg SM, et al. Use of proteomic patterns in serum to identify ovarian cancer. Lancet. 2002; 359:572–7.

30. Lopez MF, Mikulskis A, Kuzdzal S, Golenko E, Petricoin EF, Liotta LA, et al. A novel, high-throughput workflow for discovery and identification of serum carrier protein-bound peptide biomarker candidates in ovarian cancer samples. Clin Chem. 2007;53:1067–74.

31. Ye H, Sun L, Huang X, Zhang P, Zhao X. A proteomic approach for plasma biomarker discovery with 8-plex iTRAQ labeling and SCX-LC-MS/MS. Mol Cell Biochem. 2010;343:91–9.

32. Aresta A, Calvano CD, Palmisano F, Zambonin CG, Monaco A, Tommasi S, et al. Impact of sample preparation in peptide/protein profiling in human serum by MALDI-TOF mass spectrometry. J Pharm Biomed Anal. 2008;46:157–64.

33. Ye B, Cramer DW, Skates SJ, Gygi SP, Pratomo V, Fu L, et al. Haptoglobin-α subunit as potential serum biomarker in ovarian Cancer. Clin Cancer Res. 2003:9.

34. Periyasamy A, Gopisetty G, Veluswami S, Joyimallaya Subramanium M, Thangarajan R. Identification of candidate biomarker mass (m/z) ranges in serous ovarian adenocarcinoma using matrix-assisted laser desorption/ionization time-of-flight mass spectrometry profiling. Biomarkers. 2015;20:292–8.

35. Wu S, Xu K, Chen G, Zhang J, Liu Z, Xie X. Identification of serum biomarkers for ovarian cancer using MALDI–TOF-MS combined with magnetic beads. Int J Clin Oncol. 2012;17:89–95.

36. Zhang Z, Bast RC, Yu Y, Li J, Sokoll LJ, Rai AJ, et al. Three biomarkers identified from serum proteomic analysis for the detection of early stage ovarian cancer. Cancer Res. 2004;64:5882–90.

37. Li C, Li H, Zhang T, Li J, Liu L, Chang J. Discovery of Apo-A1 as a potential bladder cancer biomarker by urine proteomics and analysis. Biochem Biophys Res Commun. 2014;446:1047–52.

38. Kawahara R, Bollinger JG, Rivera C, Ribeiro ACP, Brandão TB, Leme AFP, et al. A targeted proteomic strategy for the measurement of oral cancer candidate biomarkers in human saliva. Proteomics. 2016;16:159–73.

39. Grenache DG, Heichman KA, Werner TL, Vucetic Z. Clinical performance of two multi-marker blood tests for predicting malignancy in women with an adnexal mass. Clin Chim Acta. 2015;438:358–63.

40. Bland AM, D'Eugenio LR, Dugan MA, Janech MG, Almeida JS, Zile MR, et al. Comparison of variability associated with sample preparation in two-dimensional gel electrophoresis of cardiac tissue. J Biomol Tech. 2006;17:195–9.

41. Lindemann C, Thomanek N, Hundt F, Lerari T, Meyer HE, Wolters D, et al. Strategies in relative and absolute quantitative mass spectrometry based proteomics. Biol Chem. 2017;398:687–99.

42. Schubert OT, Röst HL, Collins BC, Rosenberger G, Aebersold R. Quantitative proteomics: challenges and opportunities in basic and applied research. Nat Protoc. 2017;12:1289–94.

43. Collins BC, Hunter CL, Liu Y, Schilling B, Rosenberger G, Bader SL, et al. Multi-laboratory assessment of reproducibility, qualitative and quantitative performance of SWATH-mass spectrometry. Nat Commun. 2017;8:291.

44. Uitto PM, Lance BK, Wood GR, Sherman J, Baker MS, Molloy MP. Comparing SILAC and two-dimensional gel electrophoresis image analysis for profiling Urokinase plasminogen activator signaling in ovarian Cancer cells. J Proteome Res. 2007;6:2105–12.

45. Musrap N, Tuccitto A, Karagiannis GS, Saraon P, Batruch I, Diamandis EP. Comparative proteomics of ovarian Cancer aggregate formation reveals an increased expression of calcium-activated Chloride Channel regulator 1 (CLCA1). J Biol Chem. 2015;290:17218–27.

46. Qi D, Wang Q, Li H, Zhang T, Lan R, Kwong DWJ, et al. SILAC-based quantitative proteomics identified lysosome as a fast response target to PDT agent Gd-N induced oxidative stress in human ovarian cancer IGROV1 cells. Mol BioSyst. 2015;11:3059–67.

47. Grassi ML, Palma C de S, Thomé CH, Lanfredi GP, Poersch A, Faça VM. Proteomic analysis of ovarian cancer cells during epithelial-mesenchymal transition (EMT) induced by epidermal growth factor (EGF) reveals mechanisms of cell cycle control. J Proteome. 2017;151:2–11.

48. Westbrook JA, Noirel J, Brown JE, Wright PC, Evans CA. Quantitation with chemical tagging reagents in biomarker studies. PROTEOMICS - Clin Appl. 2015;9:295–300.

49. Kristjansdottir B, Levan K, Partheen K, Carlsohn E, Sundfeldt K. Potential tumor biomarkers identified in ovarian cyst fluid by quantitative proteomic analysis, iTRAQ. Clin Proteomics. 2013;10:4.

50. Wang L-N, Tong S-W, Hu H-D, Ye F, Li S-L, Ren H, et al. Quantitative proteome analysis of ovarian cancer tissues using a iTRAQ approach. J Cell Biochem. 2012;113:3762–72.

51. Wang L, Chen S, Zhang M, Li N, Chen Y, Su W, et al. Legumain: a biomarker for diagnosis and prognosis of human ovarian cancer. J Cell Biochem. 2012; 113:2679–86.

52. Russell MR, Walker MJ, Williamson AJK, Gentry-Maharaj A, Ryan A, Kalsi J, et al. Protein Z: a putative novel biomarker for early detection of ovarian cancer. Int J Cancer. 2016;138:2984–92.

53. Waldemarson S, Krogh M, Alaiya A, Kirik U, Schedvins K, Auer G, et al. Protein expression changes in ovarian Cancer during the transition from benign to malignant. J Proteome Res. 2012;11:2876–89.

54. Hiramatsu K, Yoshino K, Serada S, Yoshihara K, Hori Y, Fujimoto M, et al. Similar protein expression profiles of ovarian and endometrial high-grade serous carcinomas. Br J Cancer. 2016;114:554–61.

55. Sinclair J, Metodieva G, Dafou D, Gayther SA, Timms JF. Profiling signatures of ovarian cancer tumour suppression using 2D-DIGE and 2D-LC-MS/MS with tandem mass tagging. J Proteome. 2011;74:451–65.

56. Nepomuceno AI, Shao H, Jing K, Ma Y, Petitte JN, Idowu MO, et al. In-depth LC-MS/MS analysis of the chicken ovarian cancer proteome reveals conserved and novel differentially regulated proteins in humans. Anal Bioanal Chem. 2015;407:6851–63.

57. Wegdam W, Argmann CA, Kramer G, Vissers JP, Buist MR, Kenter GG, et al. Label-free LC-MSe in tissue and serum reveals protein networks underlying differences between benign and malignant serous ovarian tumors. Rota R, editor. PLoS One. 2014;e108046:9.

58. Langley SR, Mayr M. Comparative analysis of statistical methods used for detecting differential expression in label-free mass spectrometry proteomics. J Proteome. 2015;129:83–92.

59. Banazadeh A, Veillon L, Wooding KM, Zabet-moghaddam M, Mechref Y. Recent advances in mass spectrometric analysis of glycoproteins. Electrophoresis. 2017;38:162–89.

60. Mechref Y, Hu Y, Garcia A, Zhou S, Desantos-Garcia JL, Hussein A. Defining putative glycan cancer biomarkers by MS. Bioanalysis. 2012;4:2457–69.
61. Tousi F, Hancock WS, Hincapie M. Technologies and strategies for glycoproteomics and glycomics and their application to clinical biomarker research. Anal Methods. 2011;3:20–32.
62. Kim K, Ruhaak LR, Nguyen UT, Taylor SL, Dimapasoc L, Williams C, et al. Evaluation of glycomic profiling as a diagnostic biomarker for epithelial ovarian cancer. Cancer Epidemiol Biomark Prev. 2014;23:611–21.
63. Abbott KL, Lim J-M, Wells L, Benigno BB, McDonald JF, Pierce M. Identification of candidate biomarkers with cancer-specific glycosylation in the tissue and serum of endometrioid ovarian cancer patients by glycoproteomic analysis. Proteomics. 2010;10:470–81.
64. Shetty V, Hafner J, Shah P, Nickens Z, Philip R. Investigation of ovarian cancer associated sialylation changes in N-linked glycopeptides by quantitative proteomics. Clin Proteomics. 2012;9:10.
65. Kuzmanov U, Musrap N, Kosanam H, Smith CR, Batruch I, Dimitromanolakis A, et al. Glycoproteomic identification of potential glycoprotein biomarkers in ovarian cancer proximal fluids. Clin Chem Lab Med. 2013:51.
66. Saldova R, Struwe WB, Wynne K, Elia G, Duffy MJ, Rudd PM. Exploring the glycosylation of serum CA125. Int J Mol Sci. 2013;14:15636–54.
67. Liau B, Tan B, Teo G, Zhang P, Choo A, Rudd PM. Shotgun Glycomics identifies tumor-associated glycan ligands bound by an ovarian carcinoma-specific monoclonal antibody. Sci Rep. 2017;7:14489.
68. Maes E, Tirez K, Baggerman G, Valkenborg D, Schoofs L, Encinar JR, et al. The use of elemental mass spectrometry in phosphoproteomic applications. Mass Spectrom Rev. 2016;35:350–60.
69. Toss A, De Matteis E, Rossi E, Casa L, Iannone A, Federico M, et al. Ovarian Cancer: can proteomics give new insights for therapy and diagnosis? Int J Mol Sci. 2013;14:8271–90.
70. Harsha HC, Pandey A. Phosphoproteomics in cancer. Mol Oncol. 2010;4:482–95.
71. Francavilla C, Lupia M, Tsafou K, Villa A, Kowalczyk K, Rakownikow Jersie-Christensen R, et al. Phosphoproteomics of primary cells reveals Druggable kinase signatures in ovarian Cancer. Cell Rep. 2017;18:3242–56.
72. Crutchfield CA, Thomas SN, Sokoll LJ, Chan DW. Advances in mass spectrometry-based clinical biomarker discovery. Clin Proteomics. 2016;13:1.
73. Mann M, Ong SE, Grønborg M, Steen H, Jensen ON, Pandey A. Analysis of protein phosphorylation using mass spectrometry: deciphering the phosphoproteome. Trends Biotechnol. 2002;20:261–8.
74. Gustafsson JOR, Oehler MK, Ruszkiewicz A, McColl SR, Hoffmann P. MALDI imaging mass spectrometry (MALDI-IMS)-application of spatial proteomics for ovarian cancer classification and diagnosis. Int J Mol Sci. 2011;12:773–94.
75. Zhu Y, Wu R, Sangha N, Yoo C, Cho KR, Shedden KA, et al. Classifications of ovarian cancer tissues by proteomic patterns. Proteomics. 2006;6:5846–56.
76. Kim H, Wu R, Cho KR, Thomas DG, Gossner G, Liu JR, et al. Comparative proteomic analysis of low stage and high stage endometrioid ovarian adenocarcinomas. Proteomics Clin Appl. 2008;2:571–84.
77. Schwamborn K, Kriegsmann M, Weichert W. MALDI imaging mass spectrometry — from bench to bedside. Biochim Biophys Acta - Proteins Proteomics. 2016.
78. Lemaire R, Ait Menguellet S, Stauber J, Marchaudon V, Lucot J-P, Collinet P, et al. Specific MALDI imaging and profiling for biomarker hunting and validation: fragment of the 11S proteasome activator complex, Reg alpha fragment, is a new potential ovary Cancer biomarker. J Proteome Res. 2007;6:4127–34.
79. McDonnell LA, Corthals GL, Willems SM, van Remoortere A, RJM v Z, Deelder AM. Peptide and protein imaging mass spectrometry in cancer research. J Proteome. 2010;73:1921–44.
80. Kang S, Shim HS, Lee JS, Kim DS, Kim HY, Hong SH, et al. Molecular proteomics imaging of tumor interfaces by mass spectrometry. J Proteome Res. 2010;9:1157–64.
81. Everest-Dass AV, Briggs MT, Kaur G, Oehler MK, Hoffmann P, Packer NH. N-glycan MALDI imaging mass spectrometry on formalin-fixed paraffin-embedded tissue enables the delineation of ovarian Cancer tissues. Mol Cell Proteomics. 2016;15:3003–16.
82. Delcourt V, Franck J, Leblanc E, Narducci F, Robin Y-M, Gimeno J-P, et al. Combined mass spectrometry imaging and top-down microproteomics reveals evidence of a hidden proteome in ovarian Cancer. EBioMedicine. 2017;21:55–64.
83. Jayson GC, Kohn EC, Kitchener HC, Ledermann JA. Ovarian cancer. Lancet. 2014;384:1376–88.
84. O'Toole S, O'Leary J. Ovarian Cancer Chemoresistance. Encycl Cancer. 2011:2674–6.
85. Deng J, Wang L, Ni J, Beretov J, Wasinger V, Wu D, et al. Proteomics discovery of chemoresistant biomarkers for ovarian cancer therapy. Expert Rev Proteomics. 2016;13:905–15.
86. Agarwal R, Kaye SB. Ovarian cancer: strategies for overcoming resistance to chemotherapy. Nat Rev Cancer. 2003;3:502–16.
87. Yan X, Pan L, Yuan Y, Lang J, Mao N. Identification of platinum-resistance associated proteins through proteomic analysis of human ovarian Cancer cells and their platinum-resistant sublines. J Proteome Res. 2007;6:772–80.
88. Dai Z, Yin J, He H, Li W, Hou C, Qian X, et al. Mitochondrial comparative proteomics of human ovarian cancer cells and their platinum-resistant sublines. Proteomics. 2010;10:3789–99.
89. Cicchillitti L, Di Michele M, Urbani A, Ferlini C, Donat MB, Scambia G, et al. Comparative proteomic analysis of paclitaxel sensitive A2780 epithelial ovarian cancer cell line and its resistant counterpart A2780TC1 by 2D-DIGE: the role of ERp57. J Proteome Res. 2009;8:1902–12.
90. Lee DH, Chung K, Song J-A, Kim T, Kang H, Huh JH, et al. Proteomic identification of paclitaxel-resistance associated hnRNP A2 and GDI 2 proteins in human ovarian Cancer cells. J Proteome Res. 2010;9:5668–76.
91. Di Michele M, Marcone S, Cicchillitti L, Della Corte A, Ferlini C, Scambia G, et al. Glycoproteomics of paclitaxel resistance in human epithelial ovarian cancer cell lines: towards the identification of putative biomarkers. J Proteome. 2010;73:879–98.
92. Chappell NP, Teng P, Hood BL, Wang G, Darcy KM, Hamilton CA, et al. Mitochondrial proteomic analysis of cisplatin resistance in ovarian Cancer. J Proteome Res. 2012;11:4605–14.
93. Zhang S-F, Wang X-Y, Fu Z-Q, Peng Q-H, Zhang J-Y, Ye F, et al. TXNDC17 promotes paclitaxel resistance via inducing autophagy in ovarian cancer. Autophagy. 2015;11:225–38.
94. Chen X, Wei S, Ma Y, Lu J, Niu G, Xue Y, et al. Quantitative proteomics analysis identifies mitochondria as therapeutic targets of multidrug-resistance in ovarian cancer. Theranostics. 2014;4:1164–75.
95. Stewart JJ, White JT, Yan X, Collins S, Drescher CW, Urban ND, et al. Proteins associated with cisplatin resistance in ovarian Cancer cells identified by quantitative proteomic technology and integrated with mRNA expression levels. Mol Cell Proteomics. 2006;5:433–43.
96. Pan S, Cheng L, White JT, Lu W, Utleg AG, Yan X, et al. Quantitative proteomics analysis integrated with microarray data reveals that extracellular matrix proteins, catenins, and P53 binding protein 1 are important for chemotherapy response in ovarian cancers. Omi A J Integr Biol. 2009;13:345–54.
97. Li S-L, Ye F, Cai W-J, Hu H-D, Hu P, Ren H, et al. Quantitative proteome analysis of multidrug resistance in human ovarian cancer cell line. J Cell Biochem. 2010;109:n/a-n/a.
98. Shetty V, Nickens Z, Testa J, Hafner J, Sinnathamby G, Philip R. Quantitative immunoproteomics analysis reveals novel MHC class I presented peptides in cisplatin-resistant ovarian cancer cells. J Proteome. 2012;75:3270–90.
99. Yu K-H, Levine DA, Zhang H, Chan DW, Zhang Z, Snyder M. Predicting ovarian Cancer patients' clinical response to platinum-based chemotherapy by their tumor proteomic signatures. J Proteome Res. 2016;15:2455–65.
100. Maes E, Mertens I, Valkenborg D, Pauwels P, Rolfo C, Baggerman G. Proteomics in cancer research: are we ready for clinical practice? Crit Rev Oncol Hematol. 2015;96:437–48.
101. Greco V, Piras C, Pieroni L, Ronci M, Putignani L, Roncada P, et al. Applications of MALDI-TOF mass spectrometry in clinical proteomics. Expert Rev Proteomics. 2018;14789450.2018.1505510.
102. Levitsky LI, Ivanov MV, Lobas AA, Gorshkov MV. Unbiased false discovery rate estimation for shotgun proteomics based on the target-decoy approach. J Proteome Res. 2017;16:393–7.

22

Comparative study of endometrioid borderline ovarian tumor with and without endometriosis

Wen Zhang[1†], Shuangzheng Jia[1†], Yang Xiang[1], Junjun Yang[1], Congwei Jia[2] and Jinhua Leng[1*]

Abstract

Background: Synchronous endometriosis has been poorly studied in women with endometrioid borderline ovarian tumors (EBOTs). The aims of this study were to compare the clinicopathological features and prognosis of EBOTs with or without endometriosis.

Results: Of 52 patients diagnosed with EBOTs, no death was observed and only one case had successful pregnancy during the follow-up period. Older, menopausal EBOT patients, EBOT patients with small tumors and relatively low CA125 level probably had better progression-free survival (PFS) outcomes. About 1/3 of EBOTs had concomitant endometrial lesions. Approximately 1/3 of EBOTs were associated with endometriosis. Patients were divided into two groups according to the presence or not of endometriosis in this retrospective cohort study. Patients with endometriosis-associated endometrioid borderline ovarian tumor (EAEBOT) were more likely to be younger and premenopausal. Variables such as PFS outcomes, endometrial lesions did not differ statistically between groups. However, in specific EBOT patients like parous patients, patients with CA125 ≥ 140 U/ml or patients without fertility sparing surgery, coexisting endometriosis perhaps predicted worse PFS outcomes.

Conclusion: We considered EAEBOT as an entity similar to non-EAEBOT. Closely follow-up for some particular patients with concomitant endometriosis was necessary.

Keywords: Endometrioid borderline ovarian tumor, Endometriosis-associated endometrioid borderline ovarian tumor, Endometriosis

Background

Endometrioid ovarian epithelial tumors occur as endometrioid cystadenomas, endometrioid cystadenofibromas, endometrioid borderline ovarian tumors (EBOT) and endometrioid carcinomas [1]. Thereinto, endometrioid borderline ovarian tumor, second to the serous and mucinous borderline ovarian tumor (BOT), is characterized with atypical or histologically malignant endometrioid type glands or cysts without stromal invasion in accordance with WHO criteria [2].

Endometriosis is a frequent gynecological disease, which has been evaluated that 0.5–1% of the endometriosis patients are associated with neoplasia [3]. The most common endometriosis-associated malignant ovarian tumors are endometrioid carcinomas and clear cell carcinomas [4]. Endometriosis–associated borderline ovarian tumors are less common when compared with the endometriosis-associated malignant ovarian tumors [5]. Previous endometriosis history or discovery of endometriosis during the histological analysis is frequent in EBOTs [2]. Concomitant endometriosis was identified in 12 patients from 33 EBOTs in one research [6] and 16 out of 31 EBOTs had ovarian or ovarian and/or vaginal endometriosis in another research [7] which raised the major question of relationship between EBOT and endometriosis. Previous studies had demonstrated no associations between endometriosis and the prognosis of ovarian endometrioid carcinomas and ovarian clear cell carcinomas [8, 9]. However, no studies had compared endometriosis-associated EBOT (EAEBOT) with non-EAEBOT in terms of clinical

* Correspondence: lengjenny@vip.sina.com
†Wen Zhang and Shuangzheng Jia contributed equally to this work.
¹Department of Obstetrics and Gynecology, Peking Union Medical College Hospital, Chinese Academy of Medical Sciences and Peking Union Medical College, No. 1 Shuaifuyuan, Dongcheng District, Beijing 100730, China
Full list of author information is available at the end of the article

and pathological features and prognosis. Therefore, in the present study, we aimed to identify whether EAEBOT represented a heterogeneous disease distinct from other forms of EBOTs in aspects of clinical, pathological features and prognosis.

Methods

After obtaining Institutional Review Board approval for medical record review, patients with a primary histopathology diagnosis of borderline ovarian tumor of endometrioid histotype at the Peking Union Medical College Hospital were identified and included in this retrospective cohort study from 1995 to 2015. Subjects with malignant ovarian tumors or borderline ovarian tumors of other histotypes were excluded.

All patients were treated in our institution and followed up in outpatient department or by telephone. No patients had chemotherapy before the surgery. Patients had undergone either a laparotomic or a laparoscopic approach. Staging surgical procedures had been performed dependent on the surgical teams, on whether the EBOT had been diagnosed during or after the surgical procedure and on disease extension. The International Federation of Gynecology and Obstetrics (FIGO) 2013 staging system for epithelial ovarian tumors was used for determining disease stage based on the operative descriptions and pathology records [10]. Staging surgery was performed wherein all peritoneal surfaces were carefully inspected using peritoneal washing, random or oriented multiple biopsies, and infracolic omentectomy [11]. Conservative surgery was defined as fertility sparing wherein the uterus and at least part of one ovary are salvaged, whereas radical surgery was defined as bilateral salpingo-oophorectomy with or without a hysterectomy. Microscopic slides were reviewed and confirmed by two experienced gynecologic pathologists.

Patients were divided into two groups according to the detection of EBOT arising from endometriosis or not. Specifically, EAEBOT was defined as follows: [1] presence of EBOT and endometriosis in the same ovary (see Fig. 1), [2] presence of endometriosis in one ovary and of EBOT in the contralateral ovary, [3] presence of EBOT and extraovarian endometriosis. Figure 1 shows the concomitant endometriosis and EBOT in the same ovary.

Medical records were comprehensively reviewed, and variables such as patient's age, fertility status, gravidity number, symptoms, menopausal status, preoperative serum CA-125 levels, surgery date, maximal tumor diameter, cyst rupture, FIGO stage, laterality of tumor, surgical approach (laparoscopy or laparotomy), whether comprehensive staging surgery or fertility sparing surgery was performed, chemotherapy, concomitant endometriosis, date of disease progression or recurrence were collected. The simultaneous detection of endometrial cancer (EC) or endometrial intraepithelial neoplasia (EIN) in the surgical specimen was also reported, and in cases without hysterectomy uterine curettage was performed after surgery to obtain endometrial pathology. Normal upper limit of serum CA 125 was 35 U/ml and we also set another CA125 indicator of which upper limit was 140 U/ml (four times the normal value). Progression-free survival (PFS) was defined as the time interval from the date of primary surgery to the date of disease progression or recurrence.

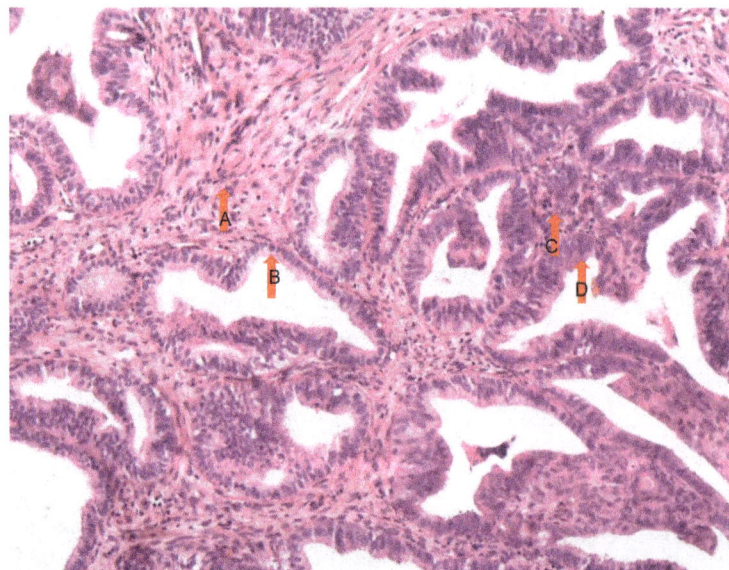

Fig. 1 Endometrioid borderline ovarian tumors (EBOT) and adjacent endometriotic lesions. Caption: **a** normal endometrial stroma; **b** normal endometrial glandular epithelia; **c** EBOT stroma; **d** EBOT glandular epithelia.

Statistical analyses were performed using SPSS version 20.0 (SPSS Inc.). Continuous variables were analyzed by t-test and categorical variables were analyzed by Chi square test or Fisher exact test to assess the significance of differences in clinical and pathological features between EAEBOTs and non-EAEBOTs. Survival analysis was obtained using the log-rank test in Kaplan–Meier method. Variables with statistical significance in univariate analyses were included in the multivariate analysis. Multivariate analysis was performed using the Cox proportional hazards regression model to identify predictors of survival. All P values reported were two tailed, and $P < 0.05$ was considered statistically significant.

Results

During the study period, a total of 52 patients met the inclusion criteria. Of them, 19(36.5%) patients were associated with endometriosis and allocated to group 1, while the other 33(63.5%) without endometriosis were assigned to group 2. Mean age ± SD at diagnosis of the entire cohort was 41.9 ± 11.6 (range 23-81 years) years old. Twelve (23.1%) were in menopause. Fifteen (29.4%) had at least 3 gravidities and 24(46.2%) were nulliparous. Distribution based on FIGO stage was 49(94.2%) for stage I, 2 for stage II, 1 for stage III, and 0 for stage IV. Forty-seven (90.4%) patients were with unilateral tumors. Twelve (23.1%) patients received chemotherapy after primary surgery. Of 52 cases, 8(15.4%) had concomitant EIN and 11(21.2%) had EC.

The clinical and pathological variables between groups are shown in Table 1. Patients with endometriosis were younger than those without endometriosis, which was statistically significant ($P = 0.040$). Consistent with age, none of the patients in group 1 and 36.4% in the group 2 were menopausal ($P = 0.002$). There was no difference between these two groups in terms of EC ($P = 0.503$) or EIN ($p = 0.694$). The most common symptom for both groups was pelvic mass, followed by vaginal bleeding. Symptoms did not differ statistically between the two groups. There were also no differences between two groups in terms of CA125 level, tumor size, FIGO stage and symptom.

After a median follow-up time of 30 months (range 6–177 months) post treatment, 9 (17.3%) disease progressions or recurrences were observed and 43 (82.7%) were censored at last follow-up in the entire study cohort. No disease-specific deaths were observed. Two cases of malignant transformation into endometrioid ovarian cancer were observed after 18 and 68 months respectively during the follow-up, of which one is EAEBOT and the other is non-EAEBOT. Of the 25 women with fertility sparing surgery, only one woman with non-EAEBOT on stage IC had two successful term births during the follow-up time and the first birth was 1 year after the

Table 1 Clinical and pathological characteristics of the patients

Characteristics	EAEBOT ($n = 19$)	Non-EAEBOT ($n = 33$)	P
Age(years)(mean ± SD)	39.9 ± 7.5	43.1 ± 13.3	0.280
Age ≥ 50 years	1(5.3%)	10(30.3%)	0.040
Nulliparous	9(47.4%)	15(45.5%)	0.894
Gravidity number > 2	4(21.1%)	11(33.3%)	0.405
Symptom			
Pelvic mass	19(100.0%)	28(84.8%)	0.145
Vaginal bleeding	2(10.5%)	7(21.2%)	0.458
Pain	1(5.3%)	5(15.2%)	0.397
Torsion	0(0.0%)	2(6.1%)	0.527
Distension	1(5.3%)	0(0.0%)	0.365
Menopause	0(0.0%)	12(36.4%)	0.002
CA125 > 35 U/ml	15(78.9%)	18(54.5%)	0.091
CA125 ≥ 140 U/ml	7(36.8%)	8(24.2%)	0.376
Maximal tumor diameter ≥ 10 cm	3(15.8%)	7(21.2%)	1.000
Cyst rupture	14(73.7%)	24(72.7%)	1.000
FIGO stage			1.000
I	18(94.7%)	31(93.9%)	
II,III,IV	1(5.3%)	2(6.1%)	
Tumor side			0.145
Unilateral	19(100.0%)	28(84.8%)	
Bilateral	0(0.0%)	5(15.2%)	
Endometrial pathology			
Endometrial cancer	5(26.3%)	6(18.2%)	0.503
EIN	2(10.5%)	6(18.2%)	0.694

EAEBOT endometriosis-associated endometrioid borderline ovarian tumor, *EIN* endometrial intraepithelial neoplasia

surgery. Median PFS was 169 months for the entire cohort. Table 2 shows the results of uni-variate and multivariate progression free survival analysis. In uni-variate analysis, age, menopause status, CA125 level (cutoff value = 140 U/ml) and tumor size were significant prognostic factors for PFS. Patients who were older than 50 years old, in menopause, with CA 125 < 140 U/ml, with maximal tumor diameter < 10 cm had better PFS outcomes and P values were 0.031, 0.023, 0.019 and 0.040, respectively. However, concomitant presence of endometriosis was not significantly associated with PFS outcomes. There were also no relationships between PFS outcomes and the following variables, like surgical approach (laparoscopy or laparotomy), whether comprehensive staging surgery was conducted, whether fertility sparing surgery was performed, cyst rupture, FIGO stage, whether patients received chemotherapy after surgery, concomitant endometrial lesion and tumor side (unilateral or bilateral). Multivariate Cox regression survival analysis has been performed in the whole cohort

Table 2 Predictors of progression-free survival in univariate and multivariate survival analysis

Characteristics		n	P(univariate analysis)	P(multivariate analysis)	P(stratified analysis)
Age	< 50 years	41(78.8%)	0.031	1.000	0.733
	≥50 years	11(21.2%)			–
Nulliparous	No	28(53.8%)	0.548	–	0.045
	Yes	24(46.2%)			0.315
Gravidity	≤2	36(70.6%)	0.746	–	0.492
	> 2	15(29.4%)			0.536
Menopause	No	40(76.9%)	0.023	0.983	0.834
	Yes	12(23.1%)			–
CA125	< 35 U/ml	15(31.3%)	0.893	–	0.336
	≥35 U/ml	33(68.7%)			0.103
CA125	< 140 U/ml	33(68.7%)	0.019	0.344	0.301
	≥140 U/ml	15(31.3%)			0.045
Maximal tumor diameter	< 10 cm	40(80.0%)	0.040	0.265	0.292
	≥10 cm	10(20.0%)			0.077
Surgical approach	Laparoscopy	22(42.3%)	0.890	–	0.480
	Laparotomy	30(57.7%)			0.120
Comprehensive staging surgery	No	23(44.2%)			0.824
	Yes	29(55.8%)	0.586	–	0.108
Fertility sparing surgery	No	27(51.9%)	0.697	–	0.019
	Yes	25(48.1%)			0.272
Cyst rupture	No	12(24.0%)	0.055	–	–
	Yes	38(76.0%)			0.517
FIGO stage	I	49(94.2%)	0.651	–	0.282
	II、III、IV	3(5.8%)			–
Chemotherapy after surgery	No	40(76.9%)	0.387	–	0.851
	Yes	12(23.1%)			0.441
Endometrial pathology	Without EIN/EC	33(63.5%)	0.830	–	0.122
	EIN	8(15.4%)			–
	EC	11(21.2%)			0.371
Tumor side	Unilateral	47(90.4%)	0.076	–	0.121
	Bilateral	5(9.6%)			–
Endometriosis	No	33(63.5%)	0.315	–	–
	Yes	19(36.5%)			–

EC endometrial cancer, *EIN* endometrial intraepithelial neoplasia

controlling for confounding factors. No factors were confirmed to be independent predictors of PFS.

Table 2 also shows the results of the differences of PFS outcomes between two groups after stratification by other confounding factors. For parous patients, patients with CA125 ≥ 140 U/ml or patients with radical surgery, EBOT patients with coexisting endometriosis had worse PFS outcomes compared with those without endometriosis and *P* values were 0.045, 0.045 and 0.019, respectively. However, for nulliparous patients, patients with CA125 < 140 U/ml or patients with fertility sparing surgery, there were no significant differences in terms of PFS outcomes between EAEBOT patients and non-EAEBOT patients.

Discussion

Our study showed that most patients with EBOTs were young, premenopausal and overwhelming majority of patients had stage I diseases. During the follow-up, 9 cases showed disease progressions or recurrences and only one woman had successful term birth. Older, menopausal patients and patients with relatively low CA125

(< 140 U/ml) and relatively small tumors (< 10 cm) probably had better PFS outcomes. Patients with EAEBOT were younger and more likely to be premenopausal. Variables such as FIGO stage, endometrial lesions did not differ statistically between the two groups. Concomitant Endometriosis was not associated with PFS outcomes. However, in some specific type of patients, like parous patients, patients with CA125 ≥ 140 U/ml or patients without fertility sparing surgery, coexisting endometriosis perhaps predicted worse PFS outcomes.

How ovarian endometriosis developed into ovarian neoplasm had been debated for decades from biological, epidemiological and clinical perspectives [12–16]. Several studies reported concomitant endometriosis in EBOTs [2, 6, 7, 17] which was in line with our results. A substantially increased risk of BOT or ovarian cancer was observed in endometriosis patients, additionally, hazard ratios associated with endometriosis were reported to be 12.4 for ovarian cancer and 5.5 for BOT [18]. Such data indicated the possibility of EBOT developed from endometriosis, possibly via the stage of atypical endometriosis [19]. While the pathogenesis of EAEBOT remained unclear, atypical endometriosis could be found in some endometriosis associated ovarian tumors and was considered to be a intermediate link during the neoplastic progression [5].

Present studies have shown that endometriosis-associated ovarian carcinoma (EAOC) might deviate from the non-EAOC [9]. However, as for EBOTs, EAEBOT and non-EAEBOT showed almost the same clinical and pathological features, as well as the PFS. In terms of clinical and pathological features, both groups showed no significant differences in most aspects except for age and menopausal status. Consistent with our study, previous studies also indicated that endometriosis-associated neoplasms were frequently found in younger women [5]. This was probably because of the symptoms of endometriosis like dysmenorrhea, dyspareunia, and/or pelvic mass so that these patients were more likely to see a doctor and then detected the ovarian tumors at earlier ages.

According to our results, prognoses of younger patients, premenopausal patients or patients with relatively high CA125 level or relatively large tumors were likely to be poor. Younger and premenopausal patients are still under the effect of sex hormone which could exert an effect of hormonal field effect. Field effect, also described as field cancerization, means a field of cellular and molecular aberrations, which predisposes to the initiation and progression of tumor [20]. Sex hormone in younger women could probably help constitute a field of susceptibility to endometriosis and endometrioid cell-type tumors, as well as the recurrence or progression of diseases, which also could account for the phenomenon

that younger and premenopausal patients have worse prognosis. What is more, patients with relatively high CA125 level or relatively large tumors were likely to have poor prognoses. One case report shows that even a slight CA125 increase can be indicative of a poor prognosis [21], which supports our results. And as described in one article that CA125 level is positively correlated with the tumor size [22], it could be deduced from the above evidences that large tumor size is probably also an indicator of poor prognosis. Up to this point, these patients should pay attention to the recurrence of EBOT during follow-up. As for the association between endometriosis and the prognosis of EBOT, on one hand, the current published articles served to demonstrate that ovarian tumors associated with endometriosis had a better prognosis than those without endometriosis [19]. On the other hand, two articles about endometrioid ovarian cancer and ovarian clear cell carcinoma demonstrated that no significant differences in overall survival or progression-free survival could be found between patients with or without endometriosis [8, 9]. While in our study, tumors with concomitant endometriosis did not show better or worse PFS outcomes when compared with those without. Nevertheless, when compared with non-EAEBOT patients, EAEBOT patients presented with worse PFS outcomes in some particular patients (parous patients, patients with CA125 ≥ 140 U/ml or with radical surgery). The above mentioned hormonal field effect could also be used to explain the phenomenon. The specific hormonal field effect predisposes to the development of endometriosis and EBOT, and endometriosis could lead to the increase of CA125. Extremely increased CA125 level and endometriosis found in the parous patients (pregnancy is usually considered be the protective factor for endometriosis) probably indicate the severe endometriosis, which may imply the stronger hormonal field effect and the strong effect could probably increase the risk for progression or recurrence of EBOT. Furthermore, for parous patients and patients with CA125 ≥ 140 U/ml, radical surgery are often suggested for them, which could indirectly lead to results that EAEBOT patients with radical surgery may have poor prognosis. Given these findings, for EAEBOT patients with the above conditions, strict follow-up would be necessary for them in case of recurrence or disease progression.

A systematic review evaluated the fertility outcome after serous and mucinous BOT management. Conservative management of early stage BOT resulted in a spontaneous pregnancy rate of 54% and 34% in advanced stage BOT [23]. However, there was only one (4%) case of successful term birth in women with conservative surgery which demonstrated a poor fertility outcome of EBOT.

It is noteworthy that about one third of EBOTs had synchronous endometrial disorders in our study. Previous studies also reported concomitant endometrial lesions such as endometrioid adenocarcinoma [2], atypical hyperplasia [6, 7], simple hyperplasia [6, 7], polyps [7, 17, 24] in EBOTs. Concerning these evidences, uterine curettage was suggested for the patients with conservative surgery and hysterectomy was advised for patients underwent radical surgery. Our article also briefly evaluated the relationship between synchronous endometrial lesion and endometriosis. Unlike the results of previous study which reported that rate of endometrial cancer diagnosis was significantly higher in women with endometriosis associated endometrioid ovarian cancer than in the other patients [8], our study did not find the association between concomitant endometriosis and synchronous endometrial disease.

The strengths of our study include the following aspects. Firstly, in order to identify whether EAEBOT represented a separated entity distinct from the non-EAEBOT, which was never had been studied, we performed comparisons between EAEBOT and non-EAEBOT patients in aspects such as clinical and pathological features, synchronous endometrial lesion and PFS. Secondly, we described the clinical and pathological characteristics of EBOT, reported information about the treatment of EBOTs, and provided the detailed follow-up data which efficiently made up the deficiencies of current studies due to the rarity of this kind of disease. Thirdly, we also focused the synchronous endometrial disorders in EBOT and explored the association between concomitant endometriosis and endometrial disorder which,to the best of our knowledge, had never been discussed. Fourthly, we reported the reproductive outcomes after conservative surgery for EBOTs, and according to our results, we distinguished the population with worse PFS outcomes in EBOT and EAEBOT women in which close follow-up should be suggested for them.

This study has, however, some limitations. Firstly, when interpreting the results of this study, one thing must be pointed out that the sample size was not sufficient which perhaps could lead to false negative results such as the inability to discover the differences between EAEBOTs and non-EAEBOTs and identify more risk factors affecting PFS, which should be considered with caution. Study with a large sample size is needed to verify our present study results or come up with novel theory. Secondly, study from a single academic institution often involved in the selection biases. Thirdly, current findings that consider EAEBOT as an entity similar to non-EAEBOT were derived mostly from the clinical results of our study, which required confirmation at the molecular level such as gene diagnosis.

Conclusions

There were no significant differences between EAEBOT and non-EAEBOT in many main aspects of clinicopathological features and prognosis, thus we considered EAEBOT as an entity similar to non-EAEBOT. Patients with EAEBOT were more likely to be younger and premenopausal. Close follow-up for some particular patients with endometriosis was necessary.

Acknowledgements
We thank all of the patients for participating in our study.

Funding
This study was supported by the National Key R&D Program of China (2017YFC1001200).

Authors' contributions
WZ, SJ and JL contributed substantially to the study conceptualization, and design, acquisition of data, analysis and interpretation of data, and manuscript writing. JY, YX, and CJ contributed to the interpretation of data and performed critical revisions of important intellectual content. All authors gave approval for the publication of the final version.

Competing interests
The authors declare that they have no competing interests.

Author details
[1]Department of Obstetrics and Gynecology, Peking Union Medical College Hospital, Chinese Academy of Medical Sciences and Peking Union Medical College, No. 1 Shuaifuyuan, Dongcheng District, Beijing 100730, China. [2]Department of Pathology, Peking Union Medical College Hospital, Chinese Academy of Medical Sciences and Peking Union Medical College, No. 1 Shuaifuyuan, Dongcheng District, Beijing 100730, China.

References
1. Norris HJ. Proliferative endometrioid tumors and endometrioid tumors of low malignant potential of the ovary. Int J Gynecol Pathol. 1993;12:134–40.
2. Uzan C, Berretta R, Rolla M, Gouy S, Fauvet R, Darai E, Duvillard P, Morice P. Management and prognosis of endometrioid borderline tumors of the ovary. Surg Oncol. 2012;21:178–84.
3. Wei JJ, William J, Bulun S. Endometriosis and ovarian cancer: a review of clinical, pathologic, and molecular aspects. Int J Gynecol Pathol. 2011;30:553–68.
4. Gurung A, Hung T, Morin J, Gilks CB. Molecular abnormalities in ovarian carcinoma: clinical, morphological and therapeutic correlates. Histopathology. 2013;62:59–70.
5. Matias-Guiu X, Stewart CJR. Endometriosis-associated ovarian neoplasia. Pathology. 2018;50:190–204.
6. Bell KA, Kurman RJ. A clinicopathologic analysis of atypical proliferative (borderline) tumors and well-differentiated endometrioid adenocarcinomas of the ovary. Am J Surg Pathol. 2000;24:1465–79.
7. Snyder RR, Norris HJ, Tavassoli F. Endometrioid proliferative and low malignant potential tumors of the ovary. A clinicopathologic study of 46 cases. Am J Surg Pathol. 1988;12:661–71.
8. Mangili G, Bergamini A, Taccagni G, Gentile C, Panina P, Vigano P, Candiani M. Unraveling the two entities of endometrioid ovarian cancer: a single center clinical experience. Gynecol Oncol. 2012;126:403–7.
9. Ye S, Yang J, You Y, Cao D, Bai H, Lang J, Chen J, Shen K. Comparative study of ovarian clear cell carcinoma with and without endometriosis in People's Republic of China. Fertil Steril. 2014;102:1656–62.

10. Pereira A, Perez-Medina T, Magrina JF, Magtibay PM, Rodriguez-Tapia A, Peregrin I, Mendizabal E, Ortiz-Quintana L. International federation of gynecology and obstetrics staging classification for cancer of the ovary, fallopian tube, and peritoneum: estimation of survival in patients with node-positive epithelial ovarian cancer. Int J Gynecol Cancer. 2015;25:49–54.

11. Cadron I, Leunen K, Van Gorp T, Amant F, Neven P, Vergote I. Management of borderline ovarian neoplasms. J Clin Oncol. 2007;25:2928–37.

12. Munksgaard PS, Blaakaer J. The association between endometriosis and ovarian cancer: a review of histological, genetic and molecular alterations. Gynecol Oncol. 2012;124:164–9.

13. Vigano P, Somigliana E, Chiodo I, Abbiati A, Vercellini P. Molecular mechanisms and biological plausibility underlying the malignant transformation of endometriosis: a critical analysis. Hum Reprod Update. 2006;12:77–89.

14. Somigliana E, Vigano P, Parazzini F, Stoppelli S, Giambattista E, Vercellini P. Association between endometriosis and cancer: a comprehensive review and a critical analysis of clinical and epidemiological evidence. Gynecol Oncol. 2006;101:331–41.

15. Sayasneh A, Tsivos D, Crawford R. Endometriosis and ovarian cancer: a systematic review. ISRN Obstet Gynecol. 2011;2011:140310.

16. Olson JE, Cerhan JR, Janney CA, Anderson KE, Vachon CM, Sellers TA. Postmenopausal cancer risk after self-reported endometriosis diagnosis in the Iowa Women's health study. Cancer. 2002;94:1612–8.

17. Roth LM, Emerson RE, Ulbright TM. Ovarian endometrioid tumors of low malignant potential: a clinicopathologic study of 30 cases with comparison to well-differentiated endometrioid adenocarcinoma. Am J Surg Pathol. 2003;27:1253–9.

18. Buis CC, van Leeuwen FE, Mooij TM, Burger CW, Group OP. Increased risk for ovarian cancer and borderline ovarian tumours in subfertile women with endometriosis. Hum Reprod. 2013;28:3358–69.

19. Schmidt D, Ulrich U. Endometriosis-related ovarian tumors. Pathologe. 2014;35:348–54.

20. Lochhead P, Chan AT, Nishihara R, Fuchs CS, Beck AH, Giovannucci E, Ogino S. Etiologic field effect: reappraisal of the field effect concept in cancer predisposition and progression. Mod Pathol. 2015;28:14–29.

21. Anastasi E, Porpora MG, Pecorella I, Bernardo S, Frati L, Benedetti Panici P, Manganaro L. May increased CA125 in borderline ovarian tumor be indicative of a poor prognosis? A case report. Tumour Biol. 2014;35:6969–71.

22. Ayhan A, Guven S, Guven ES, Kucukali T. Is there a correlation between tumor marker panel and tumor size and histopathology in well staged patients with borderline ovarian tumors? Acta Obstet Gynecol Scand. 2007;86:484–90.

23. Darai E, Fauvet R, Uzan C, Gouy S, Duvillard P, Morice P. Fertility and borderline ovarian tumor: a systematic review of conservative management, risk of recurrence and alternative options. Hum Reprod Update. 2013;19:151–66.

24. Bell DA, Scully RE. Atypical and borderline endometrioid adenofibromas of the ovary. A report of 27 cases. Am J Surg Pathol. 1985;9:205–14.

23

Is the aging human ovary still ticking?: Expression of clock-genes in luteinized granulosa cells of young and older women

Amnon Brzezinski[1]* ⓘ, A. Saada[2], H. Miller[2], NA Brzezinski-Sinai[1] and A. Ben-Meir[1]

Abstract

Background: It has been shown – mostly in animal models - that circadian clock genes are expressed in granulosa cells and in corpora luteum and might be essential for the ovulatory process and steroidogenesis.

Objective: We sought to investigate which circadian clock genes exist in human granulosa cells and whether their expression and activity decrease during aging of the ovary.

Study design: Human luteinized granulosa cells were isolated from young (age 18–33) and older (age 39–45) patients who underwent in-vitro fertilization treatment. Levels of clock genes expression were measured in these cells 36 h after human chorionic gonadotropin stimulation.

Methods: Human luteinized granulosa cells were isolated from follicular fluid during oocyte retrieval. The mRNA expression levels of the circadian genes CRY1, CRY2, PER1, PER2, CLOCK, ARNTL, ARNTL2, and NPAS2 were analyzed by quantitative polymerase chain reaction.

Results: We found that the circadian genes CRY1, CRY2, PER1, PER2, CLOCK, ARNTL, ARNTL2, and NPAS2, are expressed in cultured human luteinized granulosa cells. Among these genes, there was a general trend of decreased expression in cells from older women but it reached statistical significance only for PER1 and CLOCK genes (fold change of 0.27 ± 0.14; $p = 0.03$ and 0.29 ± 0.16; $p = 0.05$, respectively).

Conclusions: This preliminary report indicates that molecular circadian clock genes exist in human luteinized granulosa cells. There is a decreased expression of some of these genes in older women. This decline may partially explain the decreased fertility and steroidogenesis of reproductive aging.

Keywords: Circadian clock genes, Granulosa cells, Reproductive aging

Introduction

Many physiological processes and behaviors in mammals are rhythmic. These rhythms are controlled by an endogenous molecular clock within the suprachiasmatic nucleus (SCN), located in the forebrain of mammals, which is entrained by the light/dark cycle [1–4]. The SCN synchronize countless subsidiary oscillators existing in the peripheral tissues throughout the body [5, 6]. The basis for maintaining the circadian rhythm is a molecular clock consisting of interlocked transcriptional/ translational feedback loops. The proteins encoded by the genes circadian locomotor output cycles kaput (*Clock*) and brain and muscle arnt-like protein 1(*Bmal1*, also known as *ARNTL1* or *Mop3*) heterodimerize and promote the rhythmic transcription of the period (*Per1, Per2*) and cryptochrome (*Cry1, Cry2*) gene families, whereas modified PER–CRY complexes repress the activity of the CLOCK–BMAL1 complex. Over several hours, PER–CRY complexes are degraded, and the CLOCK–BMAL1 complex is eventually released from feedback inhibition [7].

There is increasing interest in the role of circadian rhythmicity in the control of reproductive function in animals and humans [2, 8]. In mammals, circulating gonadotropin luteinizing hormone (LH) and follicle-stimulating hormone (FSH) levels oscillate with a diurnal rhythm marked by afternoon surges on the day of ovulation [9, 10].

* Correspondence: amnonbrz@gmail.com
[1]Department of Obstetrics and Gynecology, The Hebrew University Hadassah Medical Center, Jerusalem, Israel
Full list of author information is available at the end of the article

Circadian rhythms and clock genes appear to be involved in optimal reproductive performance, [11]. Expression of circadian genes *Per2* and *Bmal1* was observed in corpora luteum in rat ovaries by in situ hybridization [12]. In addition, circadian clock genes *Per2* and *Clock* were found to be involved in the regulation of steroid production and cell proliferation in granulosa cells, which turn into granulosa lutein cells after ovulation [9, 13].

Most of what we currently know regarding clock function in the mammalian ovary relates to the timing of gene expression in mature or luteinized GCs from rats and mice. We therefore sought to investigate which of the clock genes are expressed in human granulosa cells and whether ovarian aging is associated with decreased expression of these genes.

Materials and methods
Subjects
Young women (33 YO or younger) and older women (39 YO or older) were asked to participate in this study. The Hadassah-Hebrew University Medical Center Institutional Review Board approved this study. All subjects gave written informed consent to participate in the study.

Luteinized granulosa cells isolation
All our subjects kept a regular and similar sleep-wake cycle. All women had standard short agonist or antagonist protocol. The treatment protocols were equally distributed in both groups (see Table 1). All samples were collected at the same time frame (between 8:30 and 10:00 am). After egg retrieval and oocyte isolation from all follicles, follicular fluid was centrifuge and top layer of pellet was collected. Granulosa cells were separated from RBCs and most WBCs by centrifuge with Lymphoprep™ (Alere Technologies, Oslo, Norway). Cells were washed two times with 1xPBS, lysed with 300 μl of RNA buffer (Zymo Research, Irvine CA, USA) and kept in −80 until RNA isolation.

Table 1 Patients characteristics in young and old groups [mean (range)]

	Young group (n = 5)	Old group (n = 5)
Age	27.9 (24–29)	40.3 (39–43)
IVF indication	Male factor or mechanical	Age-related
Day 3 FSH	6.0 (4.9–7.2)	8.6 (5.8–11.3)
No. of oocyte retrieved	16.2 (10–21)	6.8 (4–9)
Ovarian stimulation protocol		
Antagonist	3/5	2/5
Short agonist	2/5	3/5

Gene expression analysis
Gene expression analysis was performed by quantitative reverse transcription-PCR (RT-qPCR). Total RNA was isolated using Quick RNA MicroPrep (Zymo Research, Irvine CA,USA) and c-DNA was generated using qScript cDNA Synthesis kit (Quanta Biosciences, Gathersburg, MD, US). Real-time PCR (RT-PCR) was performed using Taqman Gene Expression Assays (*CRY1* Assay ID; Hs00172734_m1, *CRY2* Assay ID; Hs00323654_m1, *CLOCK* Assay ID; Hs00231857_m1, *PER1* Assay ID; Hs0001092603_m1, *PER2* Assay ID; Hs00256143_m1, *ARNTL* Hs00154147_m1, *ARNTL2* Hs00368068_m1 *NPAS2* Hs00231212_m1 from Applied Biosystems, ThermoFisher Scientific, Waltham, MA USA). Samples were run on the ABI PRISM7900HT sequence detection system (Applied Biosystems, Foster City, CA USA). Relative quantitation was calculated by the 2^{-ddCT} method relative to human housekeeping gene *POLR2A* (Assay ID; Hs.PT.58.25515089) (Integrated DNA Technologies, Inc. (Coralville, Iowa USA).

Results
Five young women and five older women were enrolled in this study. Indication for in-vitro fertilization treatment included unexplained, mechanical or male infertility. As expected, young women had lower day 3 FSH and higher number of retrieved oocytes (Table 1).

Fold changes of mRNA levels of the CLOCK genes are presented in Fig. 1. All genes are expressed in human luteinized granulosa cells. All examined genes show tendency of decrease expression with aging, but it reached statistical significance only for *PER1* and *CLOCK* genes (fold change of 0.27 ± 0.14; $p = 0.03$ and 0.29 ± 0.16; $p = 0.05$, respectively).

Discussion
Our results indicate that the circadian genes *CRY1*, *CRY2*, *PER1*, *PER2*, *CLOCK*, *ARNTL*, *ARNTL2*, and *NPAS2* are all expressed in cultured *human* luteinized granulosa cells. Among these genes, there was a general trend of decreased expression in cells from older women, but it reached statistical significance only for *PER1* and *CLOCK* genes.

In recent years much information has accumulated to support the importance of the clockwork mechanism in reproduction by using mutant mouse models with various disruptions of the molecular clockwork (3). The mammalian period paralogues Per1 and Per2 seem to be part of the molecular network involved in the repression of G1-S transition, while the circadian transcrip-tion factors BMAL1 and CLOCK take part to the molecular network that regulates G2-M transition. Per1 and Clock1involvement in the cell cycle control have been

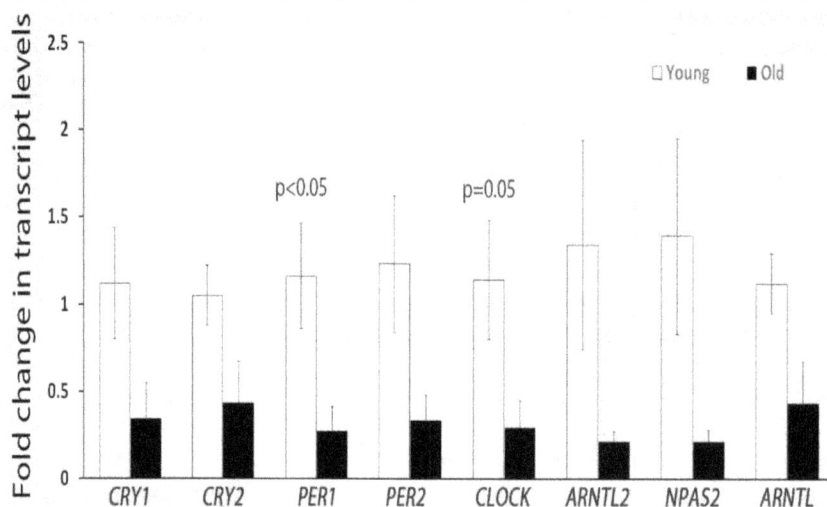

Fig. 1 Fold change in mRNA levels of genes involved in circadian rhythm in luteinized granulosa cells were normalized to young age. Transcripts encoding *CLOCK* and *PER1* genes are reduced with aging. Each sample contained a pool of granulsa cells from several follicles (young $n = 5$, old $n = 5$)

confirmed in diurnal low vertebrates such as the zebrafish.

There are other reports suggestive of interactions between clock genes and reproduction. For example, the report that estradiol and progesterone are involved in modification of circadian rhythm via direct regulation of the expression of clock genes [14], or the finding that LH surge apparently induces change in gene expression within the GCs of the preovulatory follicle [15]. It has also been reported recently [16] that the clock gene Bmal expression is affected by human chorionic gonadotropin (hCG) administration.

In spite of all these reports the extent to which the circadian timing system affects *human* reproductive performance is still not clear. There is only one report [17] that the circadian genes *CLOCK*, *PER2*, and *BMAL1* were found to be expressed in cultured *human* luteinized granulosa cells. They found that among these genes, only expression of *PER2* displayed oscillating patterns with a 16-h period. *CLOCK* and *BMAL1* did not show significant oscillating patterns. They also report that expression of the steroidal acute regulatory protein (STAR) gene showed an oscillating pattern that was similar to that of *PER2*.

In the present study we demonstrated the existence of all the known molecular circadian clocks in human granulosa cells. We observed a decreased expression of these genes in granulosa cells obtained from older

woman as compared to young women. These preliminary findings, together with the reports about the involvement of clock genes in ovarian steroidogenesis, suggest that gradual disruption of circadian rhythm with age might lead to dysregulation of steroidogenesis in corpora luteum of the human ovary and contribute to follicular dysfunction.

Acknowledgements

Not applicable.

Funding

The source of funding for this research is the local research fund of Prof. Brzezinski at Hadassah Medical Center. No external funding exist.

Authors' contributions

AB conceptualized the research and analyzed and interpreted the data. AS did the lab work and analyzed and interpreted the lab data regarding the clock genes in the granulosa cells. HM performed the lab work (The PCR for RNA of the clock genes). NABS was a major contributor in writing the manuscript. ABM contacted the patients and obtained the follicular fluid samples for retrieving the granulosa cells, and analyzed and interpreted the data. All authors read and approved the final manuscript.

Competing interests

The authors declare that they have no competing interests.

Author details

[1]Department of Obstetrics and Gynecology, The Hebrew University Hadassah Medical Center, Jerusalem, Israel. [2]Department of Genetics & Metabolism, The Hebrew University Hadassah Medical Center, Jerusalem, Israel.

References

1. Brzezinski A. Melatonin in humans. N Engl J Med. 1997;336(3):186–95.
2. Chen M, Xu Y, Miao B, Zhao H, Luo L, Shi H, Zhou C. Expression pattern of circadian genes and steroidogenesis-related genes after testosterone stimulation in the human ovary. J Ovarian Res. 2016;9(1):56.
3. Caba M, González-Mariscal G, Meza E. Circadian rhythms and clock genes in reproduction: insights from behavior and the female Rabbit's brain. Front Endocrinol (Lausanne). 2018;9:106.
4. Hastings MH. Circadian clocks. Curr Biol. 1997;7:R670–2.
5. Ko CH, Takahashi JS. Molecular components of the mammalian circadian clock. Hum Mol Genet. 2006;15:R271–7.
6. Turek FW. Circadian clocks: not your grandfather's clock. Science. 2016; 354(6315):992–3.
7. Takahashi JS, Hong HK, Ko CH, McDearmon EL. The genetics of mammalian circadian order and disorder: implications for physiology and disease. Nat Rev Genet. 2008;9:764–75.
8. Srinivasan V, Spence WD, Pandi-Perumal SR, Zakharia R, Bhatnagar KP, Brzezinski A. Melatonin and human reproduction: shedding light on the darkness hormone. Gynecol Endocrinol. 2009;25(12):779–85.
9. Shimizu T, Hirai Y, Murayama C, et al. Circadian clock genes Per2 and clock regulate steroid production, cell proliferation, and luteinizing hormone receptor transcription in ovarian granulosa cells. Biochem Biophys Res Commun. 2011;412:132–5.
10. Moenter SM, DeFazio AR, Pitts GR, Nunemaker CS. Mechanisms underlying episodic gonadotropin-releasing hormone secretion. Front Neuroendocrinol. 2003;24(2):79–93.
11. Boden MJ, Kennaway DJ. Circadian rhythms and reproduction. Reproduction. 2006;132(3):379–92.
12. Karman BN, Tischkau SA. Circadian clock gene expression in the ovary :effects of luteinizing hormone. Biol Reprod. 2006;75:624–32.
13. Yoshikawa T, Sellix M, Pezuk P, Menaker M. Timing of the ovarian circadian clock is regulated by gonadotrophins. Endocrinology. 2009;150:4338–47.
14. He PJ, Hirata M, Yamauchi N, Hattori MA. Up-regulation of Per1 expression by estradiol and progesterone in the rat uterus. J Endocrinol. 2007;194(3): 511–9.
15. Kobayashi M, Watanabe K, Matsumura R, Anayama N, Miyamoto A, Miyazaki H, Miyazaki K, Shimizu T, Akashi M. Involvement of the luteinizing hormone surge in the regulation of ovary and oviduct clock gene expression in mice. Genes Cells. 2018; (Epub ahead of print).
16. Espey LL, Richards JS. Temporal and spatial patterns of ovarian gene transcription following an ovulatory dose of gonadotropin in the rat. Biol Reprod. 2002;67(6):1662–70 Review.
17. Chen M, Xu Y, Miao B, Zhao H, Gao J, Zhou C. Temporal effects of human chorionic gonadotropin on expression of the circadian genes and steroidogenesis-related genes in human luteinized granulosa cells. Gynecol Endocrinol. 2017;33(7):570–3.

24

Intrafollicular fibroblast growth factor 13 in polycystic ovary syndrome: relationship with androgen levels and oocyte developmental competence

Yu Liu[1†], Shengxian Li[2†], Tao Tao[2], Xiaoxue Li[3,4], Qinling Zhu[3,4], Yu Liao[1], Jing Ma[2], Yun Sun[3,4] and Wei Liu[2*]

Abstract

Background: Fibroblast growth factor 13 (FGF13) is one of the most highly expressed FGF family members in adult mouse ovary. However, its precise roles in ovarian function remain largely unknown. We sought to evaluate the associations between FGF13 in follicular fluid and oocyte developmental competence in patients with polycystic ovary syndrome (PCOS).

Methods: A cross-sectional study was conducted on 43 patients with PCOS and 32 non-PCOS patients who underwent in vitro fertilization/intracytoplasmic sperm injection treatments. The highest quartiles of follicular fluid (FF)-FGF13 ($\geq$117.51 pg/mL) and FF-total testosterone (FF-TT) ($\geq$51.90 nmol/L) were defined as "elevated" FF-FGF13 levels and "elevated" FF-TT levels, respectively.

Results: The levels of FF-FGF13 were skewed, with a median of 82.97 pg/mL (59.79–117.51 pg/mL) in 75 patients. The prevalence of elevated FF-TT levels was significantly higher in the PCOS patients with elevated FF-FGF13 levels than in those without (64.3% vs. 35.7%, adjusted $P = 0.0096$). FF-TT and increased ovarian volume (> 10 mL for one or both ovaries) were positively correlated with FF-FGF13 in PCOS patients ($r = 0.37$, $P = 0.013$; $r = 0.33$, $P = 0.032$). A negative association was evident between FF-FGF13 and the MII oocyte rate in the multiple linear regression analysis ($\beta = -0.10$, SE = 0.045, adjusted $P = 0.027$). However, the associations were not evident in the non-PCOS patients.

Conclusions: Our study suggests the presence of intrafollicular FGF13 in PCOS patients and implies that FGF13 might be involved in the pathophysiological process of PCOS.

Keywords: Fibroblast growth factor 13, Testosterone, Follicular fluid, Polycystic ovary syndrome

Background

The control of ovarian function is highly complex and often involves multiple endocrine and paracrine signaling factors. In addition to pituitary gonadotrophins, several families of growth factors, such as insulin-like growth factors and transforming growth factors, play crucial roles in ovarian function [1–4].

The fibroblast growth factor (FGF) family, comprising 18 secreted proteins and four intracellular proteins (FGF11–14), participate in the regulation of ovarian function and follicular development [5, 6]. For example, FGF2 promotes granulosa cell proliferation and affects ovarian steroidogenesis [7, 8]. Furthermore, FGF18 is involved in the apoptosis of ovarian granulosa cells [9, 10].

The expression of FGF13 in the murine ovary was reported as early as 1997 [11]. In addition to FGF1 and FGF12, FGF13 is a member of the FGF family that is highly expressed in the adult mouse ovary [12]. FGF13 mRNA is detectable in the corpora lutea, theca and granulosa cells of bovine antral follicles. Moreover,

---

* Correspondence: sue_liuwei@163.com
†Yu Liu and Shengxian Li contributed equally to this work.
2Department of Endocrinology, Renji Hospital, School of Medicine, Shanghai Jiaotong University, Shanghai 200127, China
Full list of author information is available at the end of the article

FGF13 mRNA expression is upregulated in the theca cells of the bovine ovary during antral follicle development [13]. Nevertheless, the precise roles of FGF13 in ovarian physiology remain largely unknown.

To our knowledge, the data describing FGF13 expression in the adult human ovary is limited. Therefore, the objectives of our study were to detect the presence of follicular fluid (FF)-FGF13 and to evaluate the relationship between FF-FGF13 and oocyte developmental competence in patients undergoing in vitro fertilization/intracytoplasmic sperm injection (IVF/ICSI).

Materials and methods
Subjects and study design
A total of 75 patients aged 20–37 years undergoing first IVF/ICSI were recruited consecutively from Aug. 2014 to Aug. 2015 at the Center for Reproductive Medicine, Renji Hospital, School of Medicine, Shanghai Jiao Tong University. The patients had no medical history of hypertension, diabetes, hyperprolactinemia, thyroid disease, Cushing's syndrome, or congenital adrenal hyperplasia. Patients who were using insulin-sensitizing drugs, oral contraceptives, corticosteroids, anti-androgens or gonadotropin-releasing hormone agonists/antagonists or who had undergone unilateral ovariectomy were excluded. Ultimately, 43 (57.3%) cases of PCOS and 32 (42.7%) cases of tubal infertility were included in the analyses.

The study protocol was approved by the Ethics Committee of Renji Hospital with informed consent.

Collection of follicular fluid and biochemical measurements
Ovarian stimulation was performed using a GnRH antagonist protocol, and hCG (Lvzhu) was administered to trigger ovulation after adequate follicle development, as described previously [14]. Oocyte retrieval and follicular-fluid samples without blood contamination were collected under local anesthesia using vaginal ultrasound-guided punctures of follicles 36 h after hCG administration. Standard procedures were carried out for gamete-embryo handling, and embryo transfer was performed under abdominal ultrasonography guidance. The ICSI procedure was performed 4–6 h after oocyte retrieval.

Approximately 16–18 h after ICSI, the assessment of fertilization was performed. All embryos were scored as follows: Grade I, embryos with ≤5% fragmentation; Grade II, embryos with ≤20% fragmentation; Grade III, embryos with ≤50% fragmentation; and Grade IV, embryos with > 50% fragmentation [15]. On day 3, Grade I/II embryos were classified as high-quality embryos.

The levels of total testosterone (TT), estradiol (E2), progesterone (P4), luteinizing hormone (LH), follicle-stimulating hormone (FSH), and sex hormone-binding globulin (SHBG) in the follicular fluid were measured with chemiluminescence immunoassays (Elecsys autoanalyzer, Roche Diagnostics, Mannheim, Germany), and the free androgen index (FAI) was calculated with the following formula: FAI = $100 \times$ TT/SHBG (nmol/L). The levels of interleukin-6 (IL-6), FGF13 and FGF21 in the follicular fluid were measured with enzyme-linked immunosorbent assay kits (CUSABIO Biotech Co., Ltd., Newark, DE, USA). The inter- and intra-assay coefficients of variation (CV) were < 10%.

Diagnosis and definition
Polycystic ovaries were defined as follows: the presence of 12 or more follicles in each ovary measuring 2–9 mm in diameter and/or increased ovarian volume (> 10 mL for one or both ovaries) by transvaginal ultrasound. PCOS was defined when at least two of the following three criteria were met: oligo-ovulation or anovulation; clinical and/or biochemical signs of hyperandrogenism; and polycystic ovaries according to the revised Rotterdam consensus [16]. Thirty-two patients with tubal infertility who did not meet the diagnostic criteria for PCOS and had no family history of PCOS were defined as non-PCOS patients.

In the present study, "elevated" FF-FGF13 levels were defined as follicular levels in the upper quartile (i.e., ≥117.51 pg/mL). "Elevated" FF-TT levels were defined as follicular levels in the upper quartile (i.e., ≥51.90 nmol/L).

Statistical analyses
Statistical analyses were performed with SAS version 9.2 (SAS Institute, Cary, NC, USA). Continuous variables due to skewed distributions are shown as medians (interquartile range). Categorical variables are shown as absolute numbers (percentages).

The baseline characteristics of the patients with and without elevated FF-FGF13 levels were described and compared using the Kruskal-Wallis tests for continuous variables and χ^2 tests for categorical variables. Spearman correlations were performed to evaluate the relationships of FF-FGF13 to age, BMI, increased ovarian volume, FF-LH, FF-FSH, FF-TT, FF-FAI, FF-E2, FF-P4, FF-IL-6, and FF-FGF21 in the PCOS and non-PCOS patients. Spearman correlations and multiple linear regression analyses adjusted for age, BMI, FF-LH, and FF-FSH were performed to evaluate the associations between FF-FGF13 and oocyte developmental competence in the PCOS and non-PCOS patients.

Two-sided P values < 0.05 were considered statistically significant.

Results
General characteristics of the study patients
A total 75 patients with a mean age of 27.7 ± 3.7 years were enrolled. The distribution of the FF-FGF13 levels was skewed with a median of 82.97 pg/mL (interquartile

Histogram of FF-FGF13

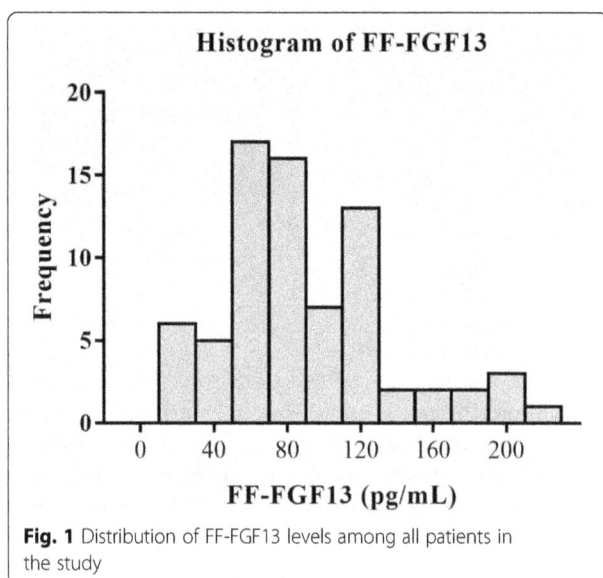

Fig. 1 Distribution of FF-FGF13 levels among all patients in the study

range 59.77–117.51 pg/mL). Figure 1 presents the histogram of the FF-FGF13 levels.

Table 1 presents the general characteristics of the patients with and without elevated FF-FGF13 levels. The patients with elevated FF-FGF13 levels had higher levels of FF-TT, FF-FAI, and FF-FGF21 than those without elevated FF-FGF13 levels (all P values < 0.05). The prevalence of increased ovarian volume was significantly higher among patients with elevated FF-FGF13 levels than among those without elevated FF-FGF13 levels (68.2% vs. 38.9%, $P = 0.021$). No significant differences

were evident in terms of age, BMI, FF-LH, FF-FSH, FF-E2, FF-P4, or FF-IL6 between the patients with and without elevated FF-FGF13 levels.

The prevalence of elevated FF-TT levels was significantly higher among PCOS patients with elevated FF-FGF13 levels than among those without elevated FF-FGF13 levels (64.3% vs. 35.7%, fully adjusted $P = 0.0096$). The prevalence of increased ovarian volume appeared to be higher among PCOS patients with elevated FF-FGF13 levels than among those without elevated FF-FGF13 levels (57.1% vs. 42.7%); however, the P value did not show a significant difference (Fig. 2).

Factors associated with FF-FGF13 in patients with and without PCOS

As shown in Table 2, FF-TT and increased ovarian volume were positively correlated with FF-FGF13 in PCOS patients ($r = 0.37$, $P = 0.013$ and $r = 0.33$, $P = 0.032$). However, no significant relationships were evident between FF-FGF13 and FF-TT or increased ovarian volume among the non-PCOS patients (both P values > 0.05).

Associations between FF-FGF13 and oocyte developmental competence in patients with and without PCOS

As shown in Table 3, Spearman correlations revealed that FF-FGF13 was significantly correlated with the MII oocyte rate in the PCOS patients ($r = -0.42$, $P = 0.0055$). The negative association persisted after the adjustments for age, BMI, FF-LH and FF-FSH in the multiple linear

Table 1 Comparison of the general characteristics of patients with and without elevated FF-FGF13

Characteristics	Elevated FF-FGF13		P values
	Yes	No	
FF-FGF13 (pg/mL)	143.22 (119.11–190.27)	70.03 (53.20–86.94)	—
n	19	56	—
Age (years)	28.0 (23.0–33.0)	27.0 (25.0–30.0)	0.69
BMI (kg/m²)	22.6 (20.2–24.0)	20.3 (19.0–23.5)	0.06
PCOS, n (%)	14 (73.7)	29 (51.8)	0.095
Increased ovarian volume, n (%)	13 (68.2)	21 (38.9)	0.021
FF-LH (IU/L)	2.73 (0.33–4.33)	0.94 (0.29–4.460)	0.57
FF-FSH (IU/L)	4.57 (3.50–6.78)	4.49 (3.36–5.55)	0.72
FF-TT (nmol/L)	51.90 (22.18–88.52)	24.71(16.32–43.44)	0.016
FF-FAI	1.86 (0.99–2.72)	0.95 (0.65–1.31)	0.014
FF-E2 (μg/L)	2028.00 (1218.00–3400.00)	1685.00 (1344.00–2353.00)	0.65
FF-P4 (mg/L)	27.62 (16.70–58.70)	39.88 (22.93–56.21)	0.21
FF-IL-6 (pg/mL)	5.39 (4.69–7.96)	5.74 (4.92–9.95)	0.71
FF-FGF21 (pg/mL)	16.48 (13.47–24.50)	13.97 (9.47–17.98)	0.023

Data are given as the median (interquartile range) for skewed variables or as the number (proportion) for categorical variables. "Elevated" FF-FGF13 levels were defined as follicular levels in the upper quartile (i.e., ≥117.51 pg/mL). P values were accessed using Kruskal-Wallis tests (continuous variables) and χ² tests (categorical variables). *FGF13* fibroblast growth factor 13; *BMI* body mass index; *PCOS* polycystic ovary syndrome; *FF* follicular fluid; *LH* luteinizing hormone; *FSH* follicle-stimulating hormone; *TT* total testosterone; *FAI* free androgen index; *E2*: estradiol; *P4*: progesterone; *IL6*: interleukin-6; *FGF21*: fibroblast growth factor 21

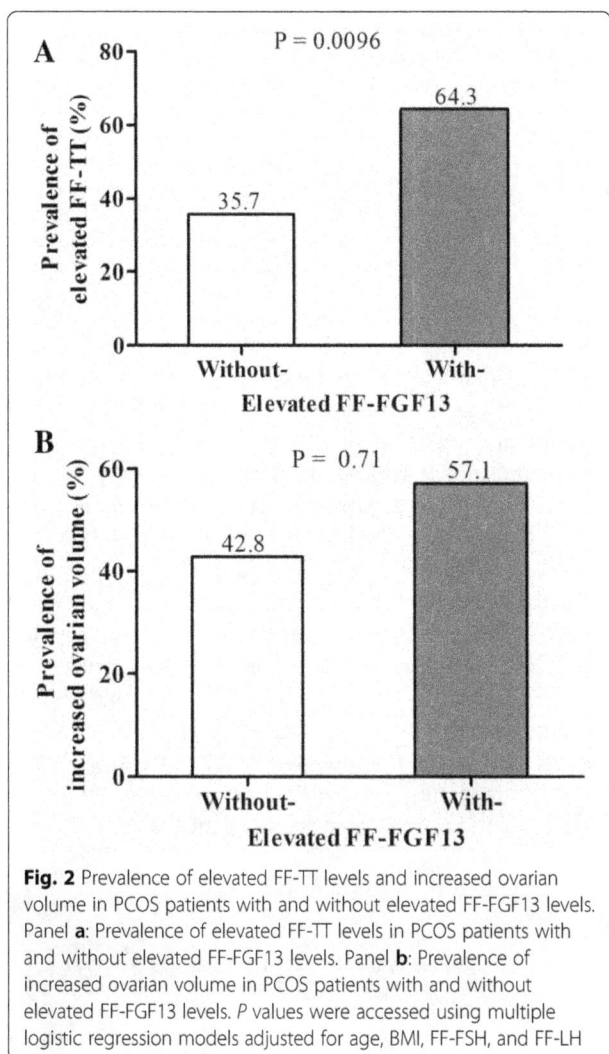

Fig. 2 Prevalence of elevated FF-TT levels and increased ovarian volume in PCOS patients with and without elevated FF-FGF13 levels. Panel **a**: Prevalence of elevated FF-TT levels in PCOS patients with and without elevated FF-FGF13 levels. Panel **b**: Prevalence of increased ovarian volume in PCOS patients with and without elevated FF-FGF13 levels. P values were accessed using multiple logistic regression models adjusted for age, BMI, FF-FSH, and FF-LH

regression analysis ($\beta = -0.10$, SE = 0.045 and $P = 0.027$). FF-FGF13 was significantly correlated with the fertilization rate in the non-PCOS patients ($r = 0.52$, $P = 0.0037$). However, the association disappeared in the multiple linear regression analysis ($\beta = 0.078$, SE = 0.099 and $P = 0.44$).

No associations were evident between FF-FGF21 and oocyte developmental competence for the PCOS patients when Spearman correlations were used (see Additional file 1).

Discussion

This study is the first to report the presence of FGF13 in the follicular fluid of women undergoing IVF/ICSI. Moreover, FF-FGF13 was significantly associated with FF-TT and the MII oocyte rate in PCOS patients undergoing first IVF/ICSI in China.

Although FGF13 has been detected in the ovaries of rodents and cows, its expression in the ovaries of other species has remained unknown. FGF13 expression was first reported in the murine ovary by Helge Hartung [11]. Thereafter, FGF13 mRNA was observed in bovine theca and granulosa cells [17]. Afterward, the above results were confirmed by I.B. Costa et al. [13]. In the present study, FGF13 was detected in the follicular fluid of women undergoing first IVF/ICSI, which has direct implications for the roles of FGF13 in human ovarian function.

Despite similarities with other secreted FGFs, FGF13 has not been regarded as a secreted protein due to its lack of N-terminal signal sequences. However, our study demonstrated the presence of FGF13 in the follicular fluid of women undergoing IVF/ICSI. Moreover, the concentrations of FF-FGF13 were much higher than the levels of IL-6 in the follicular fluid, which is one of the endocrine factors. The results raise the possibility that FGF13 might be transported to the extracellular space. If

Table 2 Spearman correlations of risk factors associated with FF-FGF13 in PCOS and non-PCOS patients

	PCOS		Non-PCOS	
	r	P values	r	P values
Age (years)	−0.038	0.81	0.090	0.62
BMI (kg/m^2)	0.10	0.50	0.37	0.041
Increased ovarian volume (YES = 1, NO = 0)	0.33	0.032	0.32	0.089
FF-LH (IU/L)	0.035	0.83	−0.0017	0.99
FF- FSH (IU/L)	−0.055	0.73	0.23	0.20
FF-TT (nmol/L)	0.37	0.013	0.035	0.85
FF-FAI	0.20	0.19	0.21	0.24
FF-E2 (μg/L)	0.14	0.3	−0.076	0.68
FF-P4 (mg/L)	−0.21	0.17	−0.20	0.27
FF-IL-6 (pg/mL)	−0.025	0.88	−0.036	0.85
FF-FGF21 (pg/mL)	0.32	0.035	0.33	0.063

r: correlation coefficient

Table 3 Correlations between FF-FGF13 and oocyte developmental competence in PCOS and non-PCOS patients

	PCOS				Non-PCOS			
	r	P values	β ± SE	P values	r	P values	β ± SE	P values
NO. of oocytes retrieved	0.100	0.52	0.021 ± 0.17	0.90	−0.12	0.54	−0.060 ± 0.23	0.78
MII oocytes rate	−0.42	0.0055	−0.10 ± 0.045	0.027	0.096	0.61	−0.054 ± 0.084	0.53
Fertilization rate	−0.16	0.30	−0.060 ± 0.054	0.27	0.52	0.0037	0.078 ± 0.099	0.44
High-quality embryos rate	−0.043	0.78	0.014 ± 0.168	0.94	0.010	0.96	−0.15 ± 0.23	0.52

P values were obtained using Spearman correlations of risk factors associated with correlation and multivariable linear regression models adjusted for age, BMI, FF-FSH, and FF-LH. Data regarding oocyte developmental competence were missing for the non-PCOS group (n = 2)
r, correlation coefficient; β, regression coefficient

so, the secretory mechanism of FGF13 might function in the same manner as that of FGF1 [18], despite the absence of a signal peptide. All of these possibilities require further investigation.

In the present study, FGF13 was associated with FF-TT in PCOS patients, raising the possibility of its essential role in the pathophysiological process of PCOS. Being different from other FGF family members, FGF13 cannot interact with FGF receptor tyrosine kinases [19]. The major downstream signaling pathways in the ovary function responsible for the association remain to be clarified. In previous research, FGF13 inhibited C2C12 cell differentiation by activating the extracellular signal-regulated kinases/mitogen-activated protein kinase (ERK/MAPK) pathway [20]. FGF13 was associated with the differential expression of the MAPK pathway in Sotos syndrome [21]. On the other hand, the MAPK pathway participated in the control of ovarian testosterone production [22]. Thus, we hypothesized that MAPK singling pathways were involved in the association between FGF13 and the testosterone secretion of the human ovary.

In addition to hyperandrogenism, the formation of ovarian interstitial fibrosis is a major cause of reproductive dysfunction in PCOS. In addition to MAPK singling pathways, the P38MAPK pathway, which is downstream of the FGF13 signaling pathway [23, 24], is involved in the expression of matrix metalloproteinase (MMP)2 and MMP9, which play important roles in extracellular matrix degradation in PCOS. Thus, FGF13 may be involved in ovarian interstitial fibrosis.

FGF21, a member of the family of secreted FGFs, is associated with insulin resistance [25, 26], an important aspect of the pathogenesis of PCOS. To explore its roles in PCOS, the levels of FGF21 in follicular fluid were examined in our study. The results showed that FGF21 was present in follicular fluid, but that it was not associated with oocyte developmental competence in PCOS patients undergoing IVF, implying that FGF21 in the follicular microenvironment might not be involved in oocyte developmental competence in PCOS patients.

The limitations of our study should be mentioned. First, the concentrations of FGF13 were examined in

infertile patients after superovulation and not under normal physiological conditions. Second, the relatively small number of patients may have influenced the statistical power, and thus, a large-scale population study is needed in the future. Third, although possible covariates were included in the adjustments, some residual or undetected confounding factors could not be ruled out.

In summary, the present study reported the presence of FGF13 in the follicular fluid of women undergoing IVF/ICSI. Moreover, the relationships between FF-FGF13 and FF-TT, ovarian morphology and oocyte developmental competence imply that FF-FGF13 might be involved in the pathophysiological process of PCOS. FGF13 might be a promising intervention target in PCOS, as long as the potential mechanisms are clarified.

Funding

This study was supported by the National Natural Science Foundation of China (Grant No. 81671518, Grant No. 81471424, Grant No. 81471029, Grant No. 81571499), Chinese National Key Basic Research Projects (Grant No. 2014CB943300) and Shanghai Municipal Education Commission-Gao feng Clinical Medicine Grant Support (Grant No. 20161413). Cultivating Funds of South Campus, Renji Hospital, School of Medicine, Shanghai Jiaotong University (Grant No. 2017PYQA05).

Authors' contributions

YL, SL: Conception and design of the study, acquisition of data, analysis and interpretation of data, draft the article. TT, XL, QZ, YL: Acquisition of data. JM: Revising the article. YS: Conception and design of the study, WL: Conception and design of the study, final approval of the version to be published.

Competing interests

The authors declared that no competing interests exist.

Author details

[1]Department of Endocrinology, South Campus, Renji Hospital, School of Medicine, Shanghai Jiaotong University, Shanghai 201112, China. [2]Department of Endocrinology, Renji Hospital, School of Medicine, Shanghai Jiaotong University, Shanghai 200127, China. [3]Center for Reproductive Medicine, Renji Hospital, School of Medicine, Shanghai JiaoTong University, Shanghai 200135, China. [4]Shanghai Key Laboratory for Assisted Reproduction and Reproductive Genetics, Shanghai 200135, China.

References

1. Law NC, Hunzicker-Dunn ME. Insulin Receptor Substrate 1, the Hub Linking Follicle-stimulating Hormone to Phosphatidylinositol 3-Kinase Activation. J Biol Chem. 2016;291:4547-60.

2. Mendes CC, Mirth CK. Stage-Specific Plasticity in Ovary Size Is Regulated by Insulin/Insulin-Like Growth Factor and Ecdysone Signaling in Drosophila. Genetics. 2016;202:703-19.

3. Mottershead DG, Sugimura S, Al-Musawi SL, Li JJ, Richani D, White MA, et al. Cumulin, an Oocyte-secreted Heterodimer of the Transforming Growth Factor-β Family, Is a Potent Activator of Granulosa Cells and Improves Oocyte Quality. J Biol Chem. 2015;290:24007-20.

4. Chen YC, Chang HM, Cheng JC, Tsai HD, Wu CH, Leung PC. Transforming growth factor-β1 up-regulates connexin43 expression in human granulosa cells. Hum Reprod. 2015;30:2190-201.

5. Parrott JA, Vigne JL, Chu BZ, Skinner MK. Mesenchymal-epithelial interactions in the ovarian follicle involve keratinocyte and hepatocyte growth factor production by thecal cells and their action on granulosa cells. Endocrinology. 1994;135:569-75.

6. Buratini J Jr, Pinto MG, Castilho AC, Amorim RL, Giometti IC, Portela VM, et al. Expression and function of fibroblast growth factor 10 and its receptor, fibroblast growth factor receptor 2B, in bovine follicles. Biol Reprod. 2007;77: 743-50.

7. Lavranos TC, Rodgers HF, Bertoncello I, Rodgers RJ. Anchorage-independent culture of bovine granulosa cells: the effects of basic fibroblast growth factor and dibutyryl cAMP on cell division and differentiation. Exp Cell Res. 1994;211:245-51.

8. Vernon RK, Spicer LJ. Effects of basic fibroblast growth factor and heparin on follicle stimulating hormone-induced steroidogenesis by bovine granulosa cells. J Anim Sci. 1994;72:2696-702.

9. Jiang Z, Guerrero-Netro HM, Juengel JL, Price CA. Divergence of intracellular signaling pathways and early response genes of two closely related fibroblast growth factors, FGF8 and FGF18, in bovine ovarian granulosa cells. Mol Cell Endocrinol. 2013;375:97-105.

10. Portela VM, Machado M, Buratini J Jr, Zamberlam G, Amorim RL, Goncalves P, et al. Expression and function of fibroblast growth factor 18 in the ovarian follicle in cattle. Biol Reprod. 2010;83:339-46.

11. Hartung H, Feldman B, Lovec H, Coulier F, Birnbaum D, Goldfarb M. Murine FGF-12 and FGF-13: expression in embryonic nervous system, connective tissue and heart. Mech Dev. 1997;64:31-9.

12. Fon Tacer K, Bookout AL, Ding X, Kurosu H, John GB, Wang L, et al. Research resource: comprehensive expression atlas of the fibroblast growth factor system in adult mouse. Mol Endocrinol. 2010;24(10):2050-64.

13. Costa IB, Teixeira NA, Ripamonte P, Guerra DM, Price C, Buratini J Jr. Expression of fibroblast growth factor 13 (Fgf13) mRNA in bovine antral follicles and corpora lutea. Anim. Reprod. 2009;6:409-15.

14. Zhu Q, Zuo R, He Y, Wang Y, Chen ZJ, Sun Y, et al. Local regeneration of cortisol by 11β-HSD1 contributes to insulin resistance of the Granulosa cells in PCOS. J Clin Endocrinol Metab. 2016;101:2168-77.

15. Brinsden PR. A textbook of in vitro fertilization and assisted reproduction: the Bourn Hall guide to clinical and laboratory practice: The Parthenon Publishing Group; 1999:196.

16. Rotterdam ESHRE/ASRM-Sponsored PCOS Consensus Workshop Group. Revised 2003 consensus on diagnostic criteria and long-term health risks related to polycystic ovary syndrome. Fertil Steril. 2004;81:19-25.

17. Buratini J, Costa I, Teixeira N, Castilho A, Price C. Fibroblast growth factor 13 gene expression in the bovine ovary. Biol Reprod. 2007;76:96.

18. Landriscina M, Bagalá C, Mandinova A, Soldi R, Micucci I, Bellum S, et al. Copper induces the assembly of a multiprotein aggregate implicated in the release of fibroblast growth factor 1 in response to stress. J Biol Chem. 2001; 276:25549-57.

19. Olsen SK, Garbi M, Zampieri N, Eliseenkova AV, Ornitz DM, Goldfarb M, et al. Fibroblast growth factor (FGF) homologous factors share structural but not functional homology with FGFs. J Biol Chem. 2003;278:34226-36.

20. Lu H, Shi X, Wu G, Zhu J, Song C, Zhang Q, et al. FGF13 regulates proliferation and differentiation of skeletal muscle by down-regulating Spry1. Cell Prolif. 2015;48:550-60.

21. Visser R, Landman EB, Goeman J, Wit JM, Karperien M. Sotos syndrome is associated with deregulation of the MAPK/ERK-signaling pathway. PLoS One. 2012;7:e49229.

22. Chabrolle C, Jeanpierre E, Tosca L, Rame C, Dupont J. Effects of high levels of glucose on the steroidogenesis and the expression of adiponectin receptors in rat ovarian cells. Reprod Biol Endocrinol. 2008;6:11.

23. Schoorlemmer J, Goldfarb M. Fibroblast growth factor homologous factors are intracellular signaling proteins. Curr Biol. 2001;11:793-7.

24. Goldfarb M. Fibroblast growth factor homologous factors: evolution, structure, and function. Cytokine Growth Factor Rev. 2005;16:215-20.

25. Jung JG, Yi SA, Choi SE, Kang Y, Kim TH, Jeon JY, et al. TM-25659-Induced Activation of FGF21 Level Decreases Insulin Resistance and Inflammation in Skeletal Muscle via GCN2 Pathways. Mol Cells. 2015;38(12):1037-43.

26. Kim KH, Jeong YT, Oh H, Kim SH, Cho JM, Kim YN, et al. Autophagy deficiency leads to protection from obesity and insulin resistance by inducing Fgf21 as a mitokine. Nat Med. 2013;19:83-92.

25

Luteolin sensitizes the antitumor effect of cisplatin in drug-resistant ovarian cancer via induction of apoptosis and inhibition of cell migration and invasion

Haixia Wang[1][*][†] ⓘ, Youjun Luo[2][†], Tiankui Qiao[2], Zhaoxia Wu[3] and Zhonghua Huang[1]

Abstract

Luteolin, a polyphenolic flavone, has been demonstrated to exert anti-tumor activity in various cancer types. Cisplatin drug resistance is a major obstacle in the management of ovarian cancer. In the present study, we investigated the chemo-sensitizing effect of luteolin in both cisplatin-resistant ovarian cancer cell line and a mice xenotransplant model. In vitro, CCK-8 assay showed that luteolin inhibited cell proliferation in a dose-dependent manner, and luteolin enhanced anti-proliferation effect of cisplatin on cisplatin-resistant ovarian cancer CAOV3/DDP cells. Flow cytometry revealed that luteolin enhanced cell apoptosis in combination with cisplatin. Western blotting and qRT-PCR assay revealed that luteolin increased cisplatin-induced downregulation of Bcl-2 expression. In addition, wound-healing assay and Matrigel invasion assay showed that luteolin and cisplatin synergistically inhibited migration and invasion of CAOV3/DDP cells. Moreover, in vivo, luteolin enhanced cisplatin-induced reduction of tumor growth as well as induction of apoptosis. We suggest that luteolin in combination with cisplatin could potentially be used as a new regimen for the treatment of ovarian cancer.

Keywords: Luteolin, Cisplatin-resistant ovarian cancer, Apoptosis, Migration, Invasion

Introduction

Ovarian cancer is one of the most common malignant tumors of gynecology, with the highest mortality compared with other gynecologic cancer because of its acute onset, rapid progress and high metastasis rate [1, 2]. Epithelial ovarian cancer (EOC) accounts for 85–90% of total ovarian carcinoma and is the most aggressive one. In early stage, surgical resection combined with chemotherapy is an effective therapy method [3]. Unfortunately, most of the patients reach advanced stage at the time of diagnosis [4, 5]. For patients with advanced EOC, platinum-based chemotherapy is the standard of care. More than 80% of ovarian tumors response to first-line platinum-based therapy [6], however, the majority of patients acquire resistance to cisplatin (CDDP)

treatment and ultimately result in relapse and poor prognosis [7, 8]. Therefore, it is necessary to develop appropriate combined reagents to solve drug resistance and enhance the sensitivity of EOC to cisplatin treatment.

Chemotherapy resistance is a key factor that limits the cure rate of ovarian cancer. The mechanisms underlying cancer cells resistance to cisplatin are not fully understood. It is acknowledged that various mechanisms are responsible for drug-resistance, including the decrease of the effective concentration of drugs in cells, the abnormalities of drug targets, and the abnormal regulation of cell apoptosis [9]. Currently, there are some ways to overcome the chemo-resistance, such as maintenance therapy, novel cytotoxic agents, modulation of apoptosis and combination therapy [10]. Natural medicine, with its small side effects and significant therapeutic effect, attracts a lot attention as a potential combination agent for cisplatin treatment.

* Correspondence: 18930819496@163.com
[†]Haixia Wang and Youjun Luo contributed equally to this work.
[1]Department of Obstetrics and Gynecology, Jinshan branch of Shanghai Sixth People's Hospital, Shanghai Jiaotong University, Shanghai, China
Full list of author information is available at the end of the article

Luteolin is one of the most common flavonoid compound that is widely existed in various plants including peppermint, rosemary, thyme, pinophyte, and pteridophyta [11]. Numerous studies suggested that luteolin possesses a variety of pharmacological properties including anti-inflammatory, antiallergic, antioxidant, antimicrobial, immune regulation and anticancer activities [11, 12]. Among all these properties, anti-tumor effect has attracted a lot of attention. Researchers have found that luteolin exerts anti-tumor activities via several mechanisms, including cell cycle arrest, apoptosis induction, angiogenesis and metastasis inhibition [13–16]. A previous study has demonstrated that luteolin can sensitize oxaliplatin-resistant colorectal cancer cells to chemotherapeutic drugs through the inhibition of the Nrf2 pathway [17]. Another study reported that luteolin can be used as a chemosensitizer to improve the therapeutic effect of tamoxifen in drug-resistant human breast cancer cells via the inhibition of cyclin E2 expression [18]. These results suggest that luteolin exhibits potential chemosensitivity property for various cancers. However, whether luteolin can increase the chemotherapy sensitivity of cisplatin-resistant ovarian cancer and the underlying mechanisms is rarely reported, which needs to be further studied.

In the current study, we investigated the synergistic effects of luteolin combined with cisplatin in drug-resistant ovarian cancer cell line CAOV3/DDP both in vitro and in vivo, and tried to explore associated molecular mechanisms.

Materials and methods
Reagents and cell lines
Luteolin was bought from Jin Sui Biological Technology (Shanghai, China). It was dissolved in DMSO as a stock of 500 mM and stored at − 20 °C. Cisplatin was purchased from QILU Pharmaceutical (Shandong, China). Human drug-resistant ovarian cancer cell line, CAOV3/DDP were obtained from the Shanghai Sixin Biotechnology company (Shanghai, China) and maintained in RPMI1640 (Gibco, Grand Island, NY, USA) containing 10% fetal bovine serum (Gibco, Grand Island, NY, USA). The cells were incubated at 37 °C in a humidified atmosphere with 5% CO_2.

Cell proliferation assay
Cell proliferation was measured using Cell Counting Kit-8 (CCK-8; Dojindo Molecular Technologies, Inc., Kumamoto,Japan). Briefly, CAOV3/DDP cells (5×10^3) were seeded into 96-well plates and allowed for adhesion overnight. Then the cells were administrated with eight treatments as follows: control (culture medium); low-dose of luteolin (10 µM); medial-dose of luteolin (50 µM); high-dose of luteolin (100 µM); CDDP (2 µg/ml); CDDP (2 µg/ml) +

low-dose of luteolin (10 µM); CDDP (2 µg/ml) + medial-dose of luteolin (50 µM); CDDP (2 µg/ml) + high-dose of luteolin (100 µM). After 48 h treatment, the culture medium was removed and CCK-8 was added according to the manufacturer's instruction. Then the cells were incubated for 1–4 h at 37 °C and the absorbance was detected at 450 nm using a microplate reader. Cell proliferation was calculated as follows:

Cell proliferation (%) = [(OD of experiment group − OD of blank) / (OD of control group − OD of blank)] × 100%.

Apoptosis analysis
Cell apoptosis was detected using Annexin V-FITC Apoptosis Detection Kit (BD Pharmingen, Franklin Lakes, NJ, USA). Cells (2×10^4) were seeded into 6-well plates and treated with various concentration of luteolin (0, 10, 50, 100 µM) or CDDP alone or in combination for 48 h. Then both the adherent and floating cells were harvested and stained according to the manufacturer's protocol. The apoptosis rate was analyzed by flow cytometry.

Wound-healing assay
Cell migration ability was measured by wound-healing assay. Briefly, cells were seeded into 6-well plates and allowed to grow to a monolayer. Subsequently, a straight scratch was generated across the plate using a 200 µl pipet tip. The cells were washed with PBS and incubated with various concentration of luteolin (0, 10, 50, 100 µM) and CDDP alone or in combination (dissolve the chemicals in serum-free culture medium). Wound healing was observed and photographed at 0 and 48 h.

Matrigel invasion assay
The Matrigel was diluted in serum-free RPMI-1640 (RPMI-1640: Matrigel = 8:1) and added into the upper chamber. After treatment with various concentrations of luteolin (0, 10, 50, 100 µM) and CDDP alone or in combination for 48 h, the cells (5×10^4) were trypsinized and collected. 5×10^4 cells in 200 µl serum-free medium were seeded into the upper chamber. The lower chamber was filled with 600 µl complete medium containing 10% FBS. After incubation for 48 h, the invaded cells were stained with crystal violet and pictured under a microscope at x100 magnification.

qRT-PCR
After treatment, the medium was removed and the cells were washed with PBS. The total RNA of each group was extracted using TRIzol (Invitrogen, California, USA). Then the RNA was reversely transcribed to cDNA using the PrimeScript™ RT Reagent kit (Takara, Dalian, China) according to the manufacturer's instruction. The qPCR was performed using a SYBR Premix Ex Taq (Tli RNaseH Plus) in Applied Biosystem 7300 (Applied

Biosystems, Foster city, CA, USA). The BCL-2 mRNA expression was analyzed using the 2-ΔΔCq method taking β-Actin as reference. The gene primer sequences were shown in Table 1.

Western blot

CAOV3/DDP cells were seeded into 6-well plates (2×10^5/well),and treated with increasing doses of luteolin (0, 10, 50, 100 μM) or cisplatin (2 μg/ml) or both for 48 h. Then, the cells were harvested, and total proteins were extracted using cell lysis buffer (1 mM PMSF, 50 mM Tris (pH 8.1), 1% SDS, sodium pyrophosphate, β-glycerophosphate, sodium orthovanadate, sodium fluoride, EDTA, leupeptin and other inhibitors) (Beyotime Biotechnology, Shanghai, China. No. P0013G). The protein concentration was detected using BCA assay (Mai Bio Co., Ltd.). 20 μg proteins of each group were separated on SDS-PAGE, and then transferred onto PVDF membranes (Millipore Corp., Bedford, MA, USA). Membranes were blocked with 5% non-fat dry milk, and probed with primary antibodies against Bax (1:4000, Cell Signaling Technology, USA), Bcl-2 (1:4000, Cell Signaling Technology, USA), and β-Actin (1:5000, ProteinTech Group, Inc., USA) at 4 °C overnight. Then the membrane was washed with PBS and incubated with HRP-conjugated secondary antibodies (1:5000) for 1 h at room temperature. Finally, the blots were imaged with ECL (EMD Millipore).

In vivo xenograft experiment

Female BALB/c nude mice (5–6 weeks old) were obtained from the Shanghai Experimental Animal Center. Animals were raised in pathogen-free conditions at 22 ° C, 50% humidity. Animal experiments were approved by the Institutional of Animal Care and Use Committee of Jinshan Hospital, Fudan University. The cisplatin resistant cell line CAOV3/DDP (5×10^6 cells) in a volume of 100 μl of PBS were inoculated in the subcutaneous tissue of the nude mice. Two weeks after implantation, the tumors were visible and the mice were randomly allocated into 8 groups (6 mice per group): (1) control group (normal saline); (2) luteolin low-dose (10 mg·kg^{-1}·d^{-1}) group; (3) luteolin medial-dose (20 mg·kg^{-1}·d^{-1}) group; (4) luteolin high-dose (40 mg·kg^{-1}·d^{-1}) group; (5) CDDP (3 mg·kg^{-1}·d^{-1}) group; (6) CDDP (3 mg·kg^{-1}·d^{-1}) plus luteolin low-dose (10 mg·kg^{-1}·d^{-1}) group; (7) CDDP (3 mg·kg^{-1}·d^{-1}) plus luteolin medial-dose

Table 1 Primer sequences for genes

Gene	Primer Sequences
BCL-2	F: 5′-AACATCGCCCTGTGGATGAC-3′
	R: 5′-AGAGTCTTCAGAGACAGCCAGGAG-3′
β-Actin	F: 5′-CATTGCCGACAGGATGCAG-3′
	R: 5′-CTCGTCATACTCCTGCTTGCTG-3′

(20 mg·kg^{-1}·d^{-1}) group; (8) CDDP (3 mg·kg^{-1}·d^{-1}) plus luteolin high-dose (40 mg·kg^{-1}·d^{-1}) group. The CDDP were intraperitoneal injected once daily, and luteolin were given by gavage once daily for 5 days. The tumor volume was measured three times a week. Three weeks after treatment, the mice were sacrificed, and the tumor volume and weight were measured. The tumor tissues were used for histopathologic examination.

TUNEL

Tumor paraffin tissue sections were processed with TUNEL assay to analyze apoptosis. The procedure was performed according to instructions of the TUNEL kit (KeyGen, Nanjing, China). The samples were observed under a microscope at × 100 magnification. The apoptotic cells were counted in three random fields for each sample, and the apoptosis percentage was calculated as follows: (Number of TUNEL-positive cells/Total number of cells in the field) × 100%.

Drug combination effect analysis

Combination effect between the luteolin and cisplatin was analyzed by the Zheng-Jun Jin method [19–21]. In this method, the combination rate was evaluated by the inhibition rate via the Q value. The formula for the Q value is: Q = Ea + b / (Ea + Eb - Ea × Eb), where Ea + b, Ea, and Eb are the inhibition rate of the combination group, drug a and drug b, respectively. Q = 1 would mean simple addition; Q > l, synergism or potentiation, Q < 1, antagonism.

Statistical analysis

All the experiments were repeated three times. The data were presented as mean ± SD. The difference between indicated groups were analyzed using Student's t-test. $P < 0.05$ was considered be statistically significant.

Results

Luteolin dose dependently enhanced the proliferation inhibition effect of cisplatin in CAOV3/DDP cells

Cells were treated with various doses of luteolin (0, 10, 50, and 100 μM), cisplatin (2 μg/ml) alone or in combination for 48 h and then cell proliferation was monitored by CCK-8 assay. As shown in Fig 1a, b, luteolin alone inhibited the cell proliferation of CAOV3/DDP cells in a concentration- dependent manner. Cells treated with combination of cisplatin (2 μg/ml) and luteolin (10, 50, 100 μM) for 48 h showed a more significant proliferation decrease in contrast with either luteolin or cisplatin alone. These results suggested that luteolin enhanced the proliferation inhibition effect of cisplatin in CAOV3/DDP cells in a concentration-dependent manner. To further investigate the nature of the combination effect between luteolin and cisplatin on CAOV3/DDP cells, the Q value was calculated based on the CCK-8 assay. As shown in Table 2, the data

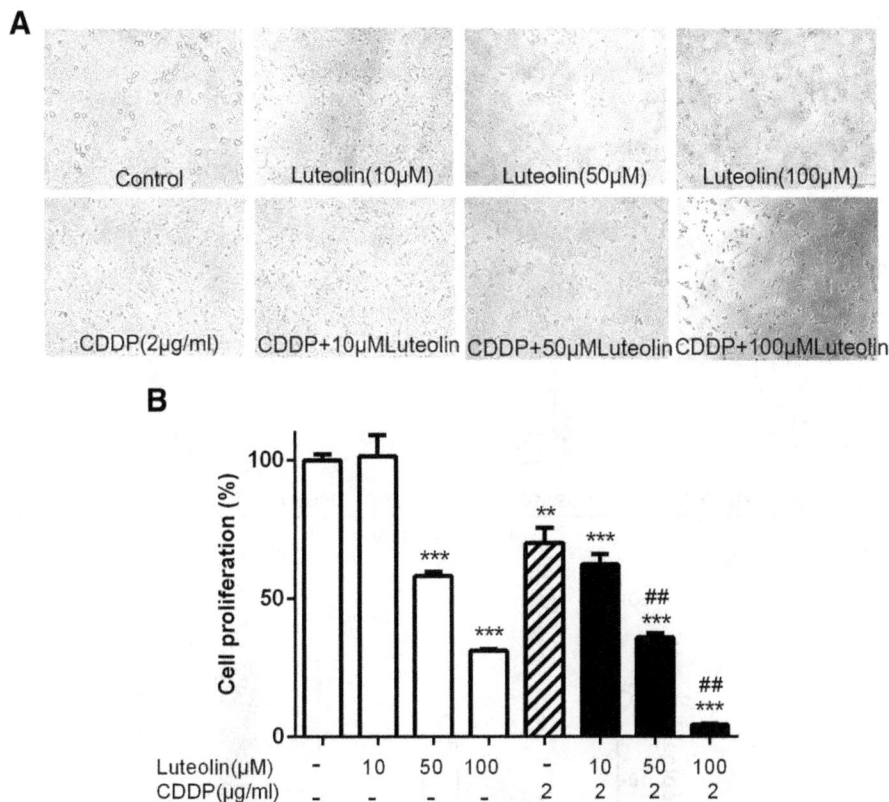

Fig. 1 Effects of luteolin and cisplatin on the proliferation of CAOV3/DDP cells. Cells were treated with indicated concentrations of luteolin or cisplatin or both for 48 h, and cell proliferation was measured by CCK-8 assay. **a** Representative morphological changes of indicated treatment at × 200 magnification; **b** Dose response curves indicated significant reduction of cell proliferation in comparison to normal control. Data were represented as mean ± standard error of three independent experiments. ** $P < 0.01$, *** $P < 0.001$, vs. control; ## $P < 0.01$ vs. cisplatin. CDDP: cisplatin

suggested that luteolin exhibited an additive or synergistic effect when combined with cisplatin.

Luteolin enhanced cisplatin induced apoptosis in CAOV3/DDP cells

As luteolin promoted cisplatin induced cell proliferation inhibition, we further determined whether the

Table 2 Luteolin increased the sensitivity of CAOV3/DDP cells to cisplatin. The Q value was calculated to evaluate the effect of the combination of the two drugs. The inhibition rates were measured by CCK-8 assay. CDDP combined with luteolin (100 μM) showed a synergistic inhibitory effect on the proliferation of CAOV3/DDP cells (Q = 1.22 ± 0.04, > 1, P < 0.01). The data were expressed as the mean ± S.D. in triplicate

Drugs	Inhibition rate (%)	Q value
Luteolin (100 μM)	69.1 ± 0.55	
Luteolin (50 μM)	42.0 ± 1.20	
Luteolin (10 μM)	−1.5 ± 6.26	
CDDP (2 μg/ml)	30.2 ± 4.54	
Luteolin (100 μM) + CDDP (2 μg/ml)	95.7 ± 0.24	1.22 ± 0.04
Luteolin (50 μM) + CDDP (2 μg/ml)	64.3 ± 1.22	1.08 ± 0.06
Luteolin (10 μM) + CDDP (2 μg/ml)	37.9 ± 3.02	1.36 ± 0.41

combination treatment could exert synergic induction on cell apoptosis. Cell apoptosis was evaluated by flow cytometry following treatment of luteolin (0, 10, 50, and 100 μM), CDDP (2 μg/ml) alone or the combined treatments. As shown in Fig. 2a-b, no significant apoptosis was observed in cells treated with 10 μM luteolin. Treatments with higher doses (50 μM and 100 μM) of luteolin induced evident cell apoptosis, and the apoptosis rates were 4.29% and 14.39% respectively. Cisplatin alone caused about 3.11% of apoptosis. When cells were treated with both luteolin and cisplatin, the apoptosis rate increased significantly. The apoptosis rates of luteolin (10 μM) + cisplatin, luteolin (50 μM) + cisplatin and luteolin (100 μM) + cisplatin group were 3.41%, 5.48% and 24.75%, respectively.

Luteolin and cisplatin decreased Bcl-2 expression synergistically

Next, to explore the underlying mechanisms involved in the sensitization effect of luteolin on cisplatin-induced apoptosis, we measured the expression level of the anti-apoptotic regulator, Bcl-2, by qRT-PCR and western blotting, and the pro-apoptotic protein Bax through

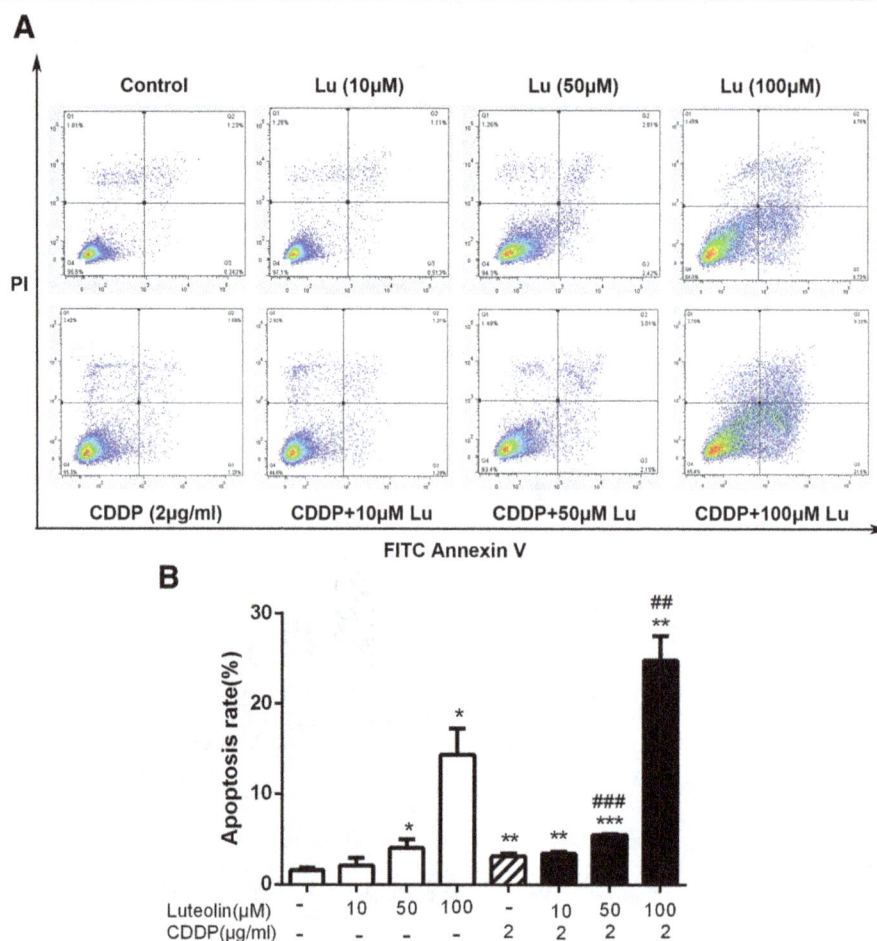

Fig. 2 Luteolin induced cell apoptosis and enhanced cisplatin-induced apoptosis of CAOV3/DDP cells. Cells were treated with luteolin or cisplatin or in combination for 48 h, and then the apoptosis was detected by Annexin V/PI. **a** Flowcytometric analysis; **b** Statistical analysis for apoptosis ratio in each group. Data were represented as mean ± SD of three independent experiments. * $P < 0.05$, ** $P < 0.01$, *** $P < 0.001$, vs. control; ## $P < 0.01$, ### $P < 0.001$ vs. cisplatin. CDDP: cisplatin. CDDP combined with luteolin (100 μM) showed a synergistic effect on the apoptosis induction of CAOV3/DDP cells (Q = 1.46 ± 0.1, > 1, $P < 0.01$)

western blotting assay. As shown in Fig. 3, luteolin at high dose of 100 μM decreased the Bcl-2 mRNA level and protein expression, and cisplatin alone also decreased the Bcl-2 level. Moreover, the Bcl-2 expression was decreased further in the combined treatment of luteolin and cisplatin. However, the Bax protein expression didn't show significant change in all the groups (data not shown). These results suggested that luteolin enhanced the antitumor response of cisplatin by modulating apoptosis pathway.

Luteolin combined with CDDP inhibited migration and invasion in CAOV3/DDP cells

To determine whether combination treatment affected cell migration and invasion ability, we then treated CAOV3/DDP cells with luteolin or cisplatin or combination of both by wound-healing assay and Matrigel invasion assay. The results (Figs. 4 and 5) showed that,

luteolin alone inhibited cell migration and invasion in a dose-dependent manner, and the combination of CDDP and luteolin evidently decreased cell migration and invasion compared with either single agent treatment. These results demonstrated that luteolin could suppress migration and invasion and enhance sensitivity to CDDP in CAOV3/DDP cell line.

Luteolin enhanced the anticancer effect of CDDP on ovarian cancer in vivo

To determine whether luteolin could enhance the cytotoxicity of CDDP in vivo, we established an ovarian cancer model in nude mice and investigated the therapeutic effects of luteolin alone or in combination with CDDP. The results showed that luteolin combined with CDDP notably impeded the tumor growth compared with cisplatin alone, exhibited as decreased tumor volume (Fig. 6a) and declined tumor weight (Fig. 6b). According

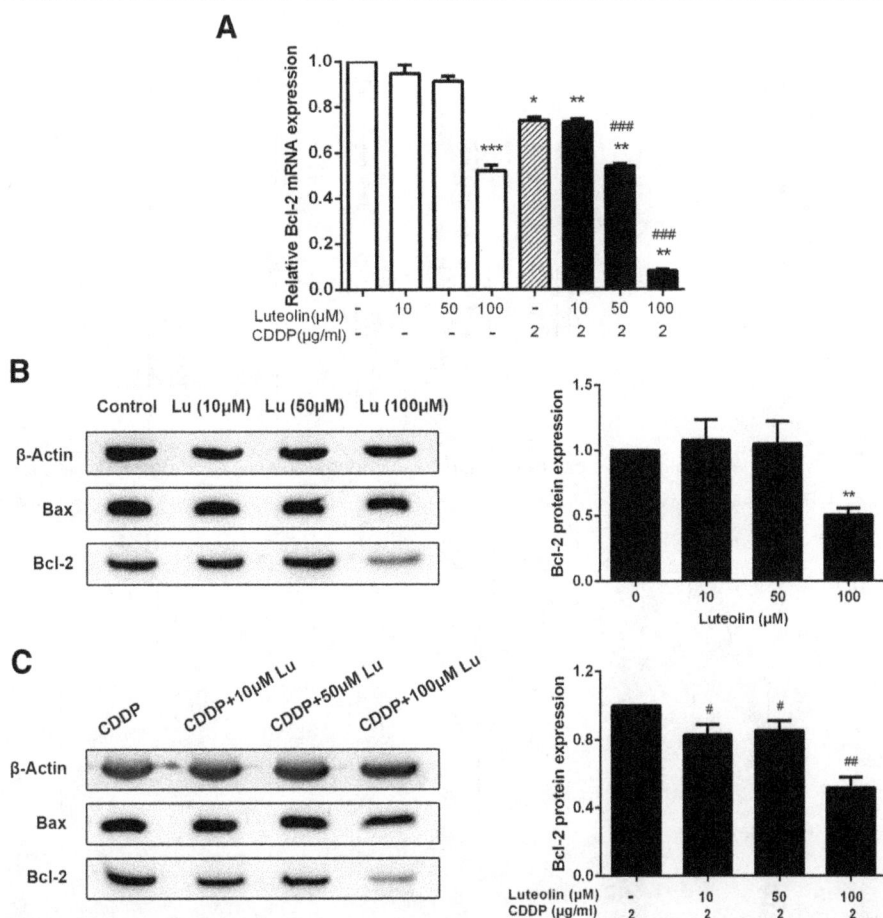

Fig. 3 Effects of luteolin in combination with cisplatin on expression of apoptosis related proteins. CAOV3/DDP cells were treated with various concentrations of luteolin or cisplatin or the combination of both for 48 h, and then the expression of Bax, Bcl-2 was assessed by qRT-PCR and western blotting. **a** Relative Bcl-2 mRNA expression was normalized to β-actin; **b** Bax and Bcl-2 protein expressions of cells treated with luteolin; **c** Bax and Bcl-2 protein expressions of cells treated with the combination of cisplatin and increasing doses of luteolin. * $P < 0.05$, ** $P < 0.01$, *** $P < 0.001$, vs. control; # $P < 0.05$, ## $P < 0.01$, ### $P < 0.001$ vs. cisplatin. CDDP: cisplatin. CDDP combined with luteolin (50, 100 μM) indicated a synergistic inhibitory effect on the Bcl-2 expression of CAOV3/DDP cells (Q = 1.43 ± 0.16 and 1.50 ± 0.09, respectively, > 1, $P < 0.01$ and $P < 0.001$, respectively)

to the tumor weight, we calculated the inhibition rate of each group, the combination tumor growth inhibition rate also showed a synergistic or additive effect (Table 3). These results were in consistent with in vitro experiments. Collectively, these results indicated that luteolin enhanced CDDP sensitivity of ovarian cancer in vivo.

Combined treatment of CDDP with luteolin increases xenograft tumor cell apoptosis

Further, we examined the effect of combined treatment of CDDP with luteolin on tumor cell apoptosis through TUNEL assay in the tumor tissues isolated from the 8 groups of mice above. As shown in Fig. 7, luteolin alone induced apoptosis at doses of 20 mg·kg^{-1}·d^{-1} and 40 mg·kg^{-1}·d^{-1} (the apoptosis rates were 0.51% and 1.70%, respectively) while the lower dose at 10 mg·kg^{-1}·d^{-1} didn't show significant effect compared with

control group (apoptosis rate: 0.24%). The results also revealed an increased apoptosis rate by combined treatment compared with cisplatin treatment alone. The apoptosis rates of CDDP, CDDP plus low dose of luteolin, CDDP plus medial dose of luteolin and CDDP plus high dose of luteolin were 1.24%, 1.59%, 3.03%, and 8.61%, respectively. This further demonstrated that luteolin enhanced antitumor effect of CDDP by increasing apoptosis of tumor cells.

Discussion

Cisplatin is one of the most effective therapeutic agents widely used in clinic for the treatment of EOC. However, drug resistance is a major problem that limits its clinical application. Therefore, combination treatment with new sensitizing agents is an effective strategy to overcome cisplatin resistance [10]. Luteolin, a flavonoid that has

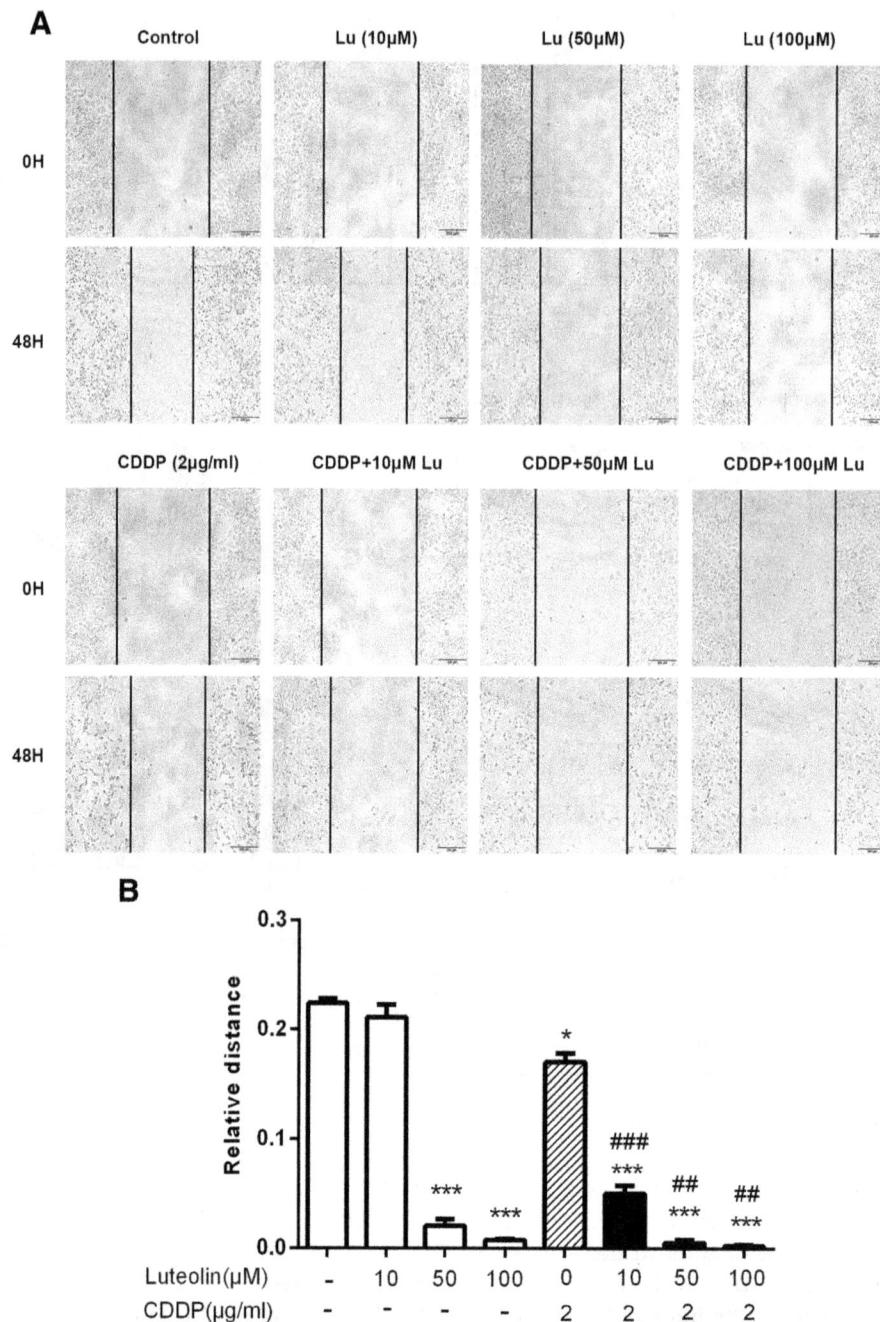

Fig. 4 Luteolin inhibited cell migration and enhanced cisplatin-induced migration suppression in CAOV3/DDP cells. Migratory ability of CAOV3/DDP cells treated with increasing doses of luteolin or cisplatin or the combination of both agents was tested using wound-healing assay. **a** The gap of indicated groups was imaged at 0 and 48 h (magnification, × 100); **b** Relative migration distance of three independent experiments. $*$ $P < 0.05$, $***$ $P < 0.001$, vs. control; ## $P < 0.01$, ### $P < 0.001$ vs. cisplatin. CDDP: cisplatin. CDDP combined with luteolin (10, 100 μM) showed a synergistic inhibitory effect on the migratory ability of CAOV3/DDP cells (Q = 2.91 ± 0.97 and 1.02 ± 0.003, respectively, > 1, $P < 0.05$ and $P < 0.01$, respectively)

been identified in many plants, has demonstrated in numbers studies to exhibit chemopreventive or chemo-sensitising properties against various human cancers. In the current study, we provide experimental evidence both in vivo and in vitro that luteolin is able to enhance the therapeutic potential of cisplatin in ovarian cancer.

In the current study, firstly, we evaluated the effect of luteolin or cisplatin or the combination of both on the cell proliferation in human cisplatin-resistant ovarian cancer CAOV3/DDP cells. We found that luteolin alone inhibited the cell proliferation in a dose-dependent manner, and co-treatment with both agents could further

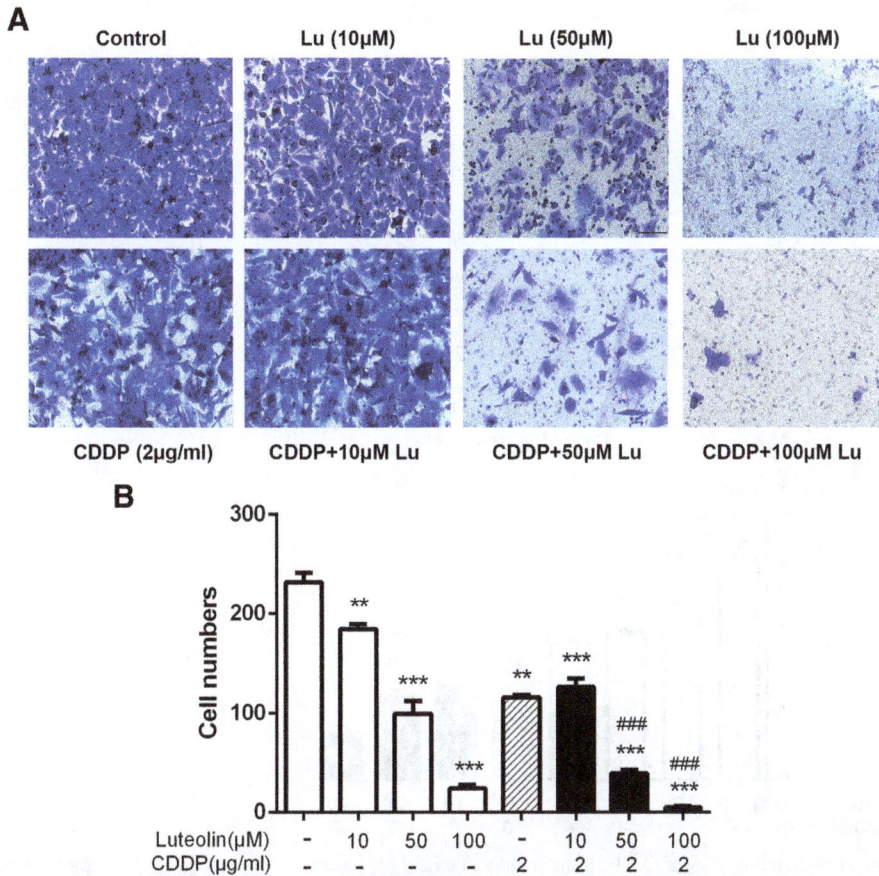

Fig. 5 Luteolin suppressed cell invasion and enhanced cisplatin-induced suppression of invasion in CAOV3/DDP cells. Invasion ability of CAOV3/DDP cells of indicated treatments was measured using Matrigel invasion assay. **a** The image of invaded cells (magnification,× 200); **b** Numbers of invaded cells in each group of three independent experiments. ** $P < 0.01$, *** $P < 0.001$, vs. control; ### $P < 0.001$ vs. cisplatin. CDDP: cisplatin. CDDP combined with luteolin (50, 100 μM) showed a synergistic inhibitory effect on the invasion of CAOV3/DDP cells ($Q = 1.06 \pm 0.02$ and 1.03 ± 0.007, respectively, > 1, $P < 0.05$ and $P < 0.01$, respectively)

decrease cell proliferation. These results suggested that luteolin could exert synergistic anti-proliferation effect with cisplatin in CAOV3/DDP cells.

Apoptosis inhibition is one of the main mechanisms responsible for the resistance of chemotherapy [22]. Cisplatin is one of the most effective drugs for the treatment of ovarian cancer, and the mechanism involved in the process of its cytotoxicity include survival inhibition and apoptosis induction. Once the apoptotic pathway is blocked, tumor cells acquire resistance to pro-apoptotic effect of cisplatin, which reduces the antitumor effect of cisplatin [23]. Therefore, inhibition of apoptosis is an effective strategy to overcome the drug resistance and promote the anti-tumor effect of cisplatin [24]. Luteolin has been reported to induce apoptosis in various cancer cells such as human cervical cancer cells [13], esophageal carcinoma cells [25] and colorectal cancer cells [26]. Our study found that the single treatment with luteolin could dose-dependently induce apoptosis in CAOV3/DDP cells, when combined with cisplatin, luteolin could

significantly enhance cisplatin-induced cell apoptosis, indicating that luteolin enhanced the sensitivity of cisplatin, in part, through apoptosis induction.

The BCL-2 protein family plays a key role in the regulation of cell apoptosis. The BCL-2 protein family can be divided into three different subfamilies, including pro-survival factions such as BCL-2, MCL1 and BCL-XL, which inhibit the apoptosis process, and two pro-apoptotic subfamilies, the death effectors BAX and BAK and the BH3-only proteins such as BID, BIM and PUMA, which contribute to cell apoptosis [27–29]. Consequently, the ratio of Bcl-2/Bax is an essential factor to determine whether a tumor cell commits apoptosis or not. Overexpression of Bcl-2 can inhibit cell apoptosis, lead to resistance to cisplatin, and result in poor prognosis of cancer patients. Recent study has demonstrated that Bcl-2 is overexpressed in ovarian cancer [30, 31] and has a significant positive correlation with sensitivity to cisplatin in ovarian cancer cells [32]. Therefore, targeting Bcl-2 may provide an effective therapeutic method

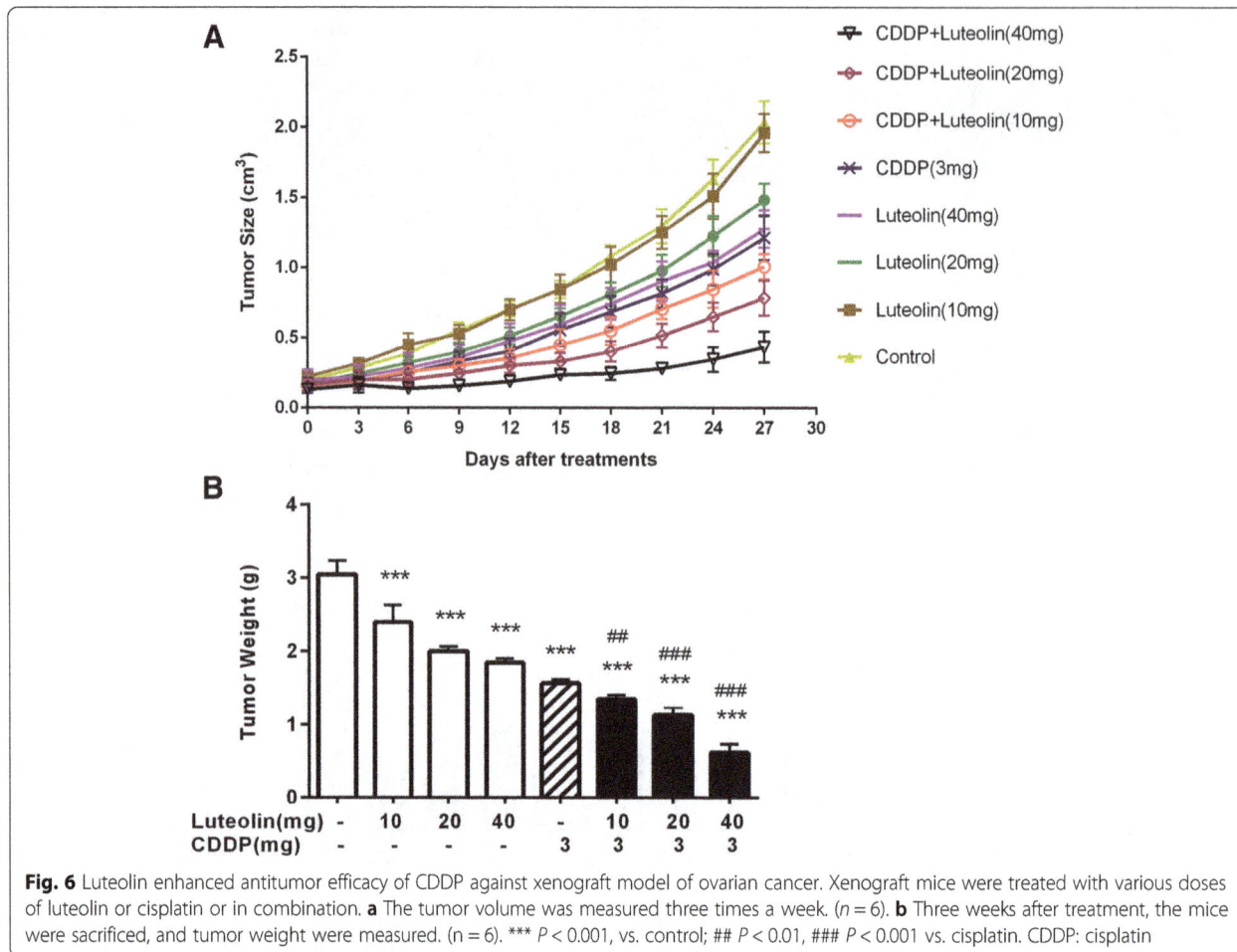

Fig. 6 Luteolin enhanced antitumor efficacy of CDDP against xenograft model of ovarian cancer. Xenograft mice were treated with various doses of luteolin or cisplatin or in combination. **a** The tumor volume was measured three times a week. ($n = 6$). **b** Three weeks after treatment, the mice were sacrificed, and tumor weight were measured. ($n = 6$). *** $P < 0.001$, vs. control; ## $P < 0.01$, ### $P < 0.001$ vs. cisplatin. CDDP: cisplatin

to solve drug resistance in ovarian cancer. It was previously reported that luteolin could decrease Bcl-2 expression in various cancer cells [33]. In the current study, results from qRT-PCR showed that luteolin at high concentration (100 μM) could significantly decrease the Bcl-2

Table 3 Luteolin increased the sensitivity of xenograft model of ovarian cancer to cisplatin. The Q value was calculated to evaluate the effect of the combination of the two drugs. The inhibition rate in each group was measured by tumor weight reduction compared to the control group. CDDP combined with luteolin (40 mg) showed a synergistic inhibitory effect on the growth of xenograft tumor ($Q = 1.16 \pm 0.03$, > 1, $P < 0.01$). The data were expressed as the mean ± S.D. in triplicate

Drugs	Inhibition rate (%)	Q value
Luteolin (40 mg)	39 ± 1.64	
Luteolin (20 mg)	34.4 ± 1.89	
Luteolin (10 mg)	21.3 ± 6.83	
CDDP (3 mg)	48.6 ± 1.55	
Luteolin (40 mg) + CDDP (3 mg)	79.8 ± 3.5	1.16 ± 0.03
Luteolin (20 mg) + CDDP (3 mg)	62.8 ± 3.09	0.95 ± 0.03
Luteolin (10 mg) + CDDP (3 mg)	55.7 ± 1.64	0.94 ± 0.05

mRNA level, and the combination of luteolin with cisplatin could evidently inhibit Bcl-2 expression compared with cisplatin alone. This suggests that the combined treatment induced cell apoptosis through the inhibition of Bcl-2 expression. The BCL-2 family proteins control the permeability of mitochondria and the release of cytochrome c to the cytoplasm, following the activation of a group of caspases, which proceeds apoptosis [27]. This suggests that mitochondrial apoptosis pathway may be involved, and further study should be focused on the pathway.

Our data also revealed the potent antitumor effect of luteolin with cisplatin in ovarian cancer in vivo. Single treatment with increasing doses of luteolin showed growth inhibition in xenograft tumor. In addition, tumor volume and weight were significantly decreased in mice of combination treatment group compared with cisplatin alone. What's more, the combination therapy synergistically induced more apoptosis than cisplatin, which is in consistent with in vitro study. These results further demonstrate that the inhibition of tumor growth was induced, in part, by the enhancement of cisplatin induced apoptosis.

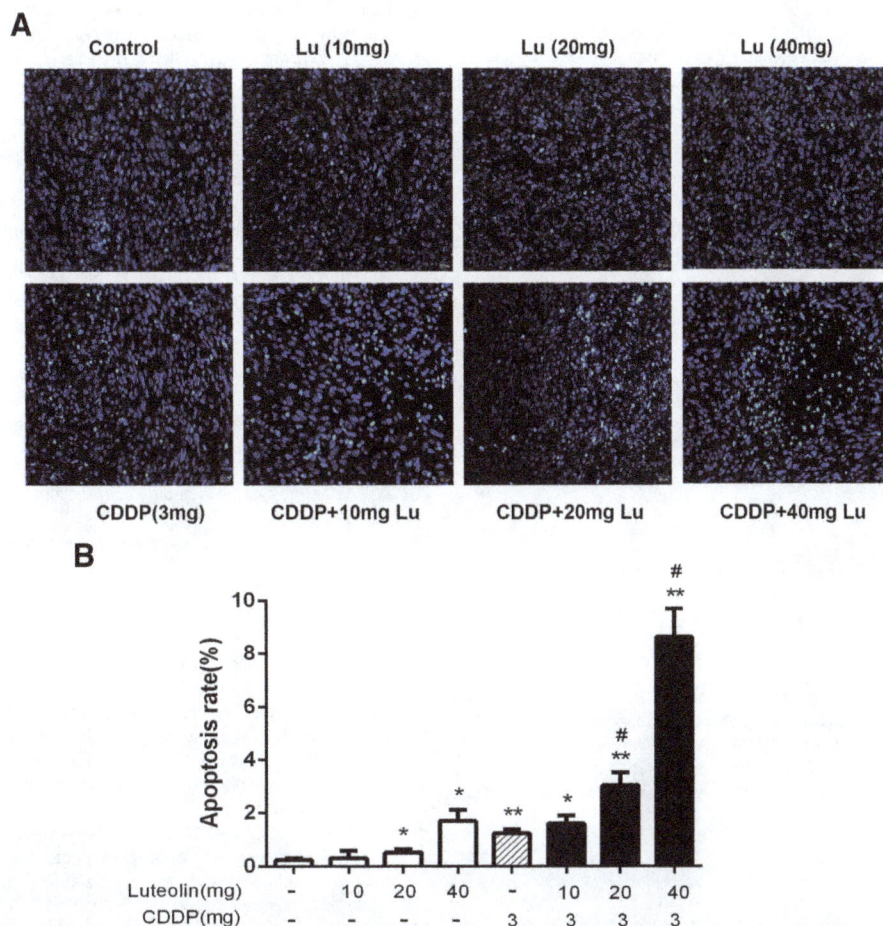

Fig. 7 Luteolin in combination with cisplatin enhanced apoptosis in vivo. Apoptosis of tumor sections were detected by TUNEL assay. **a** Representative images of apoptotic cells in each group (apoptotic cells in green and the cell nuclei in blue). **b** The tumor cell apoptosis rates of 8 groups were analyzed. * P < 0.05, ** P < 0.01, vs. control; # P < 0.05 vs. cisplatin. CDDP: cisplatin. CDDP combined with luteolin (20 mg, 40 mg) exhibited a synergistic effect on the apoptosis induction of xenograft tumor (Q = 1.73 ± 0.03 and 2.95 ± 0.16, respectively, > 1, P < 0.01 and P < 0.01, respectively)

Ovarian cancer is highly susceptible to occur metastasis in late stage. In most patients, though appearance of the lesion is still localized in the ovary, subclinical metastasis may already exist in many parts of the peritoneal or omentum [34]. In addition, chemotherapy resistance leads to the decrease of chemotherapy sensitivity in ovarian cancer cells, and also enhance its malignant degree. It suggests that the occurrence of chemotherapy resistance is closely related to the promotion of invasion and metastasis in cancer cells [35, 36]. Cancer metastasis involves several processes including adhesion, migration, and invasion. Targeting these processes provides effective strategy to enhance the chemosensitivity of cisplatin [37]. Luteolin has been proven to inhibit metastasis in various caner types such as breast cancer [38] and prostate cancer [39]. In our experiment, wound-healing assay and Matrigel invasion assay showed that luteolin exhibited a dose-dependent suppression on migration as well as invasion in CAOV3/DDP cells. Additionally, the inhibition effect became stronger when treated the cells with both increasing concentrations of luteolin and cisplatin than single agent treatment. These results indicate that the improved anticancer effect of cisplatin in CAOV3/DDP cells by luteolin is partially mediated through inhibition in cell migration and invasion.

In conclusion, our study shows that luteolin, a natural flavonoid, significantly enhances the anti-tumor effect of cisplatin in ovarian cancer both in vivo and in vitro. Combination of luteolin and cisplatin is more effective in suppressing CAOV3/DDP cell growth and metastasis. Luteolin could enhance cisplatin induced apoptosis in cisplatin-resistant ovarian cancer CAOV3/DDP cells via decreasing Bcl-2 expression. Our preliminary data provide experimental evidence for potential clinical application of luteolin as a novel chemosensitizer in the chemotherapy in ovarian cancer.

Acknowledgements

We thank Longxiang Zhou, from Department of Science and Education, Jinshan branch of Shanghai Sixth People's Hospital, Shanghai Jiaotong University, and Guiping Gan, from Department of Obstetrics and Gynecology, Jinshan branch of Shanghai Sixth People's Hospital, Shanghai Jiaotong University, for their guidance and help in our work.

Funding

This study was supported by Science and Technology Innovation Fund Program of Jinshan District (2015-3-16).

Authors' contributions

HW and YL both performed the study and wrote the manuscript, they contributed equally to this study. TQ reviewed and revised the article. ZW and ZH collected and analyzed the data. All authors read and approved the final manuscript.

Competing interests

The authors declare that they have no competing interests.

Author details

[1]Department of Obstetrics and Gynecology, Jinshan branch of Shanghai Sixth People's Hospital, Shanghai Jiaotong University, Shanghai, China. [2]Department of Oncology, Jinshan Hospital, Fudan University, Shanghai, China. [3]Department of Traditional Medicine, Jinshan branch of Shanghai Sixth People's Hospital, Shanghai Jiaotong University, Shanghai, China.

References

1. Rebecca L, Siegel M, Kimberly D, Miller M, Ahmedin Jemal DP. Cancer statistics, 2017. CA-CANCER J CLIN. 2017;67:7–30.
2. van Driel WJ, Koole SN, Sikorska K, Schagen VLJ, Schreuder H, Hermans R, et al. Hyperthermic intraperitoneal chemotherapy in ovarian Cancer. N Engl J Med. 2018;378:230–40.
3. Al RT, Lopes AD, Bristow RE, Bryant A, Elattar A, Chattopadhyay S, et al. Surgical cytoreduction for recurrent epithelial ovarian cancer. Cochrane Database Syst Rev. 2013;2:D8765.
4. Dancey J. Targeted therapies and clinical trials in ovarian cancer. Ann Oncol. 2013;24:x59–63.
5. Sundar S, Neal RD, Kehoe S. Diagnosis of ovarian cancer. BMJ. 2015;351: h4443.
6. Gad Singer RSHK. Patterns of p53 mutations separate ovarian serous borderline tumors and low- and high-grade carcinomas and provide support for a new model of ovarian carcinogenesis. Am J Surg Pathol. 2005; 29:218–24.
7. Mantia-Smaldone GM, Edwards RP, Vlad AM. Targeted treatment of recurrent platinum-resistant ovarian cancer: current and emerging therapies. Cancer Manag Res. 2011;3:25–38.
8. Matsuura K, Huang N, Cocce K, Zhang L, Kornbluth S. Downregulation of the proapoptotic pr otein MOAP-1 by the UBR5 ubiquitin ligase and its role in ovarian cancer resistance to cisplatin. Oncogene. 2016;36:1698.
9. Niero EL, Rocha-Sales B, Lauand C, Cortez BA, de Souza MM, Rezende-Teixeira P, et al. The multiple facets of drug resistance: one history, different approaches. J Exp Clin Cancer Res. 2014;33:37.
10. Agarwal R, Kaye SB. Ovarian cancer: strategies for overcoming resistance to chemotherapy. Nat Rev Cancer. 2003;3:502–16.
11. Lopez-Lazaro M. Distribution and biological activities of the flavonoid luteolin. Mini Rev Med Chem. 2009;9:31–59.
12. Lin Y, Shi R, Wang X, Shen HM. Luteolin, a flavonoid with potential for cancer prevention and therapy. Curr Cancer Drug Targets. 2008;8:634 46.
13. Horinaka M, Yoshida T, Shiraishi T, Nakata S, Wakada M, Nakanishi R, et al. Luteolin induces apoptosis via death receptor 5 upregulation in human malignant tumor cells. Oncogene. 2005;24:7180–9.
14. Fang J, Zhou Q, Shi XL, Jiang BH. Luteolin inhibits insulin-like growth factor 1 receptor signaling in prostate cancer cells. Carcinogenesis. 2006;28:713–23.
15. Song S, Su Z, Xu H, Niu M, Chen X, Min H, et al. Luteolin selectively kills STAT3 highly activated gastric cancer cells through enhancing the binding of STAT3 to SHP-1. Cell Death Dis. 2017;8:e2612.
16. Ong C, Zhou J, Ong C, Shen H. Luteolin induces G1 arrest in human nasopharyngeal carcinoma cells via the Akt–GSK-3β–cyclin D1 pathway. Cancer Lett. 2010;298:167–75.
17. Chian SLYW. Luteolin sensitizes two Oxaliplatin-resistant colorectal Cancer cell lines to chemotherapeutic drugs via inhibition of the Nrf2 pathway. Asian Pac J Cancer Prev. 2014;15:2911–6.
18. Tu S, Ho C, Liu M, Huang C, Chang H, Chang C, et al. Luteolin sensitises drug-resistant human breast cancer cells to tamoxifen via the inhibition of cyclin E2 expression. Food Chem. 2013;141:1553–61.
19. Du H, Liu Y, Chen X, Yu X, Hou X, Li H, et al. DT-13 synergistically potentiates the sensitivity of gastric cancer cells to topotecan via cell cycle arrest in vitro and in vivo. Eur J Pharmacol. 2018;818:124–31.
20. Ren Y, Zhou X, Mei M, Yuan XB, Han L, Wang GX, et al. MicroRNA-21 inhibitor sensitizes human glioblastoma cells U251 (PTEN-mutant) and LN229 (PTEN-wild type) to taxol. BMC Cancer. 2010;10:27.
21. ZJ J. About the evaluation of drug combination. Acta Pharmacol Sin. 2004; 25:146–7.
22. Baguley BC. Multiple drug resistance mechanisms in Cancer. Mol Biotechnol. 2010;46:308–16.
23. Sarosiek KA, Fraser C, Muthalagu N, Bhola PD, Chang W, McBrayer SK, et al. Developmental regulation of mitochondrial apoptosis by c-Myc governs age- and tissue-specific sensitivity to Cancer therapeutics. Cancer Cell. 2017;31:142–56.
24. Nguyen M, Marcellus RC, Roulston A, Watson M, Serfass L, Murthy MS, et al. Small molecule obatoclax (GX15-070) antagonizes MCL-1 and overcomes MCL-1-mediated resistance to apoptosis. Proc Natl Acad Sci U S A. 2007;104:19512–7.
25. Chen P, Hu T, Ma Y, Chen X, Dai L, Lei N, et al. Abstract 2808: Luteolin inhibits cell proliferation and induces cell apoptosis via down-regulation of mitochondrial membrane potential in esophageal carcinoma cells EC1 and KYSE450. Cancer Res. 2015;75:2808.
26. Xavier CPR, Lima CF, Preto A, Seruca R, Fernandes-Ferreira M, Pereira-Wilson C. Luteolin, quercetin and ursolic acid are potent inhibitors of proliferation and inducers of apoptosis in both KRAS and BRAF mutated human colorectal cancer cells. Cancer Lett. 2009;281:162–70.
27. Czabotar PE, Lessene G, Strasser A, Adams JM. Control of apoptosis by the BCL-2 protein family: implications for physiology and therapy. NAT REV MOL CELL BIO. 2014;15:49–63.
28. Inoue-Yamauchi A, Jeng PS, Kim K, Chen H, Han S, Ganesan YT, et al. Targeting the differential addiction to anti-apoptotic BCL-2 family for cancer therapy. Nat Commun. 2017;8:16078.
29. Cheng MCW EHYA. BCL-2, BCL-XL Emily H.-Y. A. Cheng,1 1 sequester BH3 domain-only molecules preventing BAX- and BAK-mediated mitochondrial apoptosis. MOL Cell. 2001;8:705–11.
30. PALMER JE, SANT CASSIA LJ, IRWIN CJ, MORRIS AG, ROLLASON TP. P53 and bcl-2 assessment in serous ovarian carcinoma. Int J Gynecol Cancer. 2008;18:241–8.
31. Fauvet R, Dufournet C, Poncelet C, Uzan C, Hugol D, Darai E. Expression of pro-apoptotic (p53, p21, bax, bak and fas) and anti-apoptotic (bcl-2 and bcl-x) proteins in serous versus mucinous borderline ovarian tumours. J Surg Oncol. 2005;92:337–43.
32. Wang H, Zhang Z, Wei X, Dai R. Small-molecule inhibitor of Bcl-2 (TW-37) suppresses growth and enhances cisplatin-induced apoptosis in ovarian cancer cells. J OVARIAN RES. 2015;8:3.
33. Zheng CH, Zhang M, Chen H, Wang CQ, Zhang MM, Jiang JH, et al. Luteolin from Flos Chrysanthemi and its derivatives: new small molecule Bcl-2 protein inhibitors. Bioorg Med Chem Lett. 2014;24:4672–7.
34. Hudson LG, Zeineldin R, Stack MS. Phenotypic plasticity of neoplastic ovarian epithelium: unique cadherin profiles in tumor progression. CLIN EXP METASTAS. 2008;25:643–55.
35. Joseph E, BRKW DL. Progression and Enhancement of metastatic potential after exposure of tumor cells to chemotherapeutic Agents1. Cancer Res. 2001;61:2857–61.
36. Yang JM, Xu Z, Wu H, Zhu H, Wu X, Hait WN. Overexpression of extracellular matrix metalloproteinase inducer in multidrug resistant cancer cells. Mol Cancer Res. 2003;1:420–7.
37. Fu X, Tian J, Zhang L, Chen Y, Hao Q. Involvement of microRNA-93, a new regulator of PTEN/Akt signaling pathway, in regulation of chemotherapeutic drug cisplatin chemosensitivity in ovarian cancer cells. FEBS Lett. 2012;586: 1279–86.

26

The value of MRI for differentiating benign from malignant sex cord-stromal tumors of the ovary: emphasis on diffusion-weighted MR imaging

Shu-Hui Zhao[1†], Hai-Ming Li[2†], Jin-Wei Qiang[2*], Deng-Bin Wang[1*] and Hua Fan[1]

Abstract

Background: To investigate MRI for differentiating benign from malignant sex cord-stromal tumors of the ovary (SCSTs) emphasizing on the value of diffusion-weighted (DW) magnetic resonance (MR) imaging.

Methods: This retrospective study included 29 benign SCSTs in 28 patients and 13 malignant SCSTs in 13 patients. DW imaging as well as conventional MR imaging was performed. Signal intensity on DW imaging was assessed and apparent diffusion coefficient (ADC) value was measured. In addition, T2 signal intensity and contrast enhancement pattern were also assessed and compared between benign and malignant SCSTs.

Results: Both of the T2 hypointensity and mild enhancement were specific to benign SCSTs. The majority of malignant SCSTs showed high signal intensity on DW imaging, whereas most benign SCSTs showed low or moderate signal intensity ($p = 0.000$). Fibromas were the tumors with the lowest observed ADC value (0.470×10^{-3} mm^2/s). Sclerosing stromal tumors were the tumors with the highest observed ADC value (2.291×10^{-3} mm^2/s). ADC value of solid component was significantly lower in malignant SCSTs ($0.825 \pm 0.129 \times 10^{-3}$ mm^2/s) than in benign SCSTs ($1.343 \pm 0.528 \times 10^{-3}$ mm^2/s) when fibromas were excluded ($p = 0.024$). T2, DCE and DW imaging has a limited value on the differential diagnosis of the benign and malignant SCSTs with an accuracy of 69.0%,71.4% and 78.1% respectively. Combination of T2, DCE and DW imaging permitted the distinction with an accuracy of 88.0%.

Conclusions: It is more helpful for distinction of the benign and malignant SCSTs by combining of T2, DCE and DW imaging than using each of the three sequences independently.

Keywords: Ovary, Sex cord-stromal tumor, Diffusion-weighted MR imaging

Background

Ovarian sex cord-stromal tumors (SCSTs) are a group of neoplasm arising from stromal cells and primitive sex cord, accounting for 8% of all ovarian tumors [1–3]. They can affect women of any age [4, 5]. Patients with SCSTs often present virilization syndromes or hyperestrogenic manifestations associated with steroid hormone overproduction [6, 7]. According to World Health Organization

(WHO) classification of the ovarian tumors (2014), SCSTs are divided into three clinicopathologic subcategories as pure stromal tumors, pure sex cord tumors and mixed sex cord-stromal tumors [3].

Morphologically, SCSTs often present as a solid mass [8–13]. On conventional MRI, some features have been found to distinguish SCSTs: Fibromas, known as the most common type of SCSTs, are characterized by very low signal intensity on T2WI and delayed mild enhancement. Sclerosing stromal tumor shows low signal intensity in peripheral area and moderate to high signal intensity in central area on T2WI with intense enhancement. Granulosa cell tumor is multiloculated cystic mass with thickened wall or mixed cystic and solid

* Correspondence: dr.jinweiqiang@163.com;
wangdengbin@xinhuamed.com.cn
†Shu-Hui Zhao and Hai-Ming Li contributed equally to this work.
²Department of Radiology, Jinshan Hospital, Fudan University, 1508 Longhang Road, Shanghai 201508, China
¹Department of Radiology, Xinhua Hospital affiliated to Shanghai Jiaotong University School of Medicine, 1665 Kongjiang Road, Shanghai 200092, China

mass [9, 10]. Sertoli-Leydig cell tumor shows as a well--defined solid mass with numerous intratumoral cysts [1]. However, it is still a challenge for radiologists to differentiate benign from malignant SCSTs based on conventional MRI preoperatively [1–3]. Diffusion-weighted MR imaging has been proved to be helpful in characterizing epithelial tumors of the ovary. To our knowledge, a comprehensive study on diffusion-weighted MR imaging features specific to SCSTs have not been reported [8]. In this study, we investigate diffusion-weighted imaging of 42 ovarian sex cord-stromal tumors in 41 patients (29 benign SCSTs in 28 patients and 13 malignant SCSTs in 13 patients) to differentiate benign from malignant sex cord-stromal tumors of the ovary. T2 signal intensity and contrast enhancement pattern were also assessed and compared between benign and malignant SCSTs.

Methods

Patient population

The institutional review board of our hospitals approved this retrospective study, and informed consent was obtained from each patient for academic use of their clinical data. Patients with suspected ovarian tumors were enrolled in an ovarian tumor MRI study project from January 2010 to November 2016 at Xinhua Hospital affiliated to Shanghai Jiaotong University School of Medicine and Obstetrics & Gynecology Hospital of Fudan University. We found a total of 41 patients with 42 primary ovarian sex cord-stromal tumors (29 benign SCSTs in 28 patients and 13 malignant SCSTs in 13 patients) (Table 1). Patients' ages ranged from 24 to 81 years (mean, 51.6 ± 16.3 years) in the benign group and 22–70 years (mean, 41.0 ± 16.2 years) in the

malignant group, with no significant difference ($p = 0.795$) (Table 1). Patients presented with abdominal swelling, irregular menstruation cycle, postmenstrual vaginal bleeding, virilization or no symptom. All patients underwent surgery within 1 week after completing the MRI scan.

MR technique

MRI was performed with a 1.5 Tesla (T) MR superconductor unit (Avanto, Siemens, Erlangen, Germany). A pelvic phased-array coil was used in each case. The patients lay in the supine position and breathed normally. The scanning range was from the inferior pubic symphysis to the renal hilum and was extended beyond the dome of tumor in the cases with huge masses.

First, the unenhanced conventional sequences were obtained as follows: axial T1-weighted imaging (T1WI) spin-echo (repetition time/echo time [TR/TE], 340 ms/ 10 ms), T2-weighted imaging (T2WI) turbo spin-echo with and without fat saturation (TR/TE, 8000 ms/83 ms and 4000 ms/98 ms), and sagittal and coronal T2WI turbo spin-echo (TR/TE, 4000 ms/98 ms).

Second, axial DW imaging was obtained using echo planar imaging sequence. The scanning parameters were as follows: TR/TE, 3200 ms/87 ms; diffusion gradient b factors, 0 and 1000 s/mm2; matrix, 128×128; field of view, 238 mm × 280 mm; ST/IG, 5.0 mm/1.5 mm; excitations, 4; acquisition time, 2 min 46 s.

Finally, the contrast enhanced T1WI flash 2D with fat saturation (TR/TE, 196 ms/2.9 ms) was performed in the axial, sagittal, and coronal planes at 30s, 60s and 90s after the intravenous administration of gadopentetate dimeglumine (Gd-DTPA, 0.1 mmol/kg of body weight, Magnevist; Bayer Schering, Guangzhou, China) injected

Table 1 Data of benign and malignant ovarian sex cord-stromal tumors

	Number (tumors/patients)	Patient age (years)	Mean size (cm)	Mean ADC value ($\times 10^{-3}$ mm^2/s)
Benign	(28/29)#			
Purely stromal tumors				
Fibroma	10	50 (24–81)	6.1	0.470 ± 0.389
Cellular fibroma	2	64 (59–68)	5.2	0.794 ± 0.159
Thecoma	7	64 (48–86)	10.2	1.207 ± 0.350
Fibrothecoma	6	55 (41–70)	11.9	1.150 ± 0.275
Sclerosing stromal tumor	4	28 (26–30)	5.2	2.291 ± 0.423
Malignant	(13/13)			
Purely sex cord tumors				
Granulosa cell tumor	7	41 (27–55)	13.2	0.694 ± 0.111
Sex cord tumor with annular tubule	1	26	2.4	0.975
Mixed Sex cord-stromal tumors				
Sertoli-leydig tumor	4	41 (22–56)	13.0	1.009 ± 0.151
Granulosathecoma	1	70	8.0	0.773

One of the 28 patients in benign group had bilateral ovarian sex cord-stromal tumors (fibroma and fibrothecoma)

at a rate of 2–3 ml/s. The scanning parameters were as follows: 5-mm slice thickness, 1.5-mm gap, 256×256 matrix, 20–25 cm $\times$ 34 cm field of view, and four excitations.

Image analysis

MR images were analyzed by S.H.Z. and H.M.L., with 10 and 8 years of experience in gynecological imaging, respectively. Their interpretations were arrived at by consensus.

1. The signal intensity (SI) of the tumor on T2W imaging was qualitatively evaluated. It was classified as hypointensity (similar signal to the muscle), isointensity (similar signal to the myometrium) and hyperintensity (higher signal than the myometrium).
2. The contrast enhancement of tumor was also qualitatively evaluated on images which acquired at 90s after administration of contrast medium. It was classified as and mild (similar to or weak than the muscles), moderate (between the muscles and the myometrium) and intense (similar to or stronger than the myometrium) enhancement.
3. The signal intensity (SI) of tumor on DW imaging was classified as low (lower than small intestine), moderate (similar to small intestine) or high (similar to the SI of nerve root). On ADC maps, a circular region of interest (ROI) of at least 1 cm^2 was placed at targeted areas in the solid components of tumor, by referring to conventional MR images including contrast-enhanced images. ROI should avoid areas such as hemorrhage, necrosis, major vascular structures, and artefacts. At least three measurements were obtained and averaged.
4. The degeneration (edema, hemorrhage, and demarcated cysts) of SCSTs was determined by analyzing unenhanced conventional MR images (T1WI, T2WI, T2FS), DW images and the contrast enhanced T1FS images.

Statistical analysis

Statistical analysis was performed using SPSS 23.0 for Mac (IBM Inc., New York, USA). Wilcoxon rank sum test was used to compare the differences of DW imaging SI between benign SCSTs and malignant SCSTs. One-way ANOVA was performed to compare the ADC values between benign SCSTs and malignant SCSTs. Wilcoxon rank sum test and chi-square test were used to compare the differences of T2 signal intensity and contrast enhancement pattern between benign SCSTs and malignant SCSTs. A p value less than 0.05 was regarded as statistically significant.

Results

Forty-two primary SCSTs were comprised of 29 benign lesions and 13 malignant lesions. The majority of malignant lesions were on stage I (FIGO) except for two lesions (granulosa cell tumors) on stage II (FIGO).

T2 signal intensity of the 42 ovarian sex cord-stromal tumors are summarized in Table 2. Malignant SCSTs showed higher T2 SI than benign SCSTs (Wilcoxon rank sum test, $p = 0.04$). T2 hypointensity was only seen in benign SCSTs with a sensitivity of 58.6% and specificity of 92.3% in diagnosing benign SCSTs which yield an accuracy of 69.0% for differential diagnosis of the two groups. All of the 10 fibromas were T2 hypointensity (Figs. 1 and 2).

Contrast enhancement pattern of the 42 ovarian sex cord-stromal tumors are summarized in Table 3. Malignant SCSTs did not show more enhancement than benign SCSTs (Wilcoxon rank sum test, $p > 0.05$). However, mild enhancement was only seen in benign SCSTs with a sensitivity of 58.6% and specificity of 100% in diagnosing benign SCSTs which yield an accuracy of 71.4% for differential diagnosis of the two groups (Figs. 1 and 2).

Fibromas were the tumors with the lowest observed ADC value (0.470×10^{-3} mm^2/s) (Table 1, Figs. 1 and 2). Sclerosing stromal tumors were the tumors with the highest observed ADC value (2.291×10^{-3} mm^2/s) (Table 1, Fig. 3).

DW imaging findings of the 42 ovarian sex cord-stromal tumors are summarized in Table 4. The solid component showed high SI in 12 of 13 (92.3%) malignant SCSTs versus in 3 of 29 (10.3%) benign SCSTs ($p = 0.000$) (Fig. 4).

Table 2 T2 signal intensity of the solid component of the 42 ovarian sex cord-stromal tumors

	Hypointensity	Isointensity	Hyperintensity
Benign	12	5	12
Purely stromal tumors			
Fibroma	10		
Cellular fibroma		1	1
Thecoma	1	1	5
Fibrothecoma	1	2	3
Sclerosing stromal tumor		1	3
Malignant	0	1	12
Purely sex cord tumors			
Granulosa cell tumor			7
Sex cord tumor with annular tubule			1
Mixed Sex cord-stromal tumors			
Sertoli-leydig tumor			4
Granulosathecoma		1	

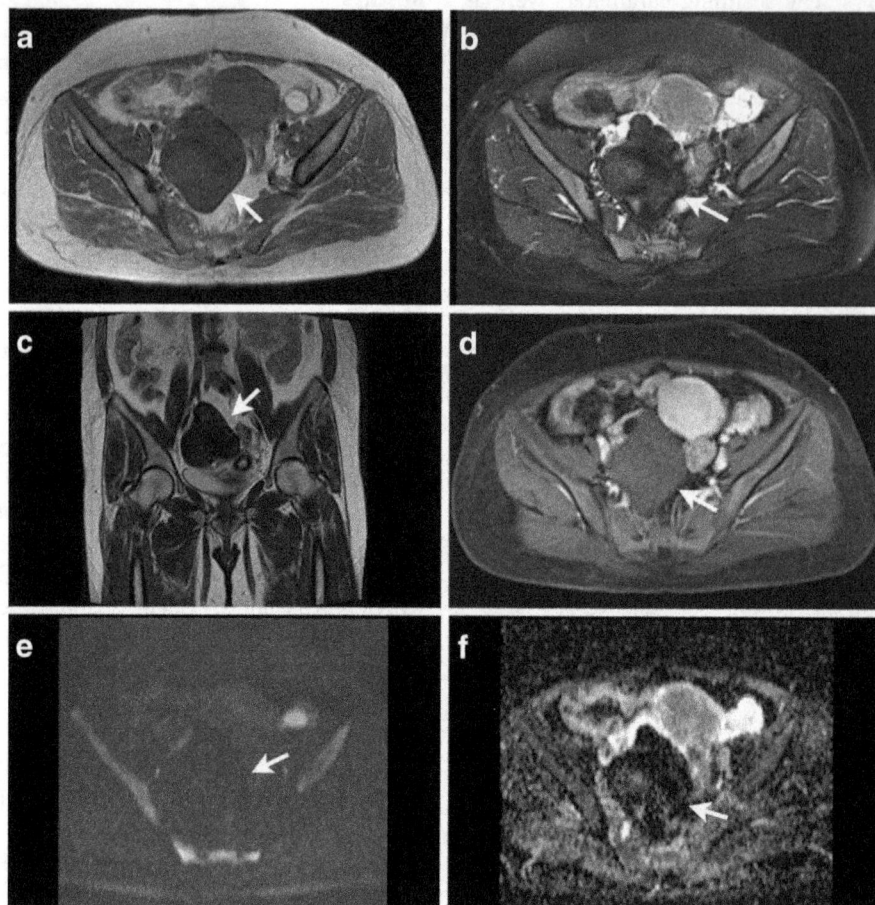

Fig. 1 A 47-year-old women with a fibroma on the right ovary(arrows). Axial T1-weighted image (**a**) shows an oval mass of low signal intensity. Axial T2-weighted with fat suppression image (**b**) and coronal T2-weighted image (**c**) shows the mass was homogenous low signal intensity. T1-weighted contrast enhanced images (**d**) shows the mass was slightly enhanced. The mass shows low signal intensity on DW imaging (**e**) and has a significant low ADC value of 0.132×10^{-3} mm^2/s (**f**)

There was no significant difference in ADC values of solid component between the two groups when fibromas were included ($p = 0.639$). However, ADC value of solid component was significantly lower in malignant SCSTs ($0.825 \pm 0.129 \times 10^{-3}$ mm^2/s) than in benign SCSTs ($1.343 \pm 0.528 \times 10^{-3}$ mm^2/s) when fibromas were excluded ($p = 0.024$) (Figs. 4 and 5). ROC curve analysis yielded an optimal ADC value threshold of 0.838×10^{-3} mm^2/s for differentiating malignant from benign tumors with a sensitivity of 61.5%, a specificity of 89.5% and an accuracy of 78.1%.

Considering each of the three sequences of T2, DCE and DW imaging has a limited value on the differential diagnosis of the benign and malignant SCSTs with an accuracy of 69.0%,71.4% and 78.1% respectively, we developed a multiparametric assessment which combined T2 with DCE and DW imaging. The assessment uses a 3-point scale based on the likelihood that the MRI findings correlates with the malignance of an ovarian sex cord-stromal tumor (Table 5). The assessment of the

ovarian sex cord-stromal tumors was categorized as: 1-benign; 2- high likelihood to be benign; 3- high likelihood to be malignant. Category 1 (benign) was defined as a lesion which has typical MRI findings of T2 hypointensity or mild enhancement (Figs. 1 and 2). In case DCE showed non-mild enhancement, the lesion is further assessed on DW imaging. Category 2 (high likelihood to be benign) was define as a lesion which has non-mild enhancement with a high ADC value(Fig. 3). When a lesion showed moderate enhancement, a lower ADC value than 0.838×10^{-3} mm^2/s uprate the lesion to category 3(high likelihood to be malignant) (Fig. 4). When a lesion showed intense enhancement, a lower ADC value than 1.000×10^{-3} mm^2/s uprate the lesion to category 3(high likelihood to be malignant).

Combination of T2, DCE and DW imaging is helpful for differential diagnosis of benign and malignant SCSTs with an accuracy of 88.0%.

Degeneration in SCSTs demonstrated as edema, hemorrhage and demarcated cysts (Table 6).

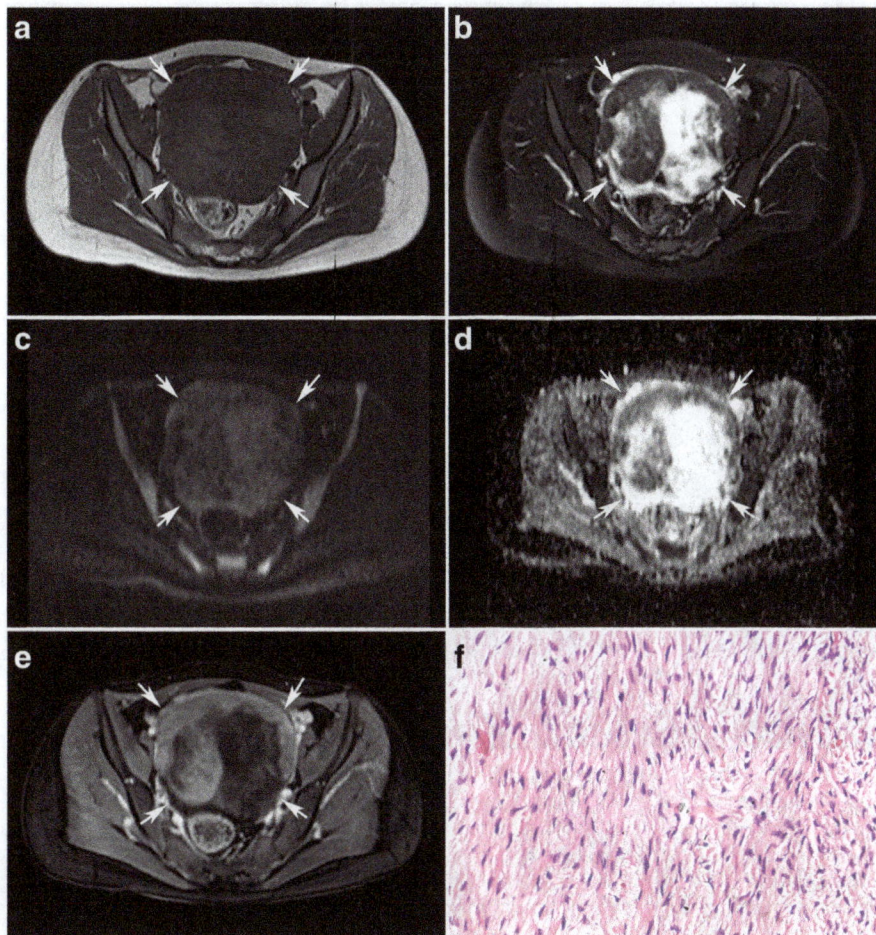

Fig. 2 A 38-year-old women with a fibroma on the right ovary(arrows). Axial T1-weighted image (**a**) shows an oval mass of low signal intensity. T2-weighted with fat suppression image (**b**) shows the mass has significant low signal intensity with edema area of high signal intensity. The mass shows low signal intensity on DW imaging (**c**) and has a significant low ADC value of 0.181×10^{-3} mm^2/s in the non-edema area (**d**). T1-weighted contrast enhanced images (**e**) shows the mass was slightly enhanced after delay. The photomicrograph (H&E, × 400) (**f**) shows abundant fibrocytes

Table 3 Contrast enhancement pattern of the 42 ovarian sex cord-stromal tumors

	Mild	Moderate	Intense
Benign	17	8	4
Purely stromal tumors			
Fibroma	9	1	
Cellular fibroma		2	
Thecoma	4	3	
Fibrothecoma	4	2	
Sclerosing stromal tumor			4
Malignant	0	9	4
Purely sex cord tumors			
Granulosa cell tumor		7	
Sex cord tumor with annular tubule		1	
Mixed Sex cord-stromal tumors			
Sertoli-leydig tumor			4
Granulosathecoma		1	

Edema and hemorrhage was only found in benign SCSTs. Edema area in lesion showed moderate signal intensity on DW imaging with a high ADC value. Hemorrhage showed high signal intensity on DW imaging with a low ADC value. Demarcated cysts were found in 14% of benign lesions versus 90% of malignant lesions. Numerous mini cysts within the solid mass were only seen in malignant lesions.

Discussion

Fibromas can be distinguished from other types of SCSTs based on the specific features on conventional MR imaging. Shinagare [14] reported that fibromas are abundant in bland spindle cells and intercellular collagen which contribute to the remarkable low signal intensity on T2WI and slight enhancement by contrast agent [15–18]. In this study, we found that T2 hypointensity is more specific than mild enhancement to fibromas. So T2WI is the dominant sequence to distinguish fibromas from the the rest of SCSTs. Also, fibromas were the

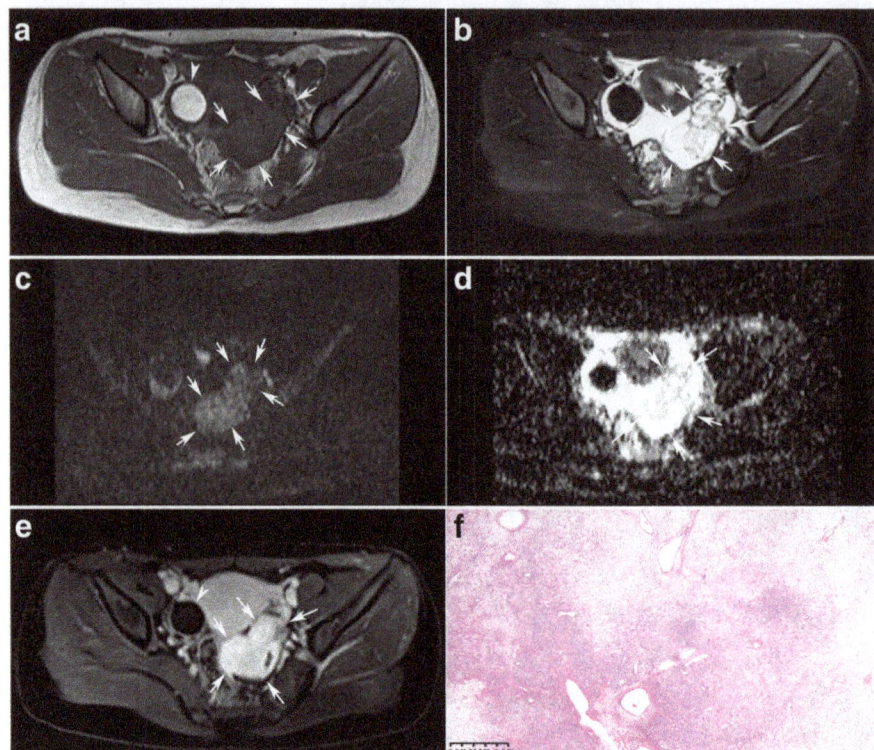

Fig. 3 A 30-year-old young women with a sclerosing stromal tumor on the left ovary (arrows) combined with a mature teratoma on the right ovary(arrow heads). Axial T1-weighted image (**a**) shows a mass of low signal intensity. T2-weighted with fat suppression image (**b**) shows the mass has heterogenous high signal intensity. The mass shows moderate signal intensity on DW imaging (**c**) and has a significant high ADC value of 2.291×10^{-3} mm^2/s (**d**). T1-weighted contrast enhanced images (**e**) showed the mass was enhanced significantly. The photomicrograph (H&E, $\times$40) (**f**) shows the pseudolobulation of the cellular areas separated by hypocellular areas of loose edematous connective tissue

tumors with the lowest ADC value. Bland spindle cells and intercellular collagen lined so densely that water molecule movement is more restricted in less intercellular space.

Although both T2 hypointensity and mild enhancement play a role in distinguishing benign SCSTs with a specificity of 100%, mild enhancement is more sensitive to benign SCSTs (Category 1). In case a lesion has a non-mild enhancement, the lesion should be further assessed on

Table 4 DW imaging signal intensity (SI) and ADC value of benign and malignant ovarian sex cord-stromal tumors

	Benign(29)	Malignant(13)	p value
SI			< 0.001
Low	11	0	
Moderate	15	1	
High	3	12	
ADC value ($\times 10^{-3}$ mm^2/s)[a]	0.951 ± 0.625	0.825 ± 0.129	0.639
ADC value ($\times 10^{-3}$ mm^2/s)[b]	1.343 ± 0.528	0.825 ± 0.129	0.024

[a]ADC values was measured and averaged in 29 benign SCSTs and 13 malignant SCSTs respectively;
[b]ADC values was measured and averaged in 19 benign SCSTs (fibromas were excluded) and 13 malignant
SCSTs respectively

DW imaging (Category 2). The ADC value threshold to uprate a lesion of Category 2 to Category 3 was 0.838×10^{-3} mm^2/s.

Sclerosing stromal tumors were the only subtype of benign SCSTs which were enhanced intensely [2, 3]. We found that sclerosing stromal tumors were the tumors with the highest observed ADC value (2.291×10^{-3} mm^2/s). The explanation may be that the tumor has a characteristic microscopic pattern with pseudolobulation of the cellular areas separated by hypocellular areas of loose edematous connective tissue. Atram [19] reported that the edematous stromal change is a constant feature of sclerosing stromal tumors of the ovary. Sertoli-leydig tumors were the subtype of malignant SCSTs which were enhanced intensely [2, 3, 20]. The mean ADC value of sertoli-leydig tumors was 1.009×10^{-3} mm^2/s. So when a lesion showed intensely enhancement, we recommended a much higher ADC value threshold of 1.000×10^{-3} mm^2/s to uprate the lesion to Category 3.

Degeneration in SCSTs is common which demonstrated as edema, hemorrhage and cyst change [14, 21]. Edema and hemorrhage were only observed in benign lesions. However, demarcated cysts were observed in benign and

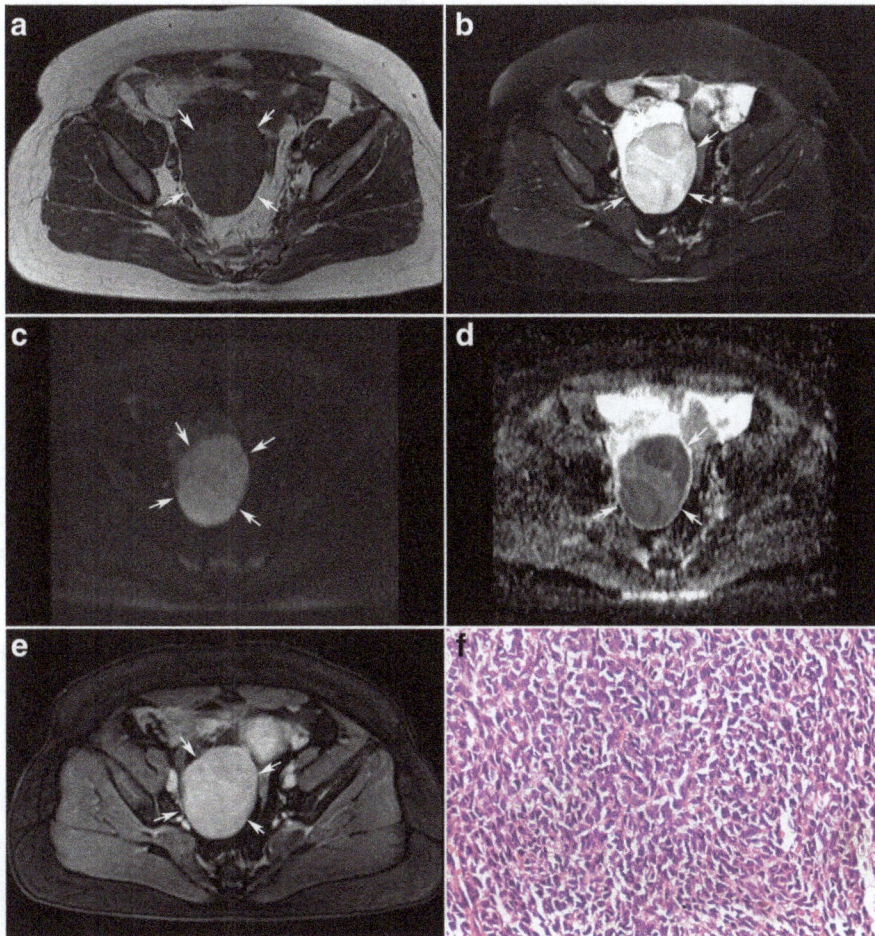

Fig. 4 A 55-year women with an adult granulosa cell tumor on the right ovary(arrows). Axial T1-weighted image (**a**) shows a solid mass of low signal intensity. Axial T2-weighted with fat suppression images (**b**) show the mass has slightly high signal intensity. The solid mass shows high signal intensity on DW imaging (**c**) and has a low ADC value of 0.588×10^{-3} mm^2/s (**d**). T1-weighted contrast enhanced images (**e**) showed the solid mass was enhanced moderately. The photomicrograph (H&E, $\times$ 400) (**f**) confirmed the diagnosis of an adult granulosa cell tumor

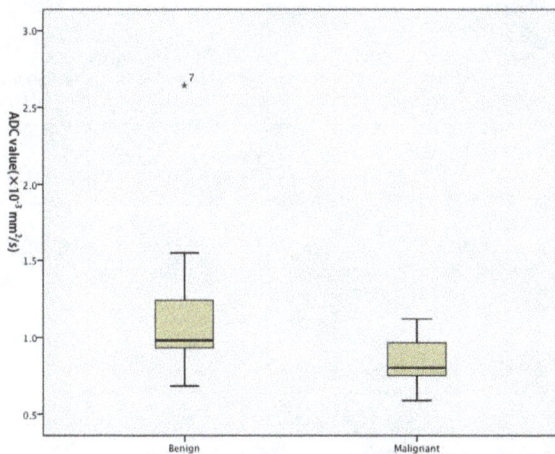

Fig. 5 Boxplot of the ADC value of sex cord-stromal tumor of the ovary. ADC value of solid component was significantly lower in malignant SCSTs ($0.825 \pm 0.129 \times 10^{-3}$ mm^2/s) than in benign SCSTs ($1.343 \pm 0.528 \times 10^{-3}$ mm^2/s) when fibromas were excluded

malignant lesions. Kato [21] reported that up to 53% of fibromas demonstrated intratumoral cysts in their study.

There are some limitations in our study. First, it is a retrospective study. We just try to discuss about differentiation between benign and malignant sex cord-stromal tumors. We did not discuss about how to differentiate SCSTs from other pathological types of ovarian solid

Table 5 Assessment of the ovarian sex cord-stromal tumors on a 3-point scale based on combination of T2 signal intensity, contrast enhancement pattern and ADC value

	T2	Enhancement	ADC value
1	hypointensity	–	–
	–	mild	
2	–	moderate	$> 0.838 \times 10^{-3}$ mm^2/s
		intense	$> 1.000 \times 10^{-3}$ mm^2/s
3	–	moderate	$\leq 0.838 \times 10^{-3}$ mm^2/s
		intense	$\leq 1.000 \times 10^{-3}$ mm^2/s

Table 6 Comparison of degeneration type and frequency between benign and malignant ovarian sex cord-stromal tumors

Degeneration	Benign(29)	Malignant(13)	p value
Edema	12 (41%)	0	< 0.001
Hemorrhage	4 (14%)	0	< 0.001
Demarcated cysts	4 (14%)	12 (90%)	0.024

tumors. Prospective large sample investigation merits further study. Secondly, completely objective measurements of ADC value are usually difficult because sex cord-stromal tumors tumors tend to be heterogeneous masses. Thirdly, the variation in ADC between the subtypes of sex cord-stromal tumors is large.

Conclusions

T2, DCE and DW imaging has a limited value on the differential diagnosis of the benign and malignant SCSTs with an accuracy of 69.0%,71.4% and 78.1% respectively. Combination of T2, DCE and DW imaging is more helpful which permit the distinction with an accuracy of 88.0%.

Abbreviations

ADC: Apparent diffusion coefficient; DW: Diffusion-weighted; MR: magnetic resonance; SCST: Sex cord-stromal tumors of the ovary

Funding

Grant from National Natural Science Foundation of China (Nos. 81501439 and 81471628); Xinhua Hospital affiliated to Shanghai Jiaotong University School of Medicine (No. 14YJ1).

Authors' contributions

ZSH conceived of the study, and participated in its design and drafted the manuscript.
LHM participated in the data analysis/data acquisition. JWQ and DBW guaranteed the integrity of entire study. FH participated in the data acquisition. All authors read and approved the final manuscript.

Competing interests

The authors declare that they have no competing interests.

References

1. Jung SE, Lee JM, Rha SE, Byun JY, Jung JI, Hahn ST. CT and MR imaging of ovarian tumors with emphasis on differential diagnosis. Radiographics. 2002; 22(6):1305–25.
2. Jung SE, Rha SE, Lee JM, Park SY, Oh SN, Cho KS, et al. CT and MRI findings of sex cord-stromal tumor of the ovary. Am J Roentgenol. 2005;185(1):207–15.
3. Horta M, Cunha TM. Sex cord-stromal tumors of the ovary: a comprehensive review and update for radiologists. Diagn Interv Radiol. 2015;21(4):277–86.
4. Kawauchi S, Tsuji T, Kaku T, Kamura T, Nakano H, Tsuneyoshi M. Sclerosing stromal tumor of the ovary: a clinicopathologic, immunohistochemical, ultrastructural, and cytogenetic analysis with special reference to its vasculature. Am J Surg Pathol. 1998;22(1):83–92.
5. Gui T, Cao D, Shen K, Yang J, Zhang Y, Yu Q, et al. A clinicopathological analysis of 40 cases of ovarian Sertoli-Leydig cell tumors. Gynecol Oncol. 2012;127(2):384–9.
6. Outwater EK, Marchetto B, Wagner BJ. Virilizing tumors of the ovary: imaging features. Ultrasound Obstet Gynecol. 2000;15(5):365–71.
7. Tanaka YO, Tsunoda H, Kitagawa Y, Ueno T, Yoshikawa H, Saida Y. Functioning ovarian tumors: direct and indirect findings at MR imaging. Radiographics. 2004;24(Suppl 1):147–66.
8. Fujii S, Kakite S, Nishihara K, Harada T, Kigawa J, Kaminou T, et al. Diagnostic accuracy of diffusion-weighted imaging in differentiating benign from malignant ovarian lesions. J Magn Reson Imaging. 2008;28(5):1149–56.
9. Ko SF, Wan YL, Ng SH, Lee TY, Lin JW, Chen WJ, et al. Adult ovarian granulosa cell tumors: spectrum of sonographic and CT findings with pathologic correlation. Am J Roentgenol. 1999;172(5):1227–33.
10. Kim SH, Kim SH. Granulosa cell tumor of the ovary: common findings and unusual appearances on CT and MR. J Comput Assist Tomogr. 2002;26(5): 756–61.
11. Scully RE. Sex cord tumor with annular tubules a distinctive ovarian tumor of the Peutz-Jeghers syndrome. Cancer. 1970;25(5):1107–21.
12. Young RH, Welch WR, Dickersin GR, Scully RE. Ovarian sex cord tumor with annular tubules: review of 74 cases including 27 with Peutz-Jeghers syndrome and four with adenoma malignum of the cervix. Cancer. 1982; 50(7):1384–402.
13. Moon WK, Kim SH, Kim WS, Kim IO, Yeon KM, Han MC. Ovarian sex cord tumor with annular tubules-imaging findings. Clin Radiol. 1995;50(8):581–2.
14. Shinagare AB, Meylaerts LJ, Laury AR, Mortele KJ. MRI features of ovarian fibroma and fibrothecoma with histopathologic correlation. Am J Roentgenol. 2012;198(3):W296–303.
15. Graef MD, Kasem Z, Batch T, Tichoux C, Maubon A, Rouanet JP. Solid black lesion of the ovary in T2 weighted sequences: do they all belong to the thecomafibroma group? Radiologist. 2003;10(4):183–91.
16. Montoriol P-F, Mons A, Ines DD, Bourdel N, Tixier L, Garcier JM. Fibrous tumours of the ovary: Aetiologies and MRI features. Clin Radiol. 2013;68(12): 1276–83.
17. Troiano RN, Lazzarini KM, Scoutt LM, Lange RC, Flynn SD, Mccarthy S. Fibroma and fibrothecoma of the ovary: MR imaging finding. Radiology. 1997;204(3):795–8.
18. Chung BM, Park SB, Lee JB, Park HJ, Kim YS, Oh YJ. Magnetic resonance imaging features of ovarian fibroma, fibrothecoma, and thecoma. Abdom Imaging. 2015;40(5):1263–72.
19. Atram M, Anshu, Sharma S, Gangane N. Sclerosing stromal tumor of the ovary. Obstet Gynecol Sci. 2014;57(5):405–8.
20. Cai SQ, Zhao SH, Qiang JW, Zhang GF, Wang XZ, Wang L. Ovarian Sertoli–Leydig cell tumors: MRI findings and pathological correlation. J Ovarian Res. 2013;6(1):73.
21. Kato H, Kanematsu M, Ono H, Yano R, Furui T, Morishige K, et al. Ovarian fibromas: MR imaging findings with emphasis on intratumoral cyst formation. Eur J Radiol. 2013;82(9):e417–21.

27

Reproductive aging and elective fertility preservation

Rani Fritz[1] and Sangita Jindal[1,2]*

Abstract

Reproductive aging is a natural process that occurs in all women, eventually leading to reproductive senescence and menopause. Over the past half century there has been a trend towards delayed motherhood. Postponing reproduction can increase the chance of a woman remaining involuntarily childless as well as an increase in pregnancy complications in those that do achieve pregnancy at advanced maternal age. Despite the well-documented decrease in fecundity that occurs as a woman ages, reproductive aged women frequently overestimate the age at which a significant decline in fertility occurs and overestimate the success of assisted reproductive technologies (ART) to circumvent infertility. Oocyte cryopreservation enables women to achieve genetically related offspring in the event that they desire to postpone their childbearing to an age after which a significant decline in fertility occurs or in circumstances in which their reproductive potential is compromised due to medical pathology. Available success rates and safety data following oocyte cryopreservation have been reassuring and is not considered experimental according to the American Society for Reproductive Medicine and the European Society for Human Reproduction and Embryology. This review article will focus on an evidence-based discussion relating to reproductive aging and oocyte cryopreservation.

Keywords: Reproductive aging- oocyte cryopreservation- reproduction

Background

Over the past several decades spanning from 1970 to 2014, the average age of first time mothers in the U.S. has increased 18.6% from 21.4–26.3 y/o [1, 2]. Alongside this trend, from 1970 to 2012 in the U.S. the percentage of women aged 35–44 y/o having children for the first time has increased more than five-fold from 2.5 to 13.3 per 1000 women [3]. Similar trends are also found in other parts of the world including Canada and Europe with one of the highest mean age of first time mothers seen in Italy at 30.6 y/o [4, 5]. These trends are likely related to an increase in women entering the workforce, obtaining advanced educational degrees, and greater use of contraceptive methods [6]. The declining birthrate is a concern for many developed countries. As birthrates in many industrialized countries fall below the replacement fertility rate of 2.1 live births per women, there is concern for future economic and social consequences including a decreased workforce to sustain the economy

and care for the elderly population [7, 8]. It has therefore been advocated in Europe that a more liberal incorporation of assisted reproductive technologies (ART) into society can assist in achieving fertility rates towards replacement levels [8].

Women are born with a finite number of oocytes reaching their peak at 20 weeks gestation with 6–7 million and decreasing to 1–2 million at birth, 300,000–500,000 at puberty, 25,000 by 37 y/o, and approximately 1000 at menopause [9, 10]. Alongside a quantitative decline in oocyte number, there is also a qualitative decline primarily attributed to an increase in aneuploidy amongst aging oocytes. A study evaluating ploidy status of over 1300 metaphase II oocytes revealed that aneuploidy rates remain relatively stable from 20 to 34 y/o ranging between 5.2–10%, increasing to 12.5–28.1% at ages 35 y/o to 40 y/o, 50% at ages 42–43 y/o, and 100% at 45 y/o [11]. A similar trend is seen in embryo aneuploidy rates, as a study evaluating over 15,000 consecutive embryo trophectoderm biopsies with comprehensive chromosomal screening revealed a dramatic increase in embryo aneuploidy rates at ages 35–37 y/o, approaching 90% at ages 43–45 y/o [12]. The increase in oocyte and

* Correspondence: SJindal@montefiore.org
[1]Department of Obstetrics, Gynecology & Women's Health, Albert Einstein College of Medicine/Montefiore Medical Center, Minneapolis, USA
[2]Montefiore's Institute for Reproductive Medicine and Health, New York, USA

embryo aneuploidy in relation to age is likely related to a disturbance in meiotic competence due to abnormal meiotic spindle formation [13, 14].

Increase aneuploidy rates with ovarian aging results in decreased fecundity, with most epidemiological studies revealing a significant decline between 35 and 37 y/o [15]. The Hutterites are one of the most frequently referenced epidemiological cohorts. They immigrated form Switzerland and settled in the Dakotas and Montana in the 1870's and detailed records were kept relating to their childbearing [16]. They did not practice contraception and were a relatively fertile population with an average childbirth rate of 9.6 children per woman and a low an infertility rate of 2.4%. In this cohort, a steep decline in fecundity was seen at 35-37y/o, with 1 in 10 woman stopping to reproduce by 35 y/o, 1 in 3 by 40 y/o and 7 in 8 by 45 y/o [16]. This trend revealing a significant decrease in fecundity at 35–37 y/o is consistent with multiple historical epidemiological studies [17]. Recent cohort studies reveal similar trends. A time to pregnancy cohort study evaluating the fecundability of 960 women aged 30–44 y/o trying to conceive 3 months or less revealed stable pregnancy rates of 82–88% after 12 menstrual cycles in women aged 30–35 y/o, decreasing to 71–76% between 36 and 39 y/o, and to 48–54% between 40-44y/o [18]. Interestingly, history of no prior pregnancy adversely affected fecundability rates. For example, in patients aged 38–39 y/o with a history of a prior pregnancy, 81% had a pregnancy after 12 cycles compared to 35% without a prior pregnancy, with similar trends seen in patients ≥40 y/o [18]. A major limitation of this study is that they did not report on live birth rates, as patients were only followed to a positive pregnancy test. With the known increase in miscarriage rates in older patient populations, live birth rates would have likely been significantly lower in the older patient populations. Other recent cohort studies reveal a similar trend with decreasing fecundability after 35 y/o [19, 20]. Limitations of the Hutterite study and other epidemiological studies are that they do not account for the possibility of decreasing sexual activity amongst aging women, however, a study evaluating intrauterine insemination (IUI) pregnancy rates using donor sperm amongst women with male partners suffering from azoospermia revealed a significant decrease in success rates after 35 y/o [21]. After 12 cycles, women 26–30 y/o had a success rate of 74.1%, whereas, women over 35 y/o had a success rate 53.6%. IUI success rates were defined as a positive pregnancy test and, as above, given the increase in miscarriage rates seen with advanced maternal age, if followed to live birth, the difference between both age groups would have likely widened. Another study evaluating pregnancy rates in 751 donor sperm cycles from couples with male infertility revealed a similar significant decline in pregnancy rates after 35 y/o [22].

Data from in vitro fertilization (IVF) cycles in the United States reveal a similar decrease in fecundity with advancing age. There is a persistent misconception that assisted reproductive technology can reverse the "aged biological clock" [23], however, IVF success rates decrease significantly as women enter their 5th decade of life. U.S data from the Centers for Disease Control in 2015 reveal live birth rates per cycle of IVF of 33.1% in woman under 35 years old, decreasing to 8.3% at 41–42 y/o, 3.2% at 43–44 y/o and 0.8% > 44 y/o [24]. Alongside these trends, there is an increase in the use of donor oocytes with advancing maternal age. Donor oocyte use is 10% or less ≤40 y/o, increasing to 18% at 41–42 y/o, 34% at 43–44 y/o and 71% over 44 y/o [24].

Involuntary childlessness is a major consequence of delayed motherhood. Psychologically and socially, involuntary childlessness is associated with higher rates of low self-esteem, depression, partner separation, and even higher rates of mortality [25]. There are also consequences of pregnancy at advanced maternal age to both the mother and newborn. Women ≥35 y/o are at increase risk for preeclampsia, gestational diabetes, placenta previa, placental abruption, operative deliveries including cesarean section, and even maternal deaths [26–29]. Women of advanced maternal age, particularly ≥40 y/o are also at increased risks of adverse neonatal outcomes including preterm birth, low birth weight, very low birth weight, neonatal intensive care unit admissions, fetal death, congenital anomalies, and increased risks of chromosomal abnormalities [26, 27, 29–32]. Spontaneous abortion, or miscarriage, also significantly increase with advance maternal age. Rates of clinical miscarriages are generally approximately 15%, however, increase to 20% by 35 y/o, and 50% by age 42 y/o [33]. Miscarriage rates in infertile populations following IVF are similar to those seen in the non-infertile population, as miscarriage rates following IVF are below 15% in women < 35 y/o, and rise to 30% at 40 y/o and 65% in women older than 44 y/o [24]. Although generally not life threatening, miscarriages may result in severe psychological burden. A survey evaluating patients with miscarriages revealed that 37% felt that they had lost a child, 47% felt guilt, 41% felt alone, and 28% felt ashamed [34]. This psychological burden may be more devastating in women of advanced maternal age struggling with infertility. Additionally, miscarriages following IVF in women of advanced maternal age may have adverse effects on the success of subsequent treatments as a delay of 6 months can cause a significant decrease in the quality and quantity of ovarian reserve.

Although it is well documented that advanced maternal age decreases a woman's chance to conceive, studies from multiple countries consistently reveal that reproductive aged women have suboptimal knowledge relating to reproductive aging, particularly underestimating age-related fertility decline, and over-estimating the success of IVF [35–42]. One of the largest surveys evaluating over 10,000 women and men from 79 countries revealed an average score of 56% on a 13 item fertility knowledge questionnaire [43]. Knowledge relating to reproductive aging and IVF success outcomes have also been shown to be suboptimal amongst obstetrics and gynecology (OB/GYN) US residents. A study evaluating 238 OB/GYN residents revealed that although approximately 73% believed that a conversation relating to fertility decline with aging should be part of a well-woman exam, 47.5% underestimated the age at which a marked decline in fertility occurs, and 78.4% over-estimated the success of IVF [44].

Premature accelerated loss of fertility, risk factors, ovarian reserve markers

Although multiple markers for ovarian reserve have been evaluated, age is likely the most predictive marker for ovarian reserve and the ability to conceive. The average age of menopause in Western countries is approximately 51 years of age [45]. Approximately 10% will experience menopause by 45 y/o, and 1% will experience primary ovarian insufficiency (POI) defined as menopause by 40 y/o [46, 47]. It is estimated that there is an accelerated decline in fertility 13 years prior to the onset of menopause, and thus approximately 10% of woman will experience an accelerated decline in fertility at around 32 y/o [46]. Ideally these patients would be easily identified so that they can be counseled on reproductive aging and the availability of elective fertility preservation, however, currently there are no optimal tests to identify these cohort of women. Obtaining an adequate medical history may identify women at risk for POI or an accelerated loss of fertility. Women diagnosed with cancer that will undergo chemotherapy or pelvic radiation, or patients that have undergone these treatments are at risk and warrant counseling with a reproductive specialist relating to elective fertility preservation. Other patients that may be at risk for accelerated fertility decline include severe endometriosis, ovarian surgery, strong smoking history, family history of early menopause, Turner Syndrome or Turner mosaic, and Fragile X pre-mutation [48–53].

Day 3 follicle stimulating hormone (FSH) alongside estradiol (E_2), antral follicle count (AFC), and anti-mullerian hormone (AMH) are all frequently utilized markers of ovarian reserve; however they cannot predict when a significant decline in fertility will begin to occur and are more predictive of ovarian response during IVF than the ability to conceive naturally [54, 55]. Early follicular FSH and E_2, generally drawn on day 3 of the menstrual cycle, require no advanced training to interpret and therefore can be obtained and interpreted by general practitioners;

however, they have significant inter-cycle and intra-cycle variability and require a functional hypothalamic pituitary ovarian axis [56]. Day 3 elevated FSH is indicative of diminished ovarian reserve and is attributed to low E_2 and inhibin B production from ovarian follicles thereby resulting in diminished hypothalamic suppression. Normal FSH levels in the presence of elevated E_2 may also be indicative of low ovarian reserve as this is related to premature follicle selection and premature elevation of E_2, thus negatively inhibiting the hypothalamus and masking diminished ovarian reserve.

AFC is the sum of all the ovarian follicles between 2 and 10 mm visualized on ultrasound. AFC count has good specificity, however, poor sensitivity for prediction of ovarian response to stimulation and pregnancy outcomes during IVF. AFC is easy to perform by a trained sonographer, however, its limitations are that it can have significant inter-observer variability and obesity can adversely affect the measurements [57].

AMH is secreted by the granulosa cells of the pre-antral and small antral follicles and likely plays a role in limiting follicular recruitment of follicles from the primordial pool, partially by attenuating their response to FSH [58]. AMH null mice reveal accelerated follicular depletion [59]. The benefits of AMH measurements are that they can be tested anytime throughout the cycle and are directly secreted form the ovary. Several studies have shown that AMH may also predict the timing of menopause [60–62]. Limitations of AMH, similar to day 3 FSH/E_2 and AFC, are that they are more reliable to predict ovarian response and IVF outcomes rather than the ability to conceive naturally, and can be falsely elevated and decreased by many reproductive, environmental, and lifestyle factors [56, 63]. One factor common to reproductive aged women is the use of oral contraception (OCP). AMH can be falsely decreased in women using OCP's and it is recommended to wait 3–4 months following discontinuation of OCP to measure AMH levels [56].

A recently published prospective time-to-pregnancy study evaluating the predictive value of AMH and Day 3 FSH in over 700 women aged 30–44 y/o, without a history of infertility, and attempting to conceive ≤3 months revealed that low AMH and elevated FSH were not predictive of the ability to conceive up to 12 menstrual cycles [64]. It is important to note that in the older age group (38–44 y/o), low AMH was also not predictive of time to pregnancy. A significant limitation of this study worth noting is that pregnancy was defined as a positive pregnancy test and if followed to live birth, it is possible that those in the low AMH/elevated FSH groups may have experienced pregnancy loss more often and therefore live birth rates may have differed.

Oocyte cryopreservation

There are no known treatments to circumvent the natural decline in fecundity that occurs with ovarian aging. Using donor oocytes is an option for women unable to conceive with their own oocytes; however, this may not be acceptable to many women and is not available and/or legal in many countries. Embryo cryopreservation and OC are available options, which may enable women to become pregnant with their own oocytes after their reproductive potential has significantly diminished. The focus of the following paragraphs will focus on OC as the majority of women that delay childbearing report lack of a partner as a reason for delay [65, 66].

The first pregnancy following OC was in 1986 [67]. Over 2 decades later, in 2012, the "experimental" label for OC was removed by the American Society for Reproductive Medicine (ASRM) and the European Society for Human Reproduction and Embryology (ESHRE) [68, 69]. Factors that led to removing the "experimental" label included improved success rates of OC and reassuring safety data relating to offspring born following OC. Since the removal of the experimental label by ASRM, OC has increased 18.6% in 1 year from 6123 cycles in 2014 to 7518 cycles in 2015 [70, 71].

Slow freeze versus Vitrification

A major advancement in OC was a shift from the slow freeze method of cryopreservation to vitrification. Vitrification is an ultra-fast cooling method for cryopreservation using high concentrations of cryoprotectants. Vitrification solidifies the oocyte to a glass-like state and minimizes ice crystal formation, more commonly seen with the slow freeze technique. The oocyte is particularly vulnerable to damage from ice crystal formation due to its high water content and its sensitive meiotic spindle apparatus [72, 73]. A randomized controlled trial reported improved oocyte survival rates, fertilization rates, and clinical pregnancy rates with vitrification compared to slow freeze [74]. Post-thaw survival rates using vitrification have been reported to be as high as 96.9% [75]. Pregnancy rates following OC have been reported to be similar to those following fresh oocyte insemination by multiple randomized controlled trials [76–78]. Although reports of high oocyte survival rates and similar pregnancy rates with OC compared to fresh insemination have been reported, these high success rates may be attributed to publication bias and therefore the success rates may not be reproducible by all centers. Data from 30,160 donor oocyte cycles reported to the Society for Assisted Reproductive Technology from 2013 to 2015 revealed that pregnancy rates from cycles following OC in donor cycles were significantly lower compared to donor cycles involving freshly inseminated oocytes [79].

Indications for oocyte cryopreservation

Aside from preventive measures for age related fertility decline, women at risk for an accelerated rate of fertility decline due to medical reasons may benefit from OC. Women diagnosed with malignant diseases that will undergo chemotherapy and/or pelvic irradiation are at significant risk for premature ovarian failure and certainly warrant counseling on OC. Women with severe endometriosis/endometriomas may be at risk for an accelerated rate of follicular decline. A study has found that ovarian cortex from ovaries with endometriomas have significantly decreased follicular densities compared to contralateral ovaries without endometriomas [53]. In a similar study, cortex from ovaries with endometriomas had significantly more atretic early follicles compared to contralateral ovaries without endometriomas [80]. Additionally, a systematic review and meta-analysis revealed that excision of endometriomas could negatively impact ovarian reserve [81]. Women with a family history of mental retardation or a known family history of Fragile X Syndrome may benefit from Fragile X carrier testing as women with premutations (55 to 200 repeats) are at increase risk of premature ovarian failure (up to 21%) and therefore could benefit from OC [52]. Other genetic disorders include patients with Turners or Turners mosaic and those with a strong family history of premature ovarian failure. Pedigree studies have shown a familial link to idiopathic premature ovarian failure as multiple genes likely play a role that are not fully understood [82]. Women undergoing female to male gender transition often undergo bilateral salpingoophorectomy and therefore should be offered OC as pregnancies have been achieved in this cohort of patients following transition [83]. Other indications for OC include inability to produce sperm at time of ooycte retrieval, ethical dilemma to producing and cryopreserving embryos, and circumventing legal implications with embryo cryopreservation in the event of divorce.

Age at which to freeze oocytes

A question frequently asked by both practitioners and patients is the ideal age at which to freeze oocytes. Although no good answer exists as every patient has unique biological and social circumstances, there is some evidence available to guide the discussion. Similar to IVF, success rates following OC may be related to the age at which the oocytes were frozen. A retrospective multicenter study spanning an 8-year time period evaluating 1468 women undergoing elective oocyte cryopreservation for reasons other than a diagnosis of cancer revealed that 191 (13%) presented to thaw and inseminate their oocytes [84]. Of those that did, the oocyte survival rate in women ≤35 y/o and ≥ 36 y/o were 94.6% vs. 82.4%, respectively [84]. Additionally, differences in live birth rates for women undergoing OC ≤ 35 y/o and ≥ 36 y/o were significantly different, with 50% and 22.9%, respectively [84]. In this study, age was associated with success even in the cohort of women undergoing OC ≤ 35 y/o, with live birth rates of 100% ≤ 29 y/o, 45% at 30–34 y/o, 28.5% at 35–39 y/o, and 3.7% at ≥40 y/o [84]. Despite a clear trend in success rates with age at which a woman undergoes OC, the majority of women that undergo elective OC are doing so after a significant decline in fertility begins to occur, with three studies revealing average ages between 36 y/o and 38 y/o [65, 84, 85].

In women considering OC, a frequent question is how many oocytes should be frozen. Although there is no precise answer to this question as every women presenting for OC will be at a different age and have different future childbearing desires, there is some data to guide a discussion. Clinical pregnancy rate per oocyte thaw have been shown to range between 4.5 and 12% [68]. A recent mathematical model based on live birth rates from a single institution from women with presumably normal ovarian reserve undergoing intracytoplasmic sperm injection (ICSI) due to male factor infertility or tubal factor infertility, revealed that for women 34, 37, and 42 y/o, they would need to freeze 10, 20, and 61 mature oocytes respectively to have a 75% likelihood of having at least 1 live birth [86]. If incorporating this or another model into a OC counseling session, it is important to discuss the possibility of needing multiple controlled ovarian hyperstimulation (COH) cycles to obtain the number of oocytes the patient desires. For example, based on the above model, a 37 y/o may feel comfortable with freezing 20 mature oocytes for a 75% chance of at least 1 live birth, however, obtaining 20 mature oocytes may require 2 or 3 COH cycles. Additionally, it must be stressed to patients undergoing OC that although mathematical models exist to guide a discussion of how many oocytes to freeze in order to assure a certain percentage of success, OC is not an 100% insurance policy to achieve a genetically related offspring and that there is a possibility of failure despite "adequate" amounts of frozen oocytes.

Cost considerations of OC

Cost of oocyte cryopreservation may vary widely from infertility center to infertility center and is an important part of a counseling session for patients desiring elective OC as this is frequently not covered by insurance for reasons other than a medical indication. Although OC incurs an expense, if performed early it may be more cost-effective and successful for women desiring to postpone their childbearing to their late 30's or early 40's. One model has shown that OC would be more cost-effective and successful if performed at 35 y/o in women looking to prolong their childbearing until 40 y/o, whereas another model

revealed that OC was most cost-effective and successful in achieving a live birth if performed by 37 y/o [87, 88]. In these models, the assumption is that the patient will return for 1 child at an older age, however, many patients may desire > 1 child. It is important to discuss with patients how many children they desire, as the more children they desire, the more cost-effective it may be to undergo OC at a younger age. Other important cost considerations that must be discussed with patients are the annual cost of storing the oocytes, cost of thawing and inseminating oocytes via ICSI, and eventual uterine transfer of the embryos. Additionally, ethical considerations of OC must be extensively discussed, documented, and consented including duration of storage of oocytes and disposition of oocytes in the event of death or incapacitation of the patient.

Risks of OC

Risks of OC must be discussed with patients undergoing the procedure. Major complications for patients are low (< 1%) and include risks during oocyte retrieval including infection, damage to organs, blood loss, ovarian torsion, and risks related to anaesthesia [89–91]. A more common risk that must be discussed is ovarian hyperstimulation syndrome (OHSS), a complication specific to COH. Although mild and moderate OHSS is burdensome for the patient, severe OHSS is potentially life-threatening and most concerning. The risk varies depending on the definition and study, but has generally been reported to be < 5% [92]. Severe OHSS is more common following COH with embryo transfer resulting in a pregnancy and is rare in the absence of pregnancy. Women undergoing OC, by definition, will not undergo a fresh embryo transfer and therefore the risk of severe OHSS is significantly less than patients undergoing IVF/ICSI with subsequent fresh embryo transfer. A study evaluating 4052 oocyte donors revealed a risk of moderate to severe OHSS of < 1%, which was eliminated with the use of a GnRH antagonist protocol and GnRH agonist trigger [93].

A frequent concern for women undergoing OC is whether there is any risk to offspring born following OC. Although data are limited and more long-term data are needed, there does not appear to be any risk to offspring related to OC. A study of 1027 children born from 804 pregnancies using vitrified oocytes compared to 1224 children from 996 pregnancies with IVF using fresh oocytes revealed no significant differences in obstetrical outcomes, gestational age at delivery, birthweight, birth defects, APGAR scores, or perinatal mortality between cryopreserved and fresh oocytes [94]. Another study evaluating 936 infants born from both vitrified and slow freeze oocytes revealed an anomaly rate of 1.3%, similar to the anomaly rate in the general population [95]. Additionally rates of embryo aneuoploidy have been reported to be similar following oocyte cryopreservation and IVF using fresh oocytes [96, 97].

Education and increasing awareness towards reproductive aging and elective OC

It is well documented that reproductive aged woman frequently underestimate the impact that increasing age has on the ability to conceive and overestimate the success of IVF to circumvent infertility. Sup-optimal physician counseling may be partly related to this as a study evaluating US OB/GYN residents reveals that they too have suboptimal knowledge relating to reproductive aging and IVF success rates [44]. A study by Hodes-Wertz et al. evaluating 183 women who underwent elective oocyte cryopreservation revealed that only 25% heard of the procedure from their OB/GYN, and 79% wished that they had undergone the procedure at an earlier age, with the most common reason for delay being unaware of the procedure or feeling that the technology was not readily available [65].

Although elective OC is generally not covered by private health insurances in the U.S. or government health policies in Europe, attitudes and policies relating to covering elective OC are shifting. Large companies such as Facebook and Apple are offering their employees elective oocyte cryopreservation [98]. Additionally, some countries such as Israel endorse elective OC for prevention of age related fertility decline and consider it "preventative medicine" [99].

Improved methods to increase awareness relating to reproductive aging and the availability of OC are warranted. A greater emphasis by OB/GYN's to counsel patients on age related fertility decline during annual exams and implementing these discussions as part of sexual education may help increase awareness. Additionally using media as a platform to discuss these important issues may be of importance as 42.3% of those that underwent elective OC in the above study by Hodes-Wertz et al. heard about the technology through media outlets [65]. Having a separate clinic to counsel women on reproductive aging may also be of benefit. A Fertility Assessment and Counseling Clinic was established in Copenhagen, Denmark, with a goal of providing pro-fertility individual assessment and guidance to women and men [100]. At the time of publication > 1200 women and men attended the clinic and filled out a survey. Ninety-nine percent of women found the clinic helpful with approximately 70% wanting to know how long they could postpone their childbearing, and after consultation, 35% of women stating that they would advance the age at which to become pregnant.

Conclusion

The adverse effect of reproductive aging on fecundity has been well documented for centuries. With delayed motherhood becoming a norm in many countries, involuntary childlessness will likely continue to rise. This may not only be detrimental to a woman's overall well-being but may also have adverse economic consequences to future generations. Despite this, reproductive aged women are frequently unaware and underestimate the effects of reproductive aging, and/or overestimate the success rates of IVF to circumvent infertility, particularly in older aged women. Increase awareness and education at earlier ages are warranted so that women can make informed decisions relating to their reproductive potential. For the first time in history, OC provides a way of increasing a woman's reproductive autonomy for those desiring genetically related children towards the end of their reproductive lifespan. The past several decades has seen an increase in effective available methods to delay childbearing including greater access to contraception and safe pregnancy terminations, however, an integral part of a woman's reproductive autonomy is pro-fertility knowledge. Discussions relating to reproductive aging and oocyte cryopreservation will enable woman to make informed decisions relating to their reproductive potential and increase their reproductive autonomy.

Abbreviations

AFC: Antral follicle count; AMH: Anti-mullerian hormone; COH: Controlled ovarian hyperstimulation; E_2: Estradiol; FSH: Follicle stimulating hormone; ICSI: Intracytoplasmic sperm injection; IUI: Intrauterine Insemination; IVF: In vitro fertilization; OB/GYN: Obstetrics and Gynecology; OCP: Oral contraception; OHSS: Ovarian hyperstimulation syndrome

Authors contributions

RF and SJ both contributed to writing and editing the manuscript. RF and SJ read and approved the final manuscript.

Competing interests

The authors declare that they have no competing interests.

References

1. Prevention CfDCa. 2002. Available from: https://www.cdc.gov/nchs/data/nvsr/nvsr51/nvsr51_01.pdf. Accessed 12/23/2017.
2. Prevention CfDCa. 2016. Available from: https://www.cdc.gov/nchs/data/databriefs/db232.pdf. Accessed 12/23/2017.
3. Prevention CfDCa. 2014. Available from: https://www.cdc.gov/nchs/data/databriefs/db152_table.pdf#1. Accessed 12/23/2017.
4. mothers. SCTDSHadocooft. 2008. Available from: https://www12.statcan.gc.ca/census-recensement/index-eng.cfm?MM=1. Accessed 31 Dec 2017.
5. Eurostat. Women in the EU gave birth to their first child at almost 29 years of age on average 2015. Available from: http://ec.europa.eu/eurostat/documents/2995521/6829228/3-13052015-CP-EN.pdf/7e9007fb-3ca9-445f-96eb-fd75d6792965. Accessed 12/31/2017.
6. Group ECW. Social determinants of human reproduction. Hum Reprod. 2001;16(7):1518–26.

7. Nargund G. Declining birth rate in developed countries: a radical policy re-think is required. Facts Views Vis Obgyn. 2009;1(3):191–3.

8. Ziebe S, Devroey P. State of ARTWG. Assisted reproductive technologies are an integrated part of national strategies addressing demographic and reproductive challenges. Hum Reprod Update. 2008;14(6):583–92.

9. Baker TG. A quantitative and cytological study of germ cells in human ovaries. Proc R Soc Lond B Biol Sci. 1963;158:417–33.

10. Block E. Quantitative morphological investigations of the follicular system in women; variations at different ages. Acta Anat (Basel). 1952;14(1–2):108–23.

11. Pellestor F, Andreo B, Arnal F, Humeau C, Demaille J. Maternal aging and chromosomal abnormalities: new data drawn from in vitro unfertilized human oocytes. Hum Genet. 2003;112(2):195–203.

12. Franasiak JM, Forman EJ, Hong KH, Werner MD, Upham KM, Treff NR, et al. The nature of aneuploidy with increasing age of the female partner: a review of 15,169 consecutive trophectoderm biopsies evaluated with comprehensive chromosomal screening. Fertility and sterility. 2014;101:3:656–63 e1.

13. Volarcik K, Sheean L, Goldfarb J, Woods L, Abdul-Karim FW, Hunt P. The meiotic competence of in-vitro matured human oocytes is influenced by donor age: evidence that folliculogenesis is compromised in the reproductively aged ovary. Hum Reprod. 1998;13(1):154–60.

14. Battaglia DE, Goodwin P, Klein NA, Soules MR. Influence of maternal age on meiotic spindle assembly in oocytes from naturally cycling women. Hum Reprod. 1996;11(10):2217–22.

15. Menken J, Trussell J, Larsen U. Age and infertility. Science. 1986;233(4771): 1389–94.

16. Tietze C. Reproductive span and rate of reproduction among Hutterite women. Fertil Steril. 1957;8(1):89–97.

17. American College of O, Gynecologists Committee on Gynecologic P, Practice C. Female age-related fertility decline. Committee Opinion No. 589. Fertility and sterility. 2014;101:3:633–4.

18. Steiner AZ, Jukic AM. Impact of female age and nulligravidity on fecundity in an older reproductive age cohort. Fertility and sterility. 2016;105:6:1584–8 e1.

19. Wesselink AK, Rothman KJ, Hatch EE, Mikkelsen EM, Sorensen HT, Wise LA. Age and fecundability in a North American preconception cohort study. American journal of obstetrics and gynecology. 2017;217:6:667 e1- e8.

20. Rothman KJ, Wise LA, Sorensen HT, Riis AH, Mikkelsen EM, Hatch EE. Volitional determinants and age-related decline in fecundability: a general population prospective cohort study in Denmark. Fertil Steril. 2013;99(7): 1958–64.

21. Schwartz D, Mayaux MJ. Female fecundity as a function of age: results of artificial insemination in 2193 nulliparous women with azoospermic husbands. Federation CECOS. N Engl J Med. 1982;306(7):404–6.

22. van Noord-Zaadstra BM, Looman CW, Alsbach H, Habbema JD, te Velde ER, Karbaat J. Delaying childbearing: effect of age on fecundity and outcome of pregnancy. BMJ. 1991;302(6789):1361–5.

23. Wyndham N, Marin Figueira PG, Patrizio P. A persistent misperception: assisted reproductive technology can reverse the "aged biological clock". Fertil Steril. 2012;97(5):1044–7.

24. Prevention CfDCa. 2017. Available from: https://www.cdc.gov/art/reports/ 2015/national-summary.html. Accessed 12/23/2017.

25. Cil AP, Turkgeldi L, Seli E. Oocyte cryopreservation as a preventive measure for age-related fertility loss. Semin Reprod Med. 2015;33(6):429–35.

26. Jacobsson B, Ladfors L, Milsom I. Advanced maternal age and adverse perinatal outcome. Obstet Gynecol. 2004;104(4):727–33.

27. Cleary-Goldman J, Malone FD, Vidaver J, Ball RH, Nyberg DA, Comstock CH, et al. Impact of maternal age on obstetric outcome. Obstet Gynecol. 2005; 105(5 Pt 1):983–90.

28. Laopaiboon M, Lumbiganon P, Intarut N, Mori R, Ganchimeg T, Vogel JP, et al. Advanced maternal age and pregnancy outcomes: a multicountry assessment. BJOG : an international journal of obstetrics and gynaecology. 2014;121(Suppl 1):49–56.

29. Gilbert WM, Nesbitt TS, Danielsen B. Childbearing beyond age 40: pregnancy outcome in 24,032 cases. Obstet Gynecol. 1999;93(1):9–14.

30. Hoffman MC, Jeffers S, Carter J, Duthely L, Cotter A, Gonzalez-Quintero VH. Pregnancy at or beyond age 40 years is associated with an increased risk of fetal death and other adverse outcomes. Am J Obstet Gynecol. 2007;196(5):e11–3.

31. Berkowitz GS, Skovron ML, Lapinski RH, Berkowitz RL. Delayed childbearing and the outcome of pregnancy. N Engl J Med. 1990;322(10):659–64.

32. Lean SC, Derricott H, Jones RL, Heazell AEP. Advanced maternal age and adverse pregnancy outcomes: A systematic review and meta-analysis. PloS one. 2017;12:10:e0186287.

33. Nybo Andersen AM, Wohlfahrt J, Christens P, Olsen J, Melbye M. Maternal age and fetal loss: population based register linkage study. BMJ. 2000; 320(7251):1708–12.

34. Bardos J, Hercz D, Friedenthal J, Missmer SA, Williams Z. A national survey on public perceptions of miscarriage. Obstet Gynecol. 2015;125(6):1313–20.

35. Chan CH, Chan TH, Peterson BD, Lampic C, Tam MY. Intentions and attitudes towards parenthood and fertility awareness among Chinese university students in Hong Kong: a comparison with western samples. Hum Reprod. 2015;30(2):364–72.

36. Peterson BD, Pirritano M, Tucker L, Lampic C. Fertility awareness and parenting attitudes among American male and female undergraduate university students. Hum Reprod. 2012;27(5):1375–82.

37. Lundsberg LS, Pal L, Gariepy AM, Xu X, Chu MC, Illuzzi JL. Knowledge, attitudes, and practices regarding conception and fertility: a population-based survey among reproductive-age United States women. Fertil Steril. 2014;101(3):767–74.

38. Bretherick KL, Fairbrother N, Avila L, Harbord SH, Robinson WP. Fertility and aging: do reproductive-aged Canadian women know what they need to know? Fertil Steril. 2010;93(7):2162–8.

39. Hashiloni-Dolev Y, Kaplan A, Shkedi-Rafid S. The fertility myth: Israeli students' knowledge regarding age-related fertility decline and late pregnancies in an era of assisted reproduction technology. Hum Reprod. 2011;26(11):3045–53.

40. Tough S, Benzies K, Newburn-Cook C, Tofflemire K, Fraser-Lee N, Faber A, et al. What do women know about the risks of delayed childbearing? Can J Public Health. 2006;97(4):330–4.

41. Adashi EY, Cohen J, Hamberger L, Jones HW Jr, de Kretser DM, Lunenfeld B, et al. Public perception on infertility and its treatment: an international survey. The Bertarelli Foundation scientific board. Hum Reprod. 2000;15(2):330–4.

42. Lampic C, Svanberg AS, Karlstrom P, Tyden T. Fertility awareness, intentions concerning childbearing, and attitudes towards parenthood among female and male academics. Hum Reprod. 2006;21(2):558–64.

43. Bunting L, Tsibulsky I, Boivin J. Fertility knowledge and beliefs about fertility treatment: findings from the international fertility decision-making study. Hum Reprod. 2013;28(2):385–97.

44. Yu L, Peterson B, Inhorn MC, Boehm JK, Patrizio P. Knowledge, attitudes, and intentions toward fertility awareness and oocyte cryopreservation among obstetrics and gynecology resident physicians. Hum Reprod. 2016; 31(2):403–11.

45. Grady D. Clinical practice. Management of menopausal symptoms. N Engl J Med. 2006;355(22):2338–47.

46. Nikolaou D, Templeton A. Early ovarian ageing: a hypothesis. Detection and clinical relevance. Hum Reprod. 2003;18(6):1137–9.

47. Coulam CB, Adamson SC, Annegers JF. Incidence of premature ovarian failure. Obstet Gynecol. 1986;67(4):604–6.

48. Barnhart K, Dunsmoor-Su R, Coutifaris C. Effect of endometriosis on in vitro fertilization. Fertil Steril. 2002;77(6):1148–55.

49. Augood C, Duckitt K, Templeton AA. Smoking and female infertility: a systematic review and meta-analysis. Hum Reprod. 1998;13(6):1532–9.

50. Cramer DW, Xu H, Harlow BL. Family history as a predictor of early menopause. Fertil Steril. 1995;64(4):740–5.

51. Schattman GL. Cryopreservation of Oocytes. Author replies. The New England journal of medicine. 2016;374:3:288.

52. Sherman SL. Premature ovarian failure in the fragile X syndrome. Am J Med Genet. 2000;97(3):189–94.

53. Kitajima M, Defrere S, Dolmans MM, Colette S, Squifflet J, Van Langendonckt A, et al. Endometriomas as a possible cause of reduced ovarian reserve in women with endometriosis. Fertil Steril. 2011;96(3):685–91.

54. Muasher SJ, Oehninger S, Simonetti S, Matta J, Ellis LM, Liu HC, et al. The value of basal and/or stimulated serum gonadotropin levels in prediction of stimulation response and in vitro fertilization outcome. Fertil Steril. 1988; 50(2):298–307.

55. Scott RT, Toner JP, Muasher SJ, Oehninger S, Robinson S, Rosenwaks Z. Follicle-stimulating hormone levels on cycle day 3 are predictive of in vitro fertilization outcome. Fertil Steril. 1989;51(4):651–4.

56. Tal R, Seifer DB. Ovarian reserve testing: A user's guide. American journal of obstetrics and gynecology. 2017;https://doi.org/10.1016/j.ajog.2017.02.027.

57. Broekmans FJ, Kwee J, Hendriks DJ, Mol BW, Lambalk CB. A systematic review of tests predicting ovarian reserve and IVF outcome. Hum Reprod Update. 2006;12(6):685–718.

58. Durlinger AL, Gruijters MJ, Kramer P, Karels B, Kumar TR, Matzuk MM, et al. Anti-Mullerian hormone attenuates the effects of FSH on follicle development in the mouse ovary. Endocrinology. 2001;142(11):4891–9.

59. Durlinger AL, Kramer P, Karels B, de Jong FH, Uilenbroek JT, Grootegoed JA, et al. Control of primordial follicle recruitment by anti-Mullerian hormone in the mouse ovary. Endocrinology. 1999;140(12):5789–96.

60. Broer SL, Eijkemans MJ, Scheffer GJ, van Rooij IA, de Vet A, Themmen AP, et al. Anti-mullerian hormone predicts menopause: a long-term follow-up study in normoovulatory women. J Clin Endocrinol Metab. 2011;96(8):2532–9.

61. Freeman EW, Sammel MD, Lin H, Boorman DW, Gracia CR. Contribution of the rate of change of antimullerian hormone in estimating time to menopause for late reproductive-age women. Fertility and sterility. 2012;98: 5:1254–9 e1–2.

62. Freeman EW, Sammel MD, Lin H, Gracia CR. Anti-mullerian hormone as a predictor of time to menopause in late reproductive age women. J Clin Endocrinol Metab. 2012;97(5):1673–80.

63. La Marca A, Sighinolfi G, Radi D, Argento C, Baraldi E, Artenisio AC, et al. Anti-Mullerian hormone (AMH) as a predictive marker in assisted reproductive technology (ART). Hum Reprod Update. 2010;16(2):113–30.

64. Steiner AZ, Pritchard D, Stanczyk FZ, Kesner JS, Meadows JW, Herring AH, et al. Association between biomarkers of ovarian reserve and infertility among older women of reproductive age. JAMA. 2017;318(14):1367–76.

65. Hodes-Wertz B, Druckenmiller S, Smith M, Noyes N. What do reproductive-age women who undergo oocyte cryopreservation think about the process as a means to preserve fertility? Fertil Steril. 2013;100(5):1343–9.

66. Hammarberg K, Clarke VE. Reasons for delaying childbearing--a survey of women aged over 35 years seeking assisted reproductive technology. Aust Fam Physician. 2005;34:3:187–8, 206.

67. Chen C. Pregnancy after human oocyte cryopreservation. Lancet. 1986; 1(8486):884–6.

68. Practice Committees of American Society for Reproductive M, Society for Assisted Reproductive T. Mature oocyte cryopreservation: a guideline. Fertility and sterility. 2013;99:1:37–43.

69. Ethics ETFo, Law, Dondorp W, de Wert G, Pennings G, Shenfield F, et al. Oocyte cryopreservation for age-related fertility loss. Human reproduction. 2012;27:5:1231–7.

70. Technologies SfAR. 2017. Available from: https://www.sartcorsonline.com/rptCSR_PublicMultYear.aspx?reportingYear=2015. Accessed 1/29/2018.

71. Technologies SfAR. 2017. Available from: https://www.sartcorsonline.com/rptCSR_PublicMultYear.aspx?reportingYear=2014. Accessed 1/229/2018.

72. Bromfield JJ, Coticchio G, Hutt K, Sciajno R, Borini A, Albertini DF. Meiotic spindle dynamics in human oocytes following slow-cooling cryopreservation. Hum Reprod. 2009;24(9):2114–23.

73. Shaw JM, Oranratnachai A, Trounson AO. Fundamental cryobiology of mammalian oocytes and ovarian tissue. Theriogenology. 2000;53(1):59–72.

74. Smith GD, Serafini PC, Fioravanti J, Yadid I, Coslovsky M, Hassun P, et al. Prospective randomized comparison of human oocyte cryopreservation with slow-rate freezing or vitrification. Fertil Steril. 2010;94(6):2088–95.

75. Cobo A, Kuwayama M, Perez S, Ruiz A, Pellicer A, Remohi J. Comparison of concomitant outcome achieved with fresh and cryopreserved donor oocytes vitrified by the Cryotop method. Fertil Steril. 2008;89(6):1657–64.

76. Cobo A, Meseguer M, Remohi J, Pellicer A. Use of cryo-banked oocytes in an ovum donation programme: a prospective, randomized, controlled, clinical trial. Hum Reprod. 2010;25(9):2239–46.

77. Parmegiani L, Cognigni GE, Bernardi S, Cuomo S, Ciampaglia W, Infante FE, et al. Efficiency of aseptic open vitrification and hermetical cryostorage of human oocytes. Reprod BioMed Online. 2011;23(4):505–12.

78. Rienzi L, Romano S, Albricci L, Maggiulli R, Capalbo A, Baroni E, et al. Embryo development of fresh 'versus' vitrified metaphase II oocytes after ICSI: a prospective randomized sibling-oocyte study. Hum Reprod. 2010; 25(1):66–73.

79. Kushnir VA, Darmon SK, Barad DH, Gleicher N. New national outcome data on fresh versus cryopreserved donor oocytes. J Ovarian Res. 2018;11:1:2.

80. Kitajima M, Dolmans MM, Donnez O, Masuzaki H, Soares M, Donnez J. Enhanced follicular recruitment and atresia in cortex derived from ovaries with endometriomas. Fertil Steril. 2014;101(4):1031–7.

81. Raffi F, Metwally M, Amer S. The impact of excision of ovarian endometrioma on ovarian reserve: a systematic review and meta-analysis. J Clin Endocrinol Metab. 2012;97(9):3146–54.

82. van Kasteren YM, Hundscheid RD, Smits AP, Cremers FP, van Zonneveld P, Braat DD. Familial idiopathic premature ovarian failure: an overrated and underestimated genetic disease? Hum Reprod. 1999;14(10):2455–9.

83. Maxwell S, Noyes N, Keefe D, Berkeley AS, Goldman KN. Pregnancy outcomes after fertility preservation in transgender men. Obstet Gynecol. 2017;129(6):1031–4.

84. Cobo A, Garcia-Velasco JA, Coello A, Domingo J, Pellicer A, Remohi J. Oocyte vitrification as an efficient option for elective fertility preservation. Fertility and sterility. 2016;105:3:755–64 e8.

85. Baldwin K, Culley L, Hudson N, Mitchell H, Lavery S. Oocyte cryopreservation for social reasons: demographic profile and disposal intentions of UK users. Reprod BioMed Online. 2015;31(2):239–45.

86. Goldman RH, Racowsky C, Farland LV, Munne S, Ribustello L, Fox JH. Predicting the likelihood of live birth for elective oocyte cryopreservation: a counseling tool for physicians and patients. Human reproduction. 2017; https://doi.org/10.1093/humrep/dex008:1-7.

87. van Loendersloot LL, Moolenaar LM, Mol BW, Repping S, van der Veen F, Goddijn M. Expanding reproductive lifespan: a cost-effectiveness study on oocyte freezing. Hum Reprod. 2011;26(11):3054–60.

88. Mesen TB, Mersereau JE, Kane JB, Steiner AZ. Optimal timing for elective egg freezing. Fertility and sterility. 2015;103:6:1551–6 e1–4.

89. Maxwell KN, Cholst IN, Rosenwaks Z. The incidence of both serious and minor complications in young women undergoing oocyte donation. Fertil Steril. 2008;90(6):2165–71.

90. Aragona C, Mohamed MA, Espinola MS, Linari A, Pecorini F, Micara G, et al. Clinical complications after transvaginal oocyte retrieval in 7,098 IVF cycles. Fertil Steril. 2011;95(1):293–4.

91. Roest J, Mous HV, Zeilmaker GH, Verhoeff A. The incidence of major clinical complications in a Dutch transport IVF programme. Hum Reprod Update. 1996;2(4):345–53.

92. Practice Committee of the American Society for Reproductive Medicine. Electronic address Aao, Practice Committee of the American Society for Reproductive M. Prevention and treatment of moderate and severe ovarian hyperstimulation syndrome: a guideline. Fertility and sterility. 2016;106:7:1634–47.

93. Bodri D, Guillen JJ, Polo A, Trullenque M, Esteve C, Coll O. Complications related to ovarian stimulation and oocyte retrieval in 4052 oocyte donor cycles. Reprod BioMed Online. 2008;17(2):237–43.

94. Cobo A, Serra V, Garrido N, Olmo I, Pellicer A, Remohi J. Obstetric and perinatal outcome of babies born from vitrified oocytes. Fertility and sterility. 2014;102:4:1006–15 e4.

95. Noyes N, Porcu E, Borini A. Over 900 oocyte cryopreservation babies born with no apparent increase in congenital anomalies. Reprod BioMed Online. 2009;18(6):769–76.

96. Cobo A, Rubio C, Gerli S, Ruiz A, Pellicer A, Remohi J. Use of fluorescence in situ hybridization to assess the chromosomal status of embryos obtained from cryopreserved oocytes. Fertil Steril. 2001;75(2):354–60.

97. Goldman KN, Kramer Y, Hodes-Wertz B, Noyes N, McCaffrey C, Grifo JA. Long-term cryopreservation of human oocytes does not increase embryonic aneuploidy. Fertil Steril. 2015;103(3):662–8.

98. Zoll M, Mertes H, Gupta J. Corporate giants provide fertility benefits: have they got it wrong? Eur J Obstet Gynecol Reprod Biol. 2015;195:A1–2.

99. Shkedi-Rafid S, Hashiloni-Dolev Y. Egg freezing for age-related fertility decline: preventive medicine or a further medicalization of reproduction? Analyzing the new Israeli policy. Fertil Steril. 2011;96(2):291–4.

100. Hvidman HW, Petersen KB, Larsen EC, Macklon KT, Pinborg A, Nyboe AA. Individual fertility assessment and pro-fertility counselling; should this be offered to women and men of reproductive age? Hum Reprod. 2015;30(1):9–15.

Permissions

The contributors of this book come from diverse backgrounds, making this book a truly international effort. This book will bring forth new frontiers with its revolutionizing research information and detailed analysis of the nascent developments around the world.

We would like to thank all the contributing authors for lending their expertise to make the book truly unique. They have played a crucial role in the development of this book. Without their invaluable contributions this book wouldn't have been possible. They have made vital efforts to compile up to date information on the varied aspects of this subject to make this book a valuable addition to the collection of many professionals and students.

This book was conceptualized with the vision of imparting up-to-date information and advanced data in this field. To ensure the same, a matchless editorial board was set up. Every individual on the board went through rigorous rounds of assessment to prove their worth. After which they invested a large part of their time researching and compiling the most relevant data for our readers.

The editorial board has been involved in producing this book since its inception. They have spent rigorous hours researching and exploring the diverse topics which have resulted in the successful publishing of this book. They have passed on their knowledge of decades through this book. To expedite this challenging task, the publisher supported the team at every step. A small team of assistant editors was also appointed to further simplify the editing procedure and attain best results for the readers.

Apart from the editorial board, the designing team has also invested a significant amount of their time in understanding the subject and creating the most relevant covers. They scrutinized every image to scout for the most suitable representation of the subject and create an appropriate cover for the book.

The publishing team has been an ardent support to the editorial, designing and production team. Their endless efforts to recruit the best for this project, has resulted in the accomplishment of this book. They are a veteran in the field of academics and their pool of knowledge is as vast as their experience in printing. Their expertise and guidance has proved useful at every step. Their uncompromising quality standards have made this book an exceptional effort. Their encouragement from time to time has been an inspiration for everyone.

The publisher and the editorial board hope that this book will prove to be a valuable piece of knowledge for researchers, students, practitioners and scholars across the globe.

List of Contributors

Guobo Quan
Yunnan Animal Science and Veterinary Institute, Jindian, Panlong county, Kunming, Yunnan province 650224, China
Department of Animal Biosciences, University of Guelph, 50 Stone Road East, Building #70, Guelph, ON N1G 2W1, Canada

Julang Li
Department of Animal Biosciences, University of Guelph, 50 Stone Road East, Building #70, Guelph, ON N1G 2W1, Canada
College of Life Science and Engineering, Foshan University, Foshan, Guangdong province, China

Xi Chen, Tao Zhu, Nanfang Liu and Aijun Yu
Department of Gynecologic Oncology, Zhejiang Cancer Hospital, 1 Banshan East Road, Zhejiang 310022, Hangzhou, China

Haiyan Sun
Department of Gynecologic Oncology, Zhejiang Cancer Hospital, 1 Banshan East Road, Zhejiang 310022, Hangzhou, China
Department of Gynecology, The First People's Hospital of Aksu, Aksu, China

Shihua Wang
Department of Cancer Biology, Wake Forest School of Medicine, Winston Salem, NC 27157, USA

Paul W. Dyce
Department of Animal Sciences, College of Agriculture, Auburn University, CASIC Building, 559 Devall Drive, Auburn, AL 36849, USA

Neil Tenn and Gerald M. Kidder
Department of Physiology and Pharmacology, The University of Western Ontario and Children's Health Research Institute, 800 Commissioners Road East, London, ON N6C 2V5, Canada

Taryne Chong, Amila Sarac, Linda Liao and Nicola Lyttle
Diagnostic Development, Ontario Institute for Cancer Research, MaRS Centre, 661 University Avenue, Suite 510, Toronto, Ontario M5G 0A3, Canada

Melanie Spears
Diagnostic Development, Ontario Institute for Cancer Research, MaRS Centre, 661 University Avenue, Suite 510, Toronto, Ontario M5G 0A3, Canada
Department of Laboratory Medicine and Pathobiology, University of Toronto, 27 King's College Circle, Toronto, Ontario M5S 1A1, Canada

John M. S. Bartlett
Diagnostic Development, Ontario Institute for Cancer Research, MaRS Centre, 661 University Avenue, Suite 510, Toronto, Ontario M5G 0A3, Canada
Department of Laboratory Medicine and Pathobiology, University of Toronto, 27 King's College Circle, Toronto, Ontario M5S 1A1, Canada
Biomarkers and Companion Diagnostics, Edinburgh Cancer Research Centre, Crewe Road South, Edinburgh EH4 2XR, UK

Cindy Q. Yao
Informatics Program, Ontario Institute for Cancer Research, MaRS Centre, 661 University Avenue, Suite 510, Toronto, Ontario M5G 0A3, Canada

Paul C. Boutros
Informatics Program, Ontario Institute for Cancer Research, MaRS Centre, 661 University Avenue, Suite 510, Toronto, Ontario M5G 0A3, Canada
Department of Medical Biophysics, University of Toronto, 101 College Street, Room 15-701, Toronto, Ontario M5G 1L7, Canada
Department of Pharmacology and Toxicology, University of Toronto, 1 King's College Circle, Room 4207, Toronto, Ontario M5S 1A8, Canada

Beili Chen and Yiran Zhou
Department of Obstetrics and Gynecology, Reproductive Medicine Center, The First Affiliated Hospital of Anhui Medical University, Meishan Road, Shushan, Hefei 230022, China

Yunxia Cao
Department of Obstetrics and Gynecology, Reproductive Medicine Center, The First Affiliated Hospital of Anhui Medical University, Meishan Road, Shushan, Hefei 230022, China
Institute of Reproductive Genetics, Anhui Medical University, Meishan Road, Shushan, Hefei 230032, China
Anhui Provincial Engineering Technology Research Center for Biopreservation and Artificial Organs, Meishan Road, Shushan, Hefei 230027, China

Binbin Wang
Department of Obstetrics and Gynecology, Reproductive Medicine Center, The First Affiliated Hospital of Anhui Medical University, Meishan Road, Shushan, Hefei 230022, China

Center for Genetics, National Research Institute for Family Planning, 12 Dahuisi Road, Haidian, Beijing 100081, China
Key Laboratory of Family planning and Reproductive Genetics, National Health and Family Planning Commission, Heb Research institute For Family Planning, Beijing 050071, People's Republic of China.

Lin Li
Central Laboratory, Beijing Obstetrics and Gynecology Hospital, Capital Medical University, Chaoyang, Beijing 100026, China

Jing Wang
Department of Medical Genetics and Developmental Biology, School of Basic Medical Sciences, Capital Medical University, No. 10 Xitoutiao, Youanmenwai, Fengtai, Beijing 100069, China

Tengyan Li, Hong Pan and Beihong Liu
Center for Genetics, National Research Institute for Family Planning, 12 Dahuisi Road, Haidian, Beijing 100081, China

Jiaheng Li and Riqiang Bao
Joint programme of Nanchang University and Queen Mary University of London, Nanchang, China

Shiwei Peng
Department of Gynecology and Obstetrics, Jiangxi Provincial People's Hospital, Nanchang, China

Chunping Zhang
Department of Cell Biology, School of Medicine, Nanchang University, Nanchang, Jiangxi 330006, People's Republic of China

Ting Zhao, Yu Shao, Yan Liu, Xiao Wang, Luyao Guan and Yuan Lu
Department of Gynecology, Obstetrics and Gynecology Hospital of Fudan University, 419 Fangxie Road, Shanghai 200011, China

Dongyan Cao, Jiaxin Yang, Ting Gui and Keng Shen
Department of Obstetrics and Gynecology, Peking Union Medical College Hospital, Chinese Academy of Medical Sciences and Peking Union Medical College, No.1 Shuaifuyuan, Dongcheng District, Beijing, China

Qianying Zhao
Department of Obstetrics and Gynecology, Peking Union Medical College Hospital, Chinese Academy of Medical Sciences and Peking Union Medical College, No.1 Shuaifuyuan, Dongcheng District, Beijing, China
Department of Gynecology and Obstetrics, West China Second University Hospital, Sichuan University, Key Laboratory of Birth Defects and Related Diseases of Women and Children (Sichuan University), Ministry of Education, Chengdu, China

Qiuhong Qian
Department of Obstetrics and Gynecology, Peking Union Medical College Hospital, Chinese Academy of Medical Sciences and Peking Union Medical College, No.1 Shuaifuyuan, Dongcheng District, Beijing, China
Department of Obstetrics and Gynecology, Qilu Hospital of Shandong University, Shandong, China

Yooyoung Lee
Division of Gynecologic Oncology, Princess Margaret Hospital Cancer Centre, Toronto, ON, Canada
Lunenfeld-Tanenbaum Research Institute at Sinai Health Systems, Mt. Sinai Hospital, 60 Murray Street, 6-10016-3, Toronto, ON M5T 3L9, Canada
Department of Obstetrics and Gynecology, University of Toronto, Toronto, ON, Canada

Taymaa May
Division of Gynecologic Oncology, Princess Margaret Hospital Cancer Centre, Toronto, ON, Canada
Department of Obstetrics and Gynecology, University of Toronto, Toronto, ON, Canada

Alexandra Kollara
Lunenfeld-Tanenbaum Research Institute at Sinai Health Systems, Mt. Sinai Hospital, 60 Murray Street, 6-10016-3, Toronto, ON M5T 3L9, Canada

Theodore J. Brown
Lunenfeld-Tanenbaum Research Institute at Sinai Health Systems, Mt. Sinai Hospital, 60 Murray Street, 6-10016-3, Toronto, ON M5T 3L9, Canada
Department of Obstetrics and Gynecology, University of Toronto, Toronto, ON, Canada

Dan Wang, Yang Xiang, Ming Wu, Keng Shen, Jiaxin Yang, Huifang Huang and Tong Ren
Department of Obstetrics and Gynecology, Peking Union Medical College Hospital, Chinese Academy of Medical Science and Peking Union Medical College, No. 1 Shuaifuyuan Road, Dongcheng District, Beijing 100730, People's Republic of China

Yuan-yuan Qin, Yang-yang Wu, Xiao-ying Xian, Jin-qiu Qin, Zhan-feng Lai, Lin Liao and Fa-quan Lin
Department of Clinical Laboratory, The First Affiliated Hospital of Guangxi Medical University, Guangxi Zhuang Autonomous Region, Nanning, China

Shunping Wang, Virginia Mensah, Warren J. Huber III and Ruben Alvero
Brown University Warren Alpert Medical School, Providence, RI 02912, USA
Women and Infants Fertility Center, Women and Infants Hospital of Rhode Island, 101 Dudley Street, Providence, RI 02905, USA

Yi Zhang
Brown University School of Public Health, Providence, RI 02912, USA

Yen-Tsung Huang
Brown University School of Public Health, Providence, RI 02912, USA
Institute of Statistical Science Academia Sinica, 128 Academia Road Sec. 2, Taipei 11529, Taiwan

Yilin Wang and Zhenyu Zhang
Department of Gynaecology and Obstetrics, Beijing Chaoyang Hospital, Capital Medical University, No. 8 South Road, workers' Stadium, Chaoyang District, Beijing 100020, China

Yanyan Wang
Department of Gynaecology and Obstetrics, Beijing Chaoyang Hospital, Capital Medical University, No. 8 South Road, workers' Stadium, Chaoyang District, Beijing 100020, China
The First Affiliated Hospital of Jinzhou Medical University, No.2, people's street, Jinzhou 121001, China

Colleen M. Britain, Andrew T. Holdbrooks and Susan L. Bellis
Department of Cell, Developmental, and Integrative Biology, University of Alabama at Birmingham, 350 McCallum Building, 1918 University Blvd, Birmingham, AL 35294, USA

Joshua C. Anderson and Christopher D. Willey
Department of Radiation Oncology, University of Alabama at Birmingham, 1700 6th Avenue South, Birmingham, AL 35233, USA

Hero A. Abdurrahman
Maternity Teaching Hospital, Kurdistan, Erbil, Iraq

Ariana Kh. Jawad
Kurdistan Board for Medical Specialists, Kurdistan, Erbil, Iraq

Shahla K. Alalalf
Department of Obstetrics and Gynecology, Hawler Medical University, College of Medicine, Kurdistan region, Erbil, Iraq

Wei Zhang, Qi Wang, Zhi-jun Yang, Sheng-bin Liao and Li Li
Department of Gynecology Oncology, Tumor Hospital of Guangxi Medical University, Nanning 530021, China

Ming-ju Huang
Department of Gynecology Oncology, Tumor Hospital of Guangxi Medical University, Nanning 530021, China

Department of Gynecology, Chongqing Three Gorges Central Hospital, Wanzhou District of Chongqing 404000, China

M. Reljič
Department for Reproductive Medicine and Gynaecological Endocrinology, Clinic for Gynecology and Perinatology, University Medical Centre Maribor, Ljubljanska 5, 2000 Maribor, Slovenia

J. Knez
Department for Reproductive Medicine and Gynaecological Endocrinology, Clinic for Gynecology and Perinatology, University Medical Centre Maribor, Ljubljanska 5, 2000 Maribor, Slovenia

Marcin Kierszk, Gieryn Katarzyna and Marek Maleńczyk
Clinical Unit of Obstetrics, Women's Disease and Gynecological Oncology, sw. Jozefa 53/59, United District Hospital, Collegium Medicum University of Nicolaus Copernicus in Toruń, Torun, Poland

Michal Migda
Clinical Unit of Obstetrics, Women's Disease and Gynecological Oncology, sw. Jozefa 53/59, United District Hospital, Collegium Medicum University of Nicolaus Copernicus in Toruń, Torun, Poland
Civis Vita Medical Center, Torun, Poland

Migda Bartosz
Department of Diagnostic Imaging, Second Faculty of Medicine with the English Division and the Physiotherapy Division, Medical University of Warsaw, Warsaw, Poland

Marian S. Migda
Civis Vita Medical Center, Torun, Poland

Wenpeng You and Ian Symonds
Adelaide Medical School, The University of Adelaide, Adelaide, SA, Australia

Maciej Henneberg
Adelaide Medical School, The University of Adelaide, Adelaide, SA, Australia
Institute of Evolutionary Medicine, University of Zürich, 8057 Zurich, Switzerland

V. N. A. Ho, T. D. Pham, A. H. Le and T. M. Ho
IVFMD, My Duc Hospital, Ho Chi Minh City, Vietnam

L. N. Vuong
IVFMD, My Duc Hospital, Ho Chi Minh City, Vietnam
Department of Obstetrics and Gynecology, University of Medicine and Pharmacy at Ho Chi Minh City, Ho Chi Minh City, Vietnam

Agata Swiatly, Szymon Plewa, Jan Matysiak and Zenon J. Kokot
Department of Inorganic and Analytical Chemistry, Poznan University of Medical Sciences, Grunwaldzka 6 Street, 60-780 Poznań, Poland

Wen Zhang, Shuangzheng Jia, Yang Xiang, Junjun Yang and Jinhua Leng
Department of Obstetrics and Gynecology, Peking Union Medical College Hospital, Chinese Academy of Medical Sciences and Peking Union Medical College, No. 1 Shuaifuyuan, Dongcheng District, Beijing 100730, China

Congwei Jia
Department of Pathology, Peking Union Medical College Hospital, Chinese Academy of Medical Sciences and Peking Union Medical College, No. 1 Shuaifuyuan, Dongcheng District, Beijing 100730, China

Amnon Brzezinski, NA Brzezinski-Sinai and A. Ben-Meir
Department of Obstetrics and Gynecology, The Hebrew University Hadassah Medical Center, Jerusalem, Israel

A. Saada and H. Miller
Department of Genetics and Metabolism, The Hebrew University Hadassah Medical Center, Jerusalem, Israel

Yu Liu and Yu Liao
Department of Endocrinology, South Campus, Renji Hospital, School of Medicine, Shanghai Jiaotong University, Shanghai 201112, China

Shengxian Li, Tao Tao, Jing Ma and Wei Liu
Department of Endocrinology, Renji Hospital, School of Medicine, Shanghai Jiaotong University, Shanghai 200127, China

Xiaoxue Li, Qinling Zhu and Yun Sun
Center for Reproductive Medicine, Renji Hospital, School of Medicine, Shanghai JiaoTong University, Shanghai 200135, China

Shanghai Key Laboratory for Assisted Reproduction and Reproductive Genetics, Shanghai 200135, China

Haixia Wang and Zhonghua Huang
Department of Obstetrics and Gynecology, Jinshan branch of Shanghai Sixth People's Hospital, Shanghai Jiaotong University, Shanghai, China

Youjun Luo and Tiankui Qiao
Department of Oncology, Jinshan Hospital, Fudan University, Shanghai, China

Zhaoxia Wu
Department of Traditional Medicine, Jinshan branch of Shanghai Sixth People's Hospital, Shanghai Jiaotong University, Shanghai, China

Shu-Hui Zhao, Deng-Bin Wang and Hua Fan
Department of Radiology, Xinhua Hospital affiliated to Shanghai Jiaotong University School of Medicine, 1665 Kongjiang Road, Shanghai 200092, China

Hai-Ming Li and Jin-Wei Qiang
Department of Radiology, Jinshan Hospital, Fudan University, 1508 Longhang Road, Shanghai 201508, China

Rani Fritz
Department of Obstetrics, Gynecology and Women's Health, Albert Einstein College of Medicine/Montefiore Medical Center, Minneapolis, USA

Sangita Jindal
Department of Obstetrics, Gynecology and Women's Health, Albert Einstein College of Medicine/Montefiore Medical Center, Minneapolis, USA
Montefiore's Institute for Reproductive Medicine and Health, New York, USA

Index

www.ingramcontent.com/pod-product-compliance
Lightning Source LLC
Chambersburg PA
CBHW080520200326
41458CB00012B/4281